PHYSICIAN ASSISTANTS IN AMERICAN MEDICINE

RODERICK S. HOOKER, PHD, PA, MBA
Associate Professor
Department of Physician Assistant Studies
University of Texas Southwestern Medical Center
Dallas, Texas

JAMES F. CAWLEY, MPH, PA-C
Professor of Prevention and Community Health
Professor of Epidemiology
School of Public Health and Health Services
Professor of Health Care Sciences
School of Medicine and Health Sciences
The George Washington University
Washington, D.C.

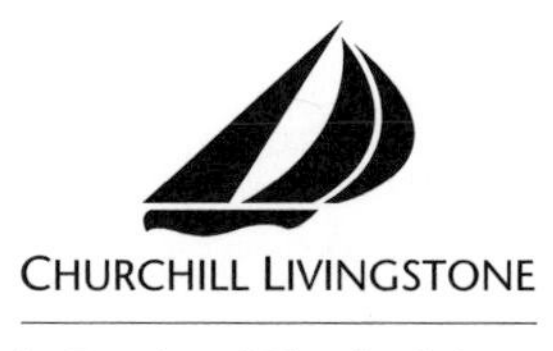

CHURCHILL LIVINGSTONE
An Imprint of Elsevier Science

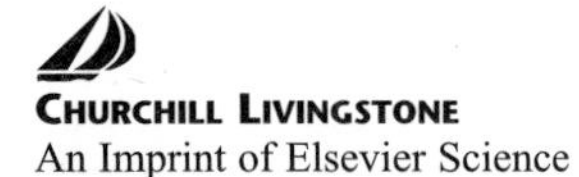

CHURCHILL LIVINGSTONE
An Imprint of Elsevier Science

11830 Westline Industrial Drive
St. Louis, Missouri 63146

PHYSICIAN ASSISTANTS IN AMERICAN MEDICINE

Distributed in the United Kingdom by Churchill Livingstone, Robert Stevenson House, 1-3 Baxter's Place, Leith Walk, Edinburgh EH1 3AF, Scotland, and by associated companies, branches, and representatives throughout the world.

Library of Congress Cataloging in Publication Data
Hooker, Roderick S.
Physician assistants in American medicine / Roderick S. Hooker, James F. Cawley.—2nd ed.
p.; cm.
Includes bibliographical references and index.
ISBN 0-443-06597-7
1. Physicians' assistants—Vocational guidance. 2. Physicians' assistants—United States.
I. Cawley, James, F. II. Title.
[DNLM: 1. Physician Assistants—United States. 2. Vocational Guidance—United States. W 21.5 H784p 2002]
R697.P45 H66 2002
610.69'53'02373—dc21

2002034995

Acquisitions Editor: Shirley Kuhn
Developmental Editor: Amy Holmes
Publishing Services Manager: John Rogers
Project Manager: Mary Turner
Designer: Paul Fry
Cover Art: Angie Chapin
Design Manager: Kathi Gosche

KI-MVY

Printed in United States of America
Last digit is the print number: 9 8 7 6 5 4 3 2

With love to my beautiful daughter, Andrea Beth.–*JFC*

To Donna, I admire you so much. To Lindsay and Tyler,
I'm proud to be your father.–*RSH*

FOREWORD

Physician Assistants in American Medicine is an extremely useful collection of the most important information available about one of the fastest-growing professions in America. It goes beyond simply providing the history, status, and promise of a new profession. Instead, it describes in detail the developments that have led to academic and clinical institutions and the establishment of more than 130 physician assistant education programs over the past three decades.

As the two leading researchers in the physician assistant field, Rod Hooker and Jim Cawley have updated their superbly researched and documented description of how significant and positive change in American health care can occur in a relatively short time. This is particularly encouraging to those of us concerned about our evolving health care system and the potential outcomes of continuing health care reform.

This book is simultaneously a history, a contemporary description, and a prospective view of one aspect of America's health care system. It demonstrates how successful change agents can be as effective and productive collaborators in a social sector. Cawley and Hooker have captured the essence and spectrum of working together as partners with physicians, other professionals, and consumers of health services that typify the physician assistant movement today.

A discussion of the profession's role in increasing access and clinical productivity while simultaneously improving cost containment is presented in balance with descriptions of the range of health care services and delivery organizations that can benefit from using physician assistants. Most importantly, the authors present data that support the growing acceptance of physician assistants as important health care team members. Consumers and physicians, as well as government and private health plans, accept physician assistants as one of the catalysts for improved access and realistic cost containment.

In a nation in which competition underpins most activities, it is a comfort to many of us that collaboration is the operative word in the past, present, and future of America's physician assistants. Cawley and Hooker describe the profession's historical roots in primary care and such partnerships with physicians, nurses, and others that improve America's health care.

The economic data presented in this book describe the improved efficiency and productivity brought to varying health care scenes when physician assistants are part of the organizational effort. It is information that communities, health professionals, administrators, and policymakers need to have as they plan for appropriate resources for access and care.

The authors are broad-based scholars. Using the disciplines of history, sociology, policy, political science, economics, anthropology, and health services research, they depict the personal adaptability and professional flexibility demonstrated in the development of physician assistants. By recounting that evolution, they describe the teamwork possible in twenty-first century health care. It is such teamwork that allows health care providers to work effectively and economically with new and emerging technologies. Ours is a culture of continuously evolving practice patterns and rapidly changing socioeconomic environments that taxes the American medical system—a system that would be lacking without physician assistants.

Richard A. Smith, MD, MPH
Director
The Medex Group
Clinical Professor
Department of Family Practice
and Community Health
John A. Burns School of Medicine
University of Hawaii, Honolulu

Foreword to the First Edition

As medical care in the United States moves forward in an environment characterized by rapid change and the realignments and adjustments related to "managed care," physician assistants have become key players. The physician assistant profession provides high-quality health care at a lower cost than does the conventional practice of using physicians exclusively. It is likely that collaborative teams containing physicians, physician assistants, and other health care professionals will emerge from the current realignments as the dominant practice model and that these teams will provide excellent and convenient care to a wider segment of our population than was possible in the past.

The physician assistant profession is still new, and regrettably, there are many who know little about its characteristics, roots, traditions, and utility across all branches and specialties of medical care. *Physician Assistants in American Medicine* will meet a real need by providing an authoritative and current source of information about the profession while reflecting its unique philosophy and relationship to the medical profession.

Although other books have been written about the profession, most have been written by physicians, educators, and/or academicians who have only observed the profession. This is a book written by individuals who were primarily educated into the profession and have practiced within it.

Each of the authors has a unique perspective, and these viewpoints fit together well for the purposes of writing a comprehensive description of the field. Both entered the profession with health care experience typical of the physician assistant practice, one in primary care and the other in specialty care. Both have pursued further education as needed for their expanded careers. Both have become leaders in the profession and are widely recognized as its spokesmen and as representatives through appointment to panels and task forces studying the profession and its relationship with other health professions. It is in this context that I have become acquainted with both authors and have come to respect their knowledge, integrity, perspective, and wisdom.

This volume is both timely and authoritative. The authors have used the remarkable data set gathered and updated each year by the American Academy of Physician Assistants. They have also extensively used sources such as the early conceptual and educational leaders of the new profession, most of whom are still alive and available, and they have included those who have not left a trail of publications. They have also consulted with a wide network of fellow physician assistants who have been willing to review and provide critical input for this volume.

Physician Assistants in American Medicine should prove to be an invaluable collection of useful and necessary information about this new and emerging field, and its authors are to be congratulated on their foresight and effort in making it available.

E. Harvey Estes, Jr., MD
Emeritus Professor of Community and Family Medicine
Duke University Medical Center
Director
Kate B. Reynolds Community Practitioner Program
North Carolina Medical Society Foundation Inc.
Raleigh, North Carolina

Preface

The form and expression of the PA profession is difficult to capture in print; it is a dynamic process that is constantly in flux. With this in mind, we set out to write the second edition with three objectives in mind. The first was to provide an interpretative history of physician assistants and their place in contemporary American medicine. A second objective was to provide a central repository of the scholarly work that documents and analyzes the role of PAs. Finally, the book should serve as a resource for understanding the place of PAs in delivering health care to a diverse society such as ours. It is important that the larger picture of health care in this country not overshadow the place where PAs reside and the contributions they make. When we wrote our first edition, we identified over 700 documents about PAs. Since that time, our collection has grown, and now almost 3000 articles, books, papers, reports, theses, and dissertations address some aspect of PA care. It is this collection, as well as our own career experiences and frequent interactions with colleagues, from which we draw.

On launching this project, it quickly became apparent that the evolution of PAs could not be fully understood without being placed in a broad social and cultural context. We were gratified to learn from the reviewers of our first edition that we got it right. What the second edition has allowed us to do is to go back to many developers of the PA model, of those who are still around, and ask them for clarification of the history and other social factors that may have been overlooked. To this end, we are grateful to a number of important people who helped us to improve the accuracy of our facts and set them in the historical place they deserve. As a consequence, the second edition was as long a journey as the first one. It is a rare privilege for historians to have the originators of a movement still around to clarify certain events. Once again we are thankful for the assistance of so many people. Their generous contributions have immeasurably enriched the final product. To Richard A. Smith, E. Harvey Estes, and Reginald Carter, we express our gratitude and enduring affection. You are among the few who are rightly considered to be the important pillars on which this profession stands. Thank you for refining our thoughts and guiding our efforts. To Marilyn Fitzgerald, Nicole Gara, Nancy Hughes, Gene Jones, Justine Strand, Leslie Kole, Ann Davis, Jeff Heinrich, Steve Crane, Richard C. Rohrs, Marshall Sinback, Glen Combs, Dennis Blessing, Richard Dehn, David Asprey, Richard Davis, Raul Cuadrado, Randy Danielsen, Bert Simon, Tony Miller, Virginia Fowkes, Ken Harbert, Ruth Ballweg, Robert McNellis, and Greg Thomas, we acknowledge their contributions to our thinking and information gathering for this book. They were the sounding boards we sought when exploring ideas and theories of why and how the profession is alive today.

Although much of the research and writing was done on personal time, both of us are full-time academics, and, as such, we are grateful to our deans and department chairs, who provided the atmosphere and indirect support to undertake such work. Our good friend P. Eugene Jones heads the Department of Physician Assistant Studies at the University of Texas Southwestern Medical Center and has supported the work of Rod for a number of years. At The George Washington University, Deans Richard Riegelman, Richard Southby, and Daniel Hoffman, Chairman Richard Windsor, and PA Program Director J. Jeffrey Heinrich have lent their support and encouragement in Jim's writing and scholarship related to the PA profession.

These professors and chairmen are scholars in their own right, and they recognize the value of supporting research, scholarship, and leadership in the PA profession. Lest we forget, to Amy Holmes and Carol O'Connell, two editors who should not have had to put up with as much as you did. Thanks for your patience.

This book is collaboration in the truest sense, and no single ownership can be claimed for any chapter. We are fused with a common mission and common ethos to be accurate in our interpretations, and each served as a counterweight to the other's writing. Consequently we take responsibility for all statements and errors.

RODERICK S. HOOKER, PHD, PA, MBA
Associate Professor
Department of Physician Assistant Studies
University of Texas Southwestern Medical Center
Dallas, Texas

JAMES F. CAWLEY, MPH, PA-C
Professor of Prevention and Community Health
Professor of Epidemiology
School of Public Health and Health Services
Professor of Health Care Sciences
School of Medicine and Health Sciences
The George Washington University
Washington, D.C.

About the Authors

Roderick S. Hooker, PhD, PA, MBA, is an associate professor in the Department of Physician Assistant Studies at the University of Texas Southwestern Medical Center in Dallas, Texas. His health care career began in the 1960s when he became a hospital corpsman in the U.S. Navy. This was followed by time as a civilian emergency room technician. He graduated from the University of Missouri with a degree in biology and briefly pursued being a tropical biologist. After working as a research assistant in Costa Rica and Missouri, he joined the Peace Corps and spent two and a half years in the Kingdom of Tonga, working as a biologist, teacher, and health care worker. Following a brief period as staff in the Peace Corps, he enrolled in the St. Louis University Physician Assistant program in the mid-1970s. After graduating as a PA, Rod joined Kaiser Permanente in Portland, Oregon, where he worked clinically in rheumatology. He also wore a second hat as a health services researcher with the Kaiser Permanente Center for Health Research. During the two decades in Portland, he obtained a master of business administration degree in health care organization and a doctorate in health policy from The Mark O. Hatfield School of Public Administration and Policy at Portland State University. In the late 1990s Rod helped start, as well as teach at, the Pacific University School of Physician Assistant Studies as an adjunct faculty. From there he joined the Department of Physician Assistant Studies at the University of Texas Southwestern Medical Center in Dallas. As a health services researcher, he has been focused on examining the role of PAs and other providers and on understanding how a mix of health care workers can improve health care organization and delivery. This work has expanded overseas through the International Medical Workforce Committee, an organization that focuses on how health care can be better employed internationally. In the end, though, he regards himself as an amateur sculptor who finds himself, through force of circumstances, trying to shape health services rather than clay.

James F. Cawley, MPH, PA-C, is the director of the Physician Assistant/Master of Public Health Program and professor of Health Care Sciences in the School of Medicine and Health Sciences at The George Washington University. He is also professor and vice chair in the Department of Prevention and Community Health in the School of Public Health and Health Services at GWU. A PA educator since 1974, Cawley has held faculty appointments at The Johns Hopkins University, State University of New York at Stony Brook, and Yale University. Since 1982 he has been on the faculty at George Washington.

Cawley earned a bachelor of arts degree in political science from St. Francis University in 1970, a bachelor of science degree and Certificate as a PA from Touro College Physician Assistant Program in New York in 1974, and a master of public health degree in infectious disease epidemiology from The Johns Hopkins University School of Public Health in 1979. He has undertaken doctoral work in health policy studies at Johns Hopkins and in the Department of Health Services Management and Policy at GWU. He was co-author with Gretchen Schafft of *Physician Assistants in a Changing Health Care Environment* (1986). Cawley has authored more than 75 peer-reviewed papers in the biomedical literature on topics spanning the PA profession, PAs in the health workforce, and preventive medicine and epidemiology. In 2003 Cawley was president of the Association of Physician Assistant Programs; other leadership roles include terms as president of the Physician Assistants Foundation, president of the Maryland Academy of Physician Assistants, and commissioner on the National Commission on Certification of Physician Assistants. He serves as a consultant to numerous educational institutions, boards, and government panels. From 1989 to 1995 he served as a member of the U.S. Public Health Service National Coordinating Committee on Clinical Preventive Services.

Contents

PHYSICIAN ASSISTANT

A TIME LINE OF THE PROFESSION

Date

1650 Feldshers, originally German military medical assistants, are introduced into Russian armies by Peter the Great in the seventeenth century.

1778 Congress provides for a number of hospital mates to assist physicians in the provision of patient care modeled after the "loblolly boys" of the British Royal Navy.

1803 Officiers de santé are introduced in France by René Fourcroy to help alleviate health personnel shortages in the military and civilian sectors. Abolished in 1892.

1891 Establishment of the first company for "medic" instruction at Fort Riley, Kansas.

1930 First "physician assistant" (PA) in the United States (urology) at Cleveland Clinic is described in the literature.

1940 Community health aids are introduced in Alaska to improve the village health status of Eskimos and other Native Americans.

1959 U.S. Surgeon General identifies shortage of medically trained personnel.

1961 Charles Hudson, in an editorial in the *Journal of the American Medical Association*, calls for a "midlevel" provider from the ranks of former military corpsmen.

World Health Organization begins introducing and promoting health care workers in developing countries (e.g., Me'decin Africain, dresser, assistant medical officer, and rural health technician).

1965 First PA class enters Duke University.

1966 Barefoot doctors in China arise in response to Chairman Mao's purge of the elite and intellectual. This action sent many physicians into the fields to work, leaving peasants without medical personnel.

Child health associate program begins at the University of Colorado. Origin of nurse practitioner (NP) profession and PA specialty.

Allied Health Professions Personnel Act (Public Law 751) promotes the development of programs to train new types of primary care providers.

1967 First class of PA graduates from Duke University.

1968 American Academy of Physician Assistants (AAPA) is established.

Health Manpower Act (Public Law 90-490) funds the training of a variety of health care providers.

Physician Assistants, Volume 1. First journal for PAs.

First conference on PA education is held at Duke University. Preceded the Association of Physician Assistant Programs (APAP).

1969 First class of graduates from the University of Colorado's Child Health Associate PA program.

1970 Kaiser Permanente becomes the first health maintenance organization (HMO) to employ a PA.

First class of graduates from the Medex Northwest program at the University of Washington.

1971 American Medical Association (AMA) recognizes the PA profession and begins work on national certification and codification of its practice characteristics.

Comprehensive Health Manpower Training Act (Public Law 92-157) contracts for PA education and deployment.

First graduates from the University of Washington Medex Northwest program.

1972 *The Physician's Assistant: Today and Tomorrow*, by Sadler, Sadler, and Bliss, is published; first book written about the PA profession.

The APAP is established.

Alderson-Broaddus College's first 4-year program graduates its first class.

"The Essentials" accreditation standards for PA programs are adopted, and the Joint Review Committee on Education Programs for the Physician Assistant (JRC-PA) is formed to evaluate compliance with the standards.

Federal support for PA education is enacted by the Health Resources Administration.

The Medex Group is established at the University of Hawaii by R. Smith. Begins developing international PA-type programs in the Pacific, Asia, Africa, and South America.

1973 First AAPA Annual Conference is held at Sheppard Air Force Base, Texas, with 275 attendees. Preceded by four smaller conferences on PA education at Duke University (1968, 1970, 1971, and 1972).

AAPA and APAP establish a joint national office in Washington, District of Columbia.

National Commission on Certification of Physician Assistants (NCCPA) is established.

National Board of Medical Examiners administers the first certifying examinations for primary care PAs.

First postgraduate program for PAs is started at Montefiore Hospital by Rosen.

1974 AAPA becomes an official organization of the JRC-PA. The committee reviews PA and surgeon assistant programs and makes accreditation recommendations to the Committee on Allied Health Education and Accreditation.

The American College of Surgeons becomes a sponsoring organization of the JRC-PA.

From 1974 to 1977, 150 PAs are recruited to work on the Alaska Pipeline. The largest scale employment of PAs in the private sector.

1975 *The Physician Assistant: A National and Local Analysis*, by Ford.

1976 Federal support of PA education continues under grants from the Health Professions Educational Assistance Act (Public Law 94-484).

1977 *The New Health Professionals: Nurse Practitioners and Physician's Assistants*, by Bliss and Cohen.

The Physician's Assistant: A Baccalaureate Curriculum, by Myers.

AAPA Education and Research Foundation (later renamed the Physician Assistant Foundation) is incorporated to recruit public and private contributions for student financial assistance and to support research on the PA profession.

Rural Health Clinic Services Act (Public Law 95-210) is passed by Congress, providing Medicare reimbursement of PA and NP services in rural clinics.

Health Practitioner (later renamed *Physician Assistant*) journal begins publication; later distributed to all PAs as the official AAPA publication.

1978 *The Physician's Assistant: Innovation in the Medical Division of Labor*, by Schneller.

AAPA House of Delegates becomes policy-making legislative body of the academy.

Air Force begins appointing PAs as commissioned officers.

1979 Graduate Medical Education National Advisory Council estimates a surplus of physicians and nonphysician providers in the near future.

1980 The AAPA Political Action Committee is established to support candidates for federal office who support the PA profession.

Formation of the Veteran's Caucus of the AAPA.

1981 *Staffing Primary Care in 1990: Physician Replacement and Cost Savings*, by Record, documents that PAs in HMO settings provide 79% of the care of a primary care physician, at 50% of the cost.

1982 *Physician Assistants: Their Contribution to Health Care*, by Perry and Breitner.

1984 *First Annual Report on Physician Assistant Educational Programs in the United States*, by Oliver and the APAP.

Alternatives in Health Care Delivery, edited by Carter and Perry.

1985 AAPA's first Burroughs Wellcome Health Policy Fellowship for PAs is created.

Membership of the AAPA surpasses the 10,000 mark. Membership categories are expanded to include physicians, affiliates, and sustaining members.

University of Colorado PA program awards a master's degree to their graduates, the first for PA education.

1986 AAPA succeeds in legislative drive for coverage of PA services in hospitals and nursing homes and for coverage of assisting in surgery under Medicare Part B (Omnibus Budget Reconciliation Act [Public Law 99-210]).

1987 National PA Day, October 6, is established, coinciding with the anniversary of the first graduating class of PAs from the Duke University PA program 20 years earlier.

Dedication of the AAPA national headquarters in Alexandria, Virginia.

AAPA publishes the *Journal of the American Academy of Physician Assistants* (JAAPA). The editor selected is the first PA hired as AAPA professional staff.

Additional Medicare coverage of PA services (in rural underserved areas) is approved by Congress.

1991 Navy PAs are commissioned.

AAPA assumes administrative responsibility of the Accreditation Review Committee on Education for the Physician Assistant (ARC-PA) (formerly the JRC-PA).

Clinician Reviews debuts, the first clinical journal to target both PAs and NPs. Created, owned, and managed by PAs.

1992 Army and Coast Guard PAs are commissioned.

The Canadian National Forces inaugurates a Canadian PA.

1993 A total of 24,600 PAs are in active practice in 50 states, territories, and the District of Columbia.

1995 *Physician Assistants in the Health Workforce, 1994* (report of the Advisory Group on Physician Assistants and the Workforce). Develops the current definition of the PA.

1996 The AMA grants observer status to the AAPA in the AMA House of Delegates.

1997 Passage of the Balanced Budget Act of 1997 (Public Law 105-33) changed level of reimbursement of PA services under Medicare.

1998 Mississippi becomes the last state to pass PA enabling legislation.

The APAP Research Institute is founded.

1999 *Perspectives on Physician Assistant Education* becomes a peer-reviewed indexed journal.

2000 The APAP determines that the master's degree is the appropriate degree for PA education.

ARC-PA becomes the independent accrediting agency for PA educational programs.

Indiana becomes the forty-seventh state to pass PA prescribing legislation.

NCCPA converts the Physician Assistant National Certification Examination (PANCE) and the Physician Assistant National Recertification Examination to computer-based administration.

2001 A record 4267 PAs sit for the PANCE (91.5% pass rate).

2002 The thirty-fifth anniversary of the first graduation of PAs. The event is chronicled in a special edition of *JAAPA*.

The AAPA estimates that there are approximately 45,000 clinically active PAs in American medicine.

Thirtieth anniversary of the APAP. The number of accredited PA programs is 134.

1

OVERVIEW OF THE PROFESSION

THE PHYSICIAN ASSISTANT PROFESSION

The concept of the physician assistant (PA) in the United States emerged in the 1960s as a strategy to cope with a shortage of primary care physicians. Giving impetus to idea, what spawned was a handful of graduates and a new profession. From those humble beginnings the new profession struggled to survive, grow, and become recognized. It was not an easy task. Now with more than three decades of growth, the PA profession is a mature and capable component of the American medical workforce. Collectively it can claim more than 50,000 graduates, a strong and stable set of educational programs, and a growing importance within the health care system.

In the decades following the origin of the profession there were many debates about the need for PAs and other nonphysician clinicians. These debates came during a prediction about a surplus of both physicians and nurses by the end of the twentieth century. Despite these predictions the PA profession has prospered. Why then has this profession prospered, and will its success and growth continue along with the new century? The answers to these and other questions about PAs are not yet clear, but it is clear that they are part of the wide and varied health care fabric that wraps around the United States. The evidence seems to point to continued growth and success for this young profession because the demand continues to exceed the supply in an American society that values choice, diversity, quality, and availability.

EVIDENCE REVIEWED: SUCCESS OF THE CONCEPT

The startling growth and success of the PA concept from its origins in the 1960s probably could not have occurred in the absence of ferment and change in the health care system, which made it possible and even necessary. Consumers of health care, existing health care professions, government, bureaucratic hierarchies, educational institutions, and accrediting bodies are all involved and have implicitly, if not explicitly, aided in the process by creating a positive political climate.

The innovation was born in the 1960s following two decades of scientific breakthroughs, development of new medical specialties and subspecialties, and overgrowth of hospitals and hospital services. Young physicians, exposed early to this exciting display of technical power, were flocking to hospital-based specialties. For the generalist physician, education and training, once the foundation of the medical workforce, had shrunk after the Korean War, and the new graduates of residencies were not replacing the general practitioners who were retiring. The consequences of this gap were not so obvious in cities with good hospitals and a strong cadre of the newly trained specialists, but in small towns and rural areas the impact was devastating.

Thus the stage was set for entry of a new alternative provider that promised improved access to health care for these areas. The country's leaders were well aware of inequities in the distribution of health care, and most were convinced that the problem was one of inadequate numbers of medical care providers. A series of actions was undertaken, at both the federal and the state level, aimed at correcting this problem. The most notable was the advent of the PA profession and the development of the nurse practitioner (NP). However, other actions were undertaken in the 1970s:

- Medical schools increased class size.
- New medical schools were created.
- The generalist physician was "revived" in the form of a new general specialty, family medicine.
- Special offices to promote medical practice in underserved areas were created in many states.
- Dispersed medical educational systems (area health education programs) were created.

An added factor in the mix was the war in Southeast Asia, which was reaching its tragic conclusion at this time. Military medical care had significantly improved by using trained medical care teams operating in combat areas and by using forward-positioned battalion aid stations. Physicians, nurses, military personnel, and corpsmen were returning home with knowledge of these improvements and the key roles played by nonphysician members of these field teams.

Yet another factor was the social climate within the country. The War on Poverty had brought to public attention the substandard conditions and deprivation of some people within the bounds of the "richest country on earth." President Lyndon Johnson's Great Society program brought an optimism that solutions might be found for these chronic social ills.

It is easy to understand why this was a favorable time for the entry of PAs on the health workforce stage. Governments, both state and federal, were willing to support some of the most far-reaching social program projects seen to that time to increase access to health care. The fact that this innovation tapped the newly available source of returning military corpsmen was an added boost.

Intertwined with these circumstances were events more directly related to the PA profession. In 1961 a prominent leader of the American Medical Association (AMA) proposed the idea of using military trained personnel as assistants to physicians. In the mid 1960s Dr. Richard Smith, then a deputy director of the Office of Equal Health Opportunity, moved into a new role in which he proposed to create a new source of health care providers for rural areas. A prominent academic pediatrician, Dr. Henry Silver, with Dr. Loretta Ford, a nurse educator, began to develop a new type of pediatric practitioner.

At Duke University the first PA program began with a small group of ex-Navy corpsmen, under the direction of Dr. Eugene Stead. As an academic physician leader, Dr. Stead had been impressed by the need for new personnel, both in the medical center and in the rural areas of his state. His previous experience with military personnel convinced him that the training period for assistants in this new program could be much shorter than that for medical students, and that close supervision by their physician employers would ensure competence and further development of skills in practice.

The history of the Medex program, another model of PA education, the Duke program, and the University of Colorado program is discussed in more detail in later chapters. At this point several unique features of the PA conceptual model should be recognized. Two have already been mentioned: the relatively brief duration of the concept and the role of the employing physician as supervisor. All of the programs were patterned after the familiar medical model: a period of basic science education followed by clinical skill development under medical instructors. The would-be PA would be trained to take a medical history, elicit symptoms, develop diagnoses, examine the patient, and take over some medical management tasks. Complicated cases or procedures were to be referred to the supervising physician. Although it was expected that the new personnel might spend more time with patient education and preventive interventions, the activities and skills would be similar to those of the physician, with the assistant assuming some but not all of the physician's tasks.

Another feature of the PA model as each developer envisioned it was the clear intention to train a generalist assistant, whose training and skill development were adequate to serve as a platform for further education and further skill development by the physician employer. The generalist assistant could work with a rural practitioner, gaining further insights and skills with time, but could also work with a narrow specialist, who would add another layer of expertise to the general education of the PA.

As might have been predicted, state and federal governmental attention was quickly achieved by three of the model PA programs (Duke University, University of Washington, and University of Colorado). Soon the government developed an interest in the regulation of this new category of health care provider. The Department of Health, Education, and Welfare sponsored a study and a series of conferences at Duke University on the regulation of practice of PAs. This activity, under the direction of Martha Ballenger, JD, and E. Harvey Estes, Jr., MD, resulted in model regulatory laws that were enacted by many states and prepared the way for the 1971 Health Manpower Act. This legislation provided funds for medical schools to increase the number of students to meet the perceived shortage of medical personnel. It also included funding for PA training programs. The availability of funding quickly increased the number of training sites, and 50 such programs were active by 1974.

In 1971 the AMA recognized the new profession and lent its name and resources to the process of national certification process, accreditation of educational programs, and codification of practice laws. This recognition did not ensure acceptance by all physicians, and occasional roadblocks to acceptance and permission to practice persisted within the jurisdiction of certain state medical components of the AMA until the 1990s.

The Physician Assistant Today

- **Graduates:** In 2002 there were more than 45,000 PAs in active clinical practice in the United States. The stability and dedication of this workforce to their profession are demonstrated by the fact that this represents almost 88% of all persons formally trained as PAs since the first class graduated in 1967. The annual attrition rate is less than 2%.
- **PA characteristics:** The mean age of PAs is 41 years; 42% are men, and 58% are women. The age reflects the relative youth of the profession and the shift in gender. The early dominance of men in the profession, related to the male gender of the former military students of the early years, has gradually changed, and young women now dominate the profession.
- **Deployment:** Forty-two percent of PAs practice in communities with a population smaller than 50,000, and 20% practice in communities smaller than 10,000. Twelve percent work in inner city clinics.
- **PA educational programs:** There were 132 accredited PA programs in 2002. Programs are accredited by the Accreditation Review Commission on Education for the Physician Assistant (ARC-PA). The typical PA program is 26 months long and usually requires a college degree and some health care experience before admission. Over half of the PA programs award a master's degree.
- **Students:** About 10,100 students are enrolled in PA programs at any one time. In 2002 more than 4500 new graduates passed the national certification examination and became eligible to practice.
- **Prescribing:** Forty-seven states, the District of Columbia, and Guam have enacted laws that authorize PA prescribing.
- **Income:** The mean total income from the main employer for PAs who are not employed by the federal government or who are not self-employed and who work full time (at least 32 hours per week) is $72,241 (standard deviation, $17,738); the median is $69,567. The comparable mean for PAs who are recent graduates is $63,168.
- **State laws:** Fifty states plus the District of Columbia and Guam have laws or regulations recognizing PA practice. All require graduation from an accredited PA program and national certification.
- **Certification:** PAs receive their national certification from the National Commission on Certification of Physician Assistants (NCCPA). Almost all states require this certification for licensure.
- **Ethnicity:** The PA profession has 10% of its members from underrepresented groups. Of those in active clinical practice, 2.8% are African Americans, 3.6% are Hispanic/Latinos, 3.2% are Asian/Pacific Islanders, and 1.1% are American Indian/Alaskan Natives. The

remaining 89% are white or do not choose to identify their racial/ethnic origin.

PAs practice in all the types of clinical settings where physician services are traditionally offered: urban neighborhoods, rural communities, hospitals, and public and private medical offices. They serve as commissioned officers in all U.S. military branches and the U.S. Public Health Service. In clinical practice most spend their time in medical office or clinic settings but some work in hospitals and divide their time among the wards and the operating and delivery rooms. In addition to roles in all the primary care specialties, PAs can be found in most non–primary care specialties. They are underrepresented in nursing home care, home health care, pathology, radiology, and some of the surgical and medical subspecialties.

The distribution of PAs in the formative years of the profession reflected the federal and state initiatives and the interest of the medical profession in extending primary care into areas of need. Early recruits were individuals with experience that enabled them to practice with minimal supervision. As the capability of PAs to fit into specialties outside primary care has become known, and as their ability and productivity have been confirmed, physicians in these specialties have successfully "outbid" the primary care specialties for their services. In comparison with physicians, PAs remain more likely to be found in primary care practice (50% of PAs, 33% of physicians) and in rural and other medically underserved areas (AMA, 2002). However, there are many influences on PA selection for a career, and these influences or factors vary at various times. Exhibit 1-1 illustrates how the primary care specialties have traded off with the non–primary care influences.

The medical model of PA education has been confirmed by the adaptability of PAs to new roles in the medical and surgical specialties. In both the primary care and the specialty care roles of the PA, the relationship between the PA and the supervising physician remains constant. The physician and the PA are a functional team. This relationship has been characterized as "negotiated performance autonomy," reflecting the continually evolving delegation of medical tasks from physician to PA based on a mutual understanding and trust in their respective professional roles. Schneller and Weiner (1978) proposed that this mutual evolution was a major determinant of clinical practice effectiveness of the PA and was advantageous to both.

The recognition and acceptance of this beneficial relationship is key to understanding the relationship between the PA and physician and to understanding the official stance of the profession: that it does *not* desire autonomy from physician supervision. Stead's early recognition

EXHIBIT 1-1

Estimated Percent Distribution of Practicing Physician Assistants by Specialty: Selected Years, 1984–2002*

Specialty	1984	1989	1990	1992	1994	1996	2000	2002
Primary care†	**55.8**	**49.3**	**45.9**	**42.8**	**45.2**	**50.8**	**47.9**	
Family medicine	42.5	37.9	33.0	31.4	33.7	39.8	36.5	32.1
General internal medicine	9.2	7.8	9.0	8.9	9.2	8.3	8.8	8.4
Pediatrics	4.1	3.6	3.0	2.5	2.3	2.7	2.6	2.6
Non–primary care‡	**44.2**	**50.7**	**55.0**	**57.2**	**48.5**	**49.2**	**52.1**	**43.1**
Obstetrics/gynecology	3.1	4.6	4.0	3.3	2.9	3.0	2.7	2.7
Surgical subspecialties	9.0	7.5	9.0	9.8	10.5	8.8	10.4	10.0
General surgery	9.2	7.9	8.0	8.0	7.7	3.1	2.7	2.5
Internal medicine subspecialties	4.8	3.8	6.0	7.1	6.3	5.8	8.1	9.4
Pediatric subspecialties	0.0	1.0	2.0	1.2	1.2	2.1	1.5	1.5
Emergency medicine	6.4	6.2	7.0	8.0	8.7	7.0	9.7	10.2
Orthopedics	4.1	5.6	6.0	7.6	7.8	6.9	7.3	9.2
Occupational medicine	4.1	3.8	5.0	3.9	3.4	3.0	3.4	3.0
Other specialties§	3.5	10.3	8.0	8.3	6.3	9.5	6.3	8.4

Unpublished data from American Academy of Physician Assistants, Alexandria, Va.
*Practicing physician assistants are figured at 85% of the total graduates.
†Primary care includes internal medicine, family/general practice, and pediatrics.
‡Includes general medicine.
§Includes correctional medicine, neurology, geriatric medicine, psychiatry, and industrial medicine.

of this principle is reflected in his prediction that PAs would gain greater freedom and growth from delegation by wise physician supervisors, who share the benefits of this growth, than from legislated autonomy.

Delegation of tasks from physician to PA is also contained in the basis of legal and regulatory authority granted to PAs in most state laws. Model legislation proposed as a result of the Duke conferences on this topic in the late 1960s permitted PAs to work in the full range of clinical practice areas: office, clinic, hospital, nursing home, or patient's home. This wide latitude was considered essential for a full range of services and effectiveness. The model legislation recognized the authority of physicians to delegate medical tasks to qualified PAs while holding them legally responsible through the doctrine of "respondeat superior." North Carolina, Colorado, and Oklahoma were among the first states to amend their medical practice acts.

These practice regulations and the supervisory relationship have also contributed to the striking versatility among the practice roles of PAs. As a result they are permitted to assist the physician in any task or function within the scope of the physician's practice but with the recognition that the responsibility and legal liability for this delegation remain with the physician in most states. This delegation is not limited to the immediate presence of the physician, but it can be extended to locations from which the supervising physician can be readily contacted for consultation and assistance, such as by beeper and telephone.

Although there has been a steadily increasing demand for PAs and steadily growing acceptance of and respect for their role as health care providers, added emphasis on cost-effectiveness under managed care has greatly augmented the importance of the profession in health care. Managed care organizations have found PAs to be capable of providing primary care at a lower cost than physicians and to be willing to move into areas in which it would not be cost-effective to place a physician. The supervising physician's role remains unchanged from that described previously. This development and the increasing demand for PAs in these settings have caused a shift of PAs away from primary care. In addition, PAs have been willing to move into various other settings that have not been popular with physicians, such as correctional health systems, substance abuse clinics, occupational health clinics, and geriatric institutions.

In summary, there has been continual evolution and enlargement of the role of PAs. In terms of employment, the near future appears to be rewarding for new graduates. What pitfalls the distant future contains cannot be anticipated.

The Physician Assistant Defined

The use of a generalist assistant, capable of mastering new skills and an enlarging role under responsible supervision of a physician partner, continues to be confirmed. The original concept has been modified and enlarged so much that periodically the American Academy of Physician Assistants (AAPA) feels it needs to develop a new definition of the profession. The last one was adopted by the AAPA House of Delegates in 1995. This definition addresses the versatility of the profession, its distribution in all geographic locations, and the various nonclinical roles that PAs might pursue.

> Physician assistants are health professionals licensed to practice medicine with physician supervision. Physician assistants are qualified by graduation from an accredited physician assistant educational program and/or certification by the National Commission on the Certification of Physician Assistants. Within the physician/PA relationship, physician assistants exercise autonomy in medical decision making and provide a broad range of diagnostic and therapeutic services. The clinical role of physician assistants includes primary and specialty care in medical and surgical practice settings in rural and urban areas. Physician assistant practice is centered on patient care and may include educational, research and administrative activities. (Frary, 1996)

Some interpretation of this definition of PAs may be required. The Professional Practices Council of the AAPA provides the following explanations.

> Physician assistants are health professionals.

This recognizes the scope of PA practice, advanced knowledge required to be a PA, exercise of discretion and judgment, use of ethical standards, and orientation toward service.

. . . licensed to practice medicine with physician supervision.

This may be of concern to PAs accustomed to the terms *certified* and *registered.* Examination of accepted definitions of occupational regulation, however, reveals that PAs are subject to *de facto* licensure regardless of terminology used by the state.

Registration is the least restrictive form of regulation. It is the process of creating an official record or list of persons, for example, voter registration. Its main purpose is not to ensure the public of its quality but to serve as a record-keeping function.

Under a certification system, practice of an activity or occupation is not directly restricted, but limits are placed on the use of certain occupational titles. The label *certified* publicly identifies persons who have met certain standards but does not prevent uncertified practitioners from engaging in the activity.

Under licensure, which is the most restrictive method of regulation, persons have no right to engage in a particular activity without permission to do so by the state. Such permission is generally conditioned on stringent requirements, such as certain educational qualifications and passage of an examination.

Because PAs must meet such standards and may not practice without state approval, *licensed* is the most appropriate way to describe the control exercised by states over PA practice. PAs are qualified to practice by graduating from an accredited PA educational program and/or by certification by the NCCPA. There are two major criteria for being a PA. The connector *and/or* is in accord with AAPA policy, which recognizes that informally trained, nationally certified PAs are an integral part of the profession.

Within the physician-PA relationship PAs exercise autonomy in medical decision making and provide a broad range of diagnostic and therapeutic services. This reinforces the concept of team practice while emphasizing the ability of PAs to think independently when making diagnoses and clinical decisions. It also refers to the broad scope of services that PAs provide.

The clinical role of PAs includes primary and specialty care in medical and surgical practice settings in rural and urban areas. PA practice is centered on patient care and may include educational, research, and administrative activities. This piece addresses the versatility of the PA profession, the distribution of the profession in all geographic regions, and the nonclinical roles that PAs may pursue.

PHYSICIAN ASSISTANT: THE NAME

The name *physician assistant* has a historical base; some of that history is outlined in Chapter 2. The name has been used since the concept originated but has not always been universally embraced.

The original concept of the PA was an assistant who would be able to handle many aspects of a physician's work. Initially the focus was on the education process and not on the name. It was not a copyrighted term such as *physical therapist* or *psychologist,* but it generally conveyed what everyone thought should be conveyed. Other names were proposed and continue to be proposed (Exhibit 1-2). It was evident that the PA's role filled a health care delivery need, but before long the movement was growing and taking on new dimensions. However, confusion arose about the label *PA,* which, after coming to public attention, was sometimes misused to describe a variety of individuals, including support personnel from physicians' offices (Fasser, Andrus, and Smith, 1984).

EXHIBIT 1-2

Historical List of Proposed Names for Assistants to Physicians
Physician assistant (PA)
Physician's assistant
Physicians' assistant
Physician associate
Physician's associate
Medex (Mx)
Child health associate (CHA)
Surgeon's assistant (SA)
Anesthesia assistant and associate
Clinical associate
Community health aide
Community health medic
Medical services assistant
Ophthalmic assistant
Orthopedic physician's assistant
Pathologist's assistant
Primex (Px)
Radiology physician's assistant
Syniatrist
Urologic physician's assistant
Flexner
Osler

The title *PA* is not a legally recognized term nationally and internationally. However, National Physician Assistant Day (October 6) is observed in most states, in the District of Columbia, and in some of the trust territories (Puerto Rico, Guam, and American Samoa). It is up to the states to protect the public health, safety, and welfare by determining how the term *PA* is used. Generally this means setting minimum standards and regulations to practice using a certain health profession or occupation. With few exceptions, most state statutes or regulations define PAs as individuals who have graduated from an accredited program and/or passed the NCCPA examination. Although this has not prevented some imposters from occasionally emerging, the known incidences are rare, and the checks and safeguards in place in most states seem sound (Fisher, 1995).

From a historical standpoint PAs themselves did not determine the title by which they would be known. Instead educators, physicians, regulators, and advocates of the concept made the first suggestions for a name. Later, PAs exerted some influence in the drive toward title uniformity when state laws were being enacted, accreditation and certification mechanisms were being established, and professional organizations were being founded. It was at this point that Stead observed, "The time has come to consider a new name for the product produced by Duke and other similar programs." Although he favored the title *physician's associate,* Stead (1971) concluded, "Agreeing on a name is the important step. What name is adopted is secondary." A number of names were advanced, including *Medex,* coined by Dr. Richard Smith at the Medex Northwest Physician Assistant Program at the University of Washington in Seattle (Smith, 1974).

Although *PA* has become the dominant title, some believe that the term *assistant* is demeaning. They argue that the term leaves the impression that PAs are mere helpers or auxiliary personnel who facilitate the work of their superior or function in a subordinate position. Inclusion of the word *assistant* leads people to draw parallels with medical assistants and nurses' aides.

Another argument for changing the title is that it does not accurately describe what PAs do. The scope of medical services and the level of care that PAs provide go beyond assisting physicians. In many underserved areas PAs are the sole or primary providers of health care. Even if the term at one time appropriately described PA practice, it is no longer accurate. The AAPA describes PAs as "practicing medicine with physician supervision."

Another point made by advocates for change is that the title is not readily understood. The word *assistant* implies entry-level knowledge, on-the-job training, or trade school education. It fails to reflect PAs' substantial clinical and didactic education and the fact that many have earned graduate degrees (Mastrangelo, 1993). Patients may be confused and may sometimes ask when the PA plans to attend medical school. Other health care providers such as nurses resist taking orders from PAs because they do not understand the PA's role. The title is not universally recognized and understood, which leads to problems with insurers, employers, and others.

Proponents of name change tend to favor the term *physician associate* because they believe it more accurately reflects the PA-physician relationship, avoids comparison with medical assistants, and is less confusing to the public. In other parts of the world *doctors' assistants* and *physician's assistants* are well-defined terms for people who support general practitioners (Fischer, 1995). Advocates point to the change from *Medex* to *PA* that occurred easily and say a change could occur again, given the relative simplicity of changing the word from *assistant* to *associate.* Other suggestions include the terms *medical practitioner, physician practitioner, clinical practitioner, assistant physician, clinical associate,* and *associative physician.*

Defenders of the title *PA* argue that replacing the term *assistant* with *associate* does not guarantee greater respect. Respect and self-esteem are gained by practicing with excellence and skill and by providing the best possible medical care to patients. These defenders find little or no dissatisfaction with the current title. For them the title correctly conveys the dependent nature of the relationship with their supervising physician.

The issue is one of semantics. Clerks and telemarketers may be called *sales associates,* whereas high government officials hold the title *special assistant to the president;* in academics, assistant professors are still referred to as *professors.*

Supporters of the current name say that time and growth, not a new name, will produce more recognition. The lack of universal recognition occurs because the profession is small and has a relatively brief history. The profession has already made an enormous investment in educating the patients and the public about the true meaning of the title *PA*. State laws define the qualifications of those who use a particular title, and once the profession abandons the title *PA*, it could be awarded to another category of health care provider, such as unlicensed medical graduates (Cornell, 1998; Anthony, 2000).

Another important observation is that the laws of all legislative jurisdictions and the federal government could not be changed simultaneously. A period of years would pass during which many different individuals would reap the benefits achieved by the PA profession by assuming the name and calling themselves PAs. In addition to the changes required by the state legislatures, licensing boards, and the federal government, other agencies would be required to make changes. Educational institutions, state and national PA organizations, and the accrediting and certifying agencies would need to be persuaded to change. Many of these organizations would have to bear significant administrative and financial costs to make the change. As the AAPA Professional Practices Council concluded

> The argument most strongly expressed by opponents of change is that this debate draws time and effort away from issues that demand urgent attention. The PA profession is at a crossroads and is faced with unprecedented opportunities to define and influence its future. The options are varied. One observer says, "it is time for PAs to dedicate themselves to achieving the greatest benefit for the greatest number of people by becoming advocates for health promotion and preventive medicine." (Tiger, 1993)

Physician Assistant-Certified

PAs who have passed the Physician Assistant National Certification Examination (PANCE) have the option of putting the word *certified* behind the title *PA*: *PA-certified* (PA-C). The intent of using *PA-C* is to distinguish formally trained PAs who are nationally certified from PAs who are informally trained and not eligible to sit for the PANCE. In the 1970s and 1980s this was thought to be important because the percentage of noncertified PAs was small but significant, and formally trained PAs felt they should have some way to show the public the difference.

Many PA observers feel that the identification of *PA-C* is unnecessary and probably confuses more people than it reassures. It is simply an indication that one has passed a test, a fact known for the most part only by the profession. The accomplishment is debatable and pales in light of other more commonly recognized letters such as *MPH*, *PhD*, and *MBA*. Adding additional letters such as *R* for *registered*, as in *RPA-C*, which is done in New York, confuses people even more. The *R* in this instance means that the PA has completed a form and sent a specified sum to an official New York address. Physicians must be licensed but do not place initials after *MD* or *DO* (e.g., *MD-L*). Nurses who have passed their boards do not use *RN-B* (Begely, 1993). If other countries adopt the term *PA*, as has Canada, the certified portion may become more divisive than intended.

Generic Terms for Nonphysician Providers

One of the more confusing evolutions of names has been the effort on the part of health services workers and medical sociologists to develop a generic term that encompasses both PAs and other workers who fill traditional physician roles such as NPs and certified nurse midwives (CNMs). One term used in the early 1970s was *new health professionals*. This was the most frequently used term for both PAs and NPs. Other terms that came into vogue were *physician extenders* and *midlevel practitioners*. These terms were never defined and remain largely meaningless: midlevel between whom? What does it mean to extend a physician? Another term carelessly used is *allied health*. *Allied health providers* is a term used rather restrictively to indicate only those occupations that are allied with the medical profession through their cooperative scheme of accreditation and certification organizations. This term has a fairly precise definition and is usually reserved for those occupations that support physician services, such as x-ray technicians, physical therapists, and medical laboratory personnel. Nurses are in an occupation that is not considered part of allied health personnel, so it is not appropriate to refer to advanced practice nurses such as NPs and CNMs as allied health, and it is not appropriate to refer to PAs as allied health.

One attempt to encompass both PAs and NPs has been the advancement of the term *affiliated clinician*. It was suggested that somehow the two professions, PAs and NPs, should merge under one title (Mittman, 1995). Not unlike the term *affiliated staff* used at Group Health Cooperative in Seattle, this effort was to counter the otherwise seemingly negative-sounding term *nonphysician provider*. The response from readers to an editorial in *Clinician Reviews* on the term *affiliate clinician* was one of disapproval. The term *nonphysician provider* was introduced in 1988 in the public health literature and seems to have been largely adopted and used by medical sociologists and the federal government. More recently, *nonphysician clinician* (NPC) has emerged in the health services research literature (Cooper, Henderson, and Dietrich, 1998). For now the easiest practice seems to be to use the terms *PAs* and *NPs* (PA/NP) and to leave the search for a generic term for another time.

THE EVOLVING ROLE

During the formative years of the PA profession many arguments were put forth about why this new health occupation was not needed or would fail. Among these arguments was the idea that PAs would be frustrated in their role and leave the field for greener pastures. The source of frustration envisioned by these critics was the stress and strain of being an "almost doctor" without the intrinsic or extrinsic rewards that our society provides for physicians. The intrinsic rewards of professional autonomy in clinical practice would not be available because of the need for close supervision by a physician (Perry, 1989).

Over the last three decades the PA occupation has helped to fill a health sector niche with highly skilled professionals. These professionals are capable of carrying out responsibilities that in the past had been within the physician's domain. Given the degree of formal training involved, the PA profession offers highly challenging and satisfying work.

The demand in the health care sector for PAs continues to exceed the available supply (Cawley et al., 2000; Hooker, 1997). The legal and bureaucratic obstacles preventing a broader scope of responsibilities in diagnosis and treatment have largely been overcome during the first two decades. The initial view held by some that PAs would be frustrated because of a narrow and limited professional role is now untenable. The intrinsic rewards are there, and the job satisfaction of PAs remains high.

A career as a PA is an attractive alternative to the years of competition, pressure, long hours, and expense required to enter and complete medical school and to finish residency training. "The career as a PA is also an alternative to the narrower scope of work and lower pay available to the nursing profession" (Perry, 1989).

PAs have the responsibility and independence most could reasonably expect. Role frustration is certainly present but does not appear to be a dominant problem (Freeborn and Hooker, 1995). Although salary levels and career advancement opportunities may be less than optimal, they are certainly not problematic enough to cause a significant exodus from the PA profession. There is a greater demand for graduates of PA programs than there are applicants entering the PA training programs.

In the first decade of the PA movement (1965 to 1975), there was considerable interest in exploring the characteristics of this new health care profession. As the profession matures, we expect to see renewed vigor for research that will shed new light on our understanding of this group of highly motivated, well-trained, compassionate health care providers. Such research should help the PA profession to become an even more dynamic force in the improvement of the quality and availability of health care in the United States.

Qualification for Practice and Legal Parameters

State medical practice statutes and regulations define the scope of practice activities, delineate the range of diagnostic and patient management tasks permitted, and set standards for professional conduct. Qualification for entry to practice as a PA in nearly all states requires that individuals possess a fairly uniform set of characteristics. This usually includes a certificate of completion verifying graduation from a PA educational program accredited by the ARC-PA and/or proof of having sat for and obtained a passing score on the PANCE. The PANCE is a standardized test of competence in primary care medicine administered annually by the NCCPA and is assembled and scored through the National Board of Medical Examiners.

The clinical professional activities and scope of practice of PAs are regulated by state licensing boards, which are often boards of medicine but in some instances comprise a separate PA licensing board. The PA profession appears to be comfortable with its dependent practice role and since its inception has not wavered in that stance. In contrast, nurse practitioners have articulated a position of practice independent from physicians. Statements by professional nursing organizations have stirred debate on the national level, with physician groups regarding the turf of primary care and related legal practice barriers and regulations. Although NPs are professionally autonomous in the performance of nursing care functions, most state medical and nursing practice regulations require that NPs work in collaboration with a physician practice, recognizing that their extended roles encompass medical diagnostic and therapeutic tasks. Thus in providing medical care tasks, most NPs work closely with physicians in a majority of clinical settings.

In contrast, the legal basis of PA practice is centered on physician supervision. Doctors are ultimately responsible for the actions of the PAs, and state laws often require that physicians clearly delineate the practice scope and supervisory arrangements of employed PAs. However, wide latitude exists within the physician's practice for the PA to exercise levels of judgment and professional autonomy in medical care decisions.

It has been noted that the level of acceptance and integration of PAs in American medicine is related to the profession's continued adherence to this position and to the PA's willingness to practice in settings, locations, and clinical care areas that physicians deem to be less preferable. Observers believe that PA use will continue as long as it extends the medical care services of physicians without competing for or challenging physician authority and autonomy.

PHYSICIAN ASSISTANTS IN AMERICAN MEDICINE: THE BOOK

We begin this book by recording the historical roots of the PA profession, incorporating the national and international medical and sociocultural trends that led to the emergence of the PA profession in the United States. In Chapter 3 we provide a broad update and overview of the current status of the PA profession and describe its major characteristics. Next, we review PA education and examine the evolution and effectiveness of curricula and deployment strategies for PAs. A major practice role for the PA has been and continues to be primary care. In Chapter 5 we give an overview of PA practice in primary care and describe PAs' accomplishments and activities in various settings in which they deliver primary care services. Another key practice area for PAs is in the hospital setting. The next chapter describes the multiple and new roles that continue to evolve for PAs in inpatient settings. While most PAs work as clinicians, there is a proportion of PAs who have elected to direct their careers toward nonclinical areas. This growing assortment of occupations and subfields continues to expand as PAs seek to use their training in areas related to medicine, such as management, publishing, politics, and the law. An impressive achievement of the PA profession has been its success in the legal and medical regulatory arena. In the next chapter we provide the fundamental legal concepts that apply to PA practice and describe PA regulatory and certification organizations and structure. In Chapter 11, a new addition to this edition, we describe the major organizations that represent PAs. Reflecting the brisk growth of the size and scope of the PA profession, the four major PA organizations—the American Academy of Physician Assistants, the Association of Physician Assistant Programs, the National Commission on Certification of Physician Assistants, and the Accreditation Review Commission on Physician Assistants—each play separate, distinct, and important public roles in the advancement of the profession. The next chapter, also a new addition to this second edition, is a chapter on PAs employed in federal service. There are deep military roots in the PA profession, and their presence remains strong in the traditional uniformed branches. Moreover, there has been expansion and increased recognition of PAs in other areas of federal services, such as the Bureau of Prisons, the Department of State, and the Department of Transportation. Finally, in the concluding chapter, we gaze into the future and analyze the likely trends and forces that will influence the future direction of PAs.

2

DEVELOPMENT OF THE PROFESSION

INTRODUCTION

When physician assistants (PAs) were introduced into medical practice in the United States in the 1960s, the principal hope was to create a new type of medical worker to assist physicians as the medical practice changed. Most believed that there was a shortage of physicians. Contributing to this shortage was the fading image of the general practitioner and the rise of the specialist physician. Organized around and continuously engaged in the early development of the PA profession, all of these collaborating partners participated in introducing and supporting the PA concept as an appropriate, timely, and useful tool for improving health care in underserved communities. PAs were envisioned as a new type of medical generalist: one whose role could build on prior medical background and experience, one who could be trained in a reasonably short period, and one who could be rapidly deployed to practice locations in medically needy areas.

The idea of using practitioners who are not physicians to provide medical care in a health system is not new. Physicians have utilized and trained, both informally and formally, a wide range of assistants and associates throughout the history of medicine. In many countries over the last two centuries health care providers who were not physicians, or nonphysician providers (a modern term), have played important roles in meeting medical service needs in many nations (Roemer, 1977; Terris, 1977). One pattern observed with new health professionals is that in certain countries at particular times they appear after some period of sociocultural change, which creates conditions ripe for their emergence. A common impetus for new types of health workers is circumstances related to changes in medical personnel need, often an undersupply or maldistribution of doctors. This may prompt societal reassessment of the roles of physicians and other providers. The use of nonphysician health professionals has been shown to be an effective health workforce measure in improving medical care delivery in the health systems of several countries in the twentieth century (Rousselot, 1971; Storey, 1972; Roemer, 1977).

The development of various types of health care professionals and occupations is an ever-evolving phenomenon in most societies' health systems. Although in the medical systems of most countries in the twentieth century physicians (those who hold the MD, DO, or MBBS degrees) are typically regarded as the "captain of the ship" and their status is thought of as the "gold standard" among health care professionals, some types of nonphysician providers assume practice roles similar to doctors, and their roles often overlap considerably.

The development of nonphysician providers has occurred in several countries after times of turmoil such as war and revolution. In some parts of the world nonphysician clinicians have established well-accepted niches in the health system. In the United States since the mid 1960s, two new types of nonphysician professions have emerged (PAs and nurse practitioners [NPs]), and one has reemerged (nurse midwives) whose clinical role includes a broad range of medical practice activities and autonomy. In this chapter we describe the forces that led to the creation and development of one type of nonphysician profession in the United States over the past half century, the PA.

CREATION OF NEW HEALTH CARE PROVIDERS

Broadly speaking, nonphysicians have fewer years of formal training than physicians, may have a regulated or physician-linked practice status, and may have roles largely defined by technology. In the case of PAs a key rationale was to create providers who could supplement and extend the delivery of medical services in a typical doctor's office. The clinical roles of PAs were founded on a strong base of medical-model education but also include perspectives imported from other health paradigms and disciplines. In such instances PA practice may not merely be substitutive of physician functions but may be expanded to encompass services that may be termed *physician complementary,* for example, health and medical services not performed by physicians (Asparantu, 2002).

The developmental experience of the PA in American medicine is in many ways unique to this system, but there are similarities to nonphysicians used in other countries and in other eras. International experience with nonphysicians parallels the formation of the PA in the United States. In analyzing the emergence of the PA in the United States, it is instructive to note the characteristics, natural history, and experiences of nonphysicians used in other countries.

PREDECESSORS OF PHYSICIAN ASSISTANTS

For centuries all over the world individuals who are not fully trained doctors have been involved in the delivery of medical care. Known by various names, given differing clinical prerogatives by societies, and discharging different functions, these types of health care providers play important roles in delivery systems, often in primary care. In the main, nonphysician health care providers and the way they function are a product of the systems and nations that have fostered their development and incorporated their roles (Cawley and Golden, 1983).

While the role of doctor as chief minister to and advocate for the person who is ill has existed since time immemorial, the role of the physician is a more recent incarnation. In the United States a wide variety of health care providers were in practice in colonial times, and some were better trained than others. By the mid 1800s the establishment of the U.S. medical profession was based on a profound European influence in training and role, the incorporation of newly developing scientific advancements, and a propensity to exert political and economic strength to define and protect professional prerogatives (Starr, 1982). During the last part of the 1800s a number of rivals popular with patients competed with allopathic physicians for acceptance and legal recognition (e.g., osteopathy, homeopathy, chiropractic, naturopathy). Allopathic physicians prevailed based largely on adherence to a philosophic and scientific approach and their ability to convince state regulatory boards to grant them authority to perform medical diagnosis and treatment, often as the sole authority.

Throughout this time physicians often trained assistants at various levels and used them in their practices. One of the few documented descriptions was written by George Crile, MD, a surgeon at the Cleveland Clinic who described what he thought was the "world's first physician assistant," an informally trained surgical provider in urology working at that institution during the 1930s and 1940s (Crile, 1987). The activities of his assistant would be a role model for a urology PA today.

INTERNATIONAL NONPHYSICIAN PROVIDERS

Throughout time many countries have used various health care workers, including nonphysician providers. Implicit in this discussion is the notion that these health care providers perform medical tasks that in some societies have been and remain in the domain of physicians. These tasks include, for example, skills in physical examination and diagnosis of common illnesses, minor surgical procedures, and knowledge and dispensing of basic medications. Countries in Africa, Asia, Oceania, and North, South, and Central America continue to employ these types of providers mainly to increase health care delivery to poorly served regions.

Various objectives underlie strategies to incorporate nonphysicians into health care systems: the need for general health care, medical assistance in times of doctor shortages, and the need for trained personnel to staff developing technology (Fulop and Roemer, 1987). Sometimes the incorporation of nonphysicians into a nation's health care system appears to be connected to social strife, and a type of health care provider emerges to fill specific health workforce policies (Exhibit 2-1) (Cawley, 1983b).

France: The Officier de Santé

In 1803 shortly after the French Revolution the eminent scientist and educator René Fourcroy submitted a report to the legislature outlining plans for a major reorganization of the French medical care system. Among his proposals was the creation of a new independent grade of health officers who would help alleviate health care personnel shortages in the military and the civilian sector, particularly in rural areas. These providers were called *officiers de santé* (health officers).

Qualifications for the grade of officier de santé in the French health care system required either a 6-year apprenticeship with a physician, a 5-year period in a hospital, or 3 years in medical school; to fully qualify as a physician one had to complete 6 years of medical school. The officiers de santé had a fairly far-reaching independent but ultimately limited scope of practice. They could not perform major operations, but they could suture, perform minor surgical procedures, prescribe medications, and practice medicine to a large degree on an independent basis. For activities within their practice scope, officiers de santé were legally liable for malpractice.

The practice of officiers de santé stirred substantial opposition from physicians. The officiers de santé came under attack from the medical profession soon after their inception and remained so almost constantly until their abolition in 1892. As French social, medical, and economic conditions improved throughout the nineteenth century, opposition to the officier created a clamor from physicians to reestablish a single qualifying degree in medicine. The argument of the entrenched physicians to the French legislature was bolstered by the reluctance of officiers to practice in rural areas. The grade of officier was attacked by physicians as sustaining "second-class practitioners" and after 1850 was considered by French physicians to have outlived its usefulness. After several legislative measures had reduced their practice privileges, officiers de santé were abolished in 1892.

EXHIBIT 2-1

Nonphysician Health Care Providers in Select Countries*

Name	Country	Time
Officier de santé	France	1803-1892
Feldsher	Russia, Eastern Europe	1600s-present
Midwife	Universal	>10,000 years ago to present
Nurse midwife	United States, Europe, others	1900-present
Village health worker	Developing countries, Alaska	1940-present
Barefoot doctor	China	1966-present
Physician assistant	United States, Canada	1965-present
Nurse practitioner	United States, Canada, Great Britain	1966-present
Community health technician	Colombia, Mexico, Peru, Guyana	1970s

*Many names denote health care workers who were modeled after the barefoot doctor. These nonphysician providers were introduced and promoted by the World Health Organization in many developing countries: dresser, medical auxiliary, health assistant, paramedic, medical aide, assistant medical officer, me'dicin Africain, and rural health technician.

> The introduction of second-class practitioners who were "good enough for the troops and the country folk" had not fulfilled the original expectations. In the long run it had done little to remedy the maldistribution of medical care between town and country. The problem of this imbalance is still with us today, affecting developed and developing countries alike in varying degree. Despite great efforts that are being made, we are still waiting for a system that will bring a satisfactory solution. (Heller, 1978)

Russia: Feldshers

The feldsher, historically, represented a link between the eras of folk cures and modern medicine. Originally feldshers (from the German *Feldscherer*) were German military assistants to the "barber surgeons" of the seventeenth century. Peter the Great introduced feldshers into the Russian armies in the 1860s. Following military service, early feldshers served as civilian clinicians and were often the only available providers for the rural peasant population. Typically, they were apprenticed to physicians for some time and provided low-cost health care for much of the Russian countryside well into the twentieth century (Sidel, 1968a, 1968b, 1969).

For many years feldshers were widely used by the armies of several eastern European countries, but eventually in most instances more highly trained personnel replaced them. In pre-Soviet Russia and throughout the existence of the Soviet Union, feldshers were extensively used as primary care providers, mainly in rural areas. In these settings, they were often the only type of trained medical personnel available and frequently functioned in an independent manner (Storey, 1972; Knaus, 1981).

For a time after the 1917 Bolshevik Revolution, it was determined that each Soviet citizen should be treated by his or her own physician, and the concept of feldsherism was considered second-class medicine. In 1936 the Soviet government reinstituted formal training for feldshers, and by the mid 1970s Russia was training approximately 30,000 feldshers annually (Condit, 1977, 1984).

While a nurse's function consists mostly of comforting the patient and carrying out physician's orders, feldshers were often independent practitioners who were trained to perform certain diagnostic and therapeutic procedures, frequently without physician supervision. Feldshers typically received between 1 and 3 years of medical education after graduation from secondary school. Length of training depends on the specialty the feldsher elects: general feldsher 2 years, midwife 2½ years, feldsher laborant 2 years, and sanitarian feldsher 1 to 1½ years. Candidates usually enter directly from secondary school. Tuition is free, stipends and living expenses are provided, and positions are guaranteed at the completion of training.

Reportedly the upper 10% of graduate feldshers are encouraged to go on to medical school. Otherwise, they can take evening study at medical school after 3 years of clinical service. Once admitted, these students are eligible for advanced placement. At one time, as many as 25% to 30% of physicians in the former Soviet Union were initially trained as feldshers.

Feldshers have had a checkered history in Russia as political and medical forces changed. For many years after the 1917 Russian Revolution, feldshers were labeled as second-class doctors and considered to be a short-term solution to health personnel shortages. As the years went by, feldshers retained their role as the enormity of the health care needs of the newly formed Soviet Union, then the largest country in the world, became apparent. At first, feldshers practiced in the rural and underserved regions of Russia and entrenched themselves as an important personnel link in the health care system: the delivery of primary care. Inevitably, as the supply of physicians began to grow in Russia, feldshers were perceived as expendable practitioners. Policy makers on one hand regarded feldshers practicing in rural areas as necessary, but only to the degree that they can be replaced by physicians (Terris, 1977; Knaus, 1981). However, an abundance of physicians did not change the distribution of medical care, and the rural areas continued to suffer limited access to health care. The role of the feldsher is basically twofold: (1) as personnel serving in the urban areas as side-by-side assistants to physicians (similar to PAs and NPs in the United States) and (2) as alternatives to physicians in underserved regions. Like PAs in the United States, physicians supervise feldshers in their clinical activities when available.

At one time an estimated 1 million feldshers were in practice (Kenyon, 1985). There have been reports that feldshers are on the wane with the breakup of the Soviet Union and restructuring of health care in these countries. Although there may be an oversupply of physicians in several of the eastern European countries, feldshers remain a type of health care personnel in the health care systems of the former Soviet Union. They play an intermediary role in medical labor with capacities in primary medical care and the ability to assume technical and specialized roles.

Although the early developers of the PA concept did not have the feldsher specifically in mind, there is some parallel between the feldsher and the American PA. With an adequate supply of doctors in the former Soviet Union many believe the occupation of feldsher is becoming obsolete. The health systems of Russia and other countries of the former Soviet Union are now plagued by problems of too many physicians, many of them specialists, and a lack of professionalism among physicians resulting from the state-enforced breakup of professional associations. Poorly trained primary care physicians, limited inpatient and outpatient diagnostic capacity, too many hospital beds, excessive use of services (particularly inpatient care), and the obsolete and poor condition of capital stock are among the litany of problems faced by the health care systems of many of these countries. In 1994 the physician/population ratios varied from 2.1 physicians per 1000 population in Tajikistan to 3.8 in Russia, with a six-country average of 3.3. This compares with an average of 2.5 in Western countries. Since 1994 these ratios have fallen slightly in all six countries except Uzbekistan. Nonetheless, the ratios throughout are still well above the European average.

Because many former Soviet bloc countries have significant health system problems, it is likely that the need for feldshers in some form as an adjunct to other medical personnel will remain.

China: Barefoot Doctors

The Chinese barefoot doctor is a health care worker once described as a "poor cousin of the Russian feldsher" and was overly romanticized in many quarters in the 1970s (Terris, 1977). A type of nonphysician health care provider, they are more like village aides than feldshers or U.S. PAs and NPs. The levels of function and training are very basic. Armed with only 3 to 6 months of medical education, barefoot doctors were created to increase the basic level of primary care delivered to China's enormous and expanding population.

Barefoot doctors emerged from the social cataclysm that marked the 1966 Cultural Revolution in China. During that period drastic reductions in medical education took place under a campaign against medical and professional elitism. This antiintellectual movement led to a massive reorganization of the system of medical education. Many medical schools were closed, with a reduction in the length of physician training and a dispersal of faculty to the rural villages. The Chinese leader Mao Ze-Dong attacked the medical status quo with a vengeance and called for the formation of a legion of primary health care workers based in the villages of China who, when not providing health care, would tend the rice fields (Wen and Hays, 1975). Barefoot doctors received only 3 months of on-the-job training in the villages in which they would serve; their roles were also oriented to the enforcement of public health measures and the prevention of common diseases (Exhibit 2-2).

In the ensuing years several million barefoot doctors were trained and deployed in China. As the fervor of the Cultural Revolution waned, the system of medical training was restored, and China has worked steadily to rebuild its system of medical education and increase its supply of physicians (Blendon, 1979). Policy assessments of the introduction of barefoot doctors note that "the program has not been a panacea; the usefulness of the barefoot doctor lies in there being a stopgap measure rather than a long-term solution to the shortage of physicians" (Hsu, 1974).

Barefoot doctors comprised a basic first tier of Chinese medicine and were the entry point to the system for peasants seeking curative services. Their numbers have declined somewhat from a high of more than 2 million in the late 1970s to about 1.2 million in 1984 (Hsiao, 1984). This reduction coincided with economic reforms in China, resulting in a decline in the cooperative medical system, the last vestige of the Cultural Revolution ideology.

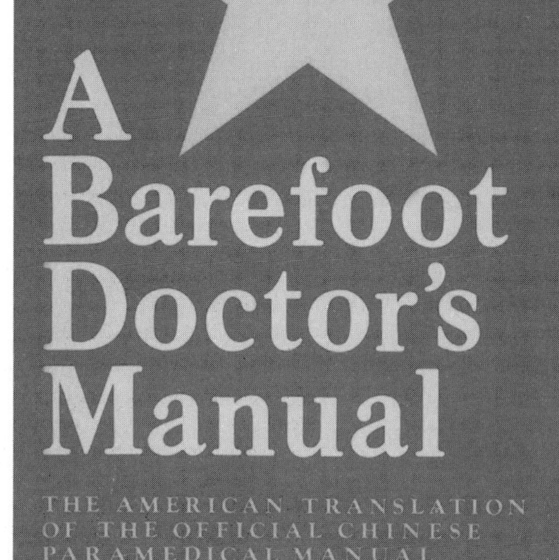

EXHIBIT 2-2 Barefoot Doctors Manual. (Reprinted with permission from *A Barefoot Doctor's Manual*, Copyright 1990, 2002 by Running Press Book Publishers, Philadelphia and London, www.runningpress.com.)

Developing Countries

The incorporation of nonphysician health providers into the health care system depends fundamentally on the extent of the needs of that country for medical services. In many developing countries, where the supply of physicians is lacking, various types of practitioners are employed to ensure delivery of essential primary care services such as prenatal care, immunization, and disease screening. In the latter half of the twentieth century many countries have successfully used nonphysicians, propelled by the increasing demand for health care services, the emphasis on primary care, and the World Health Organization (WHO) policy of "Health for All by the Year 2000" (WHO, 1980, 1987a, 1987b; Fulop, 1982).

Throughout many countries of the world, particularly in Africa (Algeria, Sudan), Asia (Burma), South America (Venezuela), and Oceania (Micronesia, Melanesia, and Polynesia), health care workers are known by many different titles (health officers, community health aides [CHAs], medical auxiliaries, health assistants, village health workers, Algerian adjoint medicaux de lasante, the Burmese health assistant, the Sudanese medical assistant, and the Venezuelan auxiliar de enfermeria) (WHO, 1968). They provide primary health care in small communities and in rural areas. These health care providers vary greatly in their backgrounds and level of clinical function (Smith, 1978).

The WHO has provided leadership in health care personnel activities in developing countries with the aim of improving primary care and other basic health care services. In the 1980s a major WHO objective in health care personnel was total population coverage for health care services. Only a rapid expansion of programs incorporating use of multipurpose auxiliary health care personnel would help developing countries achieve this goal (Storms, 1979; WHO, 1980, 1987b; Fulop, 1982).

The Pan American Health Organization has promoted other types of providers with roles similar to PAs. Peru trains and approves health care providers with professional status; this training is provided by a specialized high school education leading to a bachelor's degree in health (Acuna, 1977).

Colombia and Mexico started several experimental training programs in the 1970s for community health technicians—with components of clinical and preventive medicine, public health, and community practice—that involve postsecondary education. The modalities may vary, but the principle of incorporating the PA in the health care team is gaining acceptance (Acuna, 1977).

In the 1970s Guyana took a further step by approving the training of a full-fledged PA with the characteristics and functions similar to those of the U.S. version. Experience there has attracted the interest of neighboring countries (Acuna, 1977).

Developed Countries

A number of developed countries that are faced with the trends of increasing physician specialization and demand for primary care services have adopted different approaches in medical education to encourage primary care deployment. A major policy thrust in some industrialized countries has been to place limitations on the numbers of physicians who can become specialists. This fundamental determination in personnel ensures that a country's health care system has an adequate supply of primary care providers and precludes the need for a nonphysician provider in this role. In most countries, such as those in Europe, the use of nonphysicians to provide primary care in rural areas or similar types of health care providers in urban tertiary care centers is unheard of. Fully trained physicians deliver primary care and medical generalist services to most of the population. To be sure, roles exist for advanced practice nursing such as NPs and nurse midwives in several countries, England being the most noted. In the health care systems of most developed countries such as Sweden, however, health care personnel and primary care staffing are well established and planned by governments and key groups. In addition, the homogeneity of individual European countries' societies, the common belief that health care is a fundamental right, the smaller geographic areas of these nations, and the less entrepreneurial approach to health services' delivery systems are major reasons that most European countries have not adopted the nonphysician health care personnel concept. In Latin American countries most health care systems do not include the use of nonphysicians of any type; some countries in Latin America, as in Europe, have an oversupply of physicians, particularly in urban areas.

Canada

For a time Canada followed the U.S. model by promoting the development of the NP concept, but steady pressure from physicians over time eroded the effectiveness of NPs in the system. In the early 1980s organized medicine in Canada effectively abolished the NP concept (Spitzer, 1984) and the number of NPs steadily dwindled. Beginning in 2000 there has been a revival in the interest of certain Canadian physician groups to reintroduce NPs.

The Canadian Forces developed a PA in 1992 that is the same as the U.S. version. These are career medical assistants who receive advance training at the Canadian military base in Borden, Ontario, and then are deployed with the various services in the Canadian Forces. As of 2002 approximately 120 are in uniform and a few dozen retired military members work in the mining or oil drilling industry in remote areas. The Canada Academy of Physician Assistants is in the early stages of development and is actively working with the Royal College of Physicians and Surgeons and the Canadian Medical Association to find how to best integrate into Canadian society (Talbot, 1994; Hooker, 2002).

Alaska

The Alaska program trains local residents to provide emergency and primary care services in villages that are often hundreds of miles away from the nearest physician. Most Alaska Natives live in small villages isolated by mountain ranges, glaciers, stretches of tundra, impassable river systems, and vast distances. These individuals, called CHAs, use procedures set forth in an easy-to-read manual and consult by telephone or radio with a hospital-based physician. The foundation for the CHA program was laid in the 1940s and 1950s when in response to tuberculosis epidemics the federal government used village volunteers to dispense medicine in remote villages. These volunteers, mostly women, generally act as intermediaries between patients and hospital-based physicians. The title CHA was chosen to show the position's link to the community and to emphasize that the person in this role did not practice independently of a physician. In 1991 CHAs were serving about 45,000 Alaska Natives and handled more than 253,000 patient encounters per year. Although the program's effects have not been measured by rigorous study, available data indicate that the program has achieved substantial acceptance among the population it serves and has played a major role in improving the health status of Alaska Natives. The federal government assumes responsibility for medical malpractice claims against services provided by CHAs (General Accounting Office, 1993).

Critique of Feldsherism

Public health activist and physician Victor Sidel (1968, 1972) wrote several important papers on the past and current use of nonphysicians in various countries. These articles reflected the then widespread medical interest in new types of health care providers and in experiments with new forms of the division of medical labor. He used the term *feldsherism* to denote a country's policy of using nonphysicians to provide primary care health services (Sidel, 1968). As a strategy to deal with personnel shortages, many countries have used it, particularly when health care needs are great and physicians are in short supply. The acceptance of the policy of feldsherism depends in large part on the system of health labor organization and the needs of the population. In developing countries increasing the numbers of primary care workers is essential (Roemer, 1977; Orubuloye, 1982; WHO Study Group, 1987); their level of skill in areas of high technology may be irrelevant. Most needed are providers who can deliver basic health services referent to the acute needs of the populations of these countries, and not the advanced skills of the physician. Specifically, clinicians with knowledge of infectious diseases and their treatment, immunization, fluid-replacement therapy, prenatal care, screening for cancer, surgical and orthopedic procedures, and health education to avoid environmental health hazards are essential in providing health care services to populations (WHO, 1987a, 1987b).

In developed countries generalist physicians, rather than nonphysicians, are the principal providers of primary care. Roemer notes that this was the prevailing personnel policy in countries such as Belgium, Norway, Canada, and Australia, where directions focused on increasing the proportion of generalist physicians, limiting physician specialization, and giving priority to primary care. He suggests that the U.S. policy, coming on the worldwide trend of experimentation in health workforce in the 1960s, was a hasty expedient to shortages in primary care in America. Roemer (1977) states:

> In the world's most affluent nation, there would hardly seem to be economic justification for the use of physician extenders for primary care. U.S. policies in the 1970s were based on an unwillingness to impose social obligations on the physician (e.g., location in areas of need) and to train adequate numbers of primary care doctors. Such policies were an unfortunate acknowledgment of failure by medicine to fulfill its social mission.

Yet in America PAs have emerged as a type of primary care provider that is recognized as such by the Institute of Medicine along with NPs as important providers of primary care services (Donaldson, 1996).

Historically feldsherism was often thought of as an interim health care personnel approach. In Russia for many years feldshers were viewed as expedient providers who were necessary only until the physician supply became adequate. This view assumes a fully trained physician best delivers primary care. Yet a key revelation observed in the experience of the PA and NP professions in the United States was to show that nonphysicians could provide a large amount of primary care services. It is a poor use of medical talent to suggest that a physician need be present to deal with every human infirmity. Medical pundit Daniel Greenberg likens the Western system of medical education to putting all bus drivers through astronaut training, the point being that most physicians are overtrained for the role of the primary care generalist.

In a number of countries where nonphysicians have been used for long periods, roles have changed with advances in health care delivery and policy shifts. In Russia feldshers were employed for many years on the front lines of primary care in much of the countryside. As the health care system in the country became more sophisticated, and as the supply of physicians came into balance with the medical needs of the population, policymakers and citizens sometimes viewed feldsherism as sustaining second-class care to those already relegated to second-class health care in the system. While the PA is not formally recognized in Western Europe, the countries of the Pacific Basin, or Central or South America, in nearly all of these countries there are many discussions regarding whether they should incorporate nonphysician health care providers as the primary source of health care personnel for the future.

The use of nonphysicians has been championed as an attack on medical elitism and the professional establishment. Stead believes that the medical profession has been arrogant in its stance toward entry policies and pathways leading to medical licensure. PAs have demonstrated high levels of patient acceptance and to function on a high level with shorter training than physicians (Stead, 2001). Early critiques of PAs and NPs were that they represent a second tier of medical care. Yet nonphysicians have been shown to augment the delivery of primary care to populations like the poor, those in medically underserved areas, and other disadvantaged members of society in proportions greater than physicians. The employment of nonphysicians in various roles, spanning most primary care functions, as well as a wide swath of technical and public health and preventive medicine duties, appears to be an appropriate niche in the systems of many countries.

THE AMERICAN EXPERIENCE

Charles Hudson first suggested the concept of new types of health care personnel to extend physician services in the United States in 1961. Hudson (1961), then president of the National Board of Medical Examiners (NBME), in a speech to the House of Delegates of the American Medical Association (AMA) and in a subsequent article in *JAMA,* articulated the rationale for new health care personnel based on changing medical labor, hospital staffing personnel demands, and advancing technology.

His idea for a new type of health practitioner was to "extend the usefulness" and experience of Army and Navy corpsmen as efficient assistants who "would not be expected to exercise medical judgment, but he might well develop considerable technical skill which could be a source of satisfaction." He believed "a curriculum could be devised, consisting of 2 or 3 years of college work with certain prescribed courses" that paralleled medical school, and that these new health providers should be called *externes* in a broader sense than just *medical students.*

Hudson writes that reaction to this proposal was generally favorable, but there were some dissenting opinions. Little seems to have come from this proposal, and it was largely believed to have died in some AMA committees. People who spoke with Dr. Hudson in the early 1980s say that he was amazed at how the PA concept exceeded his imagination. Although Hudson theorized that the "goals of nursing could be redefined as part-nursing and part-medicine," thus allowing the nursing workforce to fill the role of the externe, he believed nurse leaders would frown on "the proposal of a medicine-nursing hybrid."

Duke University

It was Dr. Eugene Stead, Jr., at Duke University who transformed Hudson's prophecy into reality by developing the first PA training program. As the role developed, it hurdled nearly every obstacle Hudson had foretold. The AMA proposed the profession as an opportunity for nurses to leave their field to gain more responsibility and pay. Referencing the fact that most PAs were men and earned salaries equal to or higher than more formally educated nurses, the American Nurses Association (ANA) retorted by characterizing the new role as a bit of "government supported male chauvinism." What leaders at the respective organizations did not know was that the PA concept was the result of nearly a decade's work by Stead and others. These leaders were exploring options for training health care professionals—nurses among them—for advanced clinical role. The AMA and the ANA's dialogue on the PA was often characterized by sharp language and strong debate over the new profession. It is becoming axiomatic that miscommunication and misunderstanding between medicine and nursing caused their respective professional organizations to hinder rather than promote collaborative endeavors (Holt, 1998).

Stead was chairman of medicine at Duke University in the 1960s and recognized changing medical service and personnel needs in and around Duke University Medical Center. He was a towering figure in academic medicine and had long been interested in breaking down barriers in medical education. At Duke in the early 1960s he began experimenting with programs for new health care personnel and began this with efforts to incorporate medical training with nursing. Before coming to Duke he was a professor of medicine at Emory University during World War II and worked with very capable third-year and fourth-year medical students at a time when all of the intern staff was inducted. In spite of their limited training, on the wards the medical students gave "superb medical care" (Stead, 1979). Knowing what could be accomplished with focused training, he envisioned a new type of midlevel generalist (between the level of a doctor and a nurse), a medical clinician who could be trained in a relatively short time to assist physicians in a broad range of practice settings. Stead believed that such providers should work closely with the physician and established the role in a configuration that would not directly threaten physicians. He sought to base such a provider on a nursing background and first approached nurse Thelma Engles to undergo advanced medical training. Engles was a nursing leader at Duke who was interested in an advanced nursing or medical role. Together they began to experiment with training approaches to expand the nursing role in generalist medical care delivery.

Stead had great respect for nursing experience in patient care. After creating a prototype advanced medical training program for nurses at Duke, he concluded that nurses ". . . were very intelligent and they learned quickly, and at the end of a year we had produced a superb product, capable of doing more than any nurse I had ever met" (Stead, 1979). This program could have initiated the NP movement but was refused accreditation as an educational program by the National League of Nursing (NLN). The attempt failed because on three occasions the NLN, the agency for degree-granting nursing programs, denied accreditation on the basis that delegating medical tasks to nurses was inappropriate (Fisher, 1977). This early foray into an advanced practice nursing program was eventually phased out. Engles left Duke for the Rockefeller Foundation, and Stead was left with a conviction that people with varied backgrounds can deliver high-quality patient care if adequately trained (Christman, 1998).

During this time Stead developed and Duke University sponsored a continuing medical education (CME) program for physicians living in the region. The CME program failed because of lack of attendance. Many physicians were interested in such a program but could not attend because their patient load and the intensity of their practices were too demanding. He reasoned that if the physicians had well-trained assistants, they would be able to leave their practices for a day or two to attend CME programs (Howard, 1969).

Stead's idea of an assistant found encouragement from Amos H. Johnson, a solo general practitioner in Garland, a small rural town in North Carolina. Dr. Johnson was able to maintain his practice, as well as keep up with his CME programs and accept professional appointments such as the presidency of the American Academy of General Practice (1965 to 1966) because he had an assistant. The assistant, Henry "Buddy" Treadwell, had been trained by Johnson for his practice needs and functioned in many ways like a contemporary PA, assuming many tasks such as diagnosing and treating (Gifford, 1987a, 1987b).

Nursing and the Evolution of the PA Concept

In the 1960s organized nursing was not interested in expanding its role to one that included the medical model. What came ultimately to be known as the PA concept was less appealing to nurses because organized medicine had suggested it. Beginning with the initial proposal of Stead and Engles in 1964, and later in 1969 when the AMA suggested the recruitment of nurses to be trained as PAs, the ANA flatly rejected these ideas. This was based on the view that nursing was unwilling to be subordinate to physicians in performing professional duties and reminding medicine that it is not the prerogative of one profession to speak for another (Holt, 1998).

Ultimately, the position of the ANA became "If physicians want additional assistance, they can have it but nurses should not supply the manpower [sic]" (Holt, 1998). In spite of this attitude on nursing's part, Loretta Ford, RN, and Henry Silver, MD, started the first NP program at the University of Colorado (Silver, 1971a). Ironically when this occurred physicians were quick to suggest that NPs were practicing medicine, while nursing leaders claimed that NPs had left nursing to become handmaidens to physicians. Later nursing leaders suggested that the NP role has done much to invigorate nursing as a whole (Christman, 1998; Holt, 1998).

In creating the PA concept, Stead conceived of an entirely new category of health care professional to assist physicians. And instead of nurses, he turned to former military corpsmen. The idea was not entirely without precedent. Duke physicians had been in the military, and many were in the Reserves or were consultants in the major military hospitals in the area. In those hospitals they had observed corpsmen and medics working with physicians in direct patient care and in technical areas of diagnosis and treatment. Former military corpsmen also worked in special clinical units at Duke Hospital and other hospitals in the region (Carter and Strand, 2000). The technologic advances in medicine had put pressure on hospitals for well-trained technicians. Many of these veterans were able to assume a large portion of these tasks with little or no additional training.

In 1965 the vice provost for medical affairs at Duke University appointed an ad hoc committee to evaluate the existing programs and personnel needs at Duke's hospital. The committee concluded that two types of medical personnel were needed: (1) a very highly skilled technician limited to a specific medical discipline or specific area and (2) a more advanced specialist with a broad and basic knowledge of medicine (Stead, 1966, 1967; Estes, 1968c, 1968e; Estes and Howard, 1969; Howard, 1972).

Herbert Saltzman, a physician at Duke, applied for an NIH grant seeking support for training chamber operators in hyperbaric medicine. He cited a need for "paramedical technicians to provide the doctors with support needed in their clinical and research endeavors." Saltzman's concept of the type of personnel needed was consistent with Stead's concept of the PA. Before 1965 the National Heart Institute had not funded "nonprofessional" training programs, but Stead had recently served on the institute's study section and its members were aware of this thinking. When the grant was approved in April 1965, the successful piggybacking of the PA concept with this grant provided the initial source of funding for Stead's experiment in medical education and established the foundation for the first PA educational program in the United States.

With some federal funding support the first PA program was formed at Duke University. On October 4, 1965, four former Navy corpsmen became the first students to begin a 2-year training program. Almost by accident the new concept received nationwide publicity. *Reader's Digest* produced a series of articles entitled "Where the Jobs Are" (Velie, 1965). Even before the curriculum for the first class was planned, the *Digest* announced to its readers that the Duke faculty hoped the program would help make up for the dwindling number of rural doctors. Halfway through the training the program was portrayed in a September 6, 1966, article in *LOOK* magazine. This article, "More Than a Nurse, Less Than a Doctor," had a substantial impact and was the first airing of the concept to the general public. The article began with a paragraph implying that the social change taking place in providing the public increased access to health care services would be accomplished through "the use of mid-level providers" (Berg, 1966).

It was widely accepted at that time that the nation was experiencing a demand for physicians. The article asserted:

> There is a shortage of doctors, and it's getting worse. With the demand for medical care swelling and treatment itself growing more complex daily, the supply of physicians cannot keep up with the need for their skills. Although plans are under way to build more medical schools and expand existing ones, the experts figure it takes almost ten years from the time a medical student drops into one end of the funnel and a practicing physician emerges from the other. Sick people can't wait that long. (Berg, 1966)

In 1967 three students graduated as PAs from this new program. For 2 years they used the house staff's television lounge in the medical center hospital as their classroom, and their graduation ceremony was held in a small Durham barbecue restaurant. Within such inauspicious environments these prototype PAs began formulating a new role, one as yet uncharted.

The Duke program began to expand. In September 1967 just before the first class graduated, the training program moved from the Department of Medicine to the Department of Community Health Sciences. In 1969 Stead retired from active professional duties at Duke and the PA program was moved to the Department of Family and Community Medicine. The chair of the department, Dr. E. Harvey Estes, Jr., essentially oversaw the development of the Duke program and the dissemination of the PA concept and educational programs throughout the country. Under the leadership of Estes the Duke program continued to grow, increasing its number of students, adding the first female student, and improving its physical facilities. From the house staff television lounge the program moved to a small white trailer purchased by the newly formed American Academy of Physician Assistants (AAPA).

PA Diagnostician

One interesting point was what the role of the PA as a dependent practitioner should be. Those at Duke initially held the view that the PA would enter the medical decision-making process before and after the stages of diagnosis and prescription, but the final diagnosis and prescription would be reserved for the physician (Schneller, 1978). E. Harvey Estes, chair of the Duke University Department of Community Health Sciences in 1968, explained that practicing medicine is basically making diagnoses and prescribing treatment. The new assistant will take no part in traditional doctor functions (Estes, 1968b). Thus although Estes and colleagues in the beginning thought the role of the PA would consist of purely technical tasks, before long the PA role came to include diagnosis and patient management functions.

Early Professional Challenges

A major challenge for the new profession was how to obtain legal recognition within the medical regulatory system and at the same time avoid seeking licensure for the PA to perform any specific task. The features of physician dependency and being excluded from the diagnostic and prescriptive process were consistent with an assistant role and did not require licensure (Ballenger, 1971a, 1971b). An even more interesting fact is that the PA role has come to assume considerable diagnostic and therapeutic management responsibilities.

If the idea of the PA concept was a gleam in the eye of its creators, its success also rested squarely on the shoulders of its first students. The first PA students recall thinking that if any of them did poorly, it could be the early demise of the concept. Some physicians cooly received the idea of a PA, and only a few were initially willing to engage in the novel experiment of a formally trained assistant for doctors. Ken Ferrell, from the first Duke class, recalls that some of the physicians who would have benefited most from assistants were quite resistant to the idea. They were reluctant to relinquish any of their responsibilities, even though they were overworked (Mastrangelo, 1993).

Organized Nursing

Reception of the PA by the nursing profession was even chillier, particularly on the organizational level. Five years after the first PA program was established, the ANA charged that the AMA had designed the PA role to sabotage the ANA's efforts to define nurses as independent associates of physicians, rather than task-oriented "physician handmaidens." The fact that most PAs were men and earned salaries equal to or higher than those of more formally educated nurses was justification according to the ANA for characterizing the development of the PA as a gender-biased innovation (Holt, 1998). In an early account of nursing-PA interaction Christman describes the development of the PA concept from the nursing side and suggests that the nursing profession missed a marvelous opportunity. Christman's first acquaintance with the politics of PAs and nurses came in several debates with Stead, the first at an annual meeting of the Tennessee Medical Society in 1971 and the second in 1978 at the New York Academy of Medicine. Both debates were on the issue of nursing embracing medicine's invitation to develop NPs using the medical model. The confounding actions of the NLN to have this program be part of nursing were largely based on the league's objections to physicians teaching courses for nurses in a nursing program. Stead concluded that nurse leaders were antagonistic to innovation and said the ANA had overreacted to what he considered a constructive approach to include them in creating a more relevant type of provider. Ultimately Stead resented the nursing rejection on ideology and believed that PAs were a reality solely because nurses were not open to new and constructive concepts. Christman was also involved in the formation of the American Association of Colleges of Nursing (AACN), a liaison to the AMA. Attempts to have the AACN join up with the American Association of Medical Colleges were defeated by the strong opposition of nursing. Had this union occurred, Christman (1998) believes that NPs, not PAs, would have become the predominant type of nonphysician clinician in the U.S. system.

Other Duke Models

The idea of the PA persisted into the 1970s, and the establishment of training programs for new categories of health care professionals spread to other institutions. In 1968 a program began at Bowman-Gray School of Medicine Wake-Forest School of Medicine in Winston-Salem, North Carolina, with a curriculum similar to the Duke program. In the same year, Alderson-Broaddus College, a small private college in Phillippi, West Virginia, admitted its first class to a 4-year PA degree program. Unlike Duke, Alderson-Broaddus PA students entered training directly from high school with the intent of majoring in medical sciences and receiving a bachelor's degree at the end of a 4-year curriculum. Hu C. Meyers, MD, was a local general practice physician appointed professor and chairman of the Department of Medical Science and founded the program in 1971. As was the case with most of the pioneering PA programs, the development of the Alderson-Broaddus program was supported by grants from the Commonwealth Fund, the Robert Wood Johnson Foundation, and the then Department of Health, Education and Welfare (Meyers, 1978).

Medex Model

While credit is given to Stead and Estes at Duke for pioneering PA education, the Medex model developed by Richard Smith deserves a special place in PA history. It has remained a viable model of PA education and is often referred to as the collaborative model. The Smith concept of health care development was one in which actively involved health professions schools, local and national medical organizations, rural and urban communities, and overworked practicing physicians would come together for improvement of health care delivery. At the University of Washington in Seattle, Richard Smith, MD, MPH, professor of health sciences, began a 1-year program (later increased to 15 months and now 24 months) to augment the training of former military medical corpsmen. This was the Medex program, a contraction of the two words *medi*cine and *ex*tension. Graduates would refer to themselves as Medex and put Mx after their name. The program, which began in 1969, relied heavily on its students receiving most of their training through on-the-job preceptorships with selected physicians in rural areas of the Pacific Northwest.

The Medex curriculum was built on an individual with an enriched medical background and one willing to serve in primary care settings in rural and medically underserved areas. Smith was a physician with broad vision, a curious mind, and a wealth of experience in medical care in the Third World and in the United States. During his years in the Peace Corps in the early 1960s he was exposed to the French Africa medical officer and its Asian counterpart (the officier medicin indochinois). A brief time with Albert Schweitzer in Africa further shaped what he envisioned would be an assistant to the primary care physician. Smith returned to the United States in the mid-1960s as international health planning director for Surgeon General William Stewart. While he was a U.S. delegate to the annual WHO assembly in Geneva, he further explored the use of new health care providers with health officials from other countries. He continued to nurture the idea of the creation of a new category of health care professional, one who could work with doctors and perform tasks associated with the majority of the routine care that a physician provided.

During the 1960s Smith had become well acquainted with the same Amos Johnson from Garland, North Carolina, who had influenced Eugene Stead in gaining acceptance for his PA concept. Johnson, a country doctor, was a dominant figure in North Carolina medical politics at that time. He was president of the American Association of Family Practice and an influential figure in the AMA. He had heard of Smith's ideas, knew of Stead's work, and introduced Smith to the leadership in the AMA who provided encouragement in developing the PA concept. Johnson often mentioned the relationship he had with Buddy Treadwell and wanted Smith to develop a similar type of assistant (R. Smith, personal communication, 1996).

Dick Smith wanted his Medex program to be more than a demonstration project that was typically underwritten by the federal government and then forgotten a few years later. To succeed, he chose a state with a conservative legislature, believing that if he could sell his concept to physicians there it could succeed elsewhere. He also chose the University of Washington because he had earned his MPH at this institution and understood the politics of the university, as well as the state.

The Medex program differed from the Duke model because entering students needed to have considerable health care experience and a sponsoring physician who agreed to be their mentor for the preceptorship phase of their education. Often these physicians became their employers as well (R. Smith, personal communication, 2000). Both models built on skills obtained primarily in the military. Medical corpsmen were by far the most common applicants and students, and this background was vital to the early acceptance of the PA concept. Smith notes that it was the military medical background that was critical in gaining acceptance of the idea of the PA, Medex, and other models. Returning corpsmen had obtained extensive experience on the battlefield and were a popular and unassailable "base" on which could be built the construct of the PA. Smith firmly believes that it was difficult to underestimate the importance of having military medical corpsmen as the foundation of the PA profession (R. Smith, personal communication, 2001).

Within a few years, eight Medex programs evolved, mostly consisting of 3 to 6 months of intensive didactic work in basic and clinical sciences at the university medical center, followed by a preceptorship with a practicing primary care physician for 9 to 12 months (Exhibit 2-3). Medex programs were widely distributed from the inner city of the Watts district of Los Angeles to rural areas such as Alabama, North Dakota, and Pennsylvania. Programs also emerged at Drew University, the University of Utah, the University of South Carolina, and Dartmouth University. On completion of the preceptorship the student received a certificate (Smith, 1969).

Child Health Associate Model

The third prototype of PA education was at the University of Colorado child health associate program, which began in 1968. Under Henry Silver, a well-respected professor of pediatrics, and Loretta Ford, RN, this program recruited nurses and other applicants with diverse backgrounds for a 5-year training program (later reduced to 3 years) to assist pediatric physicians. Originally the mission was to supply preventive

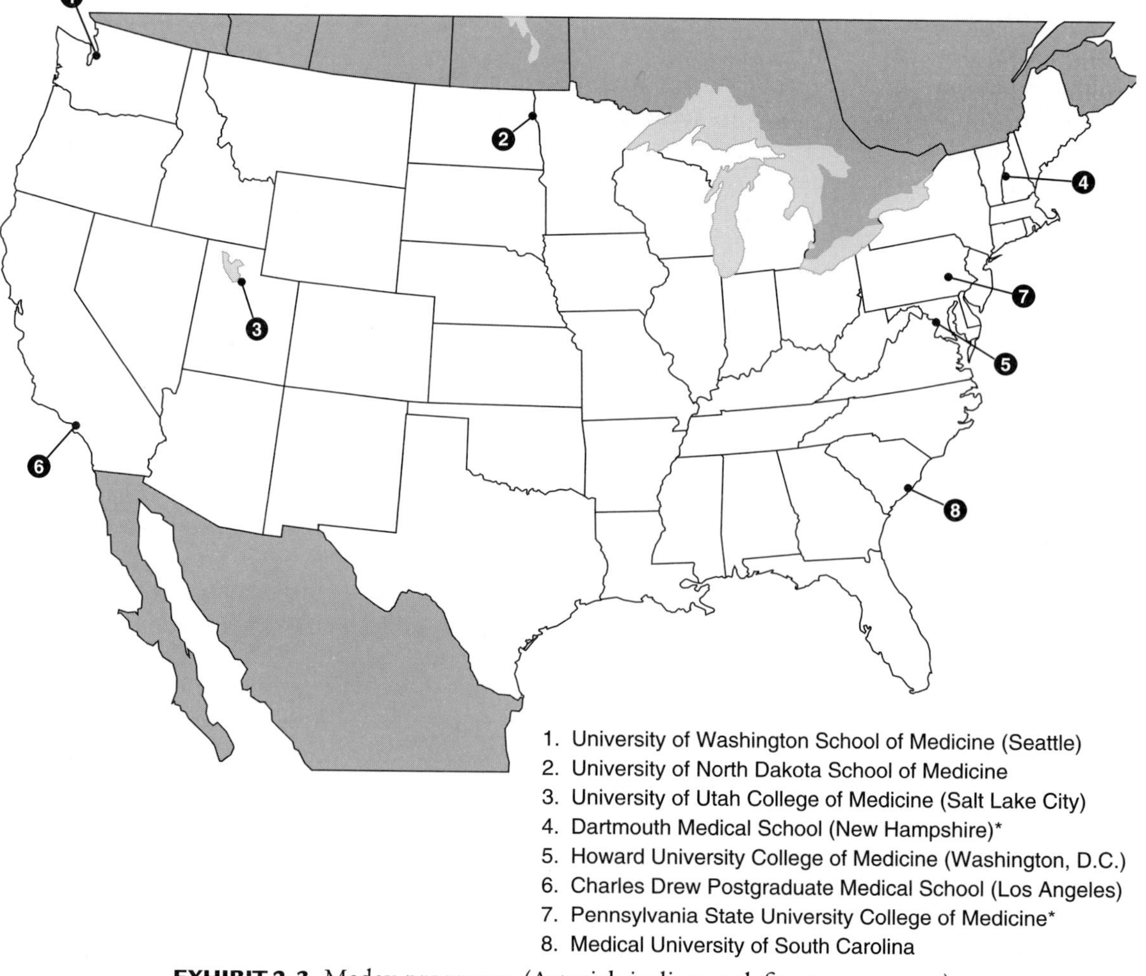

EXHIBIT 2-3 Medex programs. (Asterisk indicates defunct programs.)

and routine care to children and began as an NP program. This was later expanded to almost all areas of pediatric primary care and enrolled nonnurses (Fisher, 1977). Even though graduates of this program put *CHA* (*CHA* in this instance is child health associate and should not be confused with community health aides in Alaska) after their names, they usually take the Physician Assistant National Certification Examination (PANCE), and many are certified as pediatric PAs.

Specialty Physician Assistant Models

Other movements in specialization took place in the late 1960s as well. There was a surge of new programs to train nonphysician providers in very specific areas of care. Some of these programs include the orthopedic assistant and the urologic physician's assistant, which were 2-year programs designed to train personnel to work directly for specialists. A 4-month "health assistants" training program sponsored by Project Hope in Laredo, Texas, was launched in 1970. The program was intended to improve Hispanic health care, and the only requirement for entry was that the student had to be 18 years of age. Of the 11 students who entered the first class, 8 lacked high school equivalence and were able to earn their General Equivalency Diploma certificate on completion of the program (Sadler, 1972). Other programs sprung up of various length of training and medical specialty focus. Programs that lasted more than a year or two included gastroenterology, allergy, and dermatology. The radiology program at the University of Kentucky and the pathology program at Duke University lasted longer than most. By 1971 more than 125 programs in 35 states announced they were training "physician support personnel" (Bureau of Health Manpower Education, 1971). Yet it is interesting to note that as the concept of the primary care PA became consolidated in the early years; by 1975 the PA concept mainly survived. Most of the specialty programs expired.

Although not all programs flourished, most primary care–based ones did. A number of these programs were sponsored by academic health centers. By 1972 a total of 31 programs were in operation: 21 of the programs were federally supported by agencies such as the Office of Economic Opportunity, the Model Cities Program, the Veterans Administration, the Public Health Service, the Department of Defense, and the Department of Labor, while the remainder were financed by private foundations and institutional sources (Fisher, 1977). Throughout the 1970s private philanthropy from the Robert Wood Johnson Foundation, the Macy Foundation, and the Brunner Foundation provided start-up support for a number of PA educational programs.

Standardizing the Physician Assistant

In 1970 the National Congress on Health Manpower (sponsored by the AMA's Council on Health Manpower) sought to develop uniform terminology for the many emerging PA programs. Congress concluded that *physician's assistant* was too general to be adopted as the single generic term because PAs were receiving varied levels of training. They decided that *associate* would be a preferred term for health care workers who assume a direct and responsible role in patient care and act as colleagues to physicians, rather than as technical assistants. Congress noted that the PA terminology is often confused and used interchangeably with the established *medical assistant*, the title for the nonprofessional office helper who functions in a clerical and technical fashion (Curran, 1972). However, the AMA's House of Delegates rejected the *associate* terminology in the belief that *associate* should be applied only to physicians working in collaboration with other physicians (this criticism ignores the "*'s*," which denotes that the *associate* is not another physician). Thus no consistent position emerged from organized medicine (Sadler, 1972).

In the United States the nonphysician practitioner concept initially embodied multiple types of health care providers, PAs among them. Educational curricula designed to train a variety of PA-style health care providers were becoming abundant in the late 1960s. In 1970 the Board on Medicine of the National Academy of Sciences (NAS) unsuccessfully attempted to classify various types of PAs according to the degree of independent function in exercising medical judgment. The board report identified three levels of PAs:

Type A assistants are capable of collecting patient history and physical data and organizing and presenting them so the physician can visualize the medical problem and determine appropriate diagnostic or therapeutic steps. The assistant can assist the physician by performing diagnostic and therapeutic procedures and coordinating the roles of other more technical assistants. Functioning under the general supervision and responsibility of the physician, the assistant under defined rules may practice without the immediate surveillance of the physician. The assistant is qualified to integrate and interpret clinical findings on the basis of medical knowledge and to exercise a degree of independent judgment.

Type B assistants, although not equipped with general knowledge and skills relative to the whole range of medical care, possess exceptional technical expertise in a clinical specialty or certain procedures within such a specialty. Within a specialty area this provider may have a degree of skill beyond that of a Type A assistant and perhaps that normally possessed by physicians who are not engaged in the specialty. Because Type B assistants' knowledge and skill are limited to a particular specialty, they are less qualified for independent action.

Type C assistants are capable of performing a limited number of medical care tasks under the more direct supervision of a physician. These providers may be similar to the Type A assistants in the areas in which they can perform, but they cannot exercise the degree of independent synthesis and judgment.

Initially the NAS classification of PAs using the Type A, B, C system appeared to be helpful in attempting to define the nature of the relationship and division of duties between physicians and PAs but was soon discarded because it tended to create confusion within the hierarchy of emerging models of PA providers. The leaders of Medex programs were unhappy with this concept and that their graduates were assigned a Type C rating while Duke graduates were assigned a Type A rating, designations based on perceptions of formal training rather than on past health care experience. Although this designation was changed and refined (Estes, 1970a), eventually the entire NAS classification scheme lost relevance in attempting to capture the emerging nature of the PA-physician relationship and was abandoned.

Federal Policy

The critical role of the federal government in nurturing the development of new health care practitioners in general, and the PA in particular, came about through specific legislation. The Comprehensive Health Manpower Training Act called for the Bureau to provide support for educational programs for PAs and other nonphysicians. The act established the education grants program that was administered by the Bureau of Health Manpower under the Health Resources Administration, Department of Health, Education, and Welfare, mandated by Section 774a of the Public Health Service Act as Public Law 93-157.

Shortly thereafter assistance for 24 of the then 31 existing new provider programs and contracts with 16 developing programs were initiated. Federal support represented an investment in health professions programs to test the hypothesis that nonphysician health care professionals could provide many physician-equivalent services in primary and continuing care. The Bureau's programs were designed to carry out the intent of Congress to relieve problems of geographic and specialty maldistribution of physicians and the U.S. health care workforce. This intent was reflected in the contract process, which required each PA program to emphasize three major objectives in its demonstration:

1. Training for delivery of primary care in ambulatory settings
2. Placing graduates in medically underserved areas
3. Recruiting residents of medically underserved areas, minority groups, and women as students for these programs

Each program was free to devise various curricula and methods of instruction, but the preceding three requirements were held constant to carry out the intent of Congress (Fisher, 1977). This contributed to the demise of most Type C and B programs. They either folded in a few years because of lack of funding support or converted into primary care programs. The only survivors are the surgeon assistant, CHAs, and the pathologist assistant programs.

Naming the Profession

There was also a brief experimentation with a more appropriate name because the title *physician's assistant* was problematic by incorrectly indicated possession by the physician and was not initially well accepted by physicians and PAs alike. Silver suggested a new term, *syniatrist*, from the Greek *syn* signifying "along with" or "association" and *-iatric*, which means "relating to medicine" or a "physician" (Silver, 1971a). He proposed the syniatrist terminology by a prefix relating to each medical specialty; for example, general practice would be a general practice syniatrist associate or a general practice syniatrist aide (Sadler, 1972). Smith opted for Medex and saw his graduates placing the letters *Mx* after their names as an appropriate and distinct title. Other proposed titles in lieu of PA included *Osler, Flexner*, and *Cruzer* in honor of famous people in American medical history. The intent of these new names would be neutral and less demeaning than *PA*. Little interest in these names developed, and the title *physician assistant* remains.

Support of Organized Medicine

The PA concept would not have germinated and certainly would not have succeeded without the overt support and active involvement of major physician groups. The AMA in particular contributed substantially to confirming legitimacy and acceptance of the concept and had a strong role in the establishment of standards of PA educational program accreditation and professional credentialing organizations. Support for the development of the PA profession also came from the American College of Surgeons, the American Academy of Family Physicians, the American Academy of Pediatrics, the American College of Physicians, and other medical groups in shaping the infrastructure of the PA profession. These groups worked to build the critical components of the profession's structure, particularly legal and regulatory components. PA practice certification mechanisms were patterned to a large degree on their counterparts in the medical profession. A good example of medical collaboration was the creation of the National Commission on Certification of Physician Assistants (NCCPA). The NCCPA is the national credentialing agency for the PA profession that administers the PANCE. Physician and PA groups worked with government agencies, the NBME, the Federation of State Medical Licensing Boards, the Association of American Medical Colleges, and members of the general public to create the NCCPA, and these groups continue to comprise the governance of the organization.

EVOLUTION OF THE PHYSICIAN ASSISTANT PROFESSION

All social movements have periods of evolution, and the development of the PA profession is no exception. To appreciate the evolution of the PA profession in American medicine, we divide the history of the PA profession into five periods. These periods span the first four decades. As stages in the evolution of the PA profession, the natural history of other nonphysician professions is shown in Exhibit 2-4.

Period 1: Ideology (1961 to 1969)

When PAs were introduced into medical practice in the United States in the 1960s, the principal hope of their creators was to improve primary health care delivery, which was suffering as a result of generalist physician shortages brought about by the demise of the general practitioner. PAs were envisioned as a new type of medical generalist, one whose role would build on prior medical experiences, trained in a reasonably short time and be rapidly deployed to practice locations in medically needy areas. The assistant to the primary care physician in rural and underserved areas was idealized during this time.

Period 2: Implementation of the Concept (1966 to 1975)

Charismatic leaders and the federal government provided strong support for the creation and early development of PAs in the health care system. Domestic policy in the early 1970s sought to improve citizen access to health services by increasing the development and dispersal of health care personnel. Most policymakers believed there was a shortage of physicians overall with a decreasing proportion in general practice. Because organized medicine had not adequately addressed these issues in the past, this new federal workforce approach was composed of two major elements: expansion of physician supply by expanding medical education and promotion of the introduction of new practitioners whose roles would focus on primary care. The early 1970s was a period of intense activity and evolution for the PA concept. It was the time when the key organizations representing the profession were founded: the AAPA in 1968, the

EXHIBIT 2-4

Stages in the Development of the New Health Professionals

Stage I—Ideology

The existence of an appropriate social, medical, and political climate; medical personnel factors; and educational influences that lead to a coherent rationale and expected role necessitating the creation of a new category of health personnel. This rationale must gain the acceptance of critical existing stake holders in the health system (e.g., physicians and nurses, government health policy makers, educational institutions, medical regulators, state legislators, and health administrators). The climate in which the conceptualization of new health occupations develops helps set the stage. Stake holders must perceive a benefit. Public policy makers must be convinced that introduction of a new health profession will benefit society in improving health services, and not directly threaten existing professions.

Stage II—Implementation

Key health policy, medical education, and organizational collaboration to implement the conceptual framework, educational preparation, and professional regulation of the new profession. A variety of critical areas must be determined: length and level of training, curriculum content, scope of practice, legal status and mechanisms of regulation, sponsorship and funding, and credentialing. Academic institutions begin to develop educational programs. Organization of levels of state recognition (licensure, regulation, or certification) of practice activities for new practitioners entering medical practices. Establishment of systems of educational sponsorship, academic recognition and accreditation, professional credentialing, occupational regulation, definition of practice scope.

Stage III—Evaluation

Conduct and evaluation of organized health services research and public policy analysis designed to measure the levels of clinical performance effectiveness and practice characteristics of the new professional: measurement of levels of acceptance by patients, physicians, and other professionals; content and quality of care; cost-effectiveness; practice deployment; and role satisfaction. Also, studies begin to examine longitudinal trends of provider utilization patterns and professional demographics in the health system.

Stage IV—Incorporation

Steady growth and acceptance of the new professionals. Utilization extends from original generalist/primary care roles to include specialty areas. Clinical practice settings include private solo and group medical offices; hospitals, health facilities, and organizations; academic centers; managed care systems; long-term care facilities; and public health clinics. Legislation is promulgated in states authorizing in statute for medical licensing boards to regulate the new health professional; regulations adopted permitting new professionals in health workforce supply and requirements planning; publication of summary policy reports on impact and practice experiences.

Stage V—Maturation

Acceptance and institutionalization of the profession among the health occupations. The acceptance of educational institutions in the form of faculty appointments for PA educators. Professional utilization patterns are characterized by steady, ongoing demand for practitioners' services by both patients and physicians, and continuing utilization in a variety of medical care settings.

Association of Physician Assistant Programs (APAP) in 1971, and the NCCPA in 1973.

Also during this time the mantle of responsibility for the continuation of the development of the PA profession was passed on to the next cadre of progressive-thinking physician educators who had assumed leadership positions in medical education. These physicians were also leaders in medical and regulatory organizations. Among the most prominent of these leaders was Thomas Piemme, MD, chairman of the Department of Health Care Sciences at the George Washington University Medical Center in 1972. Piemme established the PA program at the university in that year, as well as an NP program in 1978, and was a major leader on multiple levels within the emerging PA concept during this period. He worked to define the profession's educational standards and practice qualifications by becoming the first president of the APAP and the founding president of the NCCPA. Another leading figure in the development of the PA concept was Archie Golden, MD, MPH, who helped found the health associate program at The Johns Hopkins School of Health Services in 1972 (Golden, Hagan, and Carlson, 1981). Jack Cole, MD, professor of surgery at Yale University, and Alfred Sadler, MD, founded the physician associate program at Yale University School of Medicine. Inheriting the creation of

Henry Silver, John E. Ott, MD, directed the child health associate program at the University of Colorado and performed many of the early health services research studies on child health associate performance. J. Rhodes Haverty, MD, was dean of allied health at Georgia State University and a force in the establishment of the NCCPA. Don Detmer, MD, a Duke surgeon and editor of the first PA journal, later became a leader in academic health center administration at the University of Virginia and Oxford. John Kirklin, MD, professor of surgery at the University of Alabama, founded the first surgeon assistant program; Thomas Gallager, MD, at the University of Nebraska; David Lawrence, MD, MPH, at the University of Washington; Hal Wilson, MD, at the University of Kentucky; Dennis Oliver, PhD, and Richard Rosen, MD, chairman of surgery at Montefiore Medical Center in the 1970s first used a PA in inpatient surgical units and founded the first PA postgraduate program. Their prominence as physician leaders and researchers gave a great deal of legitimacy to the development of this new profession.

Legal and Regulatory Challenges

The introduction of the PA into the American health system brought with it the necessity to consider appropriate legal and regulatory approaches to enable these and other emerging health care practitioners to enter clinical practice. Important decision points were the determination of the scope of practice of these new professionals, appropriate levels of state board recognition (licensure, registration, and certification), and stipulations for supervision and prescribing activities (Ballenger, 1971a, 1971b).

To support the entry of PAs into clinical practice the House of Delegates of the AMA in 1970 passed a resolution urging state medical licensing boards to modify health occupations statutes and regulations to permit PAs to qualify as medical practitioners. Among the first states to amend medical acts allowing PAs to practice were Colorado, North Carolina, California, and New York. On the federal level important leadership in the early nurturing of the PA concept was provided by the government in the form of grant support for PA educational programs. Initial legislative initiatives included the Allied Health Professions Personnel Act of 1966 and the Health Manpower Act of 1968. PA programs quickly sprang up in medical centers, hospitals, and colleges; state legislatures and private foundations provided support for education programs as well.

State Regulation

The legal basis of PA practice is codified in state medical practice statutes granting authorization to licensed physicians to delegate a range of medical diagnostic and therapeutic tasks to individuals who meet educational standards and practice requirements. Authority for medical task delegation is based on the legal doctrine of *respondeat superior*, which holds that it is the physician who is ultimately liable for PA practice activities and mandates that doctors who employ PAs appropriately define and supervise their clinical actions. State acts exempt PAs from the unlicensed practice of medicine with the stipulation that they function with physician supervision.

Professional activities and the scope of practice of PAs are regulated by state licensing boards, which are often boards of medicine, boards of health occupations, or in some instances separate PA licensing boards. Laws define PA qualification requirements, practice scope and professional conduct standards, and the actions of the PAs. State laws often require physicians to clearly delineate the practice scope and supervisory arrangements of PAs. Medical practice acts define the boundaries of PA practice activities but tend to vary considerably by state, particularly with regard to scope of practice, supervisory requirements, and prescribing authority. This variability has lead to barriers in practice effectiveness in a number of states (Sekscenski, 1994). Many of these barriers have largely been overcome.

As originally envisioned, the role of the PA working with physicians encompassed the full range of clinical practice areas: office, clinic, hospital, nursing home, surgical suite, or in the patient's home. Laws in many states were written to give PAs a practice scope, allowing the physician to delegate a broad range of medical tasks to PAs. This latitude allows PAs to exercise a degree of clinical judgment and autonomic decision making within the parameters of state scope of practice regulations and the supervisory relationship. This is considered essential for PAs to be fully effective in practice. Geographic practice isolation in rural and frontier settings may by necessity result in varying degrees of offsite physician supervision and require the PA to exercise some autonomy in clinical judgment, particularly when the PA is the only available onsite provider. Regulatory reluctance to support such physician-PA relationships in satellite and remote clinical settings restricts the PA in extending and providing services that might otherwise be unavailable.

Practice regulations have progressed from a delegatory model achieved by amending medical practice acts to a regulatory/authority model wherein health licensing boards are explicitly authorized to govern PA practice (Davis, 2002). Typical state regulatory acts establish PAs as agents of their supervising physicians; PAs maintain direct liability for the services they render to patients. Supervising physicians who define the standard to which PA services are held are vicariously liable for services performed by the PAs under the doctrine of *respondeat superior.*

Practice Qualification

Over a number of years and by the actions of state legislatures, a standard emerged for PA practice: qualification as a PA requires that individuals be graduates of accredited PA educational program and pass the PANCE.

PA Education

Establishment of formal accreditation standards for PA programs marked an important milestone for the PA profession. Initially established by organizations affiliated with the AMA in 1971, the Council on Education for Allied Health developed standards for PA program accreditation, promulgated as the *Essentials of an Approved Educational Program for the Assistant to the Primary Care Physician.* Authority for PA program accreditation was set within the Commission on Accreditation of Allied Health Education Programs (CAAHEP). In 2000 the Accreditation Review Committee on Education for the Physician Assistant (ARC-PA) became an independent accrediting body for the PA profession, separate and independent of the CAAHEP. Over the years the accreditation criteria underwent frequent revisions reflecting changes in educational preparation in a rapidly developing field. The *Essentials,* as they were called initially, were revised and updated in 1978, 1985, 1990, 1997, and 2000. Accreditation is necessary for PA programs to receive federal Title VII grant funding and in most states for program graduates to qualify for entry to practice. The *Standards,* as they were later referred to, define the necessary core components of PA educational programs, the nature of institutional sponsorship, the curriculum content, clinical training affiliations, basic and clinical science course offerings, faculty qualifications, and admission and selection guidelines (McCarty, 2001). Early versions of the *Standards* were written to permit PA educational programs a wide degree of latitude to create curricular configurations based on a structure awarding several types of academic degrees.

Period 3: Evaluation and Establishment (1976 to 1980)

The Comprehensive Health Manpower Act of 1973 was an important legislative milestone, marking the inclusion of PA program funding support programs. Since then, federal awards have totaled $160 million supporting PA educational programs; in fiscal year 2002, programs received $6.4 million.

A great deal of health services research was performed during the 1970s examining the impact of the introduction of PAs into medical practice. Both the PA and the NP concept and related advanced practice nursing programs were novel medical education experiments, and their outcomes were the target of intense health services research focus. After a decade of studies, over one hundred research publications revealed that PAs were well-accepted, safe and effective practitioners in medical care delivery; studies also showed that there was a high degree of patient acceptance of the PA role and that most PAs were in primary care practices in medically needy areas (Office of Technology Assessment, 1986; Hooker, 1997).

PAs can lower health care costs while providing physician-equivalent quality of care. Despite that PA cost-effectiveness has not been conclusively demonstrated in all clinical practice settings, substantial empirical and health services research supports this finding. The present increasing use and market demand for PAs in clinical practices would be unlikely if they were not to some degree cost-effective (Hooker, 2002).

Evidence indicates that the organizational setting is closely related to the productivity and possible cost benefits of PA utilization. (See Chapter 9.)

Initial PA practice distribution tended to reflect the federal and medical sector intent that PAs assume primary care roles in areas of need. Early recruits to the PA profession were often individuals with extensive levels of prior health care experience (e.g., military medical corpsmen, registered nurses, physical therapists, emergency medical technicians), factors thought to contribute to their ability to function effectively with a minimal level of physician supervision. Selection of physician preceptors in rural areas was then and still remains a goal of many of the programs. After graduation, many of these individuals select primary care physicians located in a rural or medically underserved community (Willis, 1990c).

Many of the clinical evaluations of PA use were performed in ambulatory practice and in health maintenance organization (HMO) settings. In such settings, PA clinical performance has been impressive. Their productivity (number of patient visits) has been shown to approach and sometimes exceed levels of primary care physicians (Sox, 1973; Hooker, 1993, 2002). Record (1978, 1981) carefully documented PA productivity rates in a large group model HMO. She determined that the physician/PA substitutability ratio, a measure of overall clinical efficiency, was 76%. This assumed a practice environment in which PAs were used to their maximum capacity to perform medical services (consistent with educational competency and legal scope and/or supervision), and that they worked the same number of hours per week as physicians.

By the end of the first decade of practice for PAs, experience and empiric research indicated that U.S. medicine's adoption of the PA had been generally positive (Sox, 1973; Scheffler, 1979). PAs were responsive to the public and the medical mandate to work in generalist and primary care roles in medically underserved areas. As their numbers pushed 10,000 in 1980, PAs were gaining recognition as being competent, effective, and clinically versatile health care providers (Nelson, 1975).

An important element in the acceptance and use of PAs was the development of a single pathway to licensure based not only on formal education but also on a nationally standardized certification examination. Recognizing the need for a credentialing body, which would be organizationally separate from the profession, the NCCPA was formed in 1973 and formally chartered in 1975. The NCCPA administered the first PA certifying examination in 1973 and began issuing certificates shortly thereafter. Soon the PANCE became recognized as the qualifying examination for entry to PA practice by a rapidly increasing number of state medical licensing boards. The NCCPA was established with federal and private grant support and assistance from the AMA and was closely linked to the NBME in the development of the PANCE and later the recertifying examinations for PAs. During the late 1970s and early 1980s the PANCE examination and the NCCPA certification process had become incorporated into the practice acts of most state medical practice statutes. By the 1990s successful completion of the PANCE became a universal qualification for PA practice.

Period 4: Recognition and Incorporation (1981 to 1990)

By the early 1980s PAs, as well as the other nonphysician health professions (NPs and certified nurse midwives [CNMs]), were becoming more extensively used and accepted. The cumulative results of the past decade of health services research and practical experience with PAs were overwhelmingly positive, with the specific measures being patient and health care professional acceptance, quality of care, cost-effectiveness, productivity, and clinical versatility (Carter, 1984a; Schafft, 1987a; Cawley, 1983).

For a time it appeared that the sole focus of PA practice would be primary care, although not all demand for PA services was in primary care. The PA role broadened during the 1980s when utilization extended beyond primary care into inpatient hospital settings and specialty areas. The trend toward specialization by PAs was the result, in part, of their clinical versatility and the health workforce demand. It was realized that the services of a PA could be used on inpatient hospital floors and in various other specialty settings. In 1977 the percentage of PAs working in the primary care specialties, defined as family practice, general internal medicine, and general pediatrics, was 77%. In 1981 the percentage had fallen to 62%. From 1981 to 2001 the percentage had settled at 50%. Over the same period the percentage working in surgery and the surgical subspecialties rose from 19% to 28%; PAs in emergency medicine rose from 1.3% to 10% and continues to grow.

During the early 1980s the prediction of the Graduate Medical Education National Advisory Council of a rising number of physicians in the workforce prompted questions of whether there was much of a future for PAs. Yet after a few years of doubt during which utilization was sluggish and several PA educational programs were closed (e.g., University of Indiana, Johns Hopkins University, and Stevens College), the PA profession continued to evolve and gain ground. On important levels recognition of PAs. At the federal level during the 1980s, two landmark events signaled incorporation of the occupation into the health care workforce mainstream. Perhaps the most significant of these was the congressional passage in 1986 of an amendment to the Medicare law providing reimbursement policies for PA services under Medicare Part B (Omnibus Budget Reconciliation Act, 1986). Recognition by Medicare, the largest health insurance program in the nation, indicated the legitimacy of PA services in medical care. The other event that represented a major milestone for the profession on the national and federal level was the attainment of commissioned officer status in U.S. uniformed services in 1988. Given the rich history between the military and the PA profession, this event was of particular significance and satisfaction to the profession (Hooker, 1991).

A less obvious but no less important set of events that also occurred during this time was the increasing number of states passing legislation to update medical practice acts recognizing PA practice. Lastly, on the organizational level, the building of the headquarters of the AAPA in Alexandria, Virginia (1987), marked the establishment of the PA profession as a permanent member of the health professions on the national organizational level.

Period 5: Maturation (1991 to Present)

By the 1990s the PA profession had achieved a remarkable degree of integration in U.S. medicine. Over a 35-year period, they have achieved acceptance and incorporation in health care delivery. The PA profession grew from infancy in the 1970s through a troubled adolescence during the 1980s and is now a maturing health care profession in a new millennium. Federal policies endorsed their presence in society, and they have reached a critical mass as a profession.

As a recent entrant in contrast to other new professions, the PA profession was consolidated in its representative organization early and became well stabilized. Among the notable indicators of further advancement of the profession is how often it is incorporated into national health policy projections and debate. Instead of enlarging the breadth and scope of practice the PA movement is consolidating gains. Longevity is adding depth to PA roles and status. On the federal level, PAs have been considered relevant players in health care reform under various proposals. Significant achievements in the passage of enabling legislation in all states and prescribing in 47 states, the BBA of 1997 cleared the way for Medicare reimbursement policy. States have modified their practice acts to enable PAs to practice with few barriers. Together with primary care physicians and NPs, PAs are considered essential members of America's primary care workforce (Donaldson, 1996). By the late 1990s at least half of the PA profession were practicing in primary care and the other half in surgical subspecialties and the subspecialties of internal medicine. As if to add legitimacy the largest single employer of PAs is the federal government, namely the U.S. Department of Veterans Affairs and the U.S. military.

ASSESSING THE PHYSICIAN ASSISTANT PROFESSION

The history of the PA profession is a remarkable one from a number of standpoints. Visionaries such as Charles Hudson, Eugene Stead, Richard Smith, Harvey Estes, Henry Silver, Loretta Ford, and others believed that unmet demands for improvements in health care delivery was the prime impetus for the emergence of nonphysician providers (Stanhope, 1992). Instead of the "one great man" theory that often precedes important social movements, the PA profession was founded on a few great people with remarkably similar ideas. Today though the product seems to have exceeded even the boldest imagination of its creators.

In modern American medicine, the creation of the PA marked the occurrence of physicians voluntarily deciding to share with another health care provider the key intellectual and professional functions of performing medical diagnosis and treatment. These activities were legally and functionally in the sole domain of physicians until the creation of PAs.

Some assert that curriculum revisions to increase primary care experiences for medical students should consider the approaches developed and used in PA educational programs. Innovation has flourished in PA programs partly because of their multidisciplinary design and partly because they have greater latitude in making curricular adjustments. PA programs have been pioneers in incorporating topic areas increasingly recognized as important in medical education: behavioral sciences; communication sciences; the humanities; epidemiology, preventive medicine, health promotion, and disease prevention; geriatrics; and community-based practice and community-oriented primary care. PA programs are proven innovators in leading the development of effective strategies in deploying graduates to medically underserved areas and in primary care specialties. The cumulative experiences of PA programs, including the 50 set in academic health centers and those sponsored by teaching hospitals, colleges, and universities, have been deemed to be largely successful educational endeavors. There are now 132 accredited PA programs that prepare competent and versatile generalist providers capable of handling most patient problems encountered in primary care.

To what degree has the PA profession succeeded in fulfilling a key objective of its creation: service in meeting the needs of medically needy populations? A traditional part of the social mission of medicine has been to provide health care services that meet the needs of a nation's population. U.S. medicine continues to be criticized as being overly specialized and unresponsive to the health needs of many citizens. Since the 1980s the U.S. workforce policy reform debate has centered on policy questions of the accountability of the nation's workforce to meet societal health care needs, in particular the needs of the uninsured, the rural citizens, and the medically underserved. Government study groups have concluded that America's present system of health professions education and composition seems ill fit to meet the nation's future needs for health care providers (Council on Graduate Medical Education, 1995). U.S. policymakers remain frustrated with the realization that despite the substantial expansion of physician numbers over the past two decades, as well as the long-standing federal Medicare subsidy of graduate medical education, the number and percentage of physicians who select primary care continues to dwindle. The creation of the PA and the NP professions has helped to alleviate this shortage, but demand for services continues to outstrip supply in rural and underserved areas. America has failed to produce a balanced health care workforce and has fallen short of meeting the nation's need for generalist medical care services and universal access to care.

For the creation of the PA to have occurred, the critical issue of practice autonomy had to be addressed. Medical sociologists regard autonomy as the most important defining attribute of a professional within occupations, and particularly the health occupations. Physicians, like attorneys, have long been regarded as the true professions: Doctors possess their own language and have a distinct body of knowledge, collect direct fees for their services, are autonomous in function, and are largely self-regulated. The dependent-practice role of PAs and their willingness to function within the practice of the physician and under supervision has been a critical factor in their acceptance, utilization, and success. The decision to establish the role of the PA as a dependent professional role—one characterized by a close practice relationship with a supervising physician—was a product of the collective wisdom of the profession's founders. They recognized that acceptance and use of these new providers held a direct relationship to the perceptions of physicians regarding the threat PAs may present in terms of income and professional domain. Dependent practice for PAs represented the central condition on which physician groups first accepted the PA concept. That PAs practice with supervision has always been the major factor in their acceptance and use.

There is little question that success of the U.S. experience with PAs is in large part the result of their close educational and practice relationship with physicians. There are many similarities in the medical training approaches of PAs, NPs, and primary care physicians. PAs and NPs are now well integrated into many medical practices; all PAs and most NPs work with physicians, nurses, and others on the health care team.

Conventionally defined "barriers to practice" clearly affect levels of PA clinical productivity in a broad sense. There is also evidence suggesting that differences in the delegatory styles of physicians are important determinants of PA practice effectiveness. While formalized barriers to practice effectiveness (e.g., restrictive state regulations and payment ineligibility) would appear to represent the major limiting factors in PA use, clinical practice style, overlap, and in many instances, scope of practice, professional domain ("turf") issues arise between these health professionals. Physicians now share a great deal of their medical diagnostic and therapeutic responsibilities with PAs, more than was the case in 1980 or even 1990. That they are willing to share medical functions is a result of forces affecting the evolution and the division of medical labor in the U.S. health care system.

SUMMARY

In the turbulent 1960s, a decade of change in many areas of U.S. society, a fundamental restructuring of the division of medical practice labor evolved. The introduction of the PA, as well as the NP and the rebirth of the CNM in North America, represented a major transformation in U.S. medical practice. The role of the PA was created to assume a scope of practice that included medical tasks previously reserved only for physicians. The concept developed with a medical and societal expectation focusing on extending the capabilities of doctors in the delivery of primary care, particularly to medically underserved populations or rural areas. Four decades later PAs have gained widespread recognition in nearly all aspects of medical care delivery in the United States (Mittman, Cawley, and Fenn, 2002).

In terms of its educational systems the PA profession has evolved successfully in preparing more than 45,000 PAs in active practice by 2002 and a projected 50,000 by 2005. The present model of PA education and certification gives PA graduates an opportunity to obtain employment in a primary care or generalist area or in a specialty or subspecialty area and to have clinical career-long specialty flexibility. There is strong evidence that PA educational approaches have been successful in preparing health care providers for employment in the U.S. health care system and beyond.

3

CURRENT STATUS: A PROFILE OF THE PROFESSION

INTRODUCTION

This chapter describes the characteristics of physician assistants (PAs) in the U.S. health care system. We provide a profile of PAs using contemporary data to portray their practice activities, distribution, specialties, and remuneration. The composition of the profession has changed considerably since the first graduates of those early programs, and we try to display the diverse nature of PA graduates as well. Finally, we portray some of the unique behaviors of PAs and their social standing in U.S. society.

DISTRIBUTION

As of January 2003 more than 59,000 PAs have graduated from an approved PA program. This number will exceed 65,000 by the year 2005 based on estimates of new and expanding PA program capacity. Exhibit 3-1 depicts the growth of PAs based on new graduates and the total number of graduates. A rise of the number of programs in the 1970s was followed by the decade of the 1980s where the number of annual graduates remained stable and even went down in several years. The 1990s saw a boom in annual graduate outcomes. Some of the decline was in early years as a result of closure of some programs and consolidation of others. The exact number of PA programs in the first few years is difficult to determine with precision because of different types of specialty PA programs that were in existence and were counted in different ways by different organizations.

The distribution patterns of practicing PAs by state roughly parallels that of the population, with the highest percentages located in New York (10.1%), followed by California (8.3%), Texas (6.5%), Pennsylvania (5.5%), and Florida (4.7%). Marked differences have been noted among practicing PAs with regard to their patterns of specialty and geographic location of clinical practice setting. In the western states, PAs are used mainly in office-based, ambulatory, and rural practice settings, with a concentration of primary care practice specialties (internal medicine, family practice, and general pediatrics). Such patterns differ markedly from those observed in the eastern states, where it is far more common for PAs to be employed in clinical practice roles in acute care hospital settings or in inpatient-related clinical practice specialties. More than 40% of PAs in the northeast region of the United States are employed by a hospital or perform some of their duties in a hospital setting.

The supply of PAs varies considerably from state to state (Exhibit 3-2). California and New York account for one sixth of the graduates. New York, Pennsylvania, Michigan, North Carolina, and Florida are among the states with the highest number of annual PA graduates. At the other end of the scale, low-population states such as Arkansas and Wyoming have the fewest number

EXHIBIT 3-1

Physician Assistant Graduates*

Yr	New graduates	Cumulative graduates	PA programs
1967	3	3	1
1968	17	20	2
1969	17	37	4
1970	46	83	—
1971	60	143	—
1972	277	420	—
1973	730	1,150	—
1974	1,116	2,339	—
1975	1,375	3,767	—
1976	1,552	5,354	—
1977	1,600	6,980	—
1978	1,352	8,355	—
1979	1,415	9,797	—
1980	1,437	11,258	—
1981	1,539	12,815	—
1982	1,400	14,240	—
1983	1,365	15,624	—
1984	1,228	16,884	—
1985	1,175	18,091	53
1986	1,158	19,261	51
1987	1,097	20,368	49
1988	1,051	21,420	50
1989	1,156	22,578	51
1990	1,232	23,814	51
1991	1,308	25,124	55
1992	1,565	26,690	54
1993	1,647	28,338	56
1994	1,901	30,226	63
1995	2,188	32,397	63
1996	2,570	34,696	68
1997	2,866	37,536	84
1998	3,704	41,221	94
1999	3,856	44,982	105
2000	4,668	49,636	116
2001	4,750	54,386	128
2002	4,925	59,311	132
2003	5,125†	64,431†	134
2004	5,125†	69,561†	136

Data from American Academy of Physician Assistants, Research Division.

*As of December 31.

†Estimate based on expanding PA program trend.

EXHIBIT 3-2

Distribution by State and Territory in Which PAs Practice, 2002 (N = 17,371)

State	%	State	%
Alabama	0.5	Missouri	0.7
Alaska	0.7	Montana	0.6
Arizona	1.8	Nebraska	1.4
Arkansas	0.1	Nevada	0.6
California	8.1	New Hampshire	0.6
Colorado	2.6	New Jersey	1.1
Connecticut	2.1	New Mexico	0.7
Delaware	0.3	New York	9.4
District of Columbia	0.4	North Carolina	5.1
Florida	5.7	North Dakota	0.4
Georgia	3.0	Ohio	2.4
Guam	.0	Oklahoma	1.5
Hawaii	0.2	Oregon	1.2
Idaho	0.7	Pennsylvania	5.5
Illinois	2.4	Rhode Island	0.3
Indiana	0.9	South Carolina	0.9
Iowa	1.6	South Dakota	0.8
Kansas	1.2	Tennessee	1.2
Kentucky	1.3	Texas	6.1
Louisiana	0.7	Utah	1.0
Maine	1.0	Vermont	0.3
Maryland	2.4	Virginia	1.7
Massachusetts	2.1	Washington	3.0
Michigan	4.3	West Virginia	0.8
Minnesota	1.9	Wisconsin	2.8
Mississippi	0.1	Wyoming	0.4

Data from *2002 AAPA Physician Assistant Census Report,* Alexandria, Va., 2002, American Academy of Physician Assistants.

of PAs. Although Alaska does not have a high number of PAs, the ratio of PAs per population far exceeds that of any other state.

Barriers to practice such as legislation also influence the distribution of PAs. Mississippi, with a population of 5 million, has only a handful of nonfederal PAs, reflecting the fact that there was no legislation sanctioning PA practice until 2000.

Although most of the PAs are spread throughout the United States, approximately 2% also report residencies overseas. These locations are in the U.S. territories (e.g., Guam, Virgin Islands and American Samoa), in the U.S. military (e.g., Germany, Japan, Korea, and Turkey), in private agencies that have medical facilities outside the United States (e.g., Central America, Southeast Asia, and Saudi Arabia), in the Department of State, the Central Intelligence Agency, and the Peace Corps (various countries).

The PA profession was asked by its early proponents to prove that it could provide quality care to the underserved, reduce the perceived personnel shortage in health care, and make the lives of physicians less harried. In the first 10 years all of these goals were achieved within the confines of the limited number of personnel being trained in relatively small programs. However, the criteria by which effectiveness is judged have changed, and the health care context has also shifted radically, raising new questions about the role of PAs.

About 30% of all PAs practice in communities of fewer than 50,000 people, and 13% are practicing in communities of fewer than 10,000 people (Exhibit 3-3). The community size in which PAs practice varies from the largest metropolitan areas to the most rural.

Population alone cannot account for all state variations. Mississippi, for example, is ranked 31 in population and is tied with Guam for the lowest number of PAs and the highest population/PA ratio in the country. Another important reason for the concentration of PAs in states such as New York, Texas, and California is that they also have the greatest number of PA training programs. Implicit in the location of state-supported PA programs is that many of the graduates of a program will remain in the state.

The geographic distribution of PAs in the health care workforce is probably associated with a number of factors:

- Training incentives in Title VII legislation
- Market demand and salaries
- Enabling state legislation (ability to practice and prescribe)
- Location of PA training programs (Hooker, 1992)

EXHIBIT 3-3

Practice Region, Population Base, Years as a PA, Years in Current Position, 2002

REGION WHERE EMPLOYED	
Northeast	23.7
Southeast	23.3
North Central	20.4
South Central	13.7
West	18.9
POPULATION BASE	
<5,000	6.9
5,000-9,999	5.8
10,000-24,999	7.6
25,000-49,999	8.9
50,000-99,999	13.0
100,000-249,999	16.4
250,000-499,999	10.4
500,000-999,999	10.0
1,000,000-4,999,999	14.6
>5,000,000	6.5

	No. of yr as a PA	No. of yr in current position
<1 yr	3.6	10.5
1-3 yr	22.0	49.8
4-6 yr	15.3	18.7
7-9 yr	11.9	7.6
10-12 yr	14.3	5.6
13-15 yr	12.3	3.8
16-18 yr	10.5	2.4
19 yr	9.6	1.7
Mean	9.2 yr	4.2 yr
Median	9.0 yr	2.0 yr

Data from *2002 AAPA Physician Assistant Census Report,* Alexandria, Va., 2002, American Academy of Physician Assistants, and *2002 AAPA Physician Assistant National Report.*

There are observable patterns of distribution of PAs among the states. In one cohort of more than 11,000 practicing PAs the percentage of those working in primary care specialties in the western United States was 77% versus 48% in eastern states. When percentages of PA employment levels in hospital and institutional settings were compared, only 13.9% of PAs in western states were working in such settings, compared to 45.5% in eastern states (Oliver, 1993). These practice differences appear to stem from the multiple, sometimes competing, medical marketplace demands in different geographic regions and are influenced by state licensing regulations that affect the scope of practice and prescribing authority. The preponderance of primary care PAs in western states and locations in medically underserved regions reflects one of the major policy objectives of the Title VII PA training grant program. Those PA educational programs located in the western states, which tend to have practice statutes with less physician supervisory requirements than those in eastern states, have successful track records in the deployment of PA educational graduates and have developed effective mechanisms to disperse primary health care providers among medically underserved communities (Shi et al., 1993).

PRACTICE SETTINGS

Patterns of choice of practice setting have been stable over the last decade. Almost 55% of all PAs work in either solo or group private practices, 23% in hospitals, and the remaining in settings such as public and private ambulatory clinics, health maintenance organizations (HMOs), geriatric facilities, corporate and occupational health settings, correctional systems, and other health care practices and institutions (Exhibit 3-4). Almost one tenth of PAs work in emergency medicine and another one tenth work in hospital outpatient departments. This activity has been verified by studies of patient visits using the National Ambulatory Medical Care Survey data (Hooker and McCaig, 2001).

EXHIBIT 3-4

Physician Assistant Main Employment Setting

Setting	Percent
Intensive/critical care unit of hospital	2.3
Inpatient unit of hospital	8.0
Outpatient unit of hospital	8.3
Hospital emergency room	10.0
Hospital operating room	7.8
Other unit of hospital	1.5
Federally qualified rural clinic	5.1
Other federally qualified health clinic (not rural)	1.6
Other community health center	2.6
Freestanding urgent care clinic	2.6
Freestanding surgical facility	0.3
Solo practice physician office	12.0
Single-specialty group practice	19.4
Multispecialty group practice	8.9
HMO facility	2.2
Nursing home or long-term care facility	0.8
College health facility	0.7
School-based health facility	0.3
Other outpatient facility	2.2
Correctional facility	1.4
Industrial facility	0.6
Mobile health unit	0.1
Other	1.3
TOTAL	100

Data from *2002 AAPA Physician Assistant Census Report,* Alexandria, Va., 2002, American Academy of Physician Assistants.

PRACTICE CHARACTERISTICS

The physician workforce has become increasingly specialty oriented, and there are more than 125 disciplines the American Medical Association (AMA) annually tracks. The specialty orientation of PAs seems to parallel this activity up to a point. After a decade in which PAs were largely deployed in primary care, more recent patterns reveal a trend toward PA practice in non-primary care specialties and location in urban and inpatient settings. The number of PAs in primary care specialties has fluctuated since the early 1980s (Exhibit 3-5).

Among currently practicing PAs, 43% work in the primary care clinical practice specialties, which are defined by the U.S. Department of Health and Human Services as the specialties of family practice, general internal medicine, and general pediatrics. This proportion is down from the 57% reported in 1980. In 2002, 32.1% of all PAs were working in family practice, 8.4% in general internal medicine, and 2.6% in general pediatrics (AAPA, 2002). Over the last decade, the percentages of PAs who work in the primary care specialties have declined with a corresponding increase in proportions employed in hospital-based and specialty care practices. Fluctuations in numbers may be the result of shifting trends and variations in assigning specialty categories. Primary care figures also differ depending on who is counting. The American Academy of Physician Assistants (AAPA) and some nurse practitioner (NP) organizations include gynecology as a primary care discipline. Others mention that industrial and environmental (occupational) medicine and corrections medicine are primary care disciplines that are simply under a different name.

In the last 15 years the percentage of PAs employed by hospitals has remained fairly con-

EXHIBIT 3-5

Percentage Specialty Distribution Trends of PAs for Select Years

	YR (NO.)							
Specialty	**1974 (939)**	**1978 (3,416)**	**1981 (4,312)**	**1987 (10,692)**	**1994 (12,281)**	**1996 (12,701)**	**2000 (16,547)**	**2002 (16,835)**
Family practice	43.6	52.0	49.1	38.7	37.2	39.8	36.5	32.1
General internal medicine	20.0	12.0	8.9	9.5	7.7	8.3	8.8	8.4
General pediatrics	6.2	3.3	3.4	4.0	2.5	2.7	2.6	2.6
General surgery	12.1	5.5	4.6	8.8	2.8	3.1	2.7	2.5
Surgical specialties	6.8	6.2	7.7	13.8	19.1	8.3	17.4	19.2
Medical specialties	3.9	6.3	2.7	7.1	7.4	5.8	8.11	9.4
Emergency medicine	1.3	4.9	4.5	6.5	8.4	7.0	9.7	10.2
Occupational medicine	1.8	2.7	3.1	4.1	3.1	3.0	3.5	3.0
Other specialty	4.3	7.1	16.0	7.5	7.0	9.5	6.5	8.4

Data from the Association of Physician Assistant Programs: *1981 National Survey of Physician Assistants,* Alexandria, Va., 1984, Association of Physician Assistant Programs; American Academy of Physician Assistants: *The 1984 and 1987 Masterfile Surveys of Physician Assistants,* Alexandria Va., 1985, 1987, American Academy of Physician Assistants; Oliver DR: *Eighth Annual Report on Physician Assistant Educational Programs in the United States, 1991-1992,* Alexandria, Va., Association of Physician Assistant Programs; American Academy of Physician Assistants: *General Census Data on Physician Assistants, 1996,* Alexandria, Va., 2000, American Academy of Physician Assistants; *2002 American Academy of Physician Assistants.*

stant, after rising from 14% in 1974. As the proportion of PAs in primary care practice declined, the rates of PAs working in acute care settings in medical and surgical specialties and subspecialties rose correspondingly. Key factors in expanding the role of the PA and their numbers in positions in inpatient care were hospital cutbacks in physician residency programs, curtailed availability of international medical graduates (IMGs), and cost-effectiveness in inpatient roles.

It may be argued that trends in PA use patterns since 1980 have closely mirrored those of physicians. With the physician workforce becoming increasingly specialized, and with changes in physician-determined patterns in the division of medical labor, PA use has moved to some degree toward specialty areas, a process to be expected of any developing occupation. While primary care remains the major practice thrust of the PA profession, recent trends emphasizing specialty practice in the PA profession continue. An intriguing question not known is how much primary care is provided by PAs working within specialty practices.

Setting

The largest percentage of PAs of the respondents to the AAPA census are employed by a single or multispecialty physician group practice (42%). Almost one fourth (23%) of the respondents are employed by hospitals.

Public Service

About 10% of the respondents work for a government agency. The Department of Veterans Affairs is the single largest government employer of PAs, accounting for 3% of all respondents.

Type of Community Served

PAs practice medicine in communities ranging from the most rural to the inner city. One fifth (22%) of respondents work in rural or frontier areas of the country. Approximately 9% work in inner cities.

DEMOGRAPHIC DATA

The median age at graduation from a PA program has generally declined since the 1960s and 1970s. The current age to begin a PA career is approximately 33 years. The average age, as well as the median of all practicing PAs, is 42 years. Since 1974 the trend in age of practicing PAs has risen from 30.6 (Perry, 1976) to 38 years in 1991 to 40 years and is expected to hover at this age for the next several years.

By the beginning of 2002 there were 59,000 PA graduates, of which approximately 40,000 were in active clinical practice in the United States (AAPA census data). Thus, about 85% of all persons trained as PAs are still practicing (Exhibit 3-6). The AAPA membership survey reports that the mean years in clinical practice for PAs is 9.2, with a median of 9 years. A sizable proportion of those in the profession have been in clinical practice for less than 3 years (22%), and 15% have been in clinical practice less than 6 years.

The attained educational degree is the highest degree reported. About 94% of graduates have at least a bachelor's degree. This percentage is increasing each year for two reasons. First, most PA programs are shifting from a certificate to a bachelor or master's program. This results in part from the desire to remain competitive with other programs and in response to the pressure of a competitive job market that demands at least

EXHIBIT 3-6

Estimated Number of Practicing PAs as of January 2001

	Count	% Practicing	No. practicing
AAPA fellow members in 2000	24,696	93.08*	22,986
Potential AAPA fellow members	18,761	71.73*	13,457
PAs lost to contact	1,938	0†	0
New graduates in 2000	4,684	85.81‡	4,026
TOTAL PEOPLE ELIGIBLE TO PRACTICE AS PAs	50,079	80.81	40,469

*Percentage in practice, based on 1999 AAPA census data.
†Percentage in practice assumed to be zero.
‡Percentage in practice, based on data for those who became eligible to practice as PAs in 1999.

a baccalaureate degree for professional legitimacy. The Association of Physician Assistant Programs (APAP) has also decided that a graduate degree is the appropriate entry-level document for the rigor of the coursework that students attend. Second, more and more students already have degrees (both undergraduate and graduate) when entering programs. More than 75% of the students possessed at least an undergraduate degree before entering training programs, and more than 90% have a degree of some type on graduating. The trend toward degree-granting programs and applicants with degrees already in hand is expected to continue.

Certification (the last portion of Exhibit 3-7) refers to the percentage of PAs who are nationally certified. Although certification is not a requirement everywhere, most states, federal government agencies, and private employers are requiring it as a condition of employment. Today more than 95% of clinically active PAs are certified. (The issue of certification is discussed in Chapter 4.)

EXHIBIT 3-7

Full-Time Practicing PAs, 2000*

	%	No.
Total PA graduates		49,636
Total practicing PAs	(85.6%)	42,488
Gender		
Female	55.3	
Male	44.7	
Ethnicity		
Asian/Pacific Islander	9.9	
Black (not Hispanic)	3.3	
Hispanic/Latino origin	3.5	
Native American/Alaskan Indian	1.1	
White (not Hispanic)	89.0	
Multiethnic	0.3	
Highest degree ever attained		
Certificate	7.0	
Associate	2.5	
Bachelor	39.6	
Postbachelor's PA certificate	21.1	
Master	27.5	
Doctorate	2.3	
Currently certified		
Yes	92.7	
No	7.3	

Data from *2000 AAPA Physician Assistant Census Report,* Alexandria, Va., 2000, American Academy of Physician Assistants.
*Information is self-reported at time of membership enrollment or renewal.

The profile of the PA has changed relatively quickly, compared with that of other professions. In contrast to a group of three male veterans in 1967 (Condit, 1993) the average PA graduate in the 1990s is a woman, approximately 33 years of age, and has a nonmilitary medical background.

As the national complexion of PAs changes, we can make some predictions about what the profession will look like in the future. First, the gender distribution of PAs will probably shift even more over the next decade because the PA profession is popular and the pool of applicants is largely female. While programs may be inclined to enroll their classes in roughly even numbers of men and women, they must draw upon the applicant pool presented. Currently the PA profession is very attractive to women. Second, the average age of PAs in the workforce will slowly increase in a few years to approximately 44 years and then plateau because the aging PA is remaining in the workforce (Duryea and Hooker, 2000). The average age of entrants to PA programs is relatively stable. Although little is known about the life cycle of a PA and what the average age of retirement will be, it is likely that at least three fourths of PAs will remain in their careers until the traditional retirement age between 62 and 65 years. Another relevant factor is that PAs tend to be highly satisfied with their career, which suggests some profession stability (Freeborn and Hooker, 1995). Historically, physicians have unusually long work lives; the average 35-year-old physician used to practice almost to the age of 70 years (Kletke, 1987). Whether this holds true for PAs is not clear, but our observation is that some PAs are working beyond age 65 years (Duryea and Hooker, 2000).

Age

The mean age of clinically active PAs is 41.4 years; the median is 41 years. The 41 to 45 age interval accounts for the largest group of PAs by age (23%). Relatively few PAs have reached traditional retirement age (1%), but this number is expected to triple over the next 5 years.

In a subpopulation of elder PAs (age 60 and older), the average age is 64 and the range is between 60 and 74 years. When this set of older PAs is compared with all PAs, some differences emerge. On average older PAs were in practice longer than all PAs (18.3 years and 9.2 years, respectively), had been with their current employer for 7.7 years, and had very few job changes. Three times as many of the older PAs had a doctorate degree than all PAs. And older PAs are more likely to be taking care of older patients, working in a rural area, and remaining in a rural area longer than PAs overall (Duryea and Hooker, 2000).

Gender

In 1965 the first class of PAs was all men. Women entered the third Duke University class and have been part of the PA movement ever since. Stead (1966, 1967) conceived of the PA as being composed predominantly of men because he thought they would have a greater commitment to a career and a greater willingness to meet the demands of their work. This attitude was short lived, and by 1974 the percentage of female PAs had increased to 16% (Perry, 1976). This trend did not level off, and in 1996 more than 60% of the entering class were women (Simon, 1996). Currently the composition of the PA workforce is 55% women and the class of 2003 is 65% women. This is not as surprising as it may seem at first. Women have been moving into formerly male-dominated jobs in large numbers in recent years. For example, the percentage of female lawyers and judges rose from 4% in 1972 to 15% in 1982. Over the same period the percentage of female accountants rose from 22% to 38% of the total. For economists the increase has been from 12% to 25%. These changes reflect the different educational choices recently made by young women. For example, in 1968 women received only 8% of all medical degrees and 4% of law degrees. The percentages were 41% and 39%, respectively, in 2001.

Women continue to predominate among students and graduates within the NP and nurse midwifery (CNM) professions. There is a critical shortage of entrants to nursing programs, and this issue is, perhaps, the most critical in the health workforce at present.

The shift in the gender distribution of physician and PA applicants is a particularly interesting trend in view of the concurrent trend of an overall decrease in the number of applicants to both medical schools and PA programs.

In 2002, the majority (56%) of PAs are women. This trend began in 1983, much earlier than commonly thought. At the current rate of women entering the PA profession (66% of all students), women will comprise more than two thirds of the profession by 2006.

On average, women PAs are 10 years younger than males, and the average age of male PAs is rising rapidly. The percentage of non-White PAs is increasing overall, and the proportion of women is roughly the same for men in this group. Women are more likely than men, by a small margin, to be in family practice (39%), and more likely to be in group practices than men. Both groups work in towns of less than 10,000 people at about the same rate. There is a difference in the proportion of women who are not in clinical practice (17%) versus men (5%).

It is hard to determine what effect the increasing proportion of women in the PA profession will mean. If parallels are to be appropriately drawn from the literature on women physicians, there could be a number of differences between male and female PAs. Findings on aspects of the career characteristics of women physicians may or may not apply to PAs, and there is some evidence to suggest that women PAs may exhibit a different set of career and practice patterns and characteristics than women physicians.

Women physicians are disproportionately represented in lower-paying primary care specialties such as family practice and general pediatrics as opposed to specialties such as orthopedics or cardiology. The same is not the case among PAs (Exhibit 3-8). Women physicians spend more time with patients (Cassard et al., 1997). This has also been said to be true of PAs, although the documentation of such is difficult to find.

It has also been observed that women physicians are more likely to offer preventive services to patients (Ewing et al., 1999) and to take different pathways of communications with patients (Seto et al., 1997). For women, there remains evidence of a glass ceiling in academic medicine (Bernzweig et al., 1997).

For many modern women, the PA profession represents a preferred and attractive career choice, allowing flexibility along with a high measure of clinical responsibility. Women are making a preferred choice to enter the PA profession instead of medicine. A number of young women today consider PA programs rather than pursuing medical school, even among those with academic records that would make them a virtual certainty to be accepted to medical school.

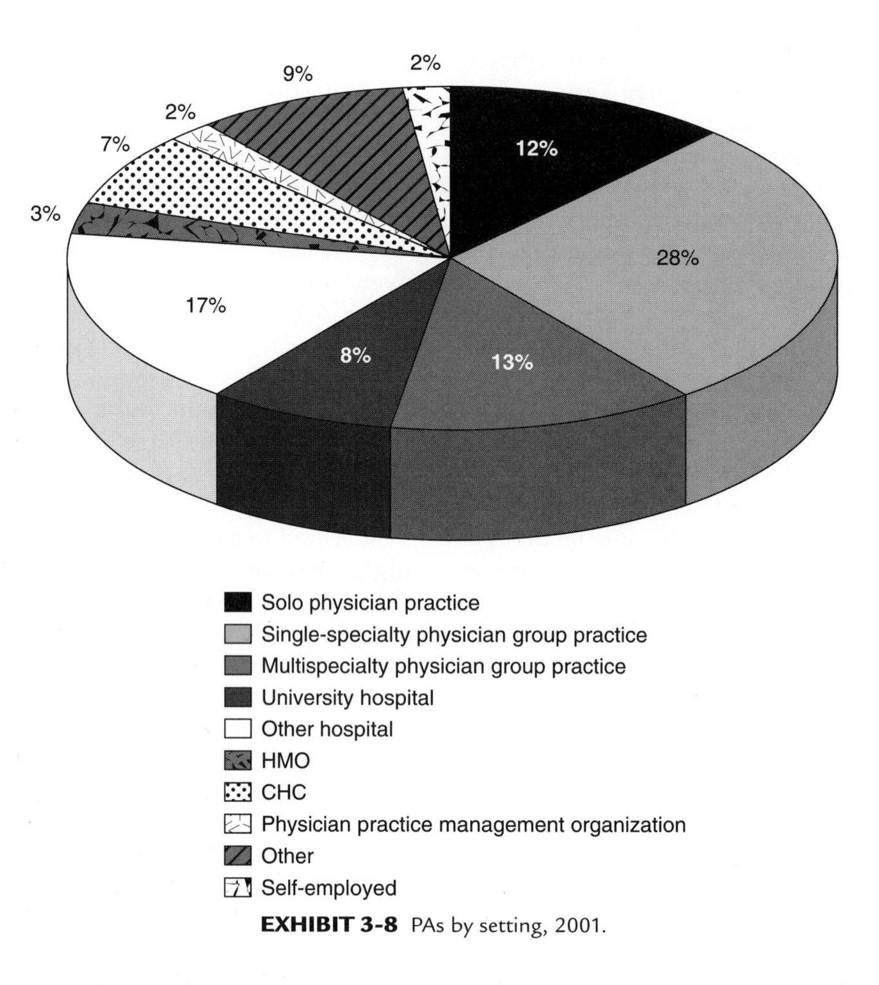

EXHIBIT 3-8 PAs by setting, 2001.

Instead, many choose to enter the PA profession over medical school ostensibly to maintain some control over their work life in a fashion that permits more lifestyle and family time and career mobility.

Gender shifts within key professions, changing perceptions of the roles and status of physicians, and system-driven forces brought about by new requirements for institutional staffing and patient care services are redefining the division of medical labor. There is also the notion of the "deprofessionalization" of medicine—the loss of overall status in society—decreasing what Paul Starr calls physician sovereignty over the health care system (Starr, 1982). Has this trend paralleled the rising profile of the status, roles, and responsibilities of nonphysical clinicians such as NPs, PAs, and CNMs? It is clear that, for many young women, the PA profession offers advantages. For some, the PA profession may be a preferable career choice vis-à-vis that of a physician, with its many demands and sacrifices. The shorter period of formal professional training, high level of clinical responsibility, increasing practice and professional autonomy, and the career flexibility options that characterize the NP and PA professions are important factors including the health career choices of many young women.

Because of the shift in the gender of certain historically male-dominated occupations, planning the future health workforce must consider a larger set of variables. Nationally, women are 11 times more likely than men to voluntarily quit a job. On average, they work 8 months in each job, while men work 3 years, and they are more likely to be part-time workers. Sustained work experience has an important affect on earnings, so these differences between men and women are relevant. Marriage also seems to affect women and men differently. Married men earn more than single men, but single women earn more than married women. This result may occur because historically marriage freed men of household duties and permitted more single-minded attention to jobs, but marriage has had the opposite effect for women. Women in their thirties who have worked without interruption since high school earn slightly more than men with the same background. Unmarried female faculty members at colleges and universities earn slightly more than unmarried male academics with similar credentials (Sowell, 1980; Ehrenberg, 1988).

In determining whether wage differences are the result of discrimination, groups of workers are compared who are equally capable, experienced, and motivated. This comparison is not easy to make given the numerous factors that affect the current earnings of any worker. Economists, taking into account easily measured factors such as age, years of schooling, region, and hours of work, found that from one half to three fourths of the gross differences in earnings between men and women can be explained by these factors (Ehrenberg, 1988). Whether the remaining differences are the result of discrimination or as yet unquantified productivity differences is and probably will continue to be a controversial issue.

Women PAs earn less than male PAs even when influencing factors such as on-call hours, years as a practicing PA, years in current practice, setting, and community size are controlled in the analysis (Carter, 1983; Willis, 1989, Oliver, 1993). Analysis by specialty also reveals that salary differences remain for family/general practice, pediatrics, obstetrics and gynecology (OB/GYN), emergency medicine, and orthopedics. However, no statistical differences emerge in the specialties of surgery, internal medicine, or occupational/industrial medicine (Willis, 1990). Other studies have found that female and male PAs that were hired at the same salary level did not have significant salary differences a few years later (Parnes, 1991).

The reasons for salary differences are not easily explained. Shortcomings of some studies have been in ignoring hourly wage, productivity (patient visits per hour), and total revenues generated by the PA. Other considerations to explain the differences may relate to initial starting salaries, the ability to negotiate for raises, participation in profit sharing, and the development of partnerships when private practices are examined.

Future studies should address whether there are different expectations between women and men in specific settings and whether employers are satisfied with the job performance of both men and women. Do male PAs ask for or receive more frequent and larger raises than women? Are there changes in the way women and men are perceived in their roles and in how they are reimbursed? What experiences discourage or block female PAs from obtaining jobs with greater potential for productivity, income, and advancement? Finally, what can women do to alter discriminatory practices (Parnes, 1990)?

Minorities

Racial and ethnic diversity is the cornerstone of U.S. culture, and adequate representation of all races and ethnic groups is essential to the viability of the PA profession. Without a heterogeneous mix of the U.S. population adequately representing the profession, meeting the cross-sectional needs of the U.S. population will fall short. The proportion of survey respondents from underrepresented minorities is rising within the profession (Exhibit 3-9). Groups showing the largest increases are Hispanics in the south central region and African Americans in the southeast (AAPA, 1996). Trend data suggest that African Americans, Native Americans, and other distinct ethnic groups are participating more than ever before in the profession; fewer than 90% of all PAs are white (Exhibit 3-10).

There are deep historical roots and organizational efforts to improve the configuration and diversity of the PA profession. Three PA training programs actively recruit a predominant student body of minority PAs, primarily African Americans. A program for Native Americans functioned for a few years in New Mexico but closed in the late 1980s. Both the Health Professions Educational Assistance Act and the Health Professions Scholarship Program are designed to attract minorities to the health care professions. Other efforts are underway such as programs to promote the sciences to minorities where they are also underrepresented.

Education

Approximately 67% of the PAs had received at least a bachelor's degree before enrolling in a PA

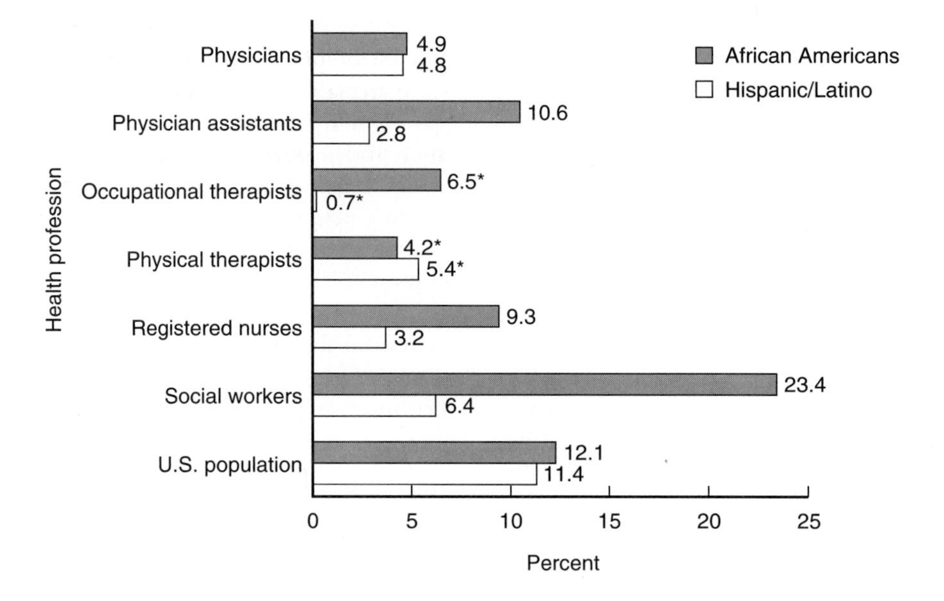

*This data includes all working therapists, which includes both pre- and post-master's degree.

EXHIBIT 3-9 Percentage of minorities represented in health professions.

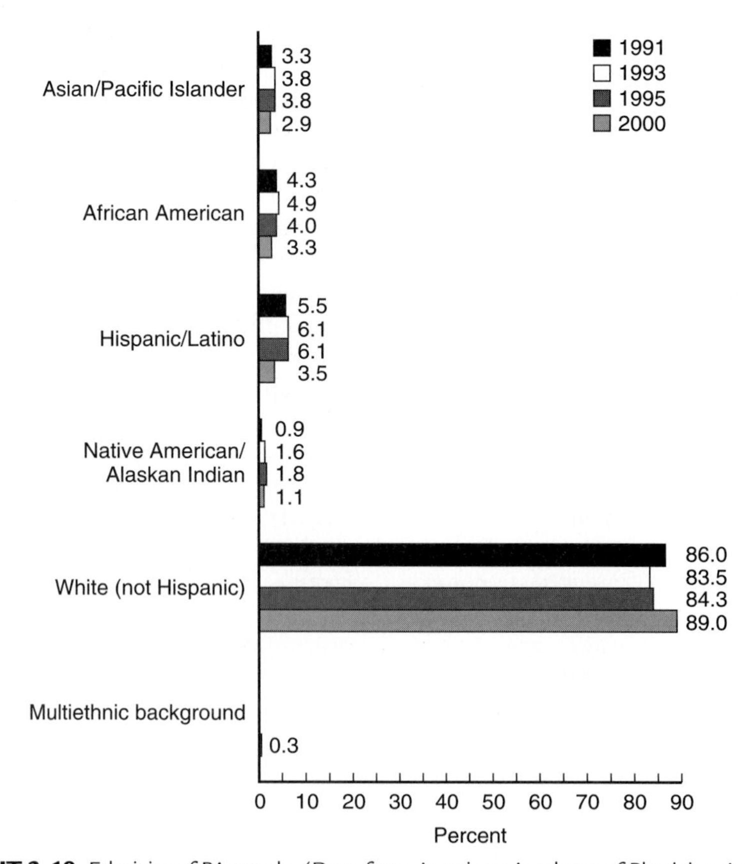

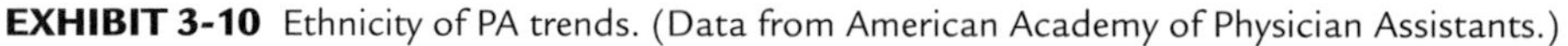
EXHIBIT 3-10 Ethnicity of PA trends. (Data from American Academy of Physician Assistants.)

program. More than half (54%) of the PAs responding received a bachelor's degree from a PA school; 11% received a master's level PA degree. Today 62% of respondents hold bachelor's degrees, 25% hold master's degrees, and 3% hold doctorate degrees. With the change to programs granting graduate degrees, these numbers will shift to more graduates with a master's degree in the workforce.

SPECIALTY

One of the more remarkable aspects of the evolution of the PA profession in U.S. medicine has been its incorporation equally into specialty as well as primary care medical practice. Although the initial mandate for PAs was to serve as primary care practitioners, half have entered specialty and subspecialty practices with equal success (Schafft and Cawley, 1987; Hooker, 1992). Exhibit 3-11 illustrates the specialty distribution of practicing PAs in 2000. The primary care specialties of family practice, general internal medicine, and general pediatrics are shown.

An important group of PAs is composed of those working in general surgery and the surgical subspecialties (22%). In this group are PAs in orthopedics (8%); PAs in surgery and the surgical subspecialties make up more than one fifth of the PA workforce. The clinical roles and activities of surgical PAs and surgeon's assistants (SAs) have been described (Mauney, 1972; Faircloth, Barker, and Hunt, 1976; Maxfield, 1976; Sonntag, Steiner, and Stein, 1977; Miller, Craver, and Hatcher, 1978; Miller and Hatcher, 1978; Perry, 1983; Beinfield, 1991.)

There is a good deal of overlap in the practice of PAs in specialties and those in primary care. For example, gynecology, geriatrics, corrections medicine, industrial and occupational medicine,

EXHIBIT 3-11

Distribution of PAs by Specialty, 2002*

Specialty	%	Specialty	%
Allergy	0.7	Pediatric general	2.9
Anesthesiology	0.4	Pediatric subspecialty	
Dermatology	2.4	Cardiology	0.1
Emergency medicine	10.2	Endocrinology	.0
Family/general medicine	32.1	Heme/oncology	0.1
Geriatrics	0.8	Nephrology	<0.1
Industrial/occupational medicine	3.0	Neurology	0.1
Orthopedics	8.9	Pulmonary	<0.1
Internal medicine, general	8.4	Neonatal perinatal	0.2
Internal medicine subspecialty		Other	0.2
Cardiology	3.0	Physical medicine and rehabilitation	0.9
Critical care	0.3	Psychiatry	1.0
Endocrinology	0.4	Public health/preventive medicine	0.2
Gastroenterology	1.3	Radiology	0.6
Hematology/immune	1.4	Surgery, general	2.5
Infectious disease	0.5	Surgery, subspecialty	
Nephrology	0.6	Cardiovascular/thoracic	4.0
Pulmonology	0.3	Colon/rectal	<0.1
Rheumatology	0.3	Hand	0.2
Other subspecialties	0.8	Neurosurgery	1.9
Neurology	0.5	Pediatric	0.1
Obstetrics and gynecology	2.7	Plastic	0.5
Ophthalmology	0.2	Oncology	0.2
Otolaryngology	0.8	Trauma	0.2
Pathology	0.1	Urology	0.8
Substance abuse	0.4	Vascular	0.5
Other medical specialty	0.8	Otorhinolaryngology	0.7
		Transplant	0.2
		Other surgical specialty	1.0

Modified from 2002 Alexandria, Va., 2002, American Academy of Physician Assistants.
*Total primary care = 43.1%; total surgery = 12.4%.

and emergency medicine are largely composed of primary care activities but may not be classified as primary care providers.

DATA SOURCES ON PHYSICIAN ASSISTANTS

There are several important sources of information on the PA profession. What is known about PAs includes the general census database of the AAPA. This is a comprehensive survey that provides detailed and timely information on socioeconomic aspects of the PA profession. The AAPA census collects continuous information as part of the annual membership renewal in the AAPA. Initially this database was used to compile data on AAPA membership, but has expanded to contain current secular trend data on a large proportion of the PA population. The AAPA membership has grown to 35,000 in 2002. About 20,000 responded to the annual census survey.

Another source of information the profession is the *Annual Report on Physician Assistant Educational Programs.* The APAP sponsors and funds this report. While the AAPA census database relies on individual responses from academy members, the annual report comprises data gathered from PA programs (Exhibit 3-12).

A third source of information is the National Commission on the Certification of Physician Assistants (NCCPA). The NCCPA registers all PA graduates who have sat for the Physician Assistant National Certification Examination, (PANCE), NCCPA, and the National Board of Medical Examiners (NBME).

Together, these three databases provide a remarkable breadth and depth of information about the profession. The APAP database provides information on students and new graduates. The NCCPA details where certified PAs are distributed, and the AAPA database collects information about what they are doing and in what type of setting. The data contained here are primarily from information collected in the membership renewal survey.

Other sources of national data on PA are obtained from time to time. Historically, this has included the National Ambulatory Medical Care Survey by the National Centers for Health Statistics and the AMA. Smaller samples of national data can be found in various surveys of managed care and other health industry reports (Hooker, 1994).

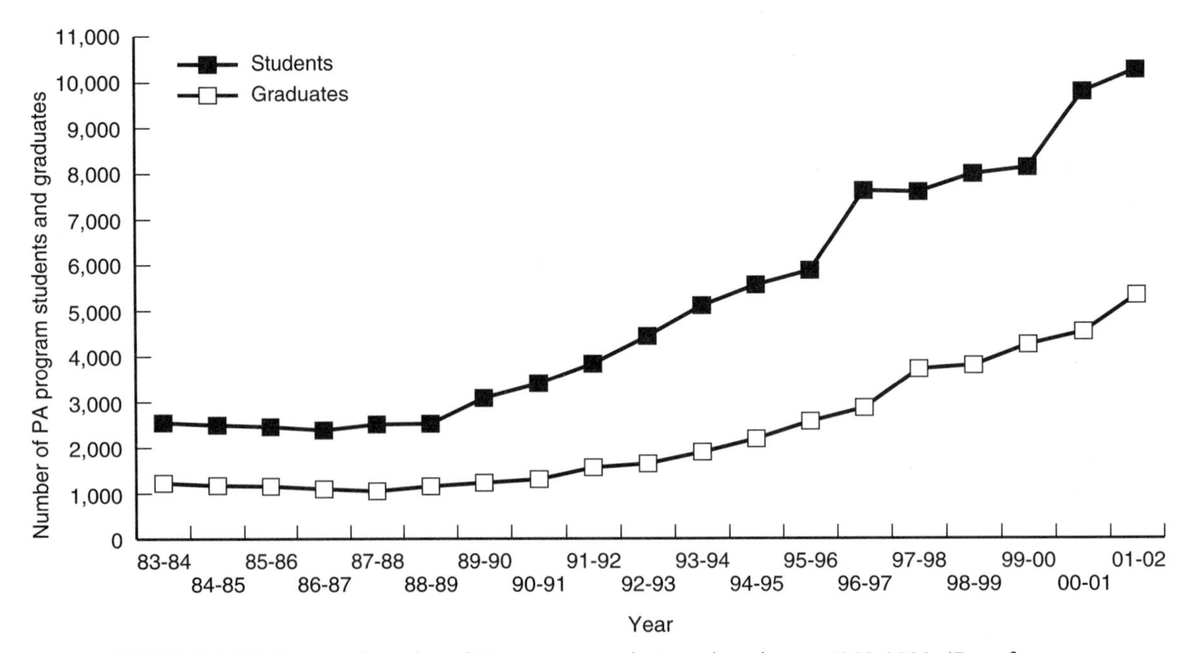

EXHIBIT 3-12 Estimated number of PA program students and graduates, 1983-2000. (Data from Simon A, Link MS, Miko AS: *Seventeenth Annual Report on Physician Assistant Educational Programs in the United States, 2000-2001*, Alexandria, Va., 2001, Association of Physician Assistant Programs.)

PRODUCTIVITY

PA productivity refers to the quantity of services PAs provide to their patients. The number of patient visits to a medical office or patients seen in the hospital are measures that capture a large proportion of overall PA use in most specialties. The time spent in practice by PAs is measured in hours per week and patients per day. On average, PAs spend 37.6 hours a week in an outpatient setting and see 19.3 patients a day (Exhibit 3-13). The total number of visits per week is a unit of productivity sometimes used for comparison among organizations because routines may be accorded to specific days of the week. In 2000 the productivity of PAs was estimated to range from 53 to 99 visits per week depending on the specialty (Exhibit 3-14). These productivity figures are similar to physicians in the same specialty.

The number of prescriptions per visit by the different specialty is also included in Exhibit 3-13. These findings suggest that prescribing is an important element of PA practice.

An inpatient practice is considered (although undefined in the survey) to exist when a PA makes a hospital and/or surgical service patient visit (often referred to as *making hospital rounds*). Exhibit 3-15 is an approximate measure of inpatient practices. Hospital use refers to the number of patients seen per day on average.

Many PAs who have an outpatient practice primarily may provide some of their work in a hospital. Likewise, many PAs working in hospitals may see only ambulatory patients.

A high percentage of PAs (72%) are based in outpatient settings. The greatest concentration of PAs outside the hospital is in multispecialty group practices (26%), followed by solo practices (11%). The high proportion of PAs in outpatient settings is consistent with the high demand for this type of medical labor.

PAs are employed by a variety of industries, agencies, and firms, the dominant employer is a physician or a group of physicians who provide outpatient primary care. How these employers perceive the benefit in employing a PA depends on the return they can achieve. These economic factors are discussed in detail in Chapter 9.

Patient Visits and Encounters

Because of the variety of work settings and specialty fields in which PAs practice, the types of patients PAs treat are quite varied. More than

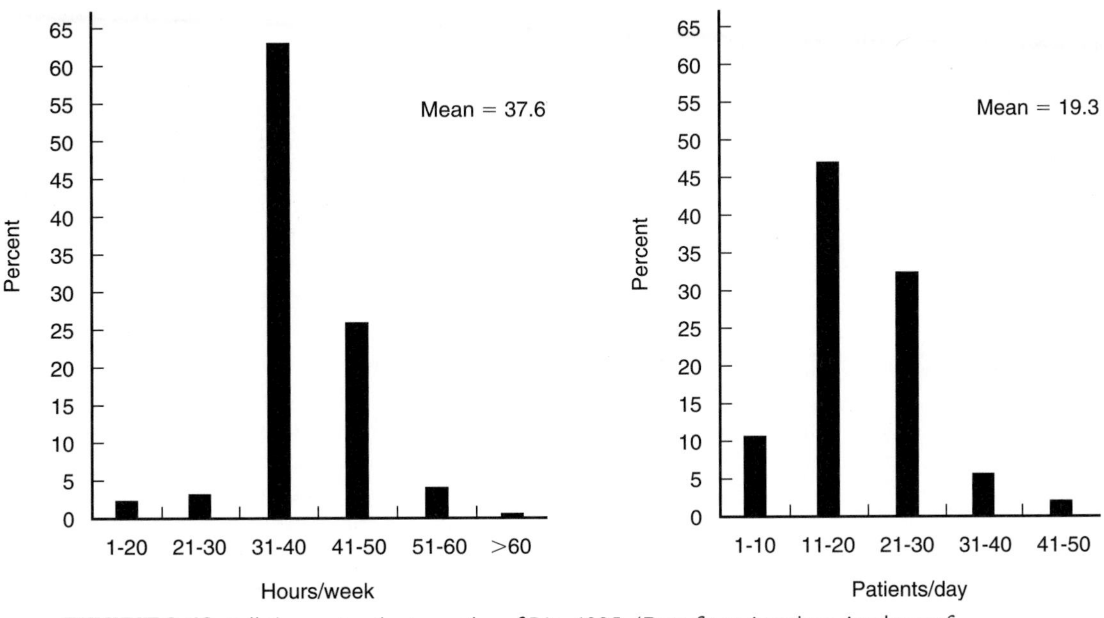

EXHIBIT 3-13 Full-time outpatient practice of PAs, 1995. (Data from American Academy of Physician Assistants, 1996.)

EXHIBIT 3-14

Estimated Number of Patient Visits and Medications Prescribed by PAs in 2000

Specialty	Average no. of visits to each PA per week*	Average no. of prescriptions per visit†
Family practice	93.7	1.34
General internal medicine	78.41	1.78
Cardiology	60.51	1.00
Other internal medicine subspecialties	59.75	1.26
Obstetrics and gynecology	64.53	1.29
Emergency medicine	93.81	1.29
General pediatrics	99.69	0.88
Pediatric subspecialty	54.16	1.18
General surgery	55.43	0.38
Cardiovascular surgery	53.13	1.37
Orthopedic surgery	78.68	0.78
Other surgical specialty	64.43	0.90
Occupational medicine	90.64	0.78
Other	77.76	1.13

Data from American Academy of Physician Assistants Marketing Research Survey, 2000, and American Academy of Physician Assistants Physician Assistant Census Survey, 2000.
*The mean number of visits per week is rounded to two decimal points; therefore, totals cannot be calculated from figures.
†Medication may be prescribed by the PA or recommended by the PA for prescribing.

90% of census respondents who work full time see outpatients in their primary job; the mean number of patient visits provided per week by PAs who see outpatients exclusively is 100.2 visits per week. Twenty-eight percent of respondents who work full-time see inpatients in their primary job; the mean number of patient encounters provided per week by respondents who see inpatients exclusively is 60. Eight percent of full-time PAs see nursing home patients in their primary job, and 5% of respondents see other types of patients.

EXHIBIT 3-15

Full-Time Inpatient Practice of PAs, 1995

Hours/ week	% (mean = 13.6)	Patients/ day	% (mean = 41.3)
1-20	3.8	1-10	40.5
21-30	1.7	11-20	40.0
31-40	39.9	21-30	13.9
41-50	37.3	31-40	4.1
51-60	14.7	41-50	1.5
>60	2.6	—	—

Data from American Academy of Physician Assistants, 1996.

COMPENSATION

Income generated by an occupation, considered either at a point in time or as a stream of revenue received over the working lifetime of an individual, strongly influences the choice of that occupation and is the most frequently mentioned attribute of an occupation.

Although the time structure of earnings is the key determinant in measuring occupational models, the annual earnings at a point in time can give a rough idea of the relative income ranking of one occupation compared with an assortment of other occupations (Exhibit 3-16).

The term *compensation* includes the combination of salaries and benefits. It is the amount the employer forgoes to retain the services of the employee. Although salary is fairly easy to calculate, benefits are more nebulous. Some benefits have a definable amount, such as the cost of dental insurance for an employee and his or her family. Other benefits are really perquisites of the job such as a cellular phone or group medical liability insurance, which the employer provides and the employee is not taxed for its use. Benefits are defined in dollar amounts and usually range from 15% to 25% of the salary.

Salary

Salary is the amount of direct compensation in money that a wage earner receives. The salary range of experienced PAs is quite wide. This is because PAs are in a wide variety of clinical settings, have many different arrangements with their employer, and have a large skill set. Results of the 2002 AAPA PA census survey indicate that the mean total income from primary employer for clinically practicing PAs working full time (32 or more hours per week) is $72,241 (standard deviation of $17,738); the median is $69,567.

Measurement of the change in the incomes reported by the same people for two periods provides a superior basis for examining the health of PA income than a comparison of the incomes reported by all PAs for two periods. The measurement of income change is important because it accounts for the complete constellation of static and dynamic factors that determine income. Conversely, the change revealed by a comparison of income reported by all PAs for two distinct periods is confounded by the income-related

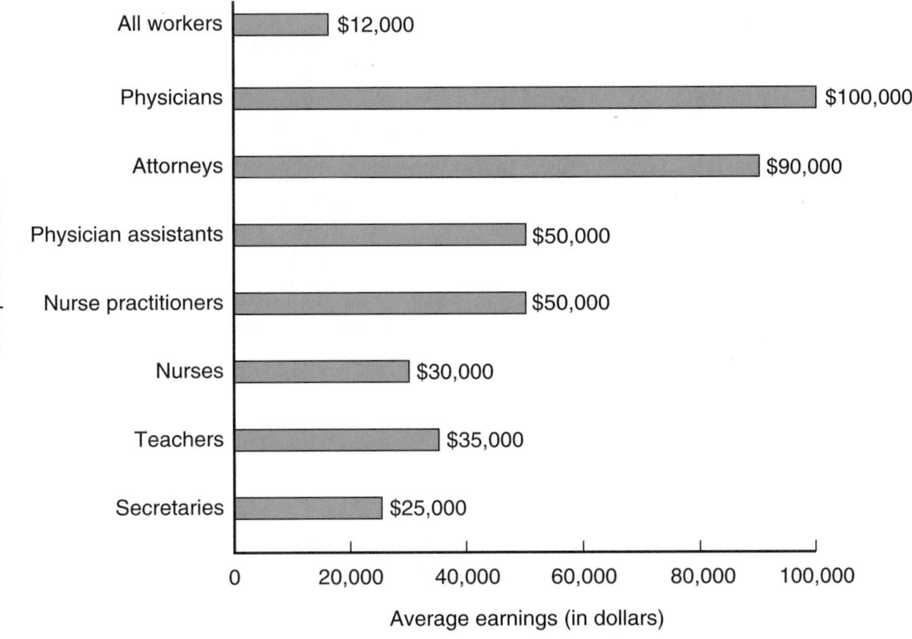

EXHIBIT 3-16 Mean full-time earnings for workers in selected occupations in 1992. (Data from Dorgan CA, Dorjan C: *Statistical Handbook of Working America: Statistics on Occupation, Careers, Employment & the Work Environment,* Gale Group, Farmington Hills, Mich., 1995.)

effects of whatever differences exist between the populations of PAs represented by each period. For example, the relative proportion of recent graduates would affect the change in each period.

As a consequence, posting an average or median salary may or may not be not useful to PAs interested in their market value on entry into the workforce. Therefore the information that follows is based on salary for recent graduates, that is, those who have graduated in or after 2000. The mean income for recent PA graduates is $63,168 (range $47,823 to $78,513), regardless of age, gender, experience before entering PA school, or specialty (Exhibit 3-17). Practice specialty, years of experience, employment setting, and city size in which a PA works all have an affect on salary.

Geographic region of the country (or even state) influences the average salary for PAs. The geographic location of PAs not only affects their salary but also may help explain why PAs locate in some areas more densely than in others. For example, salaries are high in the western United States, and there is a high prevalence of PAs in that region. Conversely, PA income is the lowest in the southeast where some states have few employed PAs. Salary also tends to increase along with the size of the city. Large metropolitan cities tend to pay PAs more than small towns. However, in some different parts of the country (i.e., the southeast and north central regions), PAs in rural areas are paid better if the region has difficulty recruiting workers. As can be seen in Exhibit 3-18, PAs starting a career in south central and western United States earn about $5000 more than those in the other regions of the country.

The variable that influences future PA salary more than others is practice specialty. Exhibit 3-19

EXHIBIT 3-17

Total Annual Income From Primary Employer for Respondents Who Work at Least 32 Hours per Week at a Nongovernment Primary Clinical Job

	All PAs*	Recent graduates†
No. of respondents	13,552	1,757
Mean	$72,241	$63,168
Standard deviation	$17,738	$15,345
10th percentile	$53,817	$50,169
25th percentile	$60,945	$55,087
Median	$69,567	$61,363
75th percentile	$80,241	$68,082
90th percentile	$93,932	$76,626

Data from American Academy of Physician Assistants, Division of Research.
*All PAs who responded to the survey in 2002.
†PAs who graduated in or after 2000.

EXHIBIT 3-18

Total Annual Income From Primary Employer for PAs Who Graduated in or After 1999

	Northeast	Southeast	North central	South central	West	Total
No. of respondents	372	326	309	161	229	1,434
Mean	$55,748	$56,911	$59,211	$60,316	$61,882	$58,297
Standard deviation	$10,397	$10,299	$8,989	$11,560	$12,995	$10,895
10th percentile	$43,375	$47,079	$50,339	$49,231	$48,612	$47,428
25th percentile	$49,304	$51,443	$53,720	$52,957	$53,817	$51,931
Median	$54,178	$55,112	$58,101	$59,041	$60,984	$56,977
75th percentile	$61,899	$61,171	$63,383	$64,031	$68,062	$63,247
90th percentile	$68,040	$68,831	$69,726	$73,374	$76,345	$71,507

Data from American Academy of Physician Assistants, Division of Research.

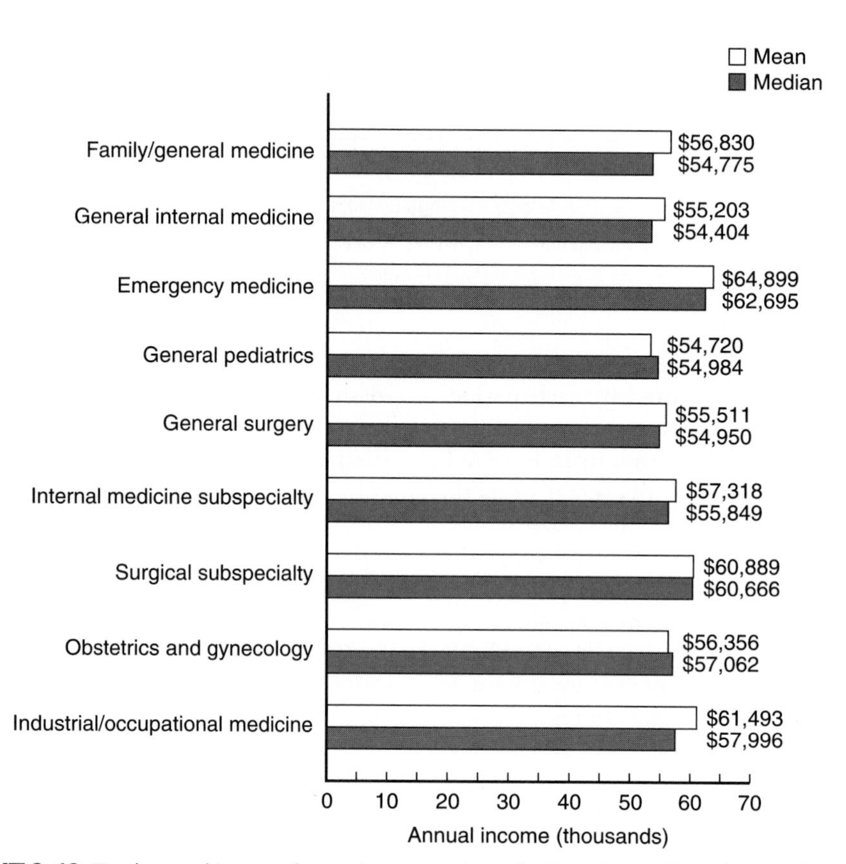

EXHIBIT 3-19 Total annual income from primary employer for PAs who graduated in or after 1999 by general specialty practiced. (Data from American Academy of Physician Assistants, Research Division, 2000.)

shows PA starting salaries for recent graduates by type of specialty. The mean starting salary in industrial and occupational medicine is approximately $61,500 versus general pediatrics in which graduates earn on average $55,000 a year.

Not surprisingly, PAs with more experience command higher salaries. When income distribution is viewed as a probability density, the data show a right-sided kurtosis. This shaped curve is classic for salary distributions and is predictable because income increases with experience at a fairly even pace. This continues until some peak density is attained and then decreases, declining exponentially at higher levels of income. The ever-diminishing tail represents the very few who for whatever entrepreneurial reasons have incomes two to four times greater than their cohorts.

As the PA-physician relationship evolves on the employer-employee level, compensation arrangements negotiated by PAs will continue to undergo change. Some forms of compensation, such as overtime, are incentive bonuses directed at driving the PA to perform more work. More commonly reported compensations range from overtime pay to event-call pay to on-call pay (such as wearing a beeper or being close to home for consultation). Increasingly, PAs are being compensated with bonuses. Almost one fifth of PAs received a bonus either because of the practice's performance or their performance in 2000.

Other arrangements include incentive pay based on productivity, as well as partnerships and percentages of revenues. Details of these partnerships are now coming to light (Barnes and Hooker, 2001).

Benefits

Surveys to determine the types of benefits that employers commonly offer to PAs done on 12,242 practicing PAs had a 56% response rate. The distribution was reported as representative of the practicing PA population by specialty, setting, population base, and gender. Aside from the base salary information, questions included areas such as insurance benefits, paid leave (vacation, continuing medical education [CME], ill time, and maternity leave), and other earnings through bonuses (Exhibit 3-20).

The average annual bonus earning is $9000, although this is a bit misleading because two thirds earned a bonus less than $5000 per year in additional revenue. More than 15% of the PAs report additional earnings ranging from $10,000 to more than $20,000.

Exhibit 3-20 also describes the findings for insurance benefits, benefits other than insurance, and the mean number of days available for various leave categories. It should be noted that the average amount of funding for CME is $1412 per year and is available to 85% of PAs who work full time.

The benefit structure of government workers, both state and federal, tends to be more encompassing than that for those in the private sector.

EXHIBIT 3-20

Breakdown of PA Benefits

Benefit	Fully funded (%)	Partially funded (%)
Individual health insurance	55	37
Family health insurance	31	43
Professional liability insurance	97	2
Dental insurance	33	38
Disability insurance	48	23
Term life insurance	44	14
Profit sharing	30	11
Retirement fund	28	52
State license fees	70	2
DEA registration fees	72	1
NCCPA fees	63	2
AAPA dues	64	2
State PA chapter dues	57	2
AAPA annual conference registration fees	58	12
Credentialing fees	71	4
Benefit	**Average/yr**	
Maternity leave	5.6 wk	
Paid vacation	17.2 days	
Sick leave	7.4 days	
Medical education leave	5.9 days	
Earnings over base	$6018	
Medical education funds available	$1412	

Data from *2002 AAPA Physician Assistant Census Report,* Alexandria, Va., 2002, American Academy of Physician Assistants.

For example, in the federal system, vacation is 30 days a year. Sick leave is generous; health, dental, and malpractice and life insurance are automatically covered. The retirement benefits of federal, state, and sometimes municipal employment make this sector particularly attractive.

Taking Call

More than one third (36%) of full-time respondents report taking call for their primary employer. The mean hours on call per month for those PAs who take some call but are not always on call is 104.

Base Pay

Eighty-two percent of respondents report receiving their base pay in the form of a salary; 17% indicate that they receive an hourly wage.

Compensation

Respondents report receiving several different forms of compensation from their primary employer. Common forms of compensation include event-call pay (9%) and overtime pay (18%). Twenty percent of respondents report receiving an incentive based on productivity or performance. Approximately two fifths (38%) of those who receive an incentive based on productivity and performance report that the incentive is based on revenue that the PA generates.

CME Funding

Eighty-eight percent of respondents report having CME funds available to them from their primary employer. For those PAs who reported the amount of CME funds available to them, the mean was $1438; the median was $1500.

Source of Funds for Expenses

More than 97% of respondents report having their employer pay 100% of their professional malpractice liability insurance. Approximately two thirds of respondents also report having their employer pay their professional (AAPA) dues (64%), state license fees (70%), NCCPA certificate maintenance fees (63%), AAPA annual conference registration fees (59%), and Drug Enforcement Administration registration fees (72%).

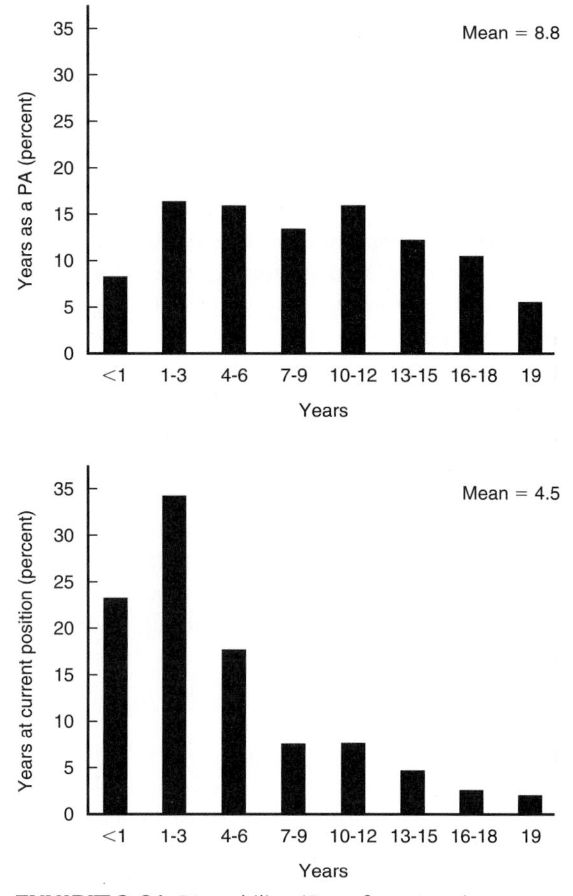

EXHIBIT 3-21 PA mobility. (Data from American Academy of Physician Assistants, 1994.)

TURNOVER AND MOBILITY

PAs are a fairly mobile occupation, meaning they tend to change jobs regularly. In workforce parlance, this is termed *turnover*. The standard method of determining the turnover rate is the number of PA clinical positions held divided by the total number of years in practice as a clinical PA. For all respondents to the 2002 membership census who practice full or part time, the rate is 0.47. On the whole, more than 60% of the profession has spent less than 3 years in their current positions (Cawley et al., 2001), and for the past few years, the percentage of PAs who have remained in the same position more than 10 years has averaged around 8% (Exhibit 3-21). Even PAs with more than 15 years of experience report that they have been with their current employer, on average, less than 3 years. This suggests PAs negotiate contracts frequently and are often active in the job market at advanced stages of their careers. Little is understood about this phenomenon other than the speculation that PA graduates tend to take their first job as entree to the workforce that may not be the most attractive, and then tend to look around for a way to raise their income and working conditions by switching employers.

ATTRITION

If career mobility is one side of the PA professional coin, attrition is the other. Attrition is the gradual and natural reduction of membership or personnel from the profession. Surveys of PAs, both on a nationwide basis and in selected populations, confirm that about 85% of all PA graduates remain working in patient care positions. This level of professional retention is higher than seen in most health professionals, though not quite as high as the level of physician retention. Only anecdotal information exists on those who are no longer practicing as PAs. Historically, at least in the early 1980s, men, former military medical corpsmen, and graduates of military PA programs had the lowest attrition rate (Perry and Redmond, 1984).

Clearly a number PAs drop out of the profession because of health, retirement, death (at least 450 PAs have died), parenting responsibilities, and career burnout. Some have used their PA background and experience to branch into related fields. Still others have acquired further formal education and used that as a stepping-stone to a different, sometimes related, career. Employment experiences and additional education have led many PAs into more complex and advanced roles in health and education. Some have shown the ability and interest to expand their horizons in the health care field by creating their own new roles and opportunities. Program alumni surveys estimate that approximately 4% of all PAs have gone on to medical, osteopathic, dental, chiropractic, or podiatric school. A considerably larger number have sought graduate education, for example, a master's degree in public health or administration, education, business administration, or public administration. One study identified 213 PAs who had a doctorate degree other than medical (e.g., PhD, DrPH, and EdD). Most of these individuals acquired their terminal degrees after graduating from a PA program (P. Eugene Jones, personal communication, 1993), a trend that has continued. However, program directors report that applicants with doctorate degrees are also applying for PA training. In 2002, 2.4% of graduates had a doctorate degree. Doctoral preparation is becoming more prominent for a career in PA education.

Employment patterns for PAs with advanced degrees are extremely varied, depending on the interests, capabilities, and personalities of the individuals. PAs have relied on their PA credential and advanced degree to achieve or enhance their positions in medical fields.

The PA credential is increasingly recognized in the health care field as representing a respected medical background that permits individuals to move into many types of expanded clinical and nonclinical roles. Attrition to some degree seems inevitable but does not appear to be a major problem for the PA profession. In any profession there will be a proportion of people who would be expected to explore new and expanding areas of opportunity, and the PA profession has appeared to be a reasonable springboard for these aspirations. Because a large number of PAs sought this profession after making one or more career changes, it seems only natural that they be afforded this view as well if they seek career latitude or an alternative role.

PART-TIME EMPLOYMENT

Part-time work is an integral part of the labor force in all parts of the United States and occurs in almost all careers. In the United States *full time* means 40 hours a week and *part time* is often defined as fewer than 32 hours a week. When all occupations (not just health care workers) are examined, women make up the bulk of part-time workers (72.2%) nationally. In the aggregate, they are often married (with the husband present) and are sometimes considered secondary wage earners. Although an age-participation profile is not available, most part-time PAs fall into this category as well because most part-time workers are women. However, apart from the fact that only 9% of PAs practice short of full time, the distinction between full-time and part-time employment from the data presented here does not differ significantly. Part-time PAs are more likely to be in primary care (71% versus 56%), but with the exception of the gender differences, the type of setting, ethnicity, and number of years in current position are only marginally different between full-time and part-time PAs. The fact that so few PAs are part time is seen as remarkable when compared with many other health care occupations, including nursing and medicine.

PUBLIC SERVICE: MILITARY, FEDERAL, AND STATE

Today about 11% of all PAs are employed in positions within the public sector. Among all PAs reported in the AAPA annual census, 7% are employed in the federal government, with 2% working for the state and 1% in local government agencies. The federal government is the single largest employer of all health care providers. Currently about 1350 of PAs serve in uniformed services branches, including 2% each in the Army and Air Force, 1.4% in the Navy, 0.1% in the Coast Guard (Department of Transportation), 3.8% in the Department of Veterans Affairs health care system, 0.5% in the Department of Justice in the Bureau of Prisons (BOP) medical system, and 0.4% in the Indian Health Service (IHS) and other agencies in the U.S. Public Health Service. PAs are also employed in the Department of State, the Department of Health and Human Services, the U.S. Customs Service, and the Department of Defense and serve at the White House.

The overall number of PAs employed by the Department of Veterans Affairs system was 1200 in 2000. PAs are also in federal service in the U.S. military and hold commissioned officer status in all branches. PAs are avidly recruited by agencies in the U.S. Public Health Service and the BOP, where the existing limitations in the available supply of PAs continue to cause ongoing vacancies in medical staffing. For example, the IHS employs 98 full-time equivalent (FTE) PAs (about one third are Native Americans). Both the IHS and other federal agencies, such as the BOP, anticipate that medical staffing requirements for PA personnel will increase substantially. This is the fastest growing federal department, and the demands for PAs and other health care workers are high in corrections medicine. The distribution of PAs in the various government agencies is shown in Exhibit 3-22.

UNDERSERVED SETTINGS

The major objective in the development of training programs for PAs was to increase the availability of health care in areas with physician shortages. These underserved areas include small communities in rural areas. The federal government defines *rural* as a county with fewer than 100,000 people and a town with fewer than 50,000 individuals. Census data classifies PAs by those that live in communities of fewer than 50,000 and 10,000 populations.

About 14% of PAs are in practice in communities of fewer than 10,000 people, with an additional 14% working in communities of 10,000 to 50,000. More PAs (29%) are working in practices in communities of fewer than 50,000 than either allopathic physicians (12%) or osteopathic physicians (15%) (Council on Graduate Medical Education [COGME], 1992; AAPA, 1996; Pasko and Seidman, 2002). The reasons for the distribution of PAs in underserved communities are multifactorial, but one of the leading reasons is the federal initiative to fund programs that serve small communities. Since the late 1970s federal statute has required that PA programs receiving grants support curricula emphasizing primary care. Programs that demonstrate successful outcomes in deployment of graduates in primary care practices and in medically underserved areas have promoted PA practice in rural communities. Until recently, a downward trend in the percentages of PAs practicing in small communities (less than 10,000 population) had been observed. Between 1981 and 1996 the percentage of PAs working in smaller communities declined from 27% to 14%. Major factors responsible for this decline include a changing medical market and the changing demography of the PA profession. Some responsible factors overlap. Nearly all rural PAs are employed in primary care practices (86%). Factors influencing PA employment trends away from both primary care and rural practice include the retirement of older male PAs (who are more likely than women to enter practices in underserved areas), the increasing proportion of women now entering the profession, and the increasingly strong demand and consequently higher remuneration levels offered to PAs in urban settings and hospital-based practices. The same negative factors that discourage physicians from working in rural areas also affect PAs (e.g., large patient care load, long hours, professional and social isolation, fewer academic centers, and lower income). However, since the 1996 low of 14% the percentages of PAs working in communities of less than 10,000 have improved. In 1992

EXHIBIT 3-22

Type of Government Employer, 2002

Employer	%
Not government employed	89.6
Air Force	0.7
Bureau of prisons	0.3
Navy	0.6
Veterans Affairs	2.7
Public Health Service	0.3
Army	1.4
Coast Guard	0.1
National Guard	0.1
Other federal government	0.5
State government	2.3
Local government	1.2

Data from American Academy of Physician Assistants, Research Division, 2002.

the figure rose to 16.5% in 1993 to 18% and in 1996 to 14%. In 2002, it remains at 14%. The effect of federal PA funding preferences on grants for PA educational programs is believed to have offset to some degree the national trend among health care professionals drifting away from rural practice (Exhibit 3-23) (Willis and Reid, 1990; Willis, 1993).

Although physicians supervise PAs, many PAs in practices in isolated rural areas often function with considerable independence. Many rural communities are dependent on a PA-staffed clinic to provide local medical care for residents. Physicians in rural communities rely on PAs to help balance patient care duties, on-call responsibilities, and leisure time, as well as to help avoid problems of social and professional isolation. PAs are cost-effective to rural practices because their salaries are about one third of physicians' salaries. Anecdotal reports suggest that most perform at productivity rates similar to those of physicians in these settings as well.

COMMUNITY AND MIGRANT HEALTH CENTERS

Shi et al. (1994) from the University of North Carolina examined the patterns and determinants of use of PAs and other nonphysician health care providers practicing in rural community and migrant health centers in all U.S. geographic regions. The primary objective of the study was to compare centers that employed PAs and other nonphysician health care providers versus those not employing such providers. Data from the 243 responses received from rural and migrant health clinics gave findings related to the use of PAs, NPs, and CNMs. Three quarters (77%) indicated that PA, NP, and CNM health care professionals were on their medical staffs. Also, 85% indicated that they were seeking to employ additional PA and NP health care providers. To meet anticipated demand for primary care providers, community and migrant health care centers would need to hire 726 physicians, 315 NPs, 218 PAs, 145 CNMs, and 169 other staff members (Samuels, 1992). A major factor in the use of PAs and other nonphysician health care providers in rural and migrant health care clinics is whether these facilities hold an affiliation with an educational program involved in the training of these providers. High proportions (77% for PAs, 67% for NPs, and 93% for CNMs) of the rural community and migrant health care centers surveyed nationally are involved in training activities of these health care professionals. Findings also suggest that the

EXHIBIT 3-23

PA Specialty and Practice Settings in Underserved Areas (%)*

Practice type	Total	High poverty	Total HPSA	Urban HPSA	Rural HPSA
Specialty					
Primary care†	42.4	36.8	66.0	41.2	87.0
Medical specialty‡	25.4	29.8	18.9	29.2	10.2
Surgical specialty§	25.4	26.1	11.0	21.9	1.8
Obstetrician-gynecologist	4.4	4.8	3.4	6.8	0.5
Other‖	2.5	2.5	0.7	0.9	0.5
Practice setting					
Group office	25.7	15.6	17.8	21.2	15.0
Clinic medical office	23.5	31.8	48.8	32.1	62.6
Private hospital	15.1	17.1	10.0	19.6	2.1
Public hospital	14.1	20.9	9.5	14.3	5.4
Solo office	12.6	7.2	11.1	7.5	14.2
HMO	8.4	7.1	2.4	5.0	0.3
Other	0.7	0.4	0.4	0.3	0.5

Data from American Academy of Physician Assistants.
**HMO*, Health maintenance organization; *HPSA*, health professional service area.
†Family/general practice, general internal medicine, and general pediatrics.
‡Allergy, dermatology, emergency medicine, geriatrics, internal medicine subspecialty, neurology, occupational medicine, pediatric subspecialty, psychiatry, and rehabilitation.
§General surgery, surgery, ophthalmology, orthopedics, and otolaryngology.
‖Anesthesiology, pathology, and radiology.

centers that actively seek to employ PAs and other nonphysician providers are more likely to establish training and employment channels with educational programs.

Working in primary care in rural community and migrant health care clinics, PAs, NPs, and CNMs tend to function in roles that are largely substitutive of physicians. A significant and inverse relationship exists between the number of physicians and the number of nonphysicians employed in these settings. Other factors shown to have an affect on patterns of use of nonphysician health care providers in these clinical settings include (1) a significant positive relationship between the number of total staff and the number of nonphysician providers employed, (2) geographic region, (3) educational program linkage, and (4) center clinical staffing policies (Shi et al., 1993).

MEDICALLY UNDERSERVED URBAN SETTINGS

For some in the PA profession, working with the impoverished is a part of their commitment to social services as health professionals. For PAs and other providers who work in urban underserved areas, there is a value placed on service to humanity and a strong sense of pride in making a difference. Focus groups of primary care providers in inner city areas reveal that they thrive on the challenge of creatively dealing with their patients' complex human needs with limited health care resources. Factors critical to survival in an underserved urban setting include a hardy personality style, a flexible but controllable work schedule, and multidisciplinary practice teams. The camaraderie and synergy of teams generate personal support and opportunities for continuing professional development (Li, Williams, and Scammon, 1995).

HMO/MANAGED CARE

PAs and primary care physicians are in stronger demand in HMOs and managed health care systems. PA use in HMOs has been slow to catch on in a number of systems, with about 8% of PAs reporting this as their primary employment, the clinical staffs of many other organizations employ a mix of physician and nonphysician health care providers in staffing. Findings from a survey of 10 HMOs nationwide and data from several other HMO studies, Weiner (1994) estimated that there are approximately 18 nonphysician health care providers (either PA or NP) per 100,000 HMO enrollees, with a range from 0 to 67 PAs and NPs. A Group Health Association of America study found that the mean number of full-time physicians per 100,000 enrollees is 142.3. The number of primary care physicians was 68.7 per 100,000 enrollees. When PAs and NPs were factored in, there was an inverse relationship (Dial et al., 1995). Our interpretation of this observation suggests that PAs and NPs are substituting for primary care physicians in these settings in underappreciated levels (Hooker and Cawley, 1995).

Other observations from this study find PAs and NPs providing direct patient care to all categories of patients (Exhibit 3-24). NPs and CNMs tend to provide more OB/GYN care than PAs, but both PAs and advance practice nurses are used extensively in primary care.

An example of the extensive integration of PAs in HMOs exists at Kaiser Permanente in Portland, Oregon. This HMO has an enrollment of more than 400,000 members, staffed by 550 FTE physicians and 150 FTE PAs and NPs within 29 clinical departments. PAs who practice in both primary care areas and specialty care roles are fully integrated as members of the health provider team. The Kaiser Permanente Center for Health Research has measured longitudinally the clinical productivity, costs, and practice characteristics of both PAs and NPs in the HMO/managed care setting (Hooker, 1993).

PAs are used extensively in major U.S. HMO systems. (The Southern California Kaiser Plan employs roughly 500 PAs and NPs; Pilgrim/Harvard Community Health Plan in Boston; Health Insurance Plan of Greater New York; Group Health Association and Partners in the District of Columbia; the Mayo Clinic in Rochester, Minnesota; Group Health Cooperative of Puget Sound in Seattle; and the Family Health Plan Systems in Utah, California, and other western states.) More than two thirds of all group-model and staff-model HMOs report that they employ PAs and/or NPs (Dial et al., 1995) (Exhibit 3-24).

EXHIBIT 3-24

Clinical Responsibilities of PAs and NPs in HMOs*

	PERCENTAGE OF HMOS	
	PAs	**NPs**
Prescriptive authority	59.5	73.3
Primary provider	70.3	68.4
Included on provider list	35.1	36.8
Provide direct access to		
Obstetrics and gynecology patients	51.5	94.7
Well adults	97.2	91.7
Chronically ill patients	91.7	91.4
Other adults	73.9	63.6
Pediatric patients	71.4	89.2
Psychiatric patients	48.4	48.4

Data from Dial: 1995 Group Health Association of America Survey of Clinical Staffing in HMOs. American Association of Health Plans, Washington, DC, 1995.
*N = 34, NPs includes certified nurse midwives.

Performance in Managed Care Systems

Major factors receiving increased attention in managed health care systems relate to the clinical capabilities and cost-effectiveness of PAs in such settings. In the HMO setting PAs and NPs have long played important roles in the clinical staffing patterns of these health care facilities. PAs and NPs have proven themselves capable of delivering most of the health care services required at physician-equivalent levels of quality of care and at lower costs than physicians (Hooker, 1993). When clinical productivity of PAs, as measured by the number of outpatient care visits per day, was compared with the patient visit rates of primary care physicians and NPs, PA clinical productivity was equal to and in some settings greater than that of the other primary care providers. In studies conducted at Kaiser Permanente Northwest, Record and colleagues (1981) compared the clinical performance of PAs with that of primary care physicians in a large HMO in handling episodes of four specific morbidities: strep throat, upper respiratory infection (URI), bursitis, and bronchitis. Outcome criteria included patient safety, as measured by the rate of adverse side effects from antibiotics and other drugs used in patient management. Over 1 year no differences in the rates between PAs and physicians were observed.

QUALITY OF CARE

PA utilization in medical practices has grown, partly a result of practice efficiency and economic advantages and a high degree of patient satisfaction with care provided by these providers. A number of health care services research studies conducted shortly after introducing a PA into practice concluded that PAs provide physician-equivalent levels of quality of patient care. Sox (1979) summarized data from more than a dozen well-conducted studies examining the clinical performance of PAs. He found that the quality of patient care delivered by PAs was at a level "indistinguishable" from that of physician care.

Patient satisfaction is a related but imperfect measure of health care provider quality of care and is a partial determinant of the use of health care personnel. High level of patient acceptance of PA services has been a consistently observed finding in many of the health care services research reports published after PAs were introduced into clinical practice (Office of Technology Assessment, 1986). These studies showed that the proportion of patients reporting acceptable to high levels of satisfaction with health care services delivered by PAs averaged between 80% and 90% among individuals not previously exposed to PA care. This figure subsequently rose more than 95% among patients surveyed after having received care from a PA (Nelson, Jacobs, and Johnson, 1974; Hooker, 1993).

Public acceptance and familiarity with PA health care providers have grown substantially, particularly over the last decade. Data from a report based on findings from a random sample of 687 adults surveyed by telephone in the Kentucky Health Survey indicated that 1 in 4 (25%) had received medical advice or treatment from a PA within the last 2 years. More than 90% of these subjects reported satisfaction with the care they received. Recipients of care from PAs did not differ from recipients of care from physicians with respect to income, education, insurance status, self-assessment of health status, or rural versus urban location (Mainous, Bertolino, and Harrell, 1992).

The quality of care provided by PAs was assessed in primary care clinics of the U.S. Air Force in which PAs delivered a considerable portion of primary care formerly provided by physicians. Quality of clinical care determinations were made on the basis of responses to predetermined diagnostic, therapeutic, and referral and disposition criteria. Therapeutic criteria included desirable actions on the part of the health care provider (e.g., prescribing the appropriate class of antibiotic for infectious otitis media at the first visit) and undesirable actions (e.g., prescribing an antibiotic for viral syndrome with gastroenteritis). On five of six such criteria, PAs performed as well as or better than physicians in identifying desirable therapeutic actions (Goldberg et al., 1981).

Kane (1978) compared the quality of clinical care performance of Medex-trained PAs to that provided by their employing and supervising physicians. Findings revealed that PAs were less likely than supervising physicians to use antibiotics in a manner judged to be inappropriate (e.g., prescribed for fevers of undetermined origin or viral URIs) and to be somewhat less likely to use systemic steroids for conditions such as contact dermatitis or asthma. This suggests that the patient care management decisions for these morbidities made by PAs were as good as or better than those of physicians (Kane, 1978b). In another study, Wright and colleagues (1977) compared the clinical performance of several types of providers of primary care services by recording decision patterns and outcome aspects of treatment by family practice residents, faculty, and PAs in two clinics staffed by health care professionals in a university family practice residency program. Activities measured in the study include patient functional outcomes, patient satisfaction, and mean cost per episode of care. Findings revealed that PAs performed as well as or better than other primary care providers in delivery of services in each of the endpoint measures (Wright et al., 1977). Duttera and Harlan (1978) evaluated the appropriateness of patient care provided by PAs in 14 rural primary care settings. They concluded that PAs were clinically competent in both diagnostic and therapeutic skills, as judged by performances observed in three specific practice circumstances: (1) when all patients were initially seen by the PA and then by a physician, (2) when undifferentiated patients were managed concurrently by physicians and PAs, and (3) when patients with specific problems were assigned to PAs. We conclude that quality care, based on the literature, does not seem to be an issue when PAs are the providers of care.

COMPARING PHYSICIAN ASSISTANTS WITH OTHER OCCUPATIONS

Over the past 15-year period, from 1987 to 2002, the income of PAs rose substantially. Thanks in part to organization of health care delivery, PAs have made significant gains in compensation when compared with other workers. This gain is in the rise of salary for PAs but is also reflected when income change is adjusted for income. As shown in Exhibit 3-25 the average salary of all PAs (full time and part time) has risen approximately 34% in 1983 dollars. Only salaries for physicians and automobile mechanics have risen higher.

MEDICAL LEGAL CONSIDERATIONS

PAs typically protect their medical legal risk, as well as their supervising physicians' malpractice liability risk, in one of two ways: by obtaining their own malpractice insurance (this varies by state and averages from $1500 to $3000 a year) or by attaching a rider to the physician's policy covering the activities of the PA. The rate of malpractice suits filed involving PAs has been quite low across a wide spectrum of practice settings and specialties (Borden, 1990). The proportionate rate of malpractice claims for PAs versus physicians as shown from data obtained from the National Practice Data Bank is that because PA practice is associated with improved patient communication and proper documentation (two leading categories of breeches prompting malpractice lawsuits), the use of a PA can mitigate a practice's medical liability risk (Cawley, Rohrs, Hooker, 1998) (see Chapter 11).

BELIEFS, BEHAVIORS, AND ATTITUDES

Understanding some of the unique characteristics of PAs is important if we are to better understand the occupation. This section lists some of

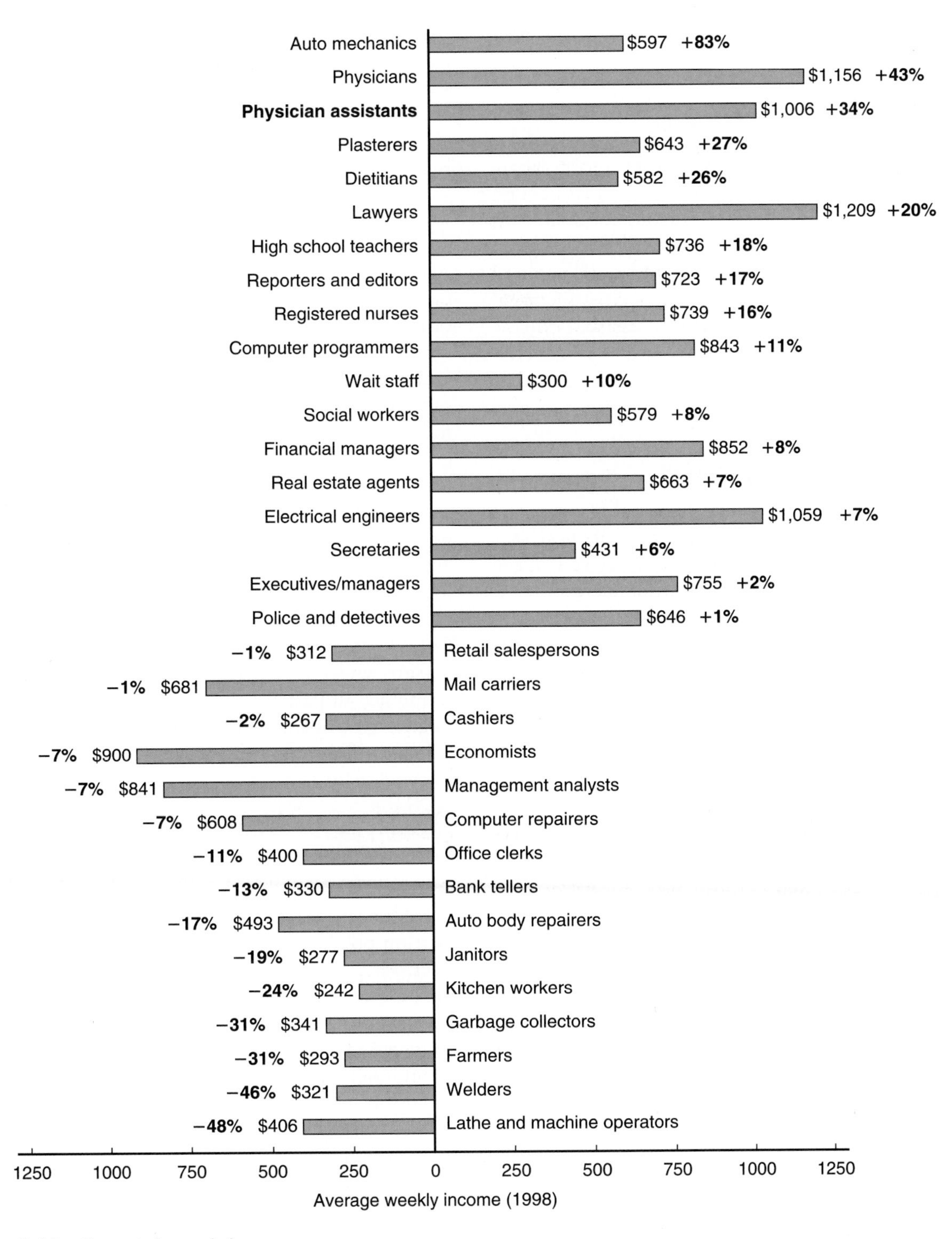

EXHIBIT 3-25 Percentage change in inflation-adjusted income, 1983-1998. (Data from Bureau of Labor Statistics, Washington, DC, 2000.)

the health beliefs and behaviors of PAs that have been reported over the last decade.

Physician-Assisted Suicide

Assisted suicide continues to be a topic of debate among health care professionals, and PAs are no exception. In a Michigan survey conducted in 1994, 48% of responding PAs tended to support provider-assisted suicide and 40% were opposed (Hayden et al., 1995). One state's cross-sectional survey, a state where physician-assisted suicide has been very controversial, cannot be generalized to PAs at large and it cannot suggest that these attitudes are static.

Hepatitis B Immunization

Recommendations by authorities seem to be important motivators for PA and medical students equally. At the University of Iowa College of Medicine, PA and medical students responded to recommendations to receive the hepatitis B immunization series at a higher rate than residents and staff physicians (Diekema, Ferguson, and Doebbeling, 1995).

Chemical Dependency

Impaired providers pose challenges to state medical boards that have the charge to protect their constituents' health and exposure to unhealthy conditions, as well as to the professional organizations that seek to protect their legal rights. Most PAs in one study were either nondrinkers or ex-drinkers. A majority of PAs (87%) reported that they rarely or never relied on drugs or medication to affect mood or to relax. Most respondents in this study reported either occasional physical activity (47%) or regular physical activity at least three times a week (47%). It found that PAs tended to be oriented more strongly toward general health matters and prevention than toward illness or sick role-related beliefs (Glazer-Waldman, 1989).

Risks for HIV/AIDS

A 1991 national survey of PAs reported that 60% thought that treating patients with human immunodeficiency virus (HIV) placed them at risk for acquired immune deficiency syndrome (AIDS). About one third thought that health care workers had a right to refuse care to patients with AIDS. However, more than 80% indicated they were willing to provide health care to patients with HIV and those considered to be in high-risk groups (Currey, 1992).

Thanatophobia

In caring for the terminally ill, a PA student's fear of death or dying (thanatophobia) may affect his or her ability to be an effective clinician and may influence his or her role as a patient advocate and educator. To assess the level and prediction of thanatophobia of PA students to that of medical students, an 80-item survey of both student groups was undertaken. Generally speaking, senior PA students scored significantly lower than senior medical students in thanatophobia, as well as in authoritarianism, machiavellianism, and depressed mood. For both student groups intolerance to clinical uncertainty was a predictor of thanatophobia. PAs might be more comfortable than doctors in treating terminally ill persons and may be better suited to caring for terminally ill patients, particularly in areas such as geriatrics, hospice, and primary care in general (Chaikin, Thornby, and Merrill, 2000).

Physician Assistant Participation in Execution

Of the 37 states with the death penalty, most use lethal injection. In 2000 the AAPA refined an existing policy on executions in its code of conduct. Although PAs can certify death (after the prisoner is officially pronounced dead), witness an execution, and relieve the acute suffering of a condemned person before the execution, they should not participate in a legally authorized execution. As a policy of statement there are no formal consequences (Knopper, 2000).

Nutrition

In a mailed survey the nutrition knowledge and attitudes of PAs in Texas were examined. The 764 PAs (54.2%) who completed the questionnaire had a mean knowledge score of 70%. Knowledge scores were significantly related to level of education, but not to other demographic and practice variables. Most of the PA respondents supported the importance of nutrition in their clinical practices, although many PAs indicated that they were not satisfied with the amount of nutrition education in their PA programs and felt that PA programs should place a greater emphasis on nutrition education (Demory-Luce and McPherson, 1999).

Patient Education

What primary care PAs and primary care physicians do in the outpatient setting has been a focus of some research. The overlap seems to be large. In other words what a PA does is largely similar to what a physician does in the same setting. One of the claims that PAs and NPs make is that they bring patient education to the medical office as an attribute of their training. The information to substantiate this is somewhat limited. Coulter, Jacobson, and Parker (2000) identified that in a series of HMOs' staff PAs and NPs who were interviewed stated they were more interested in preventive care than physicians. Harbert's work (1993) using a national survey of PAs in primary care suggests this may indeed be the case. Clearly more work is needed in this area.

Complementary and Alternative Medicine

The use of complementary and alternative medicine (CAM) is growing in the United States. Patients and their health care providers are increasingly accepting of CAM therapies (Jarski, 2001). A random sample of 250 PAs who were extensively surveyed found a high relationship between knowledge level of CAM and recommendations for CAM, although most believed that many CAM therapies exert a placebo effect (Houston et al., 2001) (Exhibits 3-26 and 3-27). PAs also have been shown to be more likely to incorporate clinical preventive services as advocated by the U.S. Prevention Services Task Force. PA practice is strongly preventive in orientation.

EXHIBIT 3-26

Respondents' Perceptions of CAM Modalities*

Categories of rating (modalities rated)	No. of respondents (%) (N = 245)
Highest rated that respondents perceived to exhibit conclusive evidence of effectiveness	
Multivitamins	50 (20)
Biofeedback	39 (16)
Antioxidants	37 (15)
Meditation	35 (14)
Chiropractic	35 (14)
Pastoral and spiritual counseling	33 (14)
Highest rated that respondents perceived to exhibit a preponderance of evidence of effectiveness	
Meditation	84 (34)
Biofeedback	77 (31)
Antioxidants	61 (25)
Pastoral and spiritual counseling	58 (24)
Massage	57 (23)
Multivitamins	52 (21)
Chiropractic	52 (21)
Highest rated that respondents perceived to exhibit growing evidence of effectiveness	
Massage	117 (48)
Saint John's wort	107 (44)
Garlic	103 (42)
Gingko	100 (41)
Meditation	100 (41)
Acupuncture	98 (40)
Acupressure	96 (39)
Highest rated that respondents perceived to exhibit no evidence of effectiveness	
Body-cleansing diets	118 (48)
Macrobiotic diets	92 (38)
Aromatherapy	87 (36)
Ergogenic aids	85 (35)
Organic food diets	84 (34)
Magnet therapy	81 (33)
Amino acids	72 (29)
Chelation therapy	72 (29)
Highest rated that respondents perceived as unfamiliar	
Rolfing	148 (60)
Guided imagery	130 (53)
Coenzyme Q10	125 (51)
Reflexology	117 (48)
Chelation therapy	115 (47)
Art therapy	109 (45)
Macrobiotic diets	106 (43)

*Only the most commonly mentioned modalities in each rating category are reported here.

SOCIAL STATUS OF PHYSICIAN ASSISTANTS

Social class or status is one of the most important variables in social research. The socioeconomic position of a person affects his or her chances for education, income, occupation, marriage, health, friends, and even life expectancy. This variable, however, has proved difficult to

EXHIBIT 3-27

Ten Most Common CAM Modalities Used by PAs

Modality	No. of respondents (%) (N = 245)
Multivitamins	68 (28)
Antioxidants	54 (22)
Massage	48 (20)
Meditation	47 (19)
Pastoral and spiritual counseling	21 (9)
Aromatherapy	19 (8)
Acupuncture	18 (7)
Organic food diets	19 (8)
Acupuncture	15 (6)
Chiropractic	15 (6)

measure in a pluralistic, egalitarian, and fluid society such as exists in the United States. Nevertheless, many researchers have tried to identify the social strata and to measure variables associated with them. Occupation has been shown to be the best single predictor of social status, and overall occupational prestige ratings have been found to be highly stable. A number of factors act in close relationship between occupation and social status. Both individual income and educational attainment correlate with occupational rank. Education is a basis for entry into many occupations, and for most persons, income is derived from occupation. House type and dwelling area constitute other highly correlated factors (Miller, 1991).

Several scales are available to determine social status, and each has its proponents and detractors. They vary in length and number of factors included in the scale. The standard Duncan Socioeconomic Index (SEI) is the most widely used and is generally considered to be superior for most survey and large-sample situations. It takes into account income, education, and occupational prestige. Another is the Siegel Prestige Score, based on subjective rankings to establish the standing of respondents in a wide variety of occupations and represents an effort to secure a "pure" prestige rating.

A third scale is the Nam-Powers, which is based on the 1970 U.S. census. It has been used as a socioeconomic status score for most occupations. Scores are based on average levels of education and income for U.S. workers in 1970. Researchers have the option of choosing the Nam-Powers socioeconomic scores if they wish to employ a measurement without prestige weights. A correlation of 0.97 is reported between the Duncan SEI and Nam-Powers socioeconomic status scores.

In Exhibit 3-28 the three social status scores are shown for the medical occupational group developed for the 1980 census. The Duncan and Nam-Powers SEI scores can take values approximately between 0 and 100 on both indexes, but because they are constructed somewhat differently, it is not appropriate to make direct comparisons. The Siegel Prestige Scores have a much smaller range, with bootblacks at the lowest (09.3) and college/university teachers at the highest (78.3).

Little is known about the social or occupational standing of PAs. The Census Bureau only started listing PAs as an occupation in 1980 as *health practitioner n.e.c.* (not elsewhere classified) but gave it a score of 96.

Of the occupations listed in Exhibit 3-28, PAs rank behind physicians, the same as marine scientists, and ahead of pharmacists, university professors, and economists.

To date, neither the Duncan SEI nor the Siegel Prestige Scores have rated PAs or NPs, although they may be considered "kindred workers" from a sociologic viewpoint. With increased examination of the profession, we expect that social scientists will modify these occupational classifications for PAs to be consistent with increased understanding of their income, status, mobility, and prestige of PAs across the spectrum of social situations.

Physician Assistants as Professionals?

PAs are individuals who practice medicine, a role traditionally considered to be among the professions, yet lacking in key attributes classically considered necessary to be regarded as a true profession. There is a tendency for newly emerging occupations to aspire to professional status in part as a means to enhance prestige and societal position. Particularly in the modern U.S. health care sector, holding the label "professional" conveys to society and other health care providers the connotation of a higher position on the ladder of occupational stratification.

Physician assistants represent a health occupation founded by medicine. PA organizations, and PAs often refer to themselves as "professional" and generally assume that PAs function in

EXHIBIT 3-28

Occupational Classification System of Three Social Status Scores for Health Care Workers, 1980

Code	Occupation	1970 Duncan SEI score	1970 Siegel Prestige score	1980 Nam-Powers (U.S. census score)
Health professional, technical, and kindred workers				
061	Chiropractors	75.0	60.0	96
062	Dentists	96.0	73.6	100
063	Optometrists	79.0	62.0	99
064	Pharmacists	81.3	60.3	95
065	Physicians (MD, DO)	92.1	81.2	100
071	Podiatrists	58.0	36.7	99
072	Veterinarians	78.0	59.7	99
073	**Physician assistants**	—	—	96
073	Nurse practitioners	—	—	96
074	Dieticians	39.0	52.1	64
075	Registered nurses	44.3	60.1	73
076	Therapists (PT, OT)	59.9	40.5	73
	Other	—	—	—
086	Clergy	52.0	69.0	70
052	Marine scientists			96
091	Economists	74.4	53.6	95
100	Social workers	64.0	52.4	75
104	Biology teachers	84.0	78.3	85
113	Health specialties teachers	84.0	78.3	85
124	Coaches, physical education teachers	64.0	53.2	74
140	College/university teachers	84.0	78.3	91
161	Surveyors	48.4	53.1	64
163	Airline pilots	79.0	70.1	93
175	Actors	60.0	55.0	76
211	Funeral directors	59.0	52.2	81
265	Insurance agents, brokers, underwriters	66.0	46.8	81
364	Receptionists	44.0	37.1	38
461	Machinists	32.9	47.7	57
802	Farm managers	36.0	43.7	54
941	Bootblack	8.0	9.3	2
964	Police officers and detectives	40.5	47.7	79

Modified from Miller DC: *Handbook of Research Design and Social Measurement,* ed. 15, Newbury Park, Calif., 1991, Sage Publications.

practice "as professionals." The question is whether or not the American PA is a true professional. Is the American PA claim to be among the ranks of other health providers recognized as professionals valid, or does the dependent nature of PA practice and the lack of a unique body of knowledge consign them to a lower rung in the health occupations pecking order? PAs represent a unique case study among the health occupations by virtue of their level of clinical responsibilities. Can PAs be legitimately classified as "professionals" in the delivery of health care, or are they, as some would assert, simply vassals of more powerful health care elite, producing wealth for their employers but not owning or controlling the means of production?

SUMMARY

Data on PAs indicate that they are improving the specialty and geographic maldistribution of the medical workforce in the United States. PAs are more likely to be working in primary care fields and in smaller communities and augment areas of medical need working with physicians. The potential for making major contributions in this area is increasing.

The average age of the employed PA is 40 years and the length of employment is approximately 9 years. The age of PA students is decreasing, now at 28 years of age. One of the problems with the work-related rewards received by PAs appears to be that they will reach an early peak in the first several years after entry into the profession and then plateau. This may be a problem for individuals who enter the PA profession early in their career who have higher career aspirations. An older individual who has been employed for some time and then makes a career move to become a PA may see this as a major career advancement.

4

PHYSICIAN ASSISTANT EDUCATION

INTRODUCTION

Physician assistant (PA) educational programs were created in the late 1960s, primarily in academic institutions preparing traditional health care professionals. The curricula of these programs were based on new concepts to prepare health care providers and represented a hybridization of existing medical and nursing educational models. In the intervening four decades PA educational programs have become well established in academic health centers and other institutions of higher education in the United States.

In their development and evolution, PA programs have helped influence concepts and trends in health professions education and have pioneered methodologies in decentralized clinical education, multidisciplinary approaches, and curriculum innovation. As PA programs have evolved, they have maintained a socially responsive tradition. Graduates of PA programs have entered practices in medically needy and rural communities to a greater degree than medical school graduates. PA educational programs have developed a reputation of providing a practically focused and multidisciplinary approach to health professions education. These programs represent innovations in medical generalist and primary care preparation, and PA education has earned a distinct identity within medical education (Carter, Emelio, and Perry, 1984; Fasser, 1987; Schafft and Cawley, 1987; Lipsky, 2001).

As of 2002 there were 132 accredited educational programs for PAs in the United States (Exhibit 4-1). These programs exist in 42 states and the District of Columbia. There is a mean of three programs per state with a range of 1 to 19. Of these programs all but two prepare PAs for roles as primary care providers; two programs prepare surgeon's assistants. Since 2001 more than 51,000 individuals have completed PA educational programs, with 83% in active clinical practice (AAPA, 2001). The United States is not alone, and PA programs exist for the Canadian military, located in Borden, Ontario, as well as in the Netherlands.

Universities, academic health centers, schools of medicine (both allopathic and osteopathic), health-related professions, and 4-year colleges sponsor PA educational programs; 50 are sponsored by academic health centers. The remainder are sponsored by college teaching hospitals, community colleges, and the U.S. military (see Appendix 5).

Accreditation

The Accreditation Review Commission on Education for the Physician Assistant (ARC-PA) defines the formal standards for PA educational programs. *The Accreditation Standards for Physician Assistant Eduction* sets the bar for PA program accreditation. The ARC had its roots in 1971 when the American Medical Association (AMA) began accrediting PA programs. The ARC became an independent accrediting body in 2000. The Board of Directors is comprised of representatives from the American Academy of Family Physicians, the American Academy of Physician Assistants (AAPA), the American College of Physicians/American Society of Internal Medicine, the American College of Surgeons, the AMA, and the Association of Physician Assistant Programs (APAP). The ARC-PA appoints site visitors, reviews applications for accreditation, and determines accreditation status (McCarty, Stuetzer, and Somers, 2001). Before 1994, PA accreditation was conducted by the ARC-PA of the Committee on Allied Health Education and Accreditation (CAHEA), a national allied health accrediting entity affiliated with the AMA. CAHEA was charged to create the Accreditation Standards for Physician Assistant Eduction, or the Standards. However, in 1994 the AMA separated from the CAHEA, and it became an independent agency, known as the Commission on Accreditation of Allied Health Education Programs (CAAHEP). There now have been five revisions of the original (1971) Standards document (1978, 1985, 1990, 1997, and 2000). Past versions of the Standards have set the tone for all aspects of PA program operation including curriculum design and content. The Standards have promoted PA program curriculum creativity and innovation, particularly in institutions that have relied on traditional modes of medical education. In the Standards, all key aspects of program operation are addressed: administration and sponsorship, personnel, financial resources, operation, curriculum, evaluation, fair practices, laboratory and library facilities, clinical affiliations, faculty qualifications, admissions processes, publications, and record keeping. Programs must demonstrate an ongoing self-study process and must undergo an onsite evaluation before the request for accreditation is approved.

Accredited PA programs are subject to periodic reviews and onsite evaluations are required for maintenance of accreditation. The ARC-PA meets semiannually to consider applications for provisional and continuing accreditation. Institutions considering accreditation for a proposed or existing program use specific guidelines in conducting a comprehensive self-analysis.

ARC accreditation is a voluntary determination; nearly all PA programs participate in the

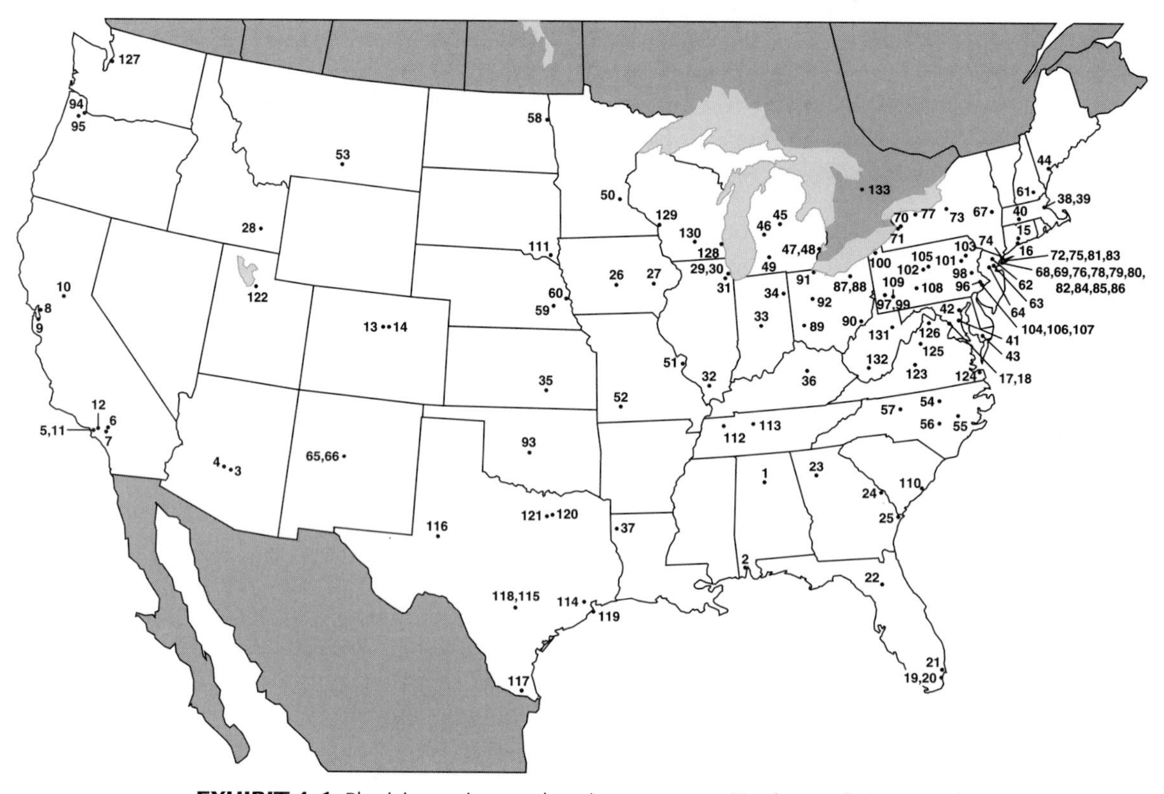

EXHIBIT 4-1 Physician assistant education programs. (See key on facing page.)

1. University of Alabama at Birmingham, Birmingham, AL
2. University of South Alabama, Mobile, AL
3. Arizona School of Health Sciences, Mesa, AZ
4. Midwestern University Glendale, Glendale, AZ
5. Charles Drew University of Medicine and Science, Los Angeles, CA
6. Loma Linda University, Loma Linda, CA
7. Riverside Community College, Moreno Valley, CA
8. Samuel Merritt College, Oakland, CA
9. Stanford University, Palo Alto, CA
10. University of California Davis, Sacramento, CA
11. University of Southern California, Los Angeles, CA
12. Western University of Health Sciences, Pomona, CA
13. Red Rocks Community College, Lakewood, CO
14. University of Colorado Health Science Center, Denver, CO
15. Quinnipiac University, Hamden, CT
16. Yale University, New Haven, CT
17. George Washington University, Washington, DC
18. Howard University, Washington, DC
19. Barry University, Miami, FL
20. Miami-Dade Community College, Miami, FL
21. Nova Southeastern University, Davie, FL
22. University of Florida, Gainesville, FL
23. Emory University, Atlanta, GA
24. Medical College of Georgia, Augusta, GA
25. South University, Savannah, GA
26. Des Moines University Osteopathic Medical Ctr., Des Moines, IA
27. University of Iowa, Iowa City, IA
28. Idaho State University, Pocatello, ID
29. Cook County Hospital/Malcolm X College, Chicago, IL
30. Finch University of Health Sciences/Chicago Medical School, North Chicago, IL
31. Midwestern University PA Program, Downers Grove, IL
32. Southern Illinois University at Carbondale, Carbondale, IL
33. Butler University/Clarian Health, Indianapolis, IN
34. University of Saint Francis, Fort Wayne, IN
35. Wichita State University, Wichita, KS
36. University of Kentucky, Lexington, KY
37. LSU Health Sciences Center, Shreveport, LA
38. Massachusetts College of Pharmacy, Boston, MA
39. Northeastern University PA Program, Boston, MA
40. Springfield College/Baystate Health System, Springfield, MA
41. Anne Arundel Community College, Arnold, MD
42. Community College of Baltimore–Essex, Baltimore, MD
43. University of MD–Eastern Shore, Princess Anne, MD
44. University of New England, Portland, ME
45. Central Michigan University, Mt. Pleasant, MI
46. Grand Valley State University, Grand Rapids, MI
47. University of Detroit Mercy, Detroit, MI
48. Wayne State University, Detroit, MI
49. Western Michigan University, Kalamazoo, MI
50. Augsburg College, Minneapolis, MN
51. Saint Louis University, Saint Louis, MO
52. Southwest Missouri State University, Springfield, MO
53. Rocky Mountain College, Billings, MT
54. Duke University Medical Center, Durham, NC
55. East Carolina University, Greenville, NC
56. Methodist College, Fayetteville, NC
57. Wake Forest University, Winston Salem, NC
58. University of North Dakota, Grand Forks, ND
59. Union College, Lincoln, NE
60. University of Nebraska Medical Center, Omaha, NE
61. Notre Dame College, Manchester, NH
62. Seton Hall University, South Orange, NJ
63. UMDNJ–Newark, Newark, NJ
64. UMDNJ and Rutgers University, Piscataway, NJ
65. University of New Mexico PA Program, Albuquerque, NM
66. University of Saint Francis, Albuquerque, NM
67. University at Albany—Hudson Valley, Albany, NY
68. Bronx Lebanon Hospital Center, Bronx, NY
69. Brooklyn Hospital/Long Island University, Brooklyn, NY
70. Daemen College, Amherst, NY
71. D'Youville College, Buffalo, NY
72. Hofstra University, Hempstead, NY
73. Le Moyne College, Syracuse, NY
74. Mercy College, Dobbs Ferry, NY
75. New York Institute of Technology, Old Westbury, NY
76. PACE University/Lenox Hill Hospital, New York, NY
77. Rochester Institute of Technology, Rochester, NY
78. Sophie Davis School of Biomedical Education, New York, NY
79. St. Vincent Catholic Medical Centers of New York, Fresh Meadows, NY
80. St. Vincent Catholic Medical Centers of New York, Staten Island, NY
81. State University of New York At Stony Brook, Stony Brook, NY
82. SUNY Downstate Medical Center, Brooklyn, NY
83. Touro College, Bay Shore, NY
84. Touro College Manhattan, New York, NY
85. Wagner College/SIU Hospital PA Program, Staten Island, NY
86. Weill Cornell University Medical College, New York, NY
87. Cuyahoga Community College, Parma, OH
88. Cuyahoga Community College, Parma, OH
89. Kettering College of Medical Arts, Kettering, OH
90. Marietta College, Marietta, OH
91. Medical College of Ohio, Toledo, OH
92. The University of Findlay, Findlay, OH
93. University of Oklahoma, Oklahoma City, OK
94. Oregon Health and Science University, Portland, OR
95. Pacific University, Forest Grove, OR
96. Arcadia University, Glenside, PA
97. Chatham College, Pittsburgh, PA
98. DeSales University, Center Valley, PA
99. Duquesne University PA Program, Pittsburgh, PA
100. Gannon University, Erie, PA
101. King's College, Wilkes Barre, PA
102. Lock Haven University of Pennsylvania, Lock Haven, PA
103. Marywood University, Scranton, PA
104. MCP Hahnemann University, Philadelphia, PA
105. Penn College of Technology, Williamsport, PA
106. Philadelphia College of Osteopathic Medicine, Philadelphia, PA
107. Philadelphia University, Philadelphia, PA
108. Saint Francis University, Loretto, PA
109. Seton Hill College, Greensburg, PA
110. Medical University of South Carolina, Charleston, SC
111. University of South Dakota, Vermillion, SD
112. Bethel College, McKenzie, TN
113. Trevecca Nazarene University, Nashville, TN
114. Baylor College of Medicine, Houston, TX
115. Interservice PA Program, Ft. Sam Houston, TX
116. Texas Tech University Health Science Center, Midland, TX
117. University of Texas Pan American PA Studies Program, Edinburg, TX
118. University of Texas Health Science Center at San Antonio, San Antonio, TX
119. University of Texas Medical Branch–Galveston, Galveston, TX
120. University of Texas/SW Medical Center, Dallas, TX
121. UNT Health Science Center, Fort Worth, TX
122. University of Utah, Salt Lake City, UT
123. College of Health Sciences, Roanoke, VA
124. Eastern Virginia Medical School, Norfolk, VA
125. James Madison University, Harrisonburg, VA
126. Shenandoah University, Winchester, VA
127. University of Washington (MEDEX), Seattle, WA
128. Marquette University, Milwaukee, WI
129. University of Wisconsin–LaCrosse Gundersen-Mayo PA Program, La Crosse, WI
130. University of Wisconsin–Madison, Madison, WI
131. Alderson-Broaddus College, Philippi, WV
132. Mountain State University, Beckley, WV
133. Canadian Forces, Borden, ON, Canada

accreditation process. Lacking ARC-PA accreditation makes one ineligible for federal grants, and their graduates may risk ineligibility for national certification or state licensure.

The Standards state the traditional philosophy of PA education while recognizing advances in medical practice.

> While the opportunity for creativity and innovation in program design remains, the Standards reflect the realization that a commonality in the core curriculum of programs has become not only desirable, but also necessary in order to offer curricula of sufficient depth and breadth to prepare PA graduates for practice in dynamic and competitive health care arena.

Historical Roots of PA Education

The creation of the PA and other types of new health care practitioners, as well as the expansion of undergraduate medical education, was a health care workforce policy approach that significantly affected medical care delivery and education during the 1970s. This policy, developed by both organized medicine and the federal government, was aimed toward the broad goals of increasing access to health care, containing costs, and improving the delivery of primary care.

The rationale for the creation of the PA profession was based on the need for a new type of health care provider who would

- Compensate for the demise of the general practitioner by augmenting physician capabilities to deliver medical care services and help alleviate the perceived shortage of primary care physicians
- Address health care access problems stemming from the geographic and specialty maldistribution of physicians
- Provide an educational means by which existing health care personnel with broad experiences could be channeled into advanced clinical roles
- Be a positive factor in helping to control health care costs and improve primary care access (Perry, 1980; Carter, Emelio, and Perry, 1984; Cawley, 1994)

Essential to the introduction of the PA was the support of the medical profession and the federal government, both who collaborated in promoting PAs. The medical profession encouraged legal efforts in recognition of PA practice, and the government granted financial support for the development of PA educational programs.

Eugene Stead and Richard Smith are generally credited as the visionaries of the PA concept in the United States. The first educational program was developed at Duke University by Stead and colleagues, soon followed by the Medex program at the University of Washington and the University of Colorado child health associate program. The Duke PA curricula comprised a 20-month, competency-based generalist program that aimed to prepare clinicians who would perform a wide range of medical diagnostic and patient management tasks previously legally done only by physicians. Duke PAs were intended to be assistants to physicians in all types and manner of practice settings and clinical specialties. The curricula built on the prior clinical experiences of medical corpsmen. The Duke curriculum not only drew its educational resources from the multiple academic and clinical departments within that particular institution but also was linked to medical practices in surrounding North Carolina communities. The initial Duke program provided 7 months of classroom instruction covering the basic and clinical medical sciences, followed by 13 months of rotating clinical clerkships, culminating in a 2-month primary care, office-based preceptorship. When its first graduates entered practice the Duke PA program received a great deal of attention in both lay and medical circles. It established a model for curriculum of many PA programs that followed.

Other PA educational programs that emerged during this time pioneered innovative approaches in health practitioner education and provided a variety of effective models in PA education. PA curricula resemble a shorter version of the structure of physician education in the generalist care specialties; maintain a competency-based approach; and draws from the biomedical, human behavioral, psychosocial, and preventive care paradigms.

Richard Smith at the University of Washington pioneered the Medex model of PA education in 1969. Individuals with extensive prior health care experience were admitted to this program who were often already matched to a physician preceptor. These physicians were often prospective employers (Smith, 1974). Medex PA students received 6 to 9 months of intensive didactic medical course work and were then assigned to serve a 12- to 15-month community-based preceptorship with a generalist physician.

Henry Silver at the University of Colorado developed the first medical specialty PA educational program in 1966. The child health associate program comprised a 3-year course of study set in a medical school that enrolled individuals with a nursing credential and prior pediatric experience (Silver, 1973b).

Another PA educational model was developed at Alderson-Broaddus College in 1969, where a PA curriculum was designed within a 4-year liberal arts college (Ippolito, 2000); this so-called 2 + 2 approach offers a curriculum that is divided into two phases. The preprofessional phase consists of courses typically taken in the first 2 years of college (e.g., liberal arts and general science courses). This is followed by a professional phase in which the final 2 years of instruction are identical in content to the aforementioned types of PA programs (Meyers, 1978).

PA educational programs tend to emphasize outpatient more than inpatient skills. For physicians most medical education takes place in the university hospital on a very select group of patients: those who have filtered through the system to what is usually a tertiary care center. In contrast, most PA education focuses on primary care and training in ambulatory care settings.

Physician Assistant Curriculum

The philosophy of PA programs is one of a broad-based approach to primary care health professions education. This focus has resulted in curricula that give PA students a strong foundation in primary care and general medicine while preparing them to enter a wide range of specialized clinical areas as well.

The format of the typical PA program is an intensive 26-month (range, 12 to 36 months) medically oriented curriculum that educates the student in primary care. Roughly 12 months are devoted to didactic instruction in the basic and clinical sciences, followed by a similar period of rotating clerkships and preceptorship in all major clinical disciplines. Didactic courses include anatomy, physiology, microbiology, biochemistry, pathology, pharmacology, and the behavioral sciences. Instruction is also provided in the clinical sciences with course work in history taking, physical examination, pathophysiology, clinical diagnosis, communication and interpersonal skills, epidemiology and preventive medicine, clinical procedures and surgical skills, and interpretation of laboratory test results and imaging studies. Courses in the basic medical sciences constitute a majority of the total didactic portion of PA curricula. Instruction devoted to the behavioral and social sciences averages more than 124 contact hours per program. The range of subjects includes health behavior, interpersonal communication skills, psychosocial dynamics, health promotion and disease prevention, bioethics, medical sociology, death and dying, and cross-cultural medicine (Exhibit 4-2).

During their second year, PA students obtain clinical training while serving on rotations, typically 4 to 8 weeks long, conducted over a wide range of inpatient and outpatient care settings. Most PA programs require students to complete rotations in core medical, pediatric, surgical, and primary care clinical disciplines. PA clinical education typically includes experiences in inpatient medicine, primary care and ambulatory medicine, surgery, pediatrics, obstetrics and gynecology, emergency medicine, and psychiatry. Clinical experiences also include elective rotations and a final preceptorship in a primary care practice setting. In serving on these clinical rotations and preceptorships, PA students are given instruction by practicing physicians, physician residents and house officers, graduate PAs, and various other health care professionals.

Innovations in Primary Care Education

The curricula of early PA programs were strongly influenced by the expectations of the founders who envisioned PAs serving as primary care and general medical providers. In many instances the specific curricular objectives of educational programs were based on addressing those clinical problems most often encountered in primary care practice. This approach differed in emphasis from traditional medical education, which often was esoteric in content. PA educators were able to develop methods of curriculum design. Federal grant funding supporting of these new curricula allowed PA educators to identify clinical and basic science faculty whose teaching focus complied with program objectives.

EXHIBIT 4-2

A Template PA Program Curriculum

Year 1 Didactic Instruction (Courses)

Basic Sciences

Anatomy
Physiology
Biochemistry
Medical Microbiology/Immunology
Pathology
Pharmacology

Clinical Sciences

Clinical Assessment (Physical Diagnosis)
Behavioral Science/Human Behavior
Clinical Medicine

Cardiology	Rheumatology	Nephrology	Hematology
Pulmonary Medicine	Dermatology	Neurology	Oncology
Gastroenterology	Allergic Disease Endocrine		
Infectious Disease	Geriatrics	Toxicology	

Pediatrics
Clinical Decision Making
Medical Genetics
Clinical Laboratory Sciences
Surgery

Otolaryngology	Urology	Vascular	Neurologic
Ophthalmology	Orthopedic	Thoracic	Trauma

Radiology/Imaging Science
Research Methods/Interpretation of the Literature
Epidemiology and Medical Statistics
Preventive Medicine and Public Health
Role of the Physician Assistant/Health Systems and Economics

Year 2 Clinical Instruction

Clinical Rotations

Family Medicine
Internal Medicine
Surgery
Pediatrics
Obstetrics and Gynecology
Emergency Medicine
Psychiatry
Medical/Surgical Subspecialties (as electives)

Preceptorship

Primary Care
Specialty Field

Curricular innovations in health professions education that have focused on the clinical preparation of providers for primary care roles originated within now prominent PA programs. PA programs using decentralized training approaches, such as those seen at the University of Washington Medex Northwest PA Program, the Stanford University Primary Care Associate Program, the University of California, Davis, and the University of Utah PA program, have paved the way for other programs in their efforts to develop effective methods in placing PA graduates in medically underserved areas.

PA programs remain sensitive to changes in the health care environment, and program curriculum undergoes regular review and modification. Experience indicates that this flexibility results in newly employed PAs who adapt more easily to many practice settings. A graduate-level educational track that aims to prepare PAs for practice in rural health care, such as the one sponsored by the Alderson-Broaddus College PA program in Philippi, West Virginia, and other rural health curricula at the University of Texas Pan-American and the Lock Haven University PA program are innovative curricula that prepare primary health care providers targeted for practices in areas with underserved populations.

Other examples of innovations of PA programs in health professions education have been the long-standing inclusion of topics such as health education, epidemiology, preventive medicine, communication skills, and biomedical ethics. These subjects have only relatively recently been regarded as important in undergraduate medical education. Areas essential to the preparation of competent primary care providers, PA programs commonly include instruction on preventive medicine, substance abuse prevention and treatment, health care for the homeless, women's health care, geriatric medicine, environmental and occupational medicine, mental health, and a practical orientation to developing skills in the delivery of clinical preventive services.

In the early 1990s a number of new models of PA education developed. These programs combined PA education with a related graduate degree program, such as the PA/master of public health program at the George Washington University, and others offered distance education master's degree programs aimed at practicing PAs.

Physician Assistant Program Support

Federal support for PA education first began in 1972 and since then has totaled more than $160 million (Exhibit 4-3). Title VII funding in the amount of $6.5 million was available for PA educational program support in fiscal year 2002. Congressional appropriation of PA educational programs through Title VII has promoted the desired boost in PA graduate output into primary care areas. Increased federal funding has supported the expansion of enrollment within existing PA programs and has provided start-up funding for more universities, academic health centers, and colleges seeking to establish new PA programs.

If there are to be increases in the enrollment capacities of PA educational programs, many programs will need to make dramatic changes. These include increasing efforts in the recruitment of new faculty members, strengthening minority recruitment and retention, and adding new clinical training sites and practice affiliations.

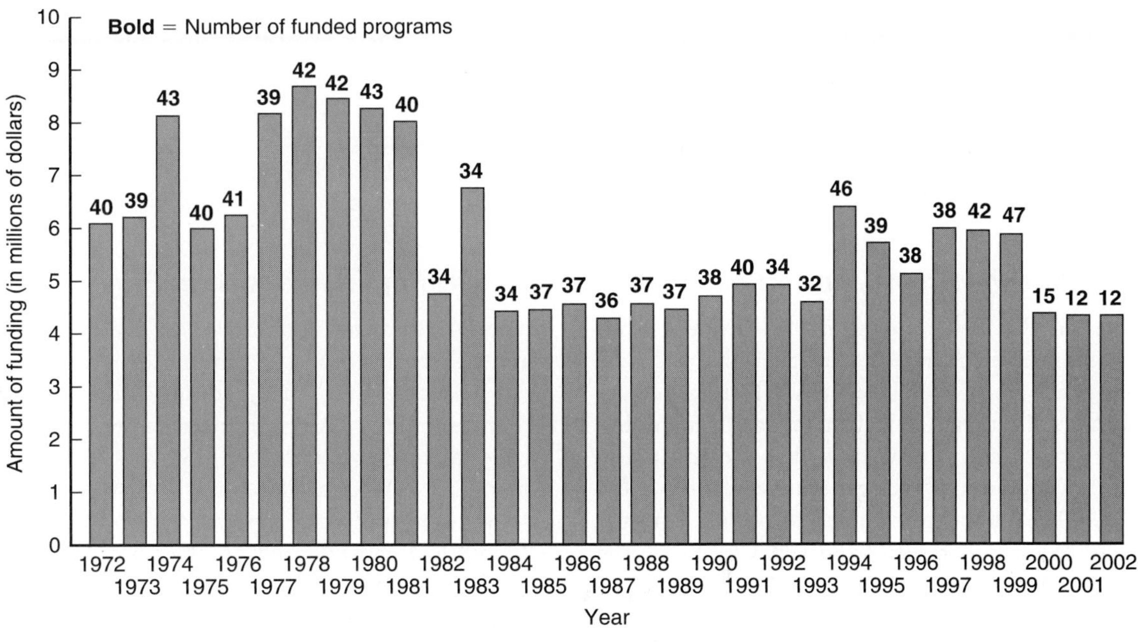

EXHIBIT 4-3 Title VII funding.

All of these efforts, linked to expanded enrollments, are dependent on increased financial support from external sources.

The level of federal support for health professions educational programs is dependent on the uncertain future of congressional appropriations related to Title VII. At times congressional health policy leaders, whose ideological adversaries are often anxious to cut discretionary federal spending categories, have shied away from continuing health professions education program subsidies. A continuing question for the PA profession is the status of the grant award support for PA programs under Title VII of the Public Health Service Act. A long-term workforce policy goal for PA professions education has been to attain Medicare-linked support for graduate clinical PA education, similar to the mechanism established for physician GME.

PHYSICIAN ASSISTANT EDUCATIONAL PROGRAMS

Data gathering on PA educational programs exist for both comparison purposes and for planning. Since 1984 the APAP has published an annual report describing the characteristics of sponsoring institutions, faculty, enrollees, and graduates of PA programs in the United States (Simon, Link, and Miko, 2001). The response rate is typically high (approximately 90%), and the data in any given report are considered an accurate description of PA education during the year the data were collected. Data contained in the APAP annual reports are used to estimate the number of PAs who have graduated and to project the number of PA graduates.

Trends in Physician Assistant Education

The gender distribution of PA students has substantially changed over the past decade. Currently more than 66% of all students are women. This change in gender has been underway since 1984. A recent trend is the admission to PA programs of younger students. From 1995 to 2001, the proportion of students younger than 25 years increased from 19.0% to 24.5%, the proportion of students ages 24 to 29 years increased from 34.0% to 38.4%, and the proportion of students older than 29 years decreased from 47.0% to 37.1%. Graduates of the last decade—predominately women—are increasingly younger than earlier cohorts. This trend will likely continue in the short term (Lillquist et al., 2000).

The average program length has increased from 24 months in 1987 to 26 months in 2002 (range 12-31 months). Didactic curriculum has increased from 1004.5 hours in 1991 to 1154.9 hours in 2000. The increases in didactic curriculum and consequent increase in total program length are more than likely related to the higher degrees granted by contemporary programs. In 1990 only three programs (6% of all programs) awarded a master's degree, which by 2002 had grown to half of all programs.

In 1999 the APAP Degree Task Force surveyed accredited programs to determine how many planned to change the academic degree in the next 5 years (Miller et al., 2001). Of the 96 responding programs, 45 indicated they were planning to change the credential awarded, and of those 45 programs, 62% said they were planning to grant a master's degree. Considering at the time 51% of programs were already awarding a master's degree, it appears that most PA programs will eventually confer a master's degree. Additionally, the APAP Degree Task Force recommended that all programs be required to graduate PAs with a master's degree by 2007. Although the task force did not address the question of enforcement, one could presume the likely mechanism would be through changing the accreditation standards to require programs to award the master's degree. It has become increasingly accepted that the academic recognition for PA education is now beyond the bachelor's degree.

Ranking Physician Assistant Programs

Since PA education has moved to the graduate degree there has been the ranking PA programs, as is the case with the graduate programs in other disciplines. PA programs are now included in the ranking conducted by *U.S. News and World Report* (USN&WR) (available at www.usnews.com/usnews/edu/grad/rankings/rankindex.htm). The USN&WR data are based on the results of surveys sent to deans, faculty, and administrators of accredited graduate programs. Respondents are asked to rate the academic quality of programs as distinguished (5 points); strong (4); good (3); adequate (2); or marginal (1), based on their own assessment of the quality of the curriculum, faculty, and graduates. Each person in the survey is asked to identify 10 schools that offer the best graduate programs in their discipline. The individuals rate the academic quality of programs based on scholarship, curriculum, and the caliber of the faculty and graduates. Scores for each school are averaged across all respondents who rated the schools.

The intent of the USN&WR ranking is to present current information on perceptions of PA programs and aid graduate school applicants in making better-informed decisions when choosing a program. The ranking of PA programs are similar to the rankings of other graduate educational programs in disciplines such as law, engineering, business, and the social sciences. The information is a combination of statistical data and perceptions of reputation. Statistical data reflect the number of students to faculty, Graduate Record Examination (GRE) scores, and other resources used in education. In the fall of 1997 the USN&WR examined 29 PA programs and ranked 16. In the fall of 1999 the USN&WR surveyed 30 master's level PA programs.

Applicants often inquire where a PA program ranks when considering a PA career. Programs typically select the best-qualified applicants based on academic grade point averages, with the expectation that academic success predicts further success. Other programs point out their success in recruiting minorities and placing graduates in federally designated health care professional shortage areas.

Programs committed to recruiting minority and rural-committed applicants argue that they may not be able to compete successfully with high academic achievers, and a ranking system could put them near the bottom of a list, thereby influencing the overall quality of applicants. Those schools affiliated with academic success argue that PA programs have evolved enough that academic scrutiny will allow competition and the quality of all programs will benefit by comparative studies.

Other arguments center on elitism and different mission statements and attempt to emulate medical and osteopathic schools that use such ranking systems. In an attempt to address the controversy of how the USN&WR conducted its survey, Blessing and colleagues (2000) surveyed 100 PA program directors seeking program attributes that should be included (Exhibit 4-4). Of 50 attributes to consider there was consensus on only three:

1. Graduation rate
2. Mean faculty full-time equivalent per student
3. Program rank should *not* be a component for graduation

They concluded that without consensus from PA programs on what to rank, the ranking should be left to disinterested parties, such as USN&WR.

ACADEMIC DEGREES FOR PHYSICIAN ASSISTANT EDUCATION

Traditionally PA education has relied on the philosophy that student performance is based on demonstration of a standard level of clinical competency and has tended to avoid assignment of a specific academic degree for what may be termed *standard* PA educational preparation. The competency-based PA educational philosophy holds that proficiency in the clinical skills identified as being necessary for future competence in primary care or generalist practice should stand as the "gold standard" of PA educational preparation, rather than necessitating adherence to institutional requirements for a specific academic degree. Allowing for variability among PA programs regarding the terminal degree or certificate awarded has proven an effective approach in preparing PA health care professionals to assume a wide range of roles in clinical practice settings and specialties. This approach has also facilitated the recruitment of individuals from diverse ethnic, cultural, and educational backgrounds into PA educational programs and represents those graduates most likely to work in primary care roles in medically needy areas (Leiken, 1985; Keene et al., 2000). The competency-based orientation of PA education has proven effective in preparing health care professionals to qualify for the national certifying examination and to meet state licensing board requirements. The generalist philosophy of PA education produces graduates who have assumed clinical

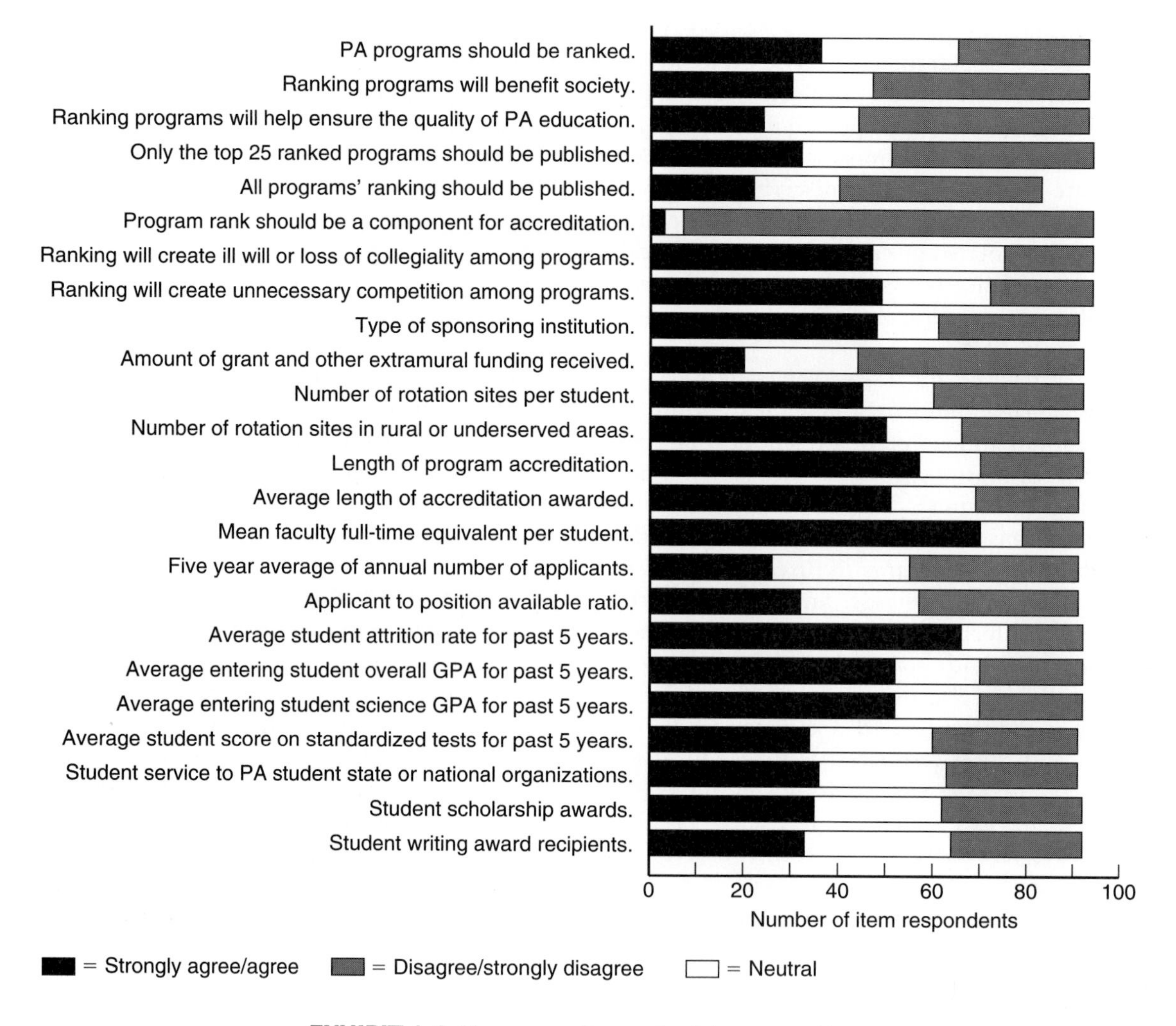

EXHIBIT 4-4 PA program directors' opinions on ranking.

practice roles in a wide range of health care settings and specialties.

Since 1985 a number of PA programs have restructured their curricula for standard PA educational preparation to be on the graduate degree level; now approximately one half of the programs offer a graduate degree (typically programs award the master of physician assistant studies, Master of health science, or master of science [MS] degrees) or another formal master's degree option. Some PA programs continue to award the bachelor's degree but also offer a master's degree option. The master's degree has been contentious, because some educators believe that the bachelor's degree should be the appropriate degree for PAs (Fowkes and Gamel, 2000; Miller et al., 2001).

The counterargument is that the most recent revision of the Standards directly reflects a graduate level of curricular intensity. Institutions that sponsor PA programs should endeavor to incorporate this higher level of academic rigor into their programs and acknowledge it with an appropriate degree. A list of the types of master's degrees is located in Exhibit 4-5.

What is the value of a master's level of education for today's practicing PA? What is the mean cost, the "going rate," for advanced-level health care professions education offered by a major academic health center? Finally, a PA master's degree must be weighed against what a more traditional degree such as a master of public health, MS, or master of business administration may mean in the medical marketplace.

EXHIBIT 4-5

Partial List of Types of Master's Degrees Granted by PA Programs

Degree initials	Description of degree
MA	Master of arts
MS	Master of science
MPH	Master of public health
MPAS	Master of physician assistant studies
MHS	Master of health sciences
MMP	Master's in medical practice
MMSc	Master's in medical science
MSCM	Master of science in clinical medicine
MSPAS	Master of science in physician assistant studies
MPA	Master's, physician assistant
MCMS	Master of clinical medicine science
MSBS	Master of science in basic science
MPAP	Master of physician assistant profession
MPSPAS	Master of professional studies in physician assistant sciences
MMSPAS	Master of medical science physician assistant studies

One argument for a master's degree lies in the philosophy that students will develop the power of critical reasoning, the capacity to generalize, and the ability to find and evaluate clinical information for themselves. The rapid growth of medical knowledge demands that evidence-based medicine is the standard that all care must follow. Using this line of reasoning, one can conclude that PA education is at a higher level than undergraduate, and that recognition as conferred by a master's degree is consistent with the quantity and quality of intellectual work to which students are subjected. The original concept for PA education was a competency-based model, consisting of 2 or 3 years of college work with certain prescribed courses plus vocational training. While this may have been appropriate in the early stages of the PA profession, the notion of competency-based education as measured by a fixed set of guidelines and no academic framework does not fit well with current standards for health care personnel. Additionally, the unique partnerships between PAs and their supervising physicians require complete trust and confidence from the physician that the PA is clinically knowledgeable in the desired areas of the physician's practice.

A tenet of PA education is contained in the Pew Health Professions Commission report, "Care delivery organizations in . . . allied health fields are looking into creating their own educational programs if the schools cannot produce graduates with the proper skills . . . educational institutions must teach skills for the 21st century" (Ballweg et al., 1998).

Growing pressure to control cost and resource use in a responsible manner requires PAs to posses advanced clinical skills and the savvy to work on interdisciplinary teams with their supervising physicians. Simple clinical competence, typically acquired in a competency-based model of undergraduate education, may be insufficient preparation given the increasing demand for cost containment, accountability, and epidemiologic-based care from a culturally competent model.

The Council on Graduate Medical Education (COGME) endorsed educational content that includes "principles of statistics and epidemiology, learning how to search efficiently for 'current best evidence,' knowing the relative value of different types of evidence, and knowing when and how to apply evidence to the care of an individual or patient group" (COGME, 1994). Achieving this degree of knowledge and clinical expertise requires a greater breadth and depth of graduate professional education than competency-based undergraduate models are typically able to accommodate. Standards of medical practice require clinicians to provide quality health care in an environment of increasing accountability.

PHYSICIAN ASSISTANT STUDENTS

Reflecting the marked expansion of PA education that took place during the late 1990s and into the twenty-first century, an estimated 5000 first-year students enrolled in 132 programs in 2002. The average size of the entering PA class in 2001 was 43 students. Historically, demographic patterns observed among PA students show a clear male predominance. However, as a result of a steady increase in the proportion of women in the PA profession since 1985, they now comprise more than half (55%) of all practicing PAs and a majority of PA students.

Among PA students enrolled in 2002, 20% were members of racial and ethnic minorities, 67% were women, and 63% were single. Furthermore 11% had been in military uniform at one time, and 74% possessed at least a bachelor's degree. The mean age of students at the time of enrollment in 2001 was 28.6 years, down from the 35.5-year figure observed in 1992 (Exhibit 4-6). The expansion of ethnic and racial minorities in PA educational programs since 1970 reflects social progress in shaping the health care professions to look more like the population at large. Percentages of minorities enrolled in PA educational programs from 1983 through 2001 averaged 18.3% per enrolled class. Expressed differently, the number of minority students has doubled from a mean of four students per program in 1983 to more than nine per program in 2001 (Simon, Link, and Miko, 2001).

Amid trends for students to come from smaller towns and have more academic preparation, PA student backgrounds are more diverse than ever before. Most students possessed substantial previous health care experience—a mean of 43 months in the class beginning in 2001 (Simon, Link, and Miko, 2001). About 10% of all individuals admitted to PA educational programs held a graduate degree (master's or doctoral degree) in 2001, 18 individuals were unlicensed graduates of international medical schools.

While typical students plan a career in health care during high school, the decision to become a PA is often made later. The majority makes the decision independently, after first ruling out medical school and researching the PA profession. Dissatisfaction with a previous health care career is a moderate motivator. Once potential students learn about the profession, it may take 3 to 4 years before beginning the enrollment process. The lag time from learning about the PA profession to starting the enrollment process results from meeting requirements, applying, being accepted, and finally enrolling. Personal contact with practicing PAs is probably the most effective recruitment tool for the profession. In the late 1980s most high school and college counselors were unaware of the profession (Todd, 2000). Anecdotal reports suggest this trend may have changed. The promulgation of information by various organizations, books on PAs in libraries, and with PAs being featured in the news has allowed the PA to be more prominent in career planning for young persons.

Only two of the accredited PA educational programs, the Howard University PA program and the PA program at the University of

EXHIBIT 4-6

Characteristics of New PA Students by Year

	1995	1997	1998	1999	2000	2001
Average age	30.4	29.7	30.3	29.0	28.6	28.7
Percent women	61	64	63	64	65	67
Percent non-white/caucasian	22	19	17	17	19	20
Married/single/other (%)	43/54/3	39/57/3	38/59/3	37/61/2	35/63/2	36/62/2
Ever in military* (%)	12	11	13	12	11	12
Bachelor's degree or higher (%)	61	70	69	70	73	74
Origins of residence of new PA students						
Inner city	—	16	13	13	15	15
Urban	—	40	34	34	35	35
Suburban	—	61	60	59	62	59
Rural	—	38	40	39	42	42
Indian reservation	—	1	1	1	1	1
Other	—	3	2	2	2	2
Characteristics of new PA students						
Student†		43	41	40	40	40
Knew PA before applying	79	86	87	88	90	90
College grade point average (mean)	3.41	3.47	3.46	3.46	3.44	3.43
Average no. of programs applied to	2.37	2.64	2.60	2.511	2.37	2.37
No. of programs accepted to	1.21	1.27	1.32	1.34	1.42	1.42
Worked in a health care field (%)	—	85	87	86	87	86

From American Academy of Physician Assistants, *Report on the Census Survey of New Students.*
*Active duty, Reserves/National Guard/Veteran.
†Full time and part time.

Maryland, Eastern Shore, are set within a historically and predominantly black college or university. Two other programs (those at Drew University and Harlem Hospital/City University of New York) enroll higher numbers of individuals from racial and ethnic minorities.

Attrition from PA programs is typically low (Simon, 2001). Overall attrition among PA students is disproportionate for racial and ethnic minority individuals (Carter, 2000; Whitman, 2000). The overall attrition rate for PA students was 4.2% in 2000; attrition was 11% for African American PA students, 6% for Hispanic/Latinos, and 6% for other racial and ethnic minorities. The attrition rate for whites and non-Hispanics was 4%. Underrepresented racial and ethnic minority persons, in particular African American women, were more likely than nonminority individuals either to be lost to attrition or to be assigned to decelerated tracks in PA programs (Whitman, 2000).

A consistent trend in PA education is a female preponderance among entering PA classes. The typical PA program received 239 applicants for the class entering the 1999 to 2000 class and 200 for the class of 2000 to 2002. On average, 43 students were accepted per program and 39 students per program were enrolled in the first-year class.

Seventy-six PA programs responded to the question about the pass rate of their graduates on the Physician Assistant National Certification Examination (PANCE) given by the National Commission on Certification of Physician Assistants (NCCPA). The mean pass rate for graduates from the responding programs was 93%. To practice as a PA, candidates are required by all states to be graduates of an accredited program and to have passed the PANCE. Programs reported that most of their recent graduates were employed in the primary care specialties of family medicine and general internal medicine. PAs traditionally have provided medical care to underserved populations, and the survey looked at the number of recent graduates who were working in such settings as rural health clinics, migrant health centers, Indian Health Service sites, and community health centers, among other settings. In 2000 a total of 61 programs reported that more than 30% of their graduates were working in underserved areas (Whitman, 2000).

Becoming a Physician Assistant

There are some data examining why aspirants seek to become PAs. Motivation is the need or desire on a person's part that causes him or her to act. Using anecdotal sources, we have compiled a list of motivators that are thought to influence individuals to apply to PA school (Exhibit 4-7). No one single motivating factor has emerged to explain why people choose a career as a PA. Some faculty believe the prime factor for young women to select a PA education over medical school is that the shortened time to achieve a professional career allows more options for family planning.

EXHIBIT 4-7

Motivations for Applying to PA School

1. Interest in medicine
2. Interest in health care but not in becoming a physician or nurse
3. Interest in helping people, the less fortunate, and contributing to the community
4. Financial reward, steady income, job security
5. Career in respected profession
6. Job satisfaction
7. Constant challenge of job
8. Preparation for medical school too long or too difficult, did not think I would be accepted
9. Personal experience (e.g., health problem in family, friend, or self)
10. Influence of family, friend, or teacher to choose a specific career
11. Draft deferment
12. Faster route to practicing medicine than medical school (shorter schooling and no residency required)
13. Less costly than medical school
14. Easier to get into PA school
15. Career advancement (i.e., I was already in a health-related field)
16. Less responsibility than becoming a physician (less legal risk and malpractice)
17. Lifestyle issues (more time for family and friends, more recreation time, fewer work hours)

Applicants to Physician Assistant Programs

In response to forces in the health care professions marketplace, PA educational programs have seen a dramatic increase in the number of program applicants in the latter part of the 1990s. Since the late 1990s this trend seems to be decreasing (Exhibit 4-8). At one time this surge in application strained the limited resources of many institutions. Because one limiting factor is funding support, and because Title VII grants for PA educational programs have remained essentially level since 1981, resources are stretched to the maximum in many programs. If programs are not funded sufficiently in the future, expansion of PA enrollment may lead to compromise in the quality of educational experiences received by students. For the class that entered in 2001, PA educational programs received more than 12,000 applications. The average of 166 applicants per program was down from the 200 figure in 2000. Thirty-eight students per program were enrolled (Simon, Link, and Miko, 2002).

Although the number of ethnic minority students enrolled in PA programs has averaged 19% since 1985, these individuals compose 10% of the practicing PA population. These figures, plus the fact that only 3.7% of all practicing PAs are African American, suggest that past federal health professions policy and program strategies supporting the recruitment and retention of ethnic minority and disadvantaged students and faculty within PA educational programs have had only partial success in increasing the number of individuals from these groups.

Selection of Physician Assistant Students

Each PA program has developed a unique set of criteria for selecting qualified students. The efficacy of selection measures for predicting successful completion of PA training has been examined. Some of these measures include the Scholastic Aptitude Test (SAT), Minnesota Multiphasic Personality Inventory (MMPI) scores, the Graduate Record Examination (GRE), transcript grade point averages, and records of length of previous health care experience. When these selection criteria are compared, test results of intellectual ability and achievement were the most efficient predictors of success in training programs. Specifically SAT scores alone predicted

EXHIBIT 4-8

Mean Number of Applicants, Percentage Enrolled, Enrollment, and Matriculants: PA Programs, 1983-2002*

Academic yr	Mean no. of applicants	Mean no. accepted	Mean no. enrolled	Mean applicant/enrollment ratio
1983-1984	—	—	24.0	—
1984-1985	98.4	30.4	24.1	4.0:1
1985-1986	101.8	44.5	24.3	4.0:1
1986-1987	86.5	31.2	24.9	3.5:1
1987-1988	84.7	30.2	25.6	3.3:1
1988-1989	86.1	30.2	25.9	3.3:1
1989-1990	90.2	33.0	26.1	3.5:1
1990-1991	106.5	35.6	29.6	3.6:1
1991-1992	133.2	36.8	32.2	4.1:1
1992-1993	203.2	40.6	35.0	5.8:1
1993-1994	275.5	39.6	37.0	7.4:1
1994-1995	379.6	44.9	41.4	9.2:1
1995-1996	419.5	44.7	42.9	9.8:1
1996-1997	383.3	45.6	39.6	9.7:1
1997-1998	338.6	46.0	40.5	8.4:1
1998-1999	290.4	48.0	42.6	6.8:1
1999-2000	238.8	42.6	39.3	6.1:1
2000-2001	199.7	48.5	40.1	5.0:1
2001-2002†	166	47.5	38.4	4.3:1

Data from Simon A, Link MS, Miko AS: *Seventeenth Annual Report on Physician Assistant Education in the United States, 2000-2001,* Alexandria, Va., 2001, Association of Physician Assistant Programs.

*The figures represent programs that had graduates and that responded to the survey.

†Estimated.

excellent or poor student performance in the program. The MMPI test results and previous health care experience had little or no significance in predicting success or failure in the program or on the PANCE (Oakes et al., 1999).

Previous Occupations

Understanding the background of PA students is important not only for recruitment purposes, but also to better understand the underlying influence on PA careers. Throughout the 1960s and 1970s, former military corpsmen and medics were viewed as the most suitable. From a predominance of veterans in the 1970s, this source had shrunk to 5% in 1994 and less than 4% in 2002. Nurses, including registered nurses, nurse practitioners (NPs), licensed practical nurses, and other types of nurses, made up almost one fifth of the 2002 student body. As can be seen in Exhibit 4-9, paramedics account for 20% of the 2001 entry-level student body and have ranged from 10% to 15% between 1990 and 2001. A wide assortment of health care professionals such as emergency medical technicians (EMTs), chiropractors, podiatrists, nutritionists, athletic trainers, audiologists, and health care educators comprise some of the past occupations of entering PA students.

EXHIBIT 4-9

Field of Prior Health Care Occupations of PA Program Enrollees, 2001

Health care field	No.	%*
Athletic trainer	222	5
Case manager	66	2
Chiropractor	18	0
Dental assistant	68	2
Emergency room technician	396	10
Emergency medical technician/paramedic	803	20
Health care administration	82	2
Health educator	222	5
Health services researcher	69	2
Home health aide	243	6
Medic/medical corpsman (military)	202	5
Medical assistant	695	17
Medical lab technician	247	6
Medical reception/records	229	6
Medical technician	155	4
Nurse practitioner	1	0
Nurse, licensed practical	82	2
Nurse, registered	208	5
Nurse, other	273	7
Nutritionist/dietitian	64	2
Operating room/surgical technician	154	4
Occupational therapist	34	1
Optometrist	5	0
Pharmacist	44	1
Phlebotomist	420	10
Physical therapist	143	4
Physician (MD/DO)	48	1
Podiatrist	5	0
Radiology technician	114	3
Respiratory technician	90	2
Social worker	55	1
Other	1187	29

From the American Academy of Physician Assistants, *Report on New Physician Assistant Enrollees, 2001.*
*Respondents were permitted to indicate multiple fields, so the sum of all fields exceeds 100%.

Prior Health Care Experience

While most programs emphasize prior health-related experience for admission the literature on this is scarce. Anecdotally students with extensive health care experience are perceived as "easier" to teach by faculty. Perhaps this may be a reflection of the early Medex and Duke programs that had minimal didactic content; those students were certainly advantaged by their extensive backgrounds. Programs are also experiencing decreased applicant pools across the profession; thus some thinking among programs are that many inexperienced but compassionate and motivated first-career people may make good PAs as well.

Most, but not all, PA programs require prior medical experience. In some programs a sizable proportion of students are matriculating from a lower division "pre-PA" curriculum in which experience was not required. Some researchers have noted that it is difficult to clearly separate the issues surrounding lack of medical background from those caused by youth and lack of life experience of those coming in halfway through their college education. A strong argument for the experience requirement is that it brings with it a degree of exposure to the "real world," usually including holding a job and the sense of responsibility that can come from that (Dehn, 2001).

A clear advantage of the experience requirement is that the applicant student is familiar with the language of medicine (i.e., medical terminology and jargon) and manner of thinking. Finally, some believe that students who enter a

PA program with significant clinical experience may find it easier to get through the clinical phase of the program.

Factors Influencing the Decision to Become a Physician Assistant

In addition to prior occupational background, a number of other factors influence a person's choice to become a PA. A list compiled by the Research Division at the AAPA, aggregates these factors (Exhibit 4-10). PAs and other professionals continue to be the dominant force influencing the majority of students to consider a PA career. However, another factor, following in a parent's footsteps, has emerged as an influence. Since 1985 dozens of adult children have followed their PA parents' careers to become PAs, sometimes enrolling at the same time. Having a family member who is a PA or a physician, or having a PA as a primary care provider is a strong influence on the decision to become a PA. Another influence seems to be visiting PAs in the classroom.

EXHIBIT 4-10

Summary Measures of Level of Influence on Decision to Become a PA of New PA Program Enrollees, 2000*

Influence factor	Score
AAPA literature	1.61
APAP literature	1.41
PA program literature	1.96
Television program	1.18
Television public service announcement	1.07
Radio program	1.07
Radio program service announcement	1.04
Cinema	1.07
Other nonwritten media	1.27
Project Access (PAs visiting schools)	1.28
AAPA staff	1.22
APAP staff	1.18
PA program faculty or staff	1.87
Family member	1.74
Career counselor or teacher (high school or college)	1.47
Physician who treated me or my family	1.78
PA who treated me or my family	1.83
Other PA acquaintance	2.33
Other health professional	2.24
Other factor	2.12

From American Academy of Physician Assistants, *Report on New Physician Enrollees, 2000.*

*The amount of influence was rated according to a 3-point scale: 1, no influence; 2, moderate influence; 3, strong influence.

Factors Influencing the Decision to Enroll in a Physician Assistant School

The factors that influence an individual's decision to become a PA (among those accepted in a PA program) are primarily "health-related work," a "PA acquaintance," or some "other health professional." These three factors account for half of all reasons for choosing a PA career and have important implications for recruitment of additional PAs (Exhibit 4-11).

Once an applicant has selected or has been selected by a PA program, two of the most influential reasons for almost half of all decisions to enroll in a particular program are "PA program location" and "program reputation." The reputation factor is interesting because there is no consensus regarding which programs have the higher reputation among applicants. Once a student has selected a program or has graduated from that program, there is an inherent belief among individuals that they made the correct educational institution decision.

EXHIBIT 4-11

Factors Influencing Decision to Enroll in PA School, 1994

Influencing factor	No. of cases	%
High school	24	0.4
College	105	1.6
Postbaccalaureate education	41	0.6
Guidance counselor	42	0.7
High school career day	21	0.3
High school library	9	0.1
High school counselor	18	0.3
High school teacher	17	0.3
College career day	85	0.7
College career library	85	1.3
College counselor	121	1.9
College professor	147	2.3
Information poster	42	0.7
Newspaper or magazine	229	3.6
Government publication	35	0.5
National PA programs directory	190	3.0
Other career guide	148	2.3
PA program brochure or catalog	583	9.2
Other media source	64	1.0
PA who treated me or my family	325	5.1
PA acquaintance	1141	17.9
Other health professional	833	13.1
Health-related work	1204	18.9
Illness/accident	217	3.4
Family member	504	7.9
Other personal experience	181	2.8

Data from American Academy of Physician Assistants, *New Students in Physician Assistant Programs, 1993 and 1994,* 1995.

Centralized Application Service to Physician Assistant Programs

A centralized application service for PA applicants (CASPA) has been established by the Association of Physician's Assistant Programs and has been operational since 2001. More than half (approximately 70) of the schools participated the first year. CASPA allows a single application to be completed electronically and sent to the PA programs of choice. CASPA enhances student choice and decreases falsifying applications. Is is expected that as more programs participate, more data characterizing the PA applicant pool will be available (Johnson et al., 1998).

Course of Instruction

PA curriculum is based on the medical school model. The average PA program spans 26 months with no breaks while the average medical school spans 48 months of instruction. A typical PA program is about 50 weeks shorter than a typical medical school program, and the primary educational objectives are similar. Both physician and PA education provide students with the theoretical knowledge and technical skills needed to perform therapeutic and diagnostic procedures accurately. Like medical schools, PA programs use a format of didactic and clinical training.

A few studies have dealt with the subject of what should be learned. Golden and Cawley (1983) found that most PA programs were teaching what had been proposed by medical school educators: the core of medicine is history taking and physical examination. Apart from the approach to the patient and certain clinical skills, this included technical skills such as urinalysis, blood analysis, electrocardiogram (ECG) interpretation, hearing and vision screening, Papanicolaou scrapings, applying and removing casts, tuberculosis skin testing, interpreting radiographs, parenteral injections, bacteriology testing, suturing, and pulmonary function testing.

A comprehensive survey of Colorado PAs found that almost all of them learned 39 common procedures (Exhibit 4-12). This formed the base for the questionnaire. Eight procedures (including reading chest and long-bone x-ray films, suturing, splinting, interpreting ECGs, and performing pelvic examinations, Papanicolaou's smears, and urinalysis) were used more than once a month by at least 50% of PAs in their practices. Three procedures (cardiopulmonary resuscitation, lumbar puncture, and suprapubic aspirations) were used less than once a year by more than 90% of PAs (Gray et al., 1995). The leading skills needed for PA practice were history taking, physical diagnosis, and patient management (Cawley et al., 2001).

In examining the content of PA clinical activities, Dehn and Hooker (1999) analyzed the results of a survey of family practice PAs in Iowa and found all provided health promotion, disease prevention, health and safety education, and prescribed drugs. The procedures reported by the respondents were the same as those performed by family medicine physicians in the

EXHIBIT 4-12

Skills Most Frequently Learned by PA Students
Procedures
Cardiopulmonary resuscitation
Electrocardiogram (perform, interpret)
Finger stick and heel stick
Fluorescein Wood's lamp examination
Parenteral injection (intradermal, subcutaneous, intramuscular)
Lumbar puncture
Suprapubic aspiration
Urethral catheterization
Venipuncture
Laboratory techniques
Agglutination test for mononucleosis (read)
Blood smear (perform, read)
Culture (streak out, read)
Gram stain (perform, read)
Sensitivity plate (read)
Stool examination for occult blood
Urinalysis (dipstick, microscopic)
Patient care
Chest radiograph (read)
Intravenous line (set up, start, monitor)
Long-bone x-ray film (read)
Papanicolaou's stain (perform)
Pelvic examination
Suturing
Wound care (burns, casts, splints)
Screening tests
Articulation screen
Denver Developmental Screening Test
Hearing screen
Vision screen

Modified from Gray J, Lacey C, Alexander S, et al.: *J Am Acad Physician Assist* 8:45-51, 1995.

same state and were considerably broader than had been surmised. The size of the community in which they practiced also made a difference: the more rural and remote the more likely the PA would perform a procedure (Dehn and Hooker, 1999).

What Makes a Good Physician Assistant?

What makes an effective PA? Is the formula of past health care experience plus an intensive medical model curriculum the most appropriate in preparing clinicians? To what degree does past health care experience determine future effectiveness as a PA? One study requested information on new PA students asking them to score their pre-PA health-related experience, rating both duration and rigor. Comparison was then made with a wide variety of parameters of self-assessed confidence and actual job use patterns (autonomy rankings). There was no statistically significant association between pre-PA health care experience and self-assessed clinical competence or use patterns of newly graduated PAs (Kelly, 2000). Extensively experienced graduates perceived their experience level as "vital" to their competence, whereas graduates with minimal to moderate experience thought that the influence of their experience was either only "helpful" or not applicable. There was no difference in perceived or self-assessed confidence in any setting or task with either group. Nor was there any difference in how supervising physicians or employers treated the graduates and in the time it took to get a first job.

Prerequisites

Jones (1994) has shown that PA program prerequisites range widely from program to program. For those programs requiring a bachelor's degree the prerequisites would likely be as follows:

- Biology
- Organic chemistry
- Genetics
- Chemistry
- English and literature
- Psychology and sociology
- Calculus/statistics

Since more than half of PA programs now offer the master's or master's option, the list of prerequisites may include additional courses.

Selection of Students

Typical selection criteria used by PA programs are those used by most other academic and clinical programs.

- Science grade point average
- Grade point average
- Personal essay
- Letters of recommendation
- Interview

How these elements are weighted in a given program depends on the mission of the PA program and factors relating to institutional preference. These criteria will change based on institutional funding, reputation, and state resident preferences (if the program is publicly funded). Some programs have well-defined goals such as Christian service (Trevecca Nazarene University, Kettering College of the Medical Arts, and Union College), a strong nursing/NP background (University of North Dakota School of Medicine, University of California, Davis), and those with a commitment for graduates to practice in a medically underserved area (many schools), or fluency in Spanish.

Applicants seeking to apply to PA programs may find some of the following ideas helpful:

- Visit the web site of the program of interest
- Visit the AAPA programs web site (www aapa.org)
- Visit the APAP web site (www.apap.org)
- *Physician Assistant Programs Directory*
- Attend a program's open house
- Speak with a faculty member
- Network with recent graduates of the program
- Communicate with students of any given PA program both by e-mail and personally at paforum.list.mc.duke.edu
- Read *Getting into the PA School of Your Choice* (Rodican, 1998), a book developed to assist the PA applicant

Predicting Success as a Physician Assistant Graduate

Without a definition about what constitutes an "effective PA," educators have turned to the only quantifiable indicator: the PANCE. Researchers have studied predictors of success in education programs to validate and improve admission requirements and course curricula. Two studies have turned to the PANCE to see if any attributes of the individual or the institution have any predictive value using the PANCE as the endpoint. Oakes and colleagues (1999) examined this among a small sample of 88 PA students and found little to predict in terms of demographics. McDowell, Clemens, and Frosch (1999) examined the PANCE scores of 38 programs in the early 1990s and found master's prepared PAs had higher average percent pass rates on the PANCE and higher average core scores, and those in programs with longer accreditation status were found to perform significantly better on the clinical skills portion of the PANCE. Hooker, Hess, and Cipher (2002) examined 18,000 test takers and also found that master's prepared graduates did slightly better on the PANCE. Program characteristics such as tuition, length of program, public versus private, medical school affiliation, and region of the country made no difference in PANCE scores. Neither did size of class, age, or gender of the student. The authors conclude that in this sample there was very little quantitative difference to predict who will pass and who will fail the PANCE in relation to academic degree.

CURRICULUM

Each PA program seeks to develop within each student a strong foundation in the basic and clinical sciences of medicine appropriate for the delivery of quality health care services. The education process may reflect a traditional medical school curriculum and even share classes with medical students, or it might introduce multidimensional assessment and decision analysis techniques that are unique to a particular PA program. Certain skills taught seem to be common to all programs (Cawley and Golden, 1983; Gray et al., 1995).

The basic science curriculum is usually structured to provide an in-depth understanding of structural features characterizing body tissues and organ systems, biochemical mechanisms regulating body metabolism, and nutrition. Next come the physiologic controls governing body system functions, pathophysiology, and behavioral alterations causing clinical manifestations of illnesses and the management of these illnesses and injuries.

By intent, there is a great deal of curricular diversity among PA programs.

The Preceptorship

The preceptorship phase of training for PA students is the final step in the professional socialization process while being a capstone experience in primary care. This process usually comes at the end of the training but varies considerably among programs. Because patient management is the essence of appropriate medical practice, PAs must learn the proper attitudes and techniques for handling this career aspect with professionalism and clinical judgment. With the science of medicine learned primarily from lectures, books, and laboratory work, the art of relating to patients is acquired through imitative role modeling, intuition, and trial and error. Views about patients will change the most during this time as students gain clinical experience and expertise.

The preceptorship is an experience shared by the physician mentor and the PA student. The physician provides a lasting role model in the memory of the student. The cardinal learning experiences of medicine—exploring, examining, and cutting into the human body; dealing with the fears, anger, sense of helplessness, and

EXHIBIT 4-13

Guidelines for PAs Working Internationally

- PAs should establish and maintain the appropriate physician/PA team.
- PAs should accurately represent their skills, training, professional credentials, identity, or service both directly and indirectly.
- PAs should provide only those services for which they are qualified via their education and/or experiences, and in accordance with all pertinent legal and regulatory processes.
- PAs should respect the culture, values, beliefs, and expectations of the patients, local health care providers, and the local health care systems.
- PAs should take responsibility for being familiar with, and adhering to, the customs, laws, and regulations of the country where they will be providing services.
- When applicable, PAs should identify and train local personnel who can assume the role of providing care and continuing the education process.

American Academy of Physician Assistants, Subcommittee on International Affairs, Statement Adopted, AAPA House of Delegates, Anaheim, Calif., May 26, 2001.

despair of patients; meeting urgent situations; accepting the limitations of medical science; and being confronted with death—will be experiences the physician will guide the PA through to professional self-actualization.

International Rotations

Increasingly PA programs are receiving requests from students to undertake some of their training in other countries. One student's experience is illustrated by a clinical rotation in the jungles of Bolivia (Pucillo, 2000). The results of a survey of 58 programs in 1999 found that 43% would consider sending or have sent their students overseas. Several schools stated that they used medical outreach groups and missionary trips to send students to international sites (Heinerich, 2000). A partial list of places where students have experienced rotations can be found in Exhibit 4-14.

Physician Assistants for Global Health (PAGH) is an official group of the AAPA. Its goal is to promote cross-cultural awareness and delivery of PA services to domestic and international health care professional shortage areas. PAGH has been involved with placing some students in overseas rotations. The APAP Committee on International PA Education provides advice to education programs outside the United States.

PROGRAM FACULTY

A wide variety of health care professionals and professional educators are used within PA educational programs. Approximately 450 PAs and 300 non-PAs were employed in PA programs nationwide in 2001. These included physicians, PAs, and masters- and doctoral-level instructors in the basic medical sciences, the behavioral and social sciences, and various other disciplines.

A PA program professional faculty composition typically consists of a full-time program director (a person increasingly likely to be a PA who holds a master's or doctorate degree), a medical director, usually a physician serving part time (0.2 to 0.5 full-time equivalent [FTE]), and an average of 4.3 FTE personnel serving in various PA faculty instructional roles (Exhibit 4-15). The total number of employees per program ranges from 3 to 13, with an average of one employee for every 7.7 students enrolled (Whitman, 2000).

Support staffs average 2.4 FTE noninstructional PA program personnel. In a mature program this averages approximately 1 faculty member to 10 students; however, in the second year, the student is often away on clinical rotations or preceptorship, and contact with the faculty may be less intense. Because many programs use part-time faculty, there are usually no more than eight students per faculty member assigned for advisement.

The mean annual salary of faculty-level personnel was $62,448 in 2001 (N = 368). Among the personnel classified as staff, those who were PAs earned a substantially higher salary than non-PAs (Exhibit 4-16). Doctoral degree–level personnel (N = 47) earned the highest salary (average, $63,208) and associate-level individuals the lowest ($53,015). The range of salaries is broad, from $56,838 for instructor rank to $79,576 for those at associate professor level (Simon, Link, and Miko, 2001).

Among PA faculty (N = 421) in PA educational programs in 2001, there were 121 (29%) in tenure-stream positions while only 31 (6.5%) held tenure. In terms of the senior ranks, only 10.2% held the rank of associate professor and 2% held

EXHIBIT 4-14

International Clinical Sites Where PA Students Have Trained

Belize	Jamaica
Bermuda	Kenya
Bolivia	Madagascar
Brazil	Mariana Islands
Canada	Netherlands
England	Papua New Guinea
Guatemala	Scotland
Haiti	Tanzania
Honduras	Trinidad
India	Other South American countries
Iran	Other African countries
Ireland	

EXHIBIT 4-15

Academic Rank of Faculty, 2002

Academic rank	No.	%
Full professor	8	2.0
Associate professor	41	10.2
Assistant professor	208	51.6
Instructor/lecture	146	36.2
TOTAL	403	100

EXHIBIT 4-16

Typical PA Program Faculty Roles and Salaries With 40 Students, 2001*

Title	Full-time equivalent	Annual salary	Range
Program director	1.0	$83,711	$50,000-$124,681
Academic coordinator or instructor	1.0	$61,408	–
Clinic coordinator or instructor	2.8	$62,830	–
Associate or assistant director	1.0	$72,313	–
Medical director	0.3	$104,355	$25,000-$200,000
Business manager	1.0	$35,000	–
Secretary or receptionist	1.4	$30,000	–
TOTAL	8.5	$449,617	–

Modified from Simon A, Link MS, Miko AS: *Eighteenth Annual Report on Physician Assistant Education in the United States, 2000-2001,* Alexandria, Va., 2002, Association of Physician Assistant Programs.
*The program may employ many part-time faculty members, and the medical director is rarely full-time.

the rank of professor (Simon, Link, and Miko, 2002).

A survey of medical directors of PA programs in 1996 found that they spend a wide range of time working with PA programs. Fifty percent have a time commitment of less than 15%, and one sixth have a time commitment of more than 50%. As to their respective programs, 100% participate in curriculum planning and committee function, most notably the admissions committee, and 100% participate in direct student instruction; rarely do they mentor students or faculty or participate in or guide research (Green, 2000).

Like other relative newcomers in health professions education, PA educational programs have experienced difficulty in identifying, recruiting, and retaining qualified faculty members. The combination of an increasing number of applicants and a growing demand for PA services has resulted in an "academic hourglass" effect. There is a bottleneck in processing PA students because there are not enough programs to train them. This is further complicated by an existing shortage of qualified educators. Rates of faculty attrition in PA programs have averaged 10% per year for the past several decades. The chief reasons cited for ending academic employment include geographic relocation (5%), career advancement (14%), return to clinical practice (25%), and termination (11%) (Simon, Link, and Miko, 2001).

Other issues include the retention and professional development of qualified faculty, particularly from underrepresented racial and ethnic minorities. As of 2002 7.4% of PA program faculty members are from underrepresented racial and ethnic minorities, 4.4% higher than the rate for medical school faculty. In most PA educational programs the need for faculty role models and mentors from underrepresented racial and ethnic groups will continue.

SATELLITE PHYSICIAN ASSISTANT PROGRAMS

A few PA programs have created satellite programs for various reasons, showing that they have matured. Some develop to reach a particular applicant pool, to take advantage of resources in the area, because PA programs are sound investments for an institution, to avoid competition for resources within their own institution, or because the state legislation wants a program developed in a region of the state. Satellite programs may remain attached to their parent institution, as in the case of the Medex Northwest PA program in Seattle, Yakima, and Spokane. Others will detach after a few years and become free-standing PA programs, as is the case of the University of Texas Medical Branch in Galveston giving rise to the University of Texas Pan American PA program in Edinburg, Texas. Another effective program is the University of Kentucky/Lexington Moorhead University PA program in eastern Kentucky. Evidence suggests that the caliber and quality of education of the satellite programs are equivalent to the primary program.

The question of the effectiveness of curriculum in satellite programs was also studied. In a comparison of the University of Washington Medex Northwest PA programs satellite programs (Seattle, Yakima, Spokane, Washington, and formerly Sitka, Alaska), there was remarkably little difference in grades and pass rates among graduates over 5 years. Because the overall academic performances in all training sites were comparable, the authors concluded that administrative and curricular controls in the home institution can achieve parity in education across their various training sites (Ballweg and Wick, 1999).

POSTGRADUATE PROGRAMS

PA postgraduate education developed in response to a perceived need for education beyond the entry level and for increased specialty training (Cultural perspectives, 2000; Jameson, 2000). It also arose because hospitals were in need of medical professionals who were inexpensive and available. The trend toward increasing specialization and autonomy has led to greater numbers of PAs seeking formal postgraduate training before entering a specialty.

Formal educational programs that offer advanced educational experiences for PAs who seek to obtain further training in a specialized area of medicine have emerged. PA postgraduate programs began with PA residency programs but include academic programs, usually at the master's degree level, which provide PAs with advanced clinical and nonclinical education. Some of these are sponsored by and located in teaching hospitals, which are typically intensive experiences that provide PA graduates advanced clinical training. Most programs are members of the Association of Postgraduate Physician Assistant Programs (APPAP). In 2002 there were 40 such programs, usually 6 to 12 months of paid clinical experiences, enrolling highly selected PA graduates (Exhibit 4-17). A number of the current PA postgraduate programs are affiliated with a physician residency program of the same type.

EXHIBIT 4-17

Types of Postgraduate PA Programs, 2002
Surgery
Orthopedics
Emergency medicine
Psychiatry
Dermatology
Urology
Pediatrics
Primary care
Family medicine
Oncology
Advanced PA studies
Neonatology
Occupational/environmental medicine
Clinical leadership
Rural primary care

The first PA postgraduate program was developed in surgery at Montefiore Hospital in New York in 1971, just 6 years after the first PA program was initiated (Rosen, 1986). Clinical disciplines represented among PA postgraduate programs include surgery, pediatrics, and emergency medicine. Most of these programs are clinically based, but a few include a lengthy phase of didactic instruction; most programs award a certificate or degree on completion.

Asprey, described postgraduate residency programs in the late 1990s (Asprey, 1999; Asprey and Helms, 1999). There are two types of PA postgraduate programs: the internship model and the academic model. The internship model includes a modest, practically oriented, didactic curriculum combined with intensive clinical rotations and educational experience. These programs tend to lead to a certificate of completion. Academic model programs combine a highly structured and formalized didactic education (through courses taken for graduate credits) with clinical rotations and lead to a master's degree (or credit toward a master's degree upon completion) (Exhibits 4-18 through 4-21).

Several groups have called for establishing standards for the PA postgraduate education process (AAPA Education Council, 2000) because of the relative lack of information on PA postgraduate programs. PA educators, policymakers, employers, and members of the profession still have relatively little systematic information on which to formulate opinions or make judgments about the value of the PA postgraduate programs. A clearly long-term outcome of postgraduate education must be undertaken and compared with outcomes of PAs who were trained on the job. To date, PA postgraduate programs have not objectively documented their value, standardized their curricula, legitimized their educational processes and outcomes

EXHIBIT 4-18

Postgraduate Residency Programs, 2001*

Program	Location
Cardiothoracic surgery	Cedars-Sinai Medical Center, Calif.
Dermatology	Northeast Regional Medical Center/Kirksville College of Osteopathic Medicine, Mo.
	University of Texas Southwestern Medical Center, Tex.
Emergency medicine	Alderson-Broaddus College, W.Va.‡
	U.S. Army Medical Department, Tex.†
	Madigan Army Medical Center, Wash.†
Orthopedic surgery	Illinois Bone and Joint Institute, Ill.
	Arrowhead Regional Medical Center, Calif.†
	U.S. Air Force Medical Service, Ohio†
Pediatrics	Norwalk Hospital/Yale University, Conn.
Advanced physician assistant studies	Arizona School of Health Sciences, Ariz.‡
Primary care	Alderson-Broaddus College, W.Va.‡
Psychiatry	University of Texas Medical Branch Correctional Managed Care, Tex.
	Cherokee Mental Health Institute, Iowa†
Surgery	Montefiore Medical Center/University Hospital for the Albert Einstein College of Medicine, N.Y.†
	Norwalk Hospital/Yale University School of Medicine, Conn.
	Spectrum Health, Mich.
Urology	Northwest Metropolitan Urology Associates, Ill.

*Military programs require that you be on active duty at the time of attending the program.
†Master's degree option available.
‡Master's degree awarded.

EXHIBIT 4-19

PA Postgraduate Program Curriculum Topics

Research methods/biostatistics/epidemiology
Advanced pharmacology
Family medicine/primary care/clinical issues
Emergency medicine/clinical training experiences
Health care systems management
Clinical ethics/clinical decision making
PA professional issues/PA studies/health services research
Health care policy/health policy analysis
Interpretation of biomedical research information
Computer applications in medicine
Medical/scientific writing/biomedical communication

EXHIBIT 4-20

Summary of All Resident Activities (Average hr/wk)

Resident educational activity	Hr/wk	% of total
Patient care	61.4	75.6
Educational activities related to patient care	10.7	13.2
Didactic education	7.4	9.1
Research-related educational activities	1.7	2.1
TOTAL	81.2	100

Data from Asprey DP, Helms L: *Perspect Physician Assist Educ* 10, 124-131, 1999.

through research, or implemented an accreditation or certification process for postgraduate education (Cawley and Jones, 1997).

Asprey found that the mean length of 17 residency programs in existence at the time was 14 months. The average academic program was approximately 8 months longer than an internship. The mean number of hours for all programs was 299.1 hours. For the 14 internship model programs the mean was 249.3 hours of didactic instruction. The three academic programs reported a mean of 531.7 hours. The mean annual stipend in 1998 was $34,902 (Asprey and Helms, 1999).

Most PAs who have entered clinical practice roles in specialty and subspecialty areas (nearly half of the profession) acquire their preparation through on-the-job experiences, learning from employer physicians within their practice or institution. Only a small percentage of PAs have completed PA residency training programs. The demonstrated capability of PAs to adapt readily

EXHIBIT 4-21

Mechanism by Which Residents Learned About PA Postgraduate Programs

Mechanism	No.	%
Information provided to me by the PA program I attended	19	41.3
From a fellow student or colleague	12	26.1
Journal advertisements	4	8.7
Other	4	8.7
By interactions with a residency graduate	3	6.5
By a mailing sent to me	2	4.3
Web site	1	2.2
Journal article about the residency	1	2.2
TOTAL	46	100

Items Influencing Residents' Decisions to Attend a Postgraduate Program

Item	Frequency of selection	%	Rank order
Increased ability to compete for a job in this specialty	41/46	89.1	1
Interest in additional clinical knowledge and skills before going into practice as a PA	39/46	84.8	2
Improved future earning potential	37/46	80.4	3
Current level of competency in this specialty area	34/46	73.9	4
Provides flexibility to change specialty area practiced	28/46	60.9	5
Obtaining an advanced degree	28/46	60.9	5
Other	4/46	8.7	7

Items Influencing Residents' Decision to Attend Their Postgraduate Program

Item	Frequency of selection	%	Rank order
Program reputation	36/46	78.3	1
Didactic component of curriculum	36/46	78.3	1
Practical clinical education component	31/46	64.4	3
Geographic location	30/46	65.2	4
Recommendation from colleague or friend	26/46	56.5	5
Degree or degree option offered	25/46	54.3	6
Recommendation from PA program faculty member	24/46	52.3	7
Impression obtained during application/interview process	24/46	52.3	7
Salary stipend	20/46	43.5	9
Benefits package	15/46	32.6	10
Other	9/46	19.6	11

Data from Asprey DP, Helms L: *Perspect Physician Assist Educ* 10, 124-131, 1999.

to and function effectively in a wide variety of clinical practice specialties is probably attributable to their broad generalist-oriented educational preparation.

Since the early 1990s newer models of PA postgraduate educational programs have emerged. These programs differ from the typical PA residency programs in that they offer an academic-oriented experience. Instead of sharpening clinical inpatient-oriented often procedural capabilities, the programs focus on skill development for graduate PAs, which spans both clinical and nonclinical areas. Included in curricula are courses in advanced work in clinical areas/clinical training, research methodology, and interpretation of the biomedical literature, computer medicine, clinical prevention, health systems management, health policy, clinical decision sciences, and medical ethics. A full-length research paper is sometimes required. Tracks for clinical, research, PA education, or health administration can be developed. The curriculum emphasizes preparation in those areas that students believe are important in expanding their professional potentials and advancement in the health care system. The prototype of this model of PA postgraduate education is the master of medical science (MMS) PA program sponsored by St. Francis University in Loretto, Pennsylvania. In operation since 1993 this program incorporates inputs from multiple clinical and nonclinical disciplines in its 33-credit curriculum.

In 1995 Alderson-Broaddus College began to enroll students in two postgraduate master's degree programs (emergency medicine and rural health). Students work in clinical settings affiliated with the Alderson-Broaddus College PA program throughout West Virginia. Many postgraduate PA programs now include distance education-based programs, such a those at the University of Nebraska, The George Washington University, the Arizona School of Health Science, and Nova Southeastern University.

PHYSICIAN ASSISTANT EDUCATIONAL COSTS

In comparison to allopathic and osteopathic medical student educational costs, the overall expense of PA training is relatively low. The average total cost for educating an allopathic medical student in 2000 and 2001 is more than $100,000 (for residents of the state) in tuition on average; the tuition cost for educating an osteopathic medical student is estimated at $45,600 (Liaison Committee on Medical Education, 2001). Findings from the APAP annual report estimate the total costs of education for PA students at $32,810 per resident student and $40,310 per nonresident student per program per year, with a range of $6,700 to $101,000 (Simon, Link, and Miko, 2001). This figure includes the costs to the student for tuition, fees, books, and equipment, but not living expenses. Costs to enrolled students vary by sponsorship (academic health center-sponsored versus nonacademic health center-sponsored programs) and by state-mandated assistance. In 2000 the first-year tuition for a PA education ranged from $3,800 in the University of Texas System to $38,000 for the PA/MPH program at George Washington University in Washington, District of Columbia (Hooker and Warren, 2001).

Tuition and fees are a major factor in the decision making of a PA applicant. A student draws the tuition from a number of sources. This may be personal income, family income, and/or financial aid. While a large number of PA students receive some type of financial aid, it is usually in the form of loans that must be repaid upon graduation.

Our knowledge of student educational expenses is limited. The annual report of PA programs provides some trend data (Simon, Link, and Miko, 2002). Among students entering PA programs in 2001, 103 programs reported that the tuition for the entire program was $28,036 (range $3900 to $80,000; average per month $895) for a resident student and $35,536 ($12,300 to $80,000; average per month $1278) for a nonresident. Books, fees, and equipment costs averaged $4774 ($800 to $47,000, average per month $170) (Simon, Link, and Miko, 2001).

The length of PA programs and the degrees offered vary widely as well. The average length of a PA program is 26.2 months, with a range of 12 to 36 months (4-year programs tend to include summer breaks) (Simon, Link, and Miko, 2001). Master's degree programs were introduced in 1988 and more than one half of the programs offered this degree at the time of this study. This trend is expected to continue.

Hooker has shown how PA programs compare in terms of tuition from the perspective of a PA applicant with complete information when seeking to assess the economic burden that PA students assume when they begin an education process. Drawing from the human capital theory, Hooker looked at individual's decisions about education and training. While educational decisions can be influenced by love of learning, desire for prestige, and a variety of other preferences and emotions, human capital theorists find it useful to analyze a schooling decision as if it were part of a business plan. The optimal length of education, from this point of view, is the number of years of school needed until the marginal revenue (in the form of increased future income) of an additional year of schooling is exactly equal to the marginal cost.

Data drawn from 126 PA programs spread over 124 institutions obtained from the eighteenth edition of the *Physician Assistant Programs Directory* (APAP, 2000), the total tuition cost of a PA education in 2000 ranged from $4370 to $69,258. The average cost of a publicly funded education was $14,366 and a private education was $38,846. At the time of this study there were 58 master's programs and 68 nonmaster's programs (bachelor's or certificate). The tuition burden of a master's program track was, on average, $32,531 (median $36,075; range $6160 to $69,258) versus $22,685 (median $23,437; range $4370 to $48,195) for a nonmaster's track. The size of the entering class differed by type of institution. Private institutions averaged 40 (median 36; range 12 to 100) students per entering class, whereas public institutions averaged 35 students (median 32; range 10 to 80).

A comparison of the length of PA programs was calculated based on the total months of a program. The average length of a PA program was 25 to 26 months, with a range of 12 to 42 months. There was little difference between public and private institutions in average program length. While the publicly financed programs tended to be shorter and the private programs tended to be longer, the median and mode for both types of programs was 24 months. A difference did emerge when programs offering a graduate degree were compared with those without a graduate degree. Master's programs are, on average, 27 months (median 27; range 24 to 36 months) compared with nonmaster's degree programs of 25 months (median 24; range 12 to 42 months).

Because private institutions are believed to have more direct costs than public institutions, we calculated the total tuition revenue stream that a PA program would generate from the entering class. The gross tuition for the entering class for all 126 PA programs for 2000 was calculated as $61,385,864. For the 57 PA programs in public institutions, this averaged $251,293 (median $220,000; range $37,493 to $1,131,429). Gross tuition for the 69 classes entering private institutions averaged $682,060 (median $620,813; range $68,000 to $1,715,000).

The cost of a PA education shows a remarkable range: almost a $65,000 difference from the least expensive tuition to the most costly. This sixteenfold difference is found between public and private institutions, with state-supported programs being less expensive, on average, than private programs. While this difference does shrink to a twelvefold difference when duration of education is held constant, the difference still demonstrates a remarkable market demand for PA education. It also represents an extraordinary differential in the expected economic return to the educational investment (Hooker and Warren, 2001). How the institutions, faculty, students, or applicants view these differences has not been explored.

The reason that states fund higher education is reflected in the policies they are trying to promote. One economic explanation lies in the established principle that by offering educational opportunities, citizens will become educated, obtain higher paying jobs, and return something to the state in the form of higher taxable revenue. Although this may be true for undergraduate education, the debt incurred during PA education in terms of the opportunity costs seems quite high for many programs. Many PA students are embarking on a second career. The return rate for some of the higher end PA educational programs may never be realized if a well-paying job is abandoned to become a PA student. Another explanation for state-supported education is that residents are more likely to attend a state-supported school and consequently remain in the state. This also offers a return to the taxpayers for their investment in higher education.

COSTS OF PHYSICIAN ASSISTANT EDUCATION TO THE STUDENT

The mean total annual budget of 101 PA educational programs in 2001 was $873,977. There were wide ranges of total budgets (range $105,598 to $2,993,000), depending on the size of the student body and the region of the country. The average cost per program to educate a PA student in 2001 was estimated to be $11,500 a year (Simon, Link, and Miko, 2001).

The primary source of internal financial support for most programs is the sponsoring institution. Based on 91 programs, they averaged $504,324 (median $476,000; SD $394,482; range $25,000 to $2,993,000). Federal grant awards to programs during 2000 ranged from $15,000 to $600,000 and averaged $154,834 per program and accounted for 18% of the total budget. Over the last decade when federal funding levels have remained constant at roughly $5 million a year, greater levels of internal support from sponsoring institutions have enabled programs to sustain operations and develop some measure of self-sufficiency. Other sources of support come from state grants (averaging $144,600 per program), research grants, program projects, hospital services, and practice plans (Simon, Link, and Miko, 2001).

Federal Support

In 2001 a total of 31 programs were awarded federal grant support under the Title VII PA Grant

Award Program. PA educational programs have been responsive to federal grant initiatives that target service in rural areas, medically underserved areas, and delivery of primary care to needy populations. Relative to other health professionals the deployment record of PAs to practices in rural communities and medically underserved areas has been impressive (Shi et al., 1993). More than half of all federally funded PA programs have developed specific curricular content addressing the health and social problems of medically underserved populations. These include people living in inner cities, remote areas, correctional systems, geriatric facilities, or rehabilitation facilities. PA curricula also typically include instruction in topics such as management of persons with human immunodeficiency virus or acquired immunodeficiency syndrome, counseling regarding the risks of adolescent pregnancy, measures to reduce infant mortality, required schedules of pediatric immunization, health behavior to lower the risk of cancer and heart disease, and skills in the management of health problems that occur disproportionately among medically underserved populations. To ensure that students receive adequate clinical opportunities to complement didactic instruction, most PA educational programs have developed links with area health education centers, rural health clinics, community/migrant health centers, and other primary health care agencies within their geographic region.

In 1992 an initiative was developed and jointly sponsored by the Health Resources and Services Administration, the National Rural Health Association, the AAPA, and APAP. The purpose of this initiative was to enhance PA clinical practice among underserved populations and in rural communities by providing support for migrant health clinic fellowships. The broad flexibility that exists within PA educational programs and a demonstrated record of responsiveness to federal incentives to increase the number of primary care providers have resulted in a number of innovative curricular approaches designed to prepare practitioners to meet future societal health care needs. The deployment of PAs to areas of medical need is largely attributed to priorities in federal Title VII grant programs. The emphasis of Title VII funding has been to promote the preparation of PAs for roles working with primary care physicians and for deployment to medically underserved areas. Incentives in Title VII grant awards have encouraged PA programs to educate practitioners with an orientation in primary care. They have also fostered methods of deployment of PA graduates to enter primary care/ambulatory practice and/or to locate in medically underserved areas. A high proportion of federally funded PA educational programs have developed curricular components that identify clinical training sites and affiliations in rural and medically underserved areas. Qualifications require students to serve a portion of clinical training in such sites.

Most educational costs for student PAs are usually borne by the individual. Students finance their education through personal funds and loans, and few are financed through the National Health Service Corps. Another well-recognized influencing force in PA education is the source of funds that PA students need to draw on to complete their education (Exhibit 4-22).

EXPANSION OF PHYSICIAN ASSISTANT EDUCATION

In the early 1990s as part of the optimistic attitudes surrounding health care reform, it was generally assumed that the need for nonphysician health care professions would continue to remain strong—an assumption justifying both the establishment of a number of new PA educational programs and the increased enrollment in existing programs. In terms of recent trends in health professions education, this has produced

EXHIBIT 4-22

Summary Measures of Rating of Amount of Funding for PA Education From Select Sources of New PA Program Enrollees by Year*

Source of funds	1997	1999	2001
Savings	1.77	1.76	1.80
Own earnings	1.29	1.28	1.39
Spouse's earnings	1.52	1.47	1.43
Other family support	1.67	1.67	1.69
Grant/scholarship	1.46	1.47	1.58
Service obligated loans	1.12	1.16	1.18
Loans	2.53	2.49	2.55

Data from American Academy of Physician Assistants, *New Students in Physician Assistant Programs.*

*Funding sources were rated according to a 3-point scale: 1, no funding; 2, moderate amount; 3, large amount.

a remarkable diversity in curriculum and degrees offered. PA programs evolved over a fairly short period to offer an education that meets the health care needs of patients today. Among the factors that led to the significant expansion of PA education in the mid 1990s was the growing public acceptance and economic attractiveness of PAs that spurred an interest among educational institutions to sponsor PA programs. During the past 5 years there has been a doubling of the number and overall output of PA programs. Program expansion has occurred as a result of increasing demand and as a response to a very strong PA applicant pool. In 1995 the average PA educational program had a mean of 420 applicants for 44 available first-year seats, a 9.8:1 applicant/acceptance ratio (Cawley and Jones, 1997). It is also possible that U.S. educational institutions may have been overly eager to expand the PA educational system. Yet several highly respected observers of the PA profession view PA workforce supply and demand in terms of a free market ideology. These free market adherents feel that the oscillations of market demand will eventually correct themselves, leading to a balance in supply and demand benefiting patients, employers, and the profession itself (Hooker, 1997). Additionally some believe workforce surpluses in desirable regions and urban communities are tolerable and will stimulate a redistribution of providers to more needy regions. In contrast to undergraduate physician education, which has had steady growth in the last decade, educational programs for PAs experienced a boom during the 1990s.

Expansion of NP Education

There has also been a boom in NP educational programs (Cooper, Laud, and Dietrich, 1998). From less than 200 in 1990 the number of educational programs training NPs has soared. According to the National Organization of Nurse Practitioner Faculties (NONPF), in 1999 there were 792 programs (master's level NP and/or combined NP-clinical nurse specialist programs) and 657 post-master's completion programs. Family NP programs constituted the largest single number of NP programs (245), followed by adult (104), pediatric (90), and smaller numbers of other track/programs, that is, school, neonatal, acute care, oncology, and others (American Association of Colleges of Nursing, 2000). It should be kept in mind that these numbers represent programs and not schools. At one institution, for instance, a school of nursing may sponsor five clinical specialty track NP programs. It should also be noted that this number appears falsely high as some of these programs/tracks may enroll only a handful of students; nonetheless, overall enrollment in NP educational programs has expanded dramatically during the past several years. For PAs the number of educational programs has more than doubled since 1994, with 132 programs now accredited and in operation. Enrollment has also markedly increased (Exhibit 4-23). In 2002 there were approximately 5000 PA graduates, in contrast to fewer than 1800 graduates in 1994. The expansion of NP and PA educational programs has come with diversity in curricular approaches. While both of these health profession's programs ostensibly aim to produce clinicians on the same level, NP and PA programs have become established in a wide variety of institutions, award a number of different academic credentials, and contain many curriculums. In contrast to physician education, which in the past was criticized as embedded in tradition and inflexible, many newly emerging PA and NP programs have created innovative and progressive educational methods.

Without question, PA educational programs have been pioneers in developing curricula focused on primary care and have demonstrated effectiveness in training competent providers who can deliver primary care services. Because PA programs are not often bound by entrenched departmental limitations, faculty members have been free to incorporate new topics such as alternative and complementary medicine, cultural sensitivity, and preventive medicine more readily. The programs also experiment with interdisciplinary approaches and adjust curricular length and content to fit specific professional needs. Along with the growth and expansion of NP and PA programs curricular diversity has been promoted because many of these programs have been established in institutions relatively new to health professions education. Although many PA and NP programs are set in academic health centers and sponsored by schools of nursing or medicine, many of the newer programs have sprung up in institutions without a long history of health professions education. One possible

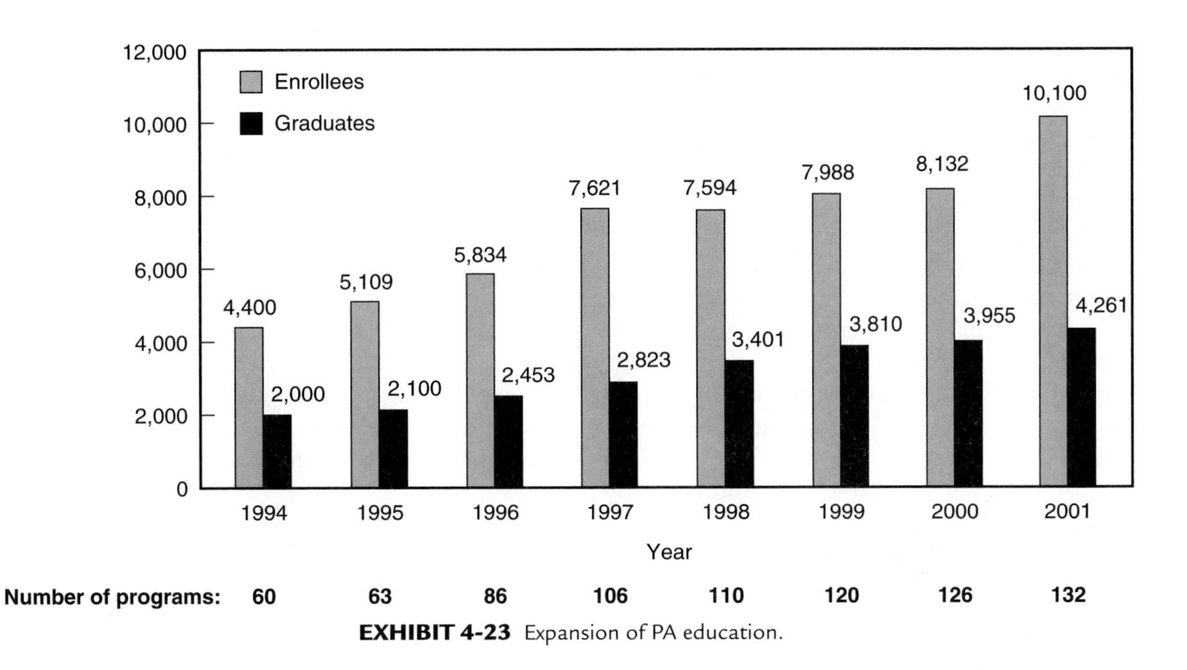

EXHIBIT 4-23 Expansion of PA education.

downside of this expansion is that it could lead to an oversupply of PAs in the medical marketplace. Should this circumstance come to pass, it would replicate past experiences observed in other professions in which a time of demand led to a period of rapid expansion of educational programs, which subsequently overshot the mark in terms of meeting supply requirements. In our society, academic institutions operate in a very competitive environment, and to survive and prosper, they must seize perceived opportunities to train needed future workers.

During the 1990s the attractiveness of the PA health professions was not lost on many university deans and vice presidents, a number of whom saw these new prospering professions as a means of rebuilding or revitalizing sagging departments or schools. Whether or not from the point of view of the nation's health workforce there was a real need for an increase in the supply of health care providers, the outcome was an uncoordinated expansion. This expansion perhaps was good for some schools in the short run but may likely be detrimental for the respective professions in the long run. The expansion of PA and NP education in the 1990s is viewed as noteworthy in terms of promotion of educational curriculum diversity innovation. It may be the beginning of a peak-trough cycle of demand for these health care professionals.

PHYSICIAN ASSISTANT GRADUATES

APAP annual reports are also useful in looking at the outcomes of the PA education process over time. Each of the reports describes the outcomes of a graduating cohort and contains the reported level of unemployment, defined as the number of graduates still looking for a job as a PA at the time of the survey. Because each survey is performed at the same time of year, this measurement is useful in tracking year-to-year changes. In the decade covered by the sixth through the seventeenth report, unemployment of the graduating class averaged 7.0%. The lowest rate of 4.5% was reported for the graduating class of 1992, and the highest was for the most recent class of 2000 at 5%.

The average starting salary for new graduates increased from $31,352 in 1989 to $68,757 in 2001. The average starting salary increased every year from 1989 to 2002, and the average annual increase was 7.6% over the last decade. The highest annual increase was from 1989 to 1990 (14.4%), and the smallest in 1997 to 1998 (1.2%)

SUMMARY

PA education entered its thirty-seventh year in 2002. It was created by several key visionaries in U.S. academic medicine and then grew and developed through the coordinated efforts of organized medicine, educational institutions, and federal government, and later the support of the PA profession's organizations. PA programs have become well established in academic health centers and other health-related institutions of higher learning across the country. This education has been characterized as a great experiment in medical education with a right to lay claim to a long string of medical curricular and provider deployment innovations, particularly in primary care. After 35 years PA educational programs in the United States have developed a well-respected system of accreditation and have been a prominent and long-term fixture in federal legislative primary care training initiatives.

One of the most dominant trends in PA education in the 1990s was the marked expansion of the numbers of programs, in addition to the graduates' recent resolution of the issue of the academic credential awarded on completion of PA studies. Yet despite these achievements and the significant recognition of the PA profession evident in U.S. medical education, there remain a number of challenges facing programs and sponsoring institutions. Some of these challenges have been brought about by the constantly changing forces in the U.S. health care delivery system and in educational institutions. The PA profession and PA education are also experiencing a significant demographic shift with most students and practicing graduates now women. This demographic has only recently taken place and will shape the PA profession and PA education to a significant degree in the coming years.

PA education has long enjoyed the support of the federal government. There is a 30-year history of inclusion in PHS Title VII funding through the PA Grant Award Program administered by the division of primary care in the BHPr of the Health Services and Resources Administration. Periodically there have been threats to the levels of federal funding for Title VII programs. Federal funding has been important to the growth and institutionalization of many PA educational programs in the United States.

Federal external support has boosted the basic operation and special activities such as creative recruitment and retention strategies, primary care training approaches, and cost-effective operation. A number of other notable trends also affect PA education, namely, falling applicant numbers. Although undoubtedly the marked recent expansion of the numbers of PA programs and available seats in PA programs help explain this trend, it may also reflect a dampening interest among the PA applicant pool. The APAP has recently established a centralized application service. Additional issues facing PA educational programs are the related forces of the loss/competition for clinical training sites, managed care, and payment for clinical student training.

There is also the institutional issue of the lack of PA faculty with tenure and senior rank appointments. In 2000 only one quarter of PA faculty were in tenure-stream positions and 6.5% held tenure. Among the senior ranks, less than 15% held the rank of associate professor and 2% held the rank of professor.

Perhaps the most significant trend within PA education is the general resolution of the issue of the academic credential to be awarded upon completion of PA studies. PA education now seems to be set at the graduate level and new programs will develop as master's programs.

The course taken by PA education will guide the fortunes of the PA profession. The PA profession will continue to travel successfully through the maze known as the U.S. health care system, and the journey will be dynamic.

5

PRIMARY CARE

INTRODUCTION

Primary care is the entry point for most people into the U.S. health care system. Not surprisingly, primary care disorders make up the vast majority of all medical conditions seen by health care providers. A substantial amount of research documents that physician assistants (PAs) are ideally suited and well qualified to deliver primary care services. PAs are trained to diagnose and treat most primary care conditions, and a substantial proportion of clinical PAs work in the primary care disciplines. In terms of medical specialties, primary care is defined as family medicine, general internal medicine, and general pediatrics. To most the term *primary care* is synonymous with ambulatory care because less than 0.5% of all conditions seen in primary care result in hospitalization.

The major focus of medical education for PA students is primary care, as is the case for medical students and most nurse practitioners (NPs). Curricula for the would-be primary care clinician are organized so that the graduate can manage most medical conditions in a typical community with a normal distributed population. Primary care forms the basis on which other areas of medicine rest. In PA education the student learns the principles and practice of primary care medicine. Those principles are often incorporated within other specialties, and in turn, specialties develop principles that are adopted in primary care. To understand this crucial role, which PAs have increasingly helped to define, we must first define *primary care.*

Primary Care Defined

Primary care is the provision of integrated accessible health care services by clinicians who are accountable for meeting most personal health care needs, developing a sustained partnership with patients, and practicing in the context of family and community. Primary care comprises medical care services that are characterized by the following attributes: (1) first-contact care, (2) longitudinality, (3) coordination, and (4) comprehensiveness (Starfield, 1993).

Evolution of Physician Assistants as Primary Care Specialists

PAs are health care professionals who assume roles in the U.S. health care system in providing primary care services. The initial mission of the creation of PAs was not specifically to become primary care providers but was to support and augment the general services of the physician, regardless of specialty. The fundamental role of the PA as a clinician was initially described as one designed to examine and gather clinical information on the patient.

For over 3 decades the federal government policies and state legislation have encouraged the use of PAs. The result has been an impressive production of health care services in the United States. Hooker and McCaig (2001) analyzed primary care physician office encounter data from the 1995 to 1999 National Ambulatory Medical Care Surveys. About one quarter of primary care office-based physicians used PAs or NPs for an average of 11% of visits. There were remarkably few differences in the types of patients, diagnoses made, and treatment rendered by the three providers. The mean age of patients seen by physicians was greater than that for PAs or NPs. NPs provided counseling and education during a higher proportion of visits than PAs or physicians. These aside, overall this study suggests that PAs and NPs are providing primary care in a way that is similar to physician care.

In the U.S. health care system, it is estimated that there were approximately 1 billion outpatient visits in 1999 (combination of federal and nonfederal medical sites, urgent and nonurgent). Approximately 60% were broadly defined as "primary care" (internal medicine, family practice, pediatrics, and obstetrics and gynecology [OB/GYN]). This care is provided in a wide variety of clinical settings. This study, consolidating 5 years of data collection, demonstrates little difference between the types of patients these providers see and the care they render. Extrapolating what is known about the productivity and distribution of PAs and NPs a conservative estimate is that they account for 11% of all U.S. ambulatory visits (Hooker and McCaig, 2001).

As the concept matured, the role of the PA transformed from merely assisting the primary care physician to one of close interdependence with the physician employer. This evolution was not planned, yet this outcome was an inevitable product of delegation and expansion of duties that occurs in almost any apprenticeship.

In the beginning the role of the PA was conceived to be one in which the PA would initially see the patient and then present the major finding to the physician. Together they would complete the patient visit. Usually the physician would be the one to decide on the final diagnosis and treatment and then delegate aspects of further diagnostic or treatment plan. The PA performs the diagnostic or treatment plan based on the PA's level of experience and skill, as well as the degree of trust between the PA and the physician. A further evolution of the PA role, now commonplace, is that the PA sees the patient without having the physician present for any part of the visit. With experience and trust, particularly in primary care practice in which the patient's problems are routine and typically straightforward, the physician-PA relationship develops. This is the point at which the physician may delegate a good portion of diagnostic and treatment responsibilities without the physician seeing or reviewing each patient.

In some instances patients will preferentially request to be seen by the PA. As the physician's confidence becomes reinforced by the skill and negotiated performance autonomy of the PA, the PA may be delegated more advanced work tasks (Schneller and Simon, 1977). In some practices PAs assume primary responsibility for the management of patients with chronic diseases such as hypertension and diabetes.

Today in many cases the PA in a practice may tend to most common primary care disorders and may have more experience with these conditions than the associated physicians in the same setting. In some instances a recently trained physician who is more familiar with hospital care than ambulatory care may employ a more experienced outpatient-based PA. In these cases there are clearly trade-offs as to who can do what better. As the PA profession and PA educational programs evolve, there will likely be increasing emphasis on independent evaluation and management of common primary care disorders by the PA.

Federal Policy

The intent of federal health policy was and continues to be to utilize PAs in primary care. The initial conceptualization of PAs was that they would work with either generalists or specialists in augmenting physician services. Evidence to date shows that this has been a policy device that is accomplishing its goals. PAs are helping to ease the maldistribution of physicians by delivering primary care to many areas in which access is difficult and physicians are not likely to practice.

Some of the early PA programs focused on supporting the generalist physician in rural areas such as the Medex program and the PA program at Alderson-Broaddus College while others prepared PAs for broader roles. At the other end of the spectrum were programs whose mission included training PAs to meet the needs of specialist physicians and in hospital settings. However, in 1973 federal incentives were established to provide training in primary care, and that policy has shaped many PA programs.

The deployment of PAs in primary care continues to be a sound policy to many observers. In the 1970s most PAs were employed in some type of primary care practice or ambulatory setting and seemed to be fulfilling the ideals of their creators (Lawrence, 1978; Steinwachs et al., 1986). Some of the early studies of PAs in communities in which they served demonstrated improvement in the health status of patients beyond what was present before their arrival. Other benefits of PA employment appeared because studies suggested health care costs were cheaper and the financial viability of the clinic's office improved (Greenfield et al., 1978; Hooker, 2000).

In 1978 the Institute of Medicine (IOM) issued a major report on primary care. This report recommended that PAs and NPs be given an important role in the delivery of primary care. The IOM study was wide sweeping and included recommendations on a number of important issues such as PA prescriptive practices, third-party reimbursement, and enabling legislation (Peterson, 1980). These findings were endorsed by the American College of Physicians and were reiterated in many health care policy reports over the next few years (Burnett, 1980; Record, 1981a).

By the early 1980s the differences in roles between PAs and physicians in primary care were blurring. Both seemed to be providing similar services in many settings such as rural practices, health maintenance organizations (HMOs), and public health clinics (Nelson, 1982; Repicky, Mendenhall, and Neville, 1982; Hooker, 1986; Steinwachs et al., 1986). Based on the observations the following health care policy question arose: What is the appropriate balance of the primary health care workforce between family practice physicians, PAs, and NPs? These studies all examined the use and contributions that PAs and NPs can make in primary care practices. One idea emanating from these studies is the estimate of primary care staffing that PAs can provide. Compared with the physician service in question, PA/NP staffing ratios ranged from 20% in pediatric services to 50% in adult services (Salmon and Stein, 1986; Steinwachs et al., 1986; Synowiez, 1986; Johnson, Hooker, and Freeborn, 1988; Hooker, 2000). These researchers believed that PAs could be substituted for a physician in a practice for 20% to 50% of services.

How much of the clinical primary care function can a PA assume? Record et al. (1981) examined a representative population of patients managed by physicians and PAs in primary care in a large HMO. Using a number of conservative assumptions, she determined that PAs could manage at least 83% of all primary care encounters (Record et al., 1981). Follow-up investigations by Hooker (1986) and Hooker and Freeborn (1991) found that based on diagnoses rendered, there was a 90% overlap in types of patients managed by physicians and PAs in the departments of internal medicine and family practice.

Additional evidence showed that PAs could assume a wide variety of medical care services that had been the traditional domain of primary care physicians. By the 1990s there was compelling evidence not only that PAs could expand the delivery of primary care services going unfilled by physicians, but also that national policies should be promulgated to promote this trend (Schroeder, 1992; Osterweis and Garfinkel, 1993). This was never more clearly expressed than in President Clinton's attempt to reform health care and improve primary care delivery in the mid 1990s (Health Security Act of 1993). The intent of this legislation was to expand the role of primary care PAs, NPs, and certified nurse midwives (CNMs).

Primary care is a raison d'être of the PA profession. A focus on primary care was in large part responsible for the profession's development and remains a major theme of PA education. In 2001 approximately half of PAs in practice are in the federally designated primary care specialties of internal medicine, general and family medicine, and general pediatrics. Some argue that many primary care services are provided by PAs who are working in clearly defined specialty areas such as correctional medicine and public health. If the percentages of PAs in clinical practice working in emergency medicine (10.1%), women's health care (2.5%), industrial medicine and occupational medicine (3.6%), and geriatrics (1%) are included, the percentage of PAs engaged to some degree in primary care clinical activities approaches two thirds (Exhibit 5-1).

The most frequently reported principal diagnoses in primary care are featured in Exhibit 5-2. These data are drawn from a national study on the content of ambulatory visits undertaken in 1999. The first 20 diagnoses are those most frequently observed in ambulatory care and

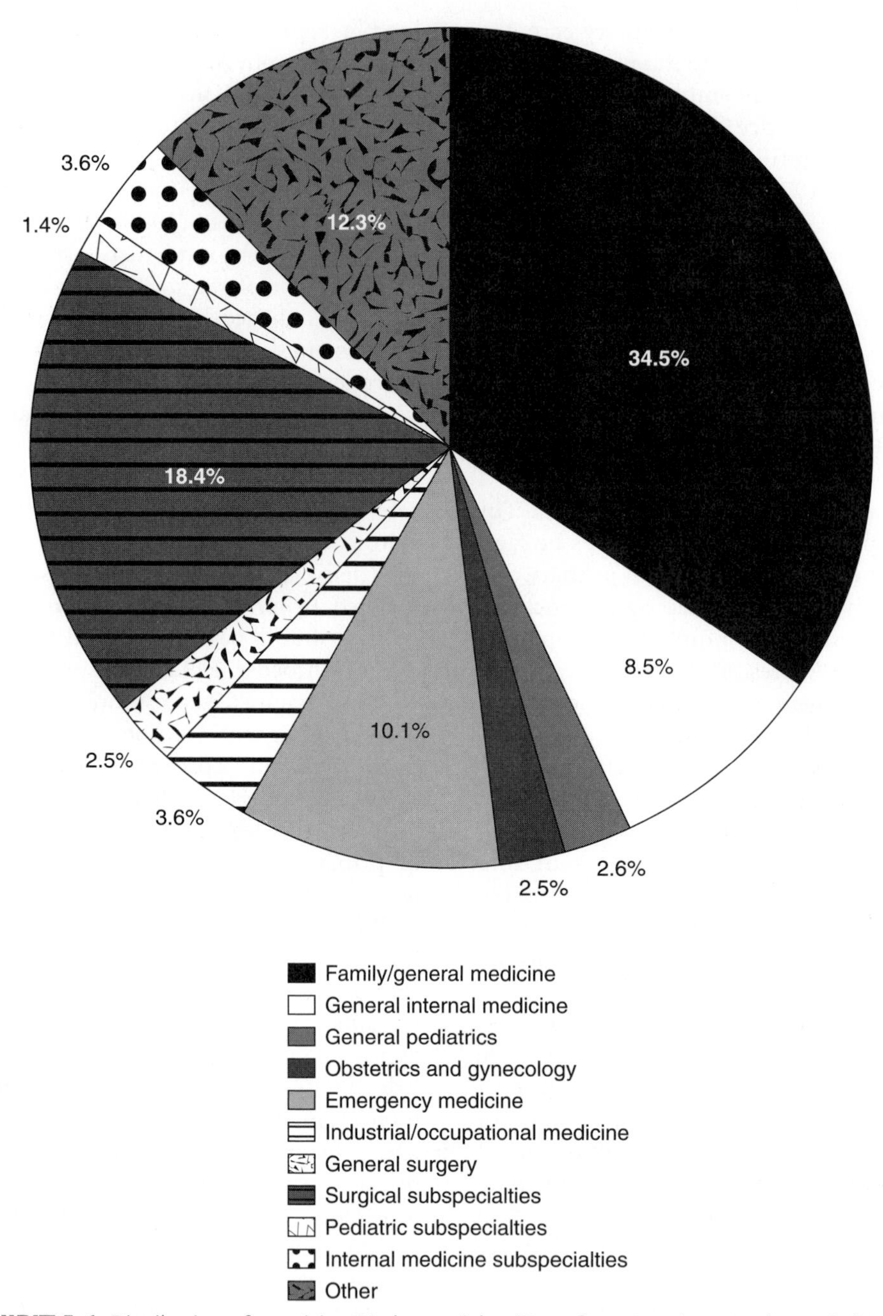

EXHIBIT 5-1 Distribution of practicing PAs by specialty. (Data from American Academy of Physician Assistants, *AAPA Physician Assistant Census Report,* 2001.)

account for 37.4% of all office visits made during 2000 (Cherry and Woodwell, 2002).

PAs are commonly used in roles as primary care providers by a wide variety of health care organizations and in various settings such as the following:

- Multispecialty group practices expanding primary care service delivery
- Managed care organizations expanding primary care capacities
- Private rural systems of care delivery and small community hospitals seeking to extend ambulatory care and primary care services
- Public health clinic settings, community and migrant health centers, and rural health clinics (RHCs)

EXHIBIT 5-2

Distribution of Office Visits by the Most Common Principal Diagnosis Groups, United States, 2000

Rank	Most common principal diagnosis	Percentage
1	Essential hypertension	4.2
2	Acute upper respiratory infections, excluding pharyngitis	3.8
3	Arthropathies and related disorders	3.1
4	Routine infant or child health check	3.0
5	Diabetes mellitus	2.6
6	Dorsopathies	2.3
7	Allergic rhinitis	2.2*
8	Normal pregnancy	2.2
9	Rheumatism, excluding back	2.2
10	Malignant neoplasms	2.0
11	Otitis media and eustachian tube disorders	1.9
12	Follow-up examination	1.8
13	General medical examination	1.8
14	Cataract	1.5
15	Chronic sinusitis	1.4
16	Heart disease, excluding ischemic	1.3
17	Ischemic heart disease	1.3
18	Potential health hazards related to personal and family history	1.3
19	Asthma	1.3
20	Benign and uncertain neoplasms	1.2
	All other diagnoses	57.9

Data from Cherry DK, Woodwell DA: *The National Ambulatory Medical Care Survey of 2000,* Hyattsville, MD, 2002, National Center for Health Statistics.

* Figure does not meet standard of reliability or precision.

- Clinical settings in which they may provide clinical preventive services, and wellness and preventive care (i.e., private clinics)
- Geriatric facilities, occupational and work site health settings
- Correctional health systems
- University and college student health facilities
- Residency programs

Physician Assistants as Primary Care Providers: Making the Case

PAs have clearly become a part of the U.S. primary care workforce. To what degree will they be the providers in future health care delivery scenarios? Central to any discussion of health care system policy is the question of workforce supply, distribution, and use. The imbalance of specialist physicians, the growth of managed care, and the issues affecting various types of health care personnel take on greater importance in a changing market-driven environment. All of this has spurred a critical reexamination of the roles, accountability, cost-effectiveness, and social responsibility of our nation's health care professionals.

A number of interacting influences in the health care workforce explain why the practices of PAs differ so much. One reason is that the demand for PA services is related to external factors such as state licensing and regulation policy, which affect both the scope of practice and the prescribing authority. Primary care PAs working in states where legislation enables wider latitude with regard to physician supervisory requirements may be used more effectively (Sekscenski et al., 1994). Another influence is the market forces that shape the demand for PAs to assume different roles than those for which one was originally trained (Hooker, 1992).

The Council on Graduate Medical Education defines primary care as "characterized by first-contact care for patients with undifferentiated health concerns; patient-centered comprehensive care that is not organ-specific or problem-specific; continuous, longitudinal patient care; and coordination of necessary medical, social, mental, and other services through appropriate consultation and referral" (Cawley, 1995). While there is contention about who should provide primary care, there is also debate regarding the range and content of the clinical activities and tasks specific to primary care practice. Some believe that primary care is more than just a set of specialty-defined clinical tasks; it involves an integrated system of health care services delivery. Such care comprises most of the health care services required by various populations (Starfield, 1993). In the mid 1990s, a study of primary care in the United States, by the IOM Committee on the Future of Primary Care, proposed an alternative definition of primary care.

> Effectiveness of primary care delivery depends, at least in part, on using the correct mix of health care personnel. Starfield (1993) has shown that this maximizes the clinical capabilities of health care professionals. In primary care practice, it is neither necessary nor particularly efficient for each patient to be seen by a physician (Perry, 1985). Since PAs are, by definition, physician-supervised clinicians, the very nature of their clinical role is to work with physicians in collaborative interdisciplinary settings (Donaldson et al., 1996b).

A number of physician and nonphysician health care professional groups have laid claim to the title of primary care (such as obstetricians and NPs, asserting that they should be included as primary care providers). Attempts to answer the question of which types of physicians should be defined as primary care providers have prompted systematic analyses of the competencies of various physician specialists to provide the range of medical and preventive care services required (Mullan, Rivo, and Politzer, 1993). The conclusion was that only the disciplines of general or family practice, internal medicine, and general pediatrics fulfilled all of the criteria to be considered primary care disciplines.

Using these same criteria the competency of PAs to provide primary care was assessed by Hooker and Cawley (1997). A matrix identified educational preparation, clinical practice, and professional certification measures of competency in the provision of primary care. Four national data sources were used as indicators of PA clinical practice performance and competency in primary care: educational preparation, national certification examination content, profession-defined role delineation, and actual data on use. The data overwhelmingly indicate that PAs are educated well enough to function as primary care providers and are successfully performing a large proportion of tasks typically required in primary care (Mullan, Rivo, and Politzer, 1993).

DELINEATION OF THE ROLE OF THE PHYSICIAN ASSISTANT

PAs are aware of the need to communicate what goes on in clinical practice with the designers of educational programs and the certification examinations. As a new profession, it requires particularly strong self-evaluation to determine how it has evolved from the original concept. This is accomplished by role delineation studies. Through role delineation studies the PA profession became codified and set into a structured framework of rules and regulations to convince those early innovators that taking an assistant into the physician's practice would be safe and convenient and would not threaten patient confidence.

Role delineation studies are a fundamental way in which information about the professional activity of an occupation is gathered and analyzed. Nine general clusters of activities are common to PA practice across specialty lines:

- Gathering data
- Seeing common problems and diseases
- Conducting laboratory and diagnostic studies
- Performing management activities
- Performing surgical procedures
- Managing emergency situations
- Conducting health promotion and disease prevention activities
- Prescribing medications
- Using interpersonal skills

Role Delineation for the New Century

In 1998 the National Commission on Certification of Physician Assistants (NCCPA) conducted a detailed study of the knowledge, skills, and abilities important for safe and effective PA practice. The purpose of the NCCPA's Practice Analysis was to update and revalidate the content blueprints for NCCPA certifying and recertifying examinations. Results of the study (1) revealed the tasks and essential knowledge and skills that are representative of the actual clinical practice roles of PAs; (2) identified differences in the practices of entry-level PAs and seasoned professionals; and (3) determined the tasks, knowledge, skills, and abilities that are specific to PA practice in primary care and in specialty areas. This work continues the efforts by the National Board of Medical Examiners, which conducted early role delineation studies in the beginning of the 1970s and by the American Academy of Physician Assistants (AAPA) in 1979 and 1985.

The NCCPA's study was based on a sample of practicing PAs and examined their professional roles and functions. It also examined the frequency of specific medical activities and determined the required knowledge and skills deemed most important to PA clinical practice.

The distribution of responses (47%) by demographic variables and by clinical specialty and setting indicates that survey respondents reflect the same profile observed in other national surveys of PAs. Two thirds (66%) of survey respondents were in practice as a PA for more than 6 years, 21% practiced between 3 and 6 years, and 13% practiced up to 2 years. More than one fourth (28%) worked in three or more specialty areas.

Results identified the domains of knowledge most important for PAs:

- Subjective data gathering
- Assessment
- Objective data gathering
- Formulation and implementation of plans
- Clinical intervention procedures
- Health promotion and disease prevention
- Ancillary professional responsibilities

Overall, survey responses showed few differences in the tasks performed by PAs based on the length of time worked in the profession. Response patterns differing across specialties were noted, particularly in the areas of cardiovascular and thoracic surgery, general surgery, and orthopedic surgery. The knowledge and skill areas rated most highly by practicing PAs were as follows:

- Skill in identifying pertinent physical findings
- Knowledge of signs and symptoms of medical conditions
- Skill in recognizing conditions that constitute medical emergencies
- Skill in performing physical examinations
- Skill in conducting a patient interview (Exhibit 5-3)
- Knowledge of conditions that constitute medical emergencies
- Skill in associating current complaints with presenting history and identifying pertinent factors
- Knowledge of physical examination directed to a specific condition
- Knowledge of physical examination techniques
- Skill in effective communication

Results of the NCCPA study reveal that PAs engage in and highly value those tasks essential for clinical practice. There were consistently high ratings in terms of both frequency and importance for the bread-and-butter functions of PA clinicians: history taking and physical diagnosis. The expected knowledge areas required for practice are consistent with competencies identified in previous surveys. PAs also value additional skills required in the practice of clinical medicine: diagnostic acumen and judgment and knowledge in the development of an effective management plan. The consistency and high ratings of these findings suggest that there is a central core of medical knowledge, tasks, and skills valued that is performed often and consistently by practicing PAs. This core of knowledge and skills appears to apply to virtually all specialties and settings.

This work reveals a picture of PAs as professionals who have a great deal in common with physicians in terms of obtaining subjective and objective patient data, reviewing and interpreting diagnostic tests, formulating diagnoses, establishing or implementing treatment plans,

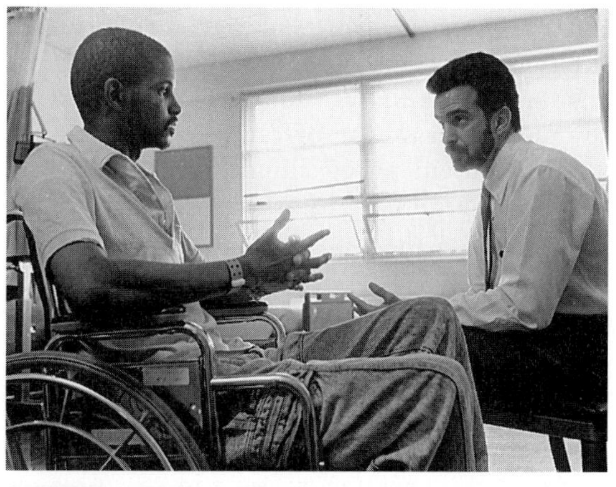

EXHIBIT 5-3 Conducting a patient interview. (Courtesy American Academy of Physician Assistants.)

prescribing certain medications, and providing patient education, counseling, and follow-up care. PAs also engage in many specialized practice activities. There are wide individual differences in the specific clinical interventions and procedures performed by PAs in different practice settings. PAs perform procedures in widely varied practice domains, but it is clear that all PAs do not perform procedures in all areas. However, PAs rated the knowledge and skills required for clinical procedures and interventions as important (except for knowledge of advanced surgical equipment). This may reflect PA willingness to be trained in and to perform whatever procedures are appropriate and required by the particular physician or practice setting (Cawley et al., 2001).

Clinical Practice Guidelines

At times, protocols have been developed in an attempt to standardize the performance of the PA and to ensure physicians and patients that medical treatment provided by the new health care practitioner would be adequate. These protocols were written statements that began with the patient's presenting complaint and follow step-by-step through the questions that should be asked, the tests that should be run, and the medications that should be prescribed. There cannot be a protocol for every situation, but hundreds were written by PA educators and physicians and were used extensively in training and practice. With time these protocols have been replaced by practice guidelines.

Clinical practice guidelines have become standard fare for many medical providers as managed care and corporate interests transform the U.S. health care system. Along with guidelines come corporate mandates for efficient use of resources, assessment of provider productivity, and measurement of clinical outcomes. The courts are beginning to ask providers to justify their medical decisions matched against published clinical guidelines.

Guidelines for providing medical care are not a new idea. The experiences of individual physicians and opinions of professors in medical schools, medical textbooks, clinical journals, and clinical trials have guided the practice of medicine for most of the twentieth century. This tendency toward standardization is not necessarily a bad idea. The medical community has always standardized medical care to some degree to provide what it thought was the best care, efficiently use resources, satisfy patients, and withstand third-party scrutiny. The level of standardization in today's guidelines is relatively new. When predicated on sound medical and scientific data, these guidelines can lessen provider variability in treatment and diagnosis. Evidence-based medicine and standardization improves measurement of resources used and assessment of benefits obtained. These guidelines can be particularly effective when applied to high-prevalence, high-cost diseases or conditions.

Guidelines come from many sources, including professional medical societies, health-related associations, and governmental authorities. In the U.S. health care system, among the most prominent organizations that promulgate clinical practice guidelines is the Practice Guidelines Partnership (PGP), composed of 13 national medical specialties societies, the American Medical Association, the Agency for Healthcare Research and Quality (AHRQ), the American Hospital Association (AHA), the Joint Commission on Accreditation of Healthcare Organizations (JCAHO), and the Center for Medicare and Medicaid Services (CMS) (www.ama-assn.org/ama/pub/category/2936.html).

For PAs in practice, it is neither desirable nor common for them to practice strictly according to written practice protocols. Practice management systems can serve as an initial "security blanket" in the PA's clinical practice until the supervising physician's confidence is sufficient to allow the PA to develop competent clinical skills and judgment. As the physician becomes comfortable with the PA's performance, there appears to be less concern with the external supports that inform the assistant of correct procedures. Consequently, the PA develops a necessary sense of clinical judgment and critical thinking, particularly knowing when the patient needs to be referred to the physician.

FAMILY MEDICINE

More PAs identify their practice as family medicine than any other. In 2001 more than one third of PAs who responded to the AAPA Census identified family or general practice as the specialty they practiced for their primary employer. No studies have been done to identify all the specific activities of PAs in family medicine. PAs enjoy strong support from family physicians, as evidenced by past statements by the American Academy of Family Practice (AAFP) affirming PA capabilities working with physicians in the delivery of primary care services. Recently several postgraduate training programs have emerged for PAs in family practice, so-called PA residencies, providing graduate PAs an additional year of clinical education in this specialty.

GENERAL INTERNAL MEDICINE

In 2002 approximately one tenth of all PAs in clinical practice identified general internal medicine as the specialty they work in for their primary employer. Internal medicine physician groups, as expressed in published statements of the American College of Physicians (ACP), support the role of PAs working in general internal medicine. Like internists, PAs in internal medicine have practices skewed toward geriatrics.

PEDIATRICS

General pediatrics is considered one of the three specialties that comprise primary care, but attention to pediatrics in this arena is often overshadowed by adult primary care. The role of PAs in child care has a rich history, much of it derived from the child health associate (CHA) program at the University of Colorado. This program was developed by Henry K. Silver and Loretta Ford in the 1960s.

In the 1970s Silver, among others, conducted studies examining the roles and capabilities of the pediatric PA in general and the CHA in particular. They found that CHAs provided a wide range of diagnostic, preventive, and therapeutic services in pediatrics. CHAs and pediatric PAs demonstrated knowledge and skill to care for more than 90% of patients seen in a pediatric practice (Fine and Silver, 1973; Silver, 1973a; Fine, 1977a, 1977b; Fine and Scriven, 1977). When compared with pediatric residents and medical students, CHA students demonstrated a comparable level of factual knowledge in the pertinent basic sciences and clinical pediatrics (Fine and Machotka, 1973; Machotka et al., 1973; Ott et al., 1974). Patient acceptance and the quality of care associated with pediatric PAs and CHAs are high (Wallen et al., 1982) (Exhibit 5-4).

One study of CHA care reported favorable marks by all mothers surveyed. Almost all (90%) indicated a desire to have their children cared for by a CHA (Dungy, 1975). In spite of the research that demonstrates that pediatric PAs and NPs are widely accepted by the parents of patients and can perform well when compared with

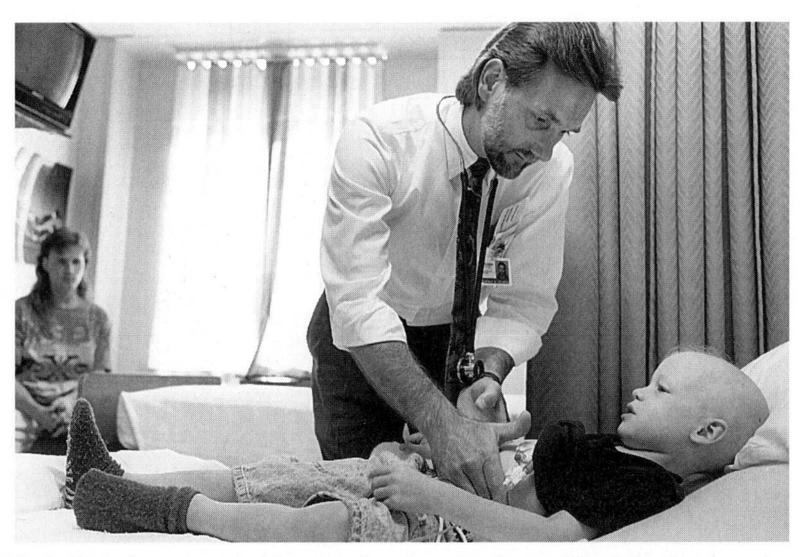

EXHIBIT 5-4 Clinical assessment. (Courtesy American Academy of Physician Assistants.)

physicians, the physicians are still slow to accept them as additions to their pediatric staff (Dungy and Silver, 1977; Silver et al., 1981).

As of 2000 there does not appear to be any increase in numbers of pediatricians being trained. To confront the challenges of providing quality health care services to more children with more diverse and difficult problems, pediatricians will increasingly have to rely on PAs and NPs to perform many of these tasks (Stone, 1995). This may give rise to more collaborative teams of pediatricians and PAs and/or NPs, along with more involvement of nurses. Shifting of pediatric services to family medicine will also continue.

WOMEN'S HEALTH

Some researchers include the field of OB/GYN as part of primary care. PAs have practiced in teams with physicians for more than 30 years, providing a broad range of OB/GYN and primary care services to women in outpatient and inpatient settings. In 2002 nearly 1200 PAs practice exclusively in the field of OB/GYN. Thousands of other PAs across the spectrum of medical and surgical specialties provide primary and specialty care to women. Studies have shown that these PAs provide cost-effective physician-quality medical care with high levels of productivity and patient acceptance. PAs' general medical education orientation allows them to provide the primary care services many obstetricians and gynecologists seek to offer their patients in this era of proliferating managed care. Many PAs work in practices in which women would be likely to receive their primary medical care.

Most OB/GYN PAs practice in outpatient settings. About 81% of OB/GYN PAs see outpatients exclusively; another 14% see outpatients and inpatients. The remaining 5% see only inpatients. PAs in OB/GYN work in family planning centers, solo physician offices, group practices, rural clinics, urban clinics, community health centers, hospital outpatient clinics, urgent care centers, HMOs, and other settings where care is delivered (AAPA, 2001).

The work of PAs in outpatient women's health or OB/GYN settings is as diverse as the work of OB/GYN physicians. PAs provide both obstetric and gynecologic care, including comprehensive annual gynecologic examinations. PAs evaluate and manage common gynecologic conditions, including contraception, vaginal infections, sexually transmitted diseases, and menopausal problems. Many PAs are commonly included on teams that evaluate and treat infertility. They provide prenatal, intrapartum, and postpartum care. In addition to direct patient examination and treatment, PAs provide patient education and counseling on contraception, breast self-examination, prenatal care, childbirth, postnatal care and lactation, and other OB/GYN topics.

PAs also perform many procedures in OB/GYN, including but not limited to ultrasound, colposcopy, cryotherapy, intrauterine device insertion and removal, Norplant insertion and removal, insemination, endometrial and vulvar biopsies, and loop excision electrocoagulation procedure. In addition, many OB/GYN PAs who work in ambulatory practices have hospital privileges to first assist in surgeries, such as hysterectomies and cesarean sections.

With the growth of managed care plans, many obstetricians and gynecologists are providing more primary care. PAs are ideally suited to provide not only treatment of ambulatory gynecologic problems, but also primary care for women. Because they are educated as generalists, PAs are well prepared to handle conditions such as respiratory infections, headaches, mild hypertension, diabetes, and urinary tract infections, as well as to provide health promotion, disease prevention, and screening for women in all stages of life.

Use of PAs in obstetric practices also can be an effective way to keep the schedule on track when deliveries would otherwise disrupt the physician's schedule. PAs often share night and weekend call for deliveries, particularly in rural practices in which there may be only one physician to serve an entire community.

The success of teams providing cost-effective care depends not only on the support of management and providers but also on the support of patients. Numerous studies of patients reveal a high level of satisfaction with care provided by PAs.

In a 1994 study specific to OB/GYN practices, the Collaborative Practice Advisory Group of the American College of Obstetricians and Gynecologists surveyed 3257 patients in 10 practice settings to ascertain their satisfaction level with care provided in practices that use both physicians and PAs, NPs, CNMs or clinical nurse specialists. Patients felt these team practices provided quicker appointments (80.6%), more time with their provider (82.2%), and more health information (86%). "Few differences were evident in their perceptions of the care provided by physicians and nonphysicians." Patients perceived nonphysicians as being less rushed and spending more time with them than physicians. However, they perceived physicians as providing more complete information (Hankins et al., 1996).

HEALTH MAINTENANCE ORGANIZATIONS

HMOs have usually been quick to seize innovative, cost-containing measures. Their experience with nonphysician providers sharing and offsetting traditional physician responsibilities dates from the 1950s when optometrists began assuming the role of refraction from ophthalmologists, nurse anesthetists began assisting for anesthesiologists, and psychiatrists began shifting mental health patients to psychologists. It was not surprising that when PAs came along, HMOs embraced them.

Background of HMOs

Although HMOs have existed in the United States in some form since the first capitated plan was set up in Elk City, Oklahoma, in 1929, it has only been since the early 1970s that substantial numbers of U.S. citizens have had access to this alternative to traditional fee-for-service health care. Sidney Garfield, a physician hired by the industrialist Henry Kaiser in the 1930s, started the first prepaid group practice. Kaiser wanted to provide care to workers in the California desert building aqueducts to reach southern California communities. When World War II broke out, Dr. Garfield was recruited to provide the same type of worker health benefit to the Kaiser shipbuilders in Walnut Creek, California. A similar program was incorporated in the Kaiser shipyards of Vancouver, Washington (near Portland), under Dr. Ernest Saward. In 1945 with the cessation of the war and the release of workers to other jobs, the two Kaiser plans opened enrollment to the public.

In 1970 there were 39 prepaid group practices operating in the United States. At this time, most of the legal and political battles against this managed care option had been fought, yet few U.S. citizens had access to this kind of plan. The Health Maintenance Act of 1973 is generally credited to have been the impetus for an explosion of growth of HMOs. As a result, by 1985 there were 323 HMOs, and by 2000 there were more than 700. The number of preferred provider organizations today is almost double this amount (more than 1200) and growing. Beginning in the new century more than 100 million U.S. citizens are in some form of managed care plan. As HMOs have developed, several variations on their basic structure have evolved. The primary organizational type is the staff model, which is composed of salaried employees and providers and a group of beneficiaries whose health care is provided by the HMO. An example is Group Health Cooperative of Puget Sound. Similar in structure is the group model, which is organized by a prepaid population of patients; but the physicians are in a separate structure, usually as shareholders, which contract with the parent structure. Kaiser Permanente is the prototypical group model HMO. A third model, the network model, has characteristics of both of the other types.

Physician Assistants in HMOs

The first HMO to hire a formally trained PA was Kaiser Permanente, based in Portland, Oregon. In 1970 a Duke graduate PA was employed by the Department of Internal Medicine not only to assist in staffing but also to gain experience for future staffing needs (Lairson, Record, and James, 1974). This organization had experience with nurse midwives, psychologists, and nurse anesthetists and believed that PAs and NPs could be useful adjuncts to the primary care physician staff. Within a decade, 10 departments had incorporated a PA or NP, and 30 years from their first hire, more than 180 PAs and NPs work alongside 600 physicians to serve more than 450,000 members in this institution alone. Other Kaiser Permanente regions have similar staffing arrangements, and other classical model HMOs have followed suit.

In some HMOs the nonphysician providers are organized as a separate department such as the Department of Physician Assistants at the LaGuardia Medical Group in Queens, New York (Goldberg, 1983), or the Department of Physician Extenders at Geisinger Medical Center in Pennsylvania (Regan and Harbert, 1991), or as affiliated staff at Group Health Cooperative of Puget Sound. In others, they are incorporated within the departments that employ them and are considered representative members of that department (Hooker, 1993; Jacobson, Parker, and Coulter, 1998; Coulter, Jacobson, and Parker, 2000).

Various organizational theories have been postulated why HMOs employ PAs and NPs. The most reasonable explanation is HMOs and other types of managed care systems have strong incentives to contain personnel costs, and their structure and size provide the opportunity to capitalize on the economy of scale and division of labor that the use of PAs and NPs can offer.

Based on a 1994 survey of medium-sized plans (45,000 to 100,000 enrollees) and large plans (more than 100,000) by the Group Health Association of America (GHAA), a surprisingly high number of PAs and NPs were used in a representative number of group and staff model HMOs (Dial et al., 1995). In Exhibit 5-5 the median number of physicians ranges from 119 to 123 per 100,000 enrollees. In addition, the PA and NP ratios range from 10.6 to 15 per 100,000 enrollees. The PA/NP staffing ratios of about 30 per 100,000 must be taken into consideration when physician ratios are extrapolated as national requirements (Weiner, 1994).

Studies also show that NPs and PAs perform at rates of clinical productivity in a manner in which quality of care is maintained at levels that are "indistinguishable" from those of physician care. Their practice orientation tends to show an emphasis on interpersonal skills, patient education, and preventive care (IOM, 1978).

EXHIBIT 5-5

Full-Time Equivalent Provider per 100,000 Enrollees in Group/Staff Model HMOs

	NO. OF ENROLLEES	
Providers	**45,000-100,000 (12 plans)**	**More than 100,000 (16 plans)**
Total physicians	118.7	122.6
Primary care physicians	68.8	59.1
Specialty care physicians	49.9	63.5
Physician assistants	10.6	11.2
Nurse practitioners	15.0	14.6
Other advanced practice nurses	6.3	2.3

Data from Dial TH, Palsbo SE, Bergsten C, et al.: *J Am Acad Physician Assist* 14:168-180, 1995.

A number of studies have shown that a PA or NP can assume approximately 81% to 91% of the medical care in a primary care setting in an HMO (Record, 1981b; Hooker, 1993; Frampton and Wall, 1994; Hummel and Pirzada, 1994). Steinwachs and colleagues (1986) demonstrated that in one HMO, PAs and NPs tended to manage more acute diseases than chronic diseases. A study a decade later, however, showed that patients managed by PAs and physicians in adult primary care settings had a 90% overlap of diagnoses (Hooker, 1986).

Because PAs are cost-effective in the delivery of primary care services, two of the largest employers of PAs—the federal government and HMOs—have incorporated PAs and similar health care providers in clinical staffing. Managed care health delivery systems using PAs and similar providers gain certain economic advantages by using a team approach. HMOs are ideally suited to employ PAs and NPs because of the nature of preventive care, by stressing health education and disease prevention, and by carefully integrating both primary care and specialty care.

RURAL HEALTH

Access to health care in rural areas in the United States depends on a sufficient supply and distribution of primary care physicians, PAs, NPs, dentists, and a host of allied health care professions. Although physician supply and distribution have been the focus of this problem, in the late 1980s attention began shifting to the PA and NP as alternatives when it became apparent that many of them were successfully filling these rural provider roles (Office of Technology Assessment [OTA], 1990).

Approximately one third of PAs practice in communities with populations of 50,000 or less, and 18% are in rural areas with 10,000 or fewer people. Even so, more PAs are needed in these areas. The National Health Service Corps believes that PAs and NPs are critical to an effort to staff rural areas and has identified a number of strategies to employ more physicians, PAs, and NPs in primary care and rural areas.

Primary care and rural health were the two driving reasons for developing the PA concept, and PAs continue to be a vital part of the health care infrastructure that supports ambulatory and institutional care in rural areas. In 1977 the U.S. Congress enacted the Rural Health Clinics Act (Public Law [PL] 95-210) to encourage the use of nonphysician providers such as PAs, NPs, and CNMs in rural areas. This decision was based on a growing realization that many small communities could no longer support a sufficient number of physicians. PL 95-210 facilitated this goal by entitling various health providers to receive reimbursement from Medicare and Medicaid on a cost basis.

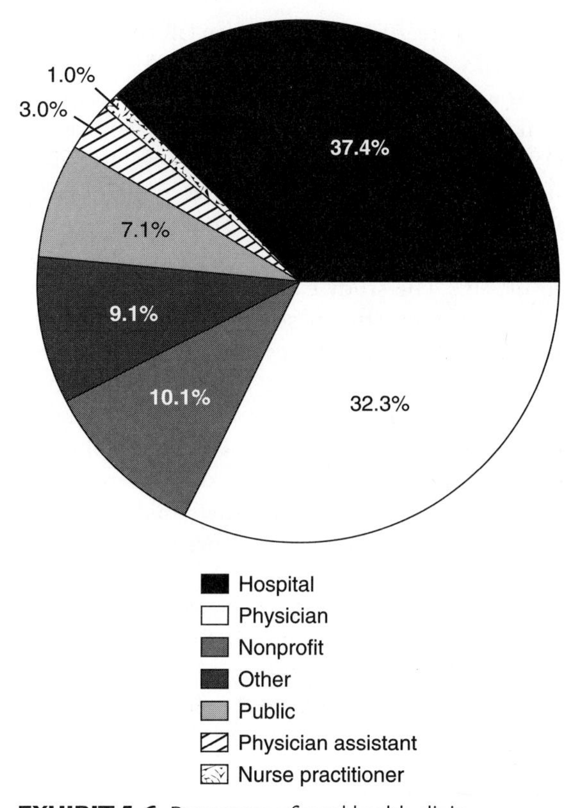

EXHIBIT 5-6 Percentage of rural health clinic ownership. (Modified from Rural Health Clinics First National Survey, 1994, Summary Report. Washington, DC, National Association of Rural Health Clinics.)

Rural Health Clinics

Certified RHCs are usually located in a health professional shortage area, a medically underserved area, or a governor-designated shortage area. Federally certified "independent" RHCs are reimbursed on a cost basis for their Medicare and Medicaid patients. Currently, RHCs make up one of the largest outpatient primary care programs for rural underserved communities and one of the fastest growing Medicare programs. By law they must be staffed by PAs, NPs, or CNMs at least half the time the clinic is open (www.narhc.org/legislative%20info.htm).

Physician-owned RHCs make up 32% of the clinics. Mostly hospitals and public and private companies own the rest (Exhibit 5-6). Sixty-six percent of RHCs employ one or more PAs, and 42% of them employ at least one NP.

Although RHCs are required to employ a PA, NP, or CNM, they may receive a waiver of this requirement for up to 1 year. Almost 19% of clinics have operated without a PA, NP, or CNM for some period. More than 18% of clinics had some problem keeping a PA, NP, or CNM. However, at the same time, more than 35% reported they had problems retaining health care professionals in general.

More recently evidence has emerged that PAs who remain in rural areas may differ from urban-based PAs. These studies indicate that PAs practicing in rural areas place considerably more importance on autonomy in selecting the location of their practice than other PAs, perhaps because they spend more time away from their supervising physician. They also have a significantly higher level of satisfaction with role and professional acknowledgment than urban-based PAs (Pan et al., 1996; Singer and Hooker, 1996; Larson, Hart, and Ballweg, 2000).

Another important issue to rural PAs is favorable reimbursement policy. Because state-to-state variability in compensation and Medicaid reimbursement laws affects PA deployment, increased efforts should be directed toward tailoring state policies to compensate PAs adequately (Pan et al., 1996).

As long as recruitment and retention of physicians in sparsely populated areas remains difficult, PAs will be sought in greater numbers to help fill this growing void, particularly in primary care. Federal and state initiatives are likely to increase recruitment of PAs to fill the needs of medically underserved America.

The retention of PAs in rural practices is quite striking. In a survey by Larson and colleagues (1999), PAs listed all the places they had practiced since completing their PA training, making it possible to classify the career histories of PAs as "all rural," "all urban," "urban to rural," or "rural to urban." The study examined the retention of PAs in rural practice at several levels: in the first practice, in rural practice overall, and by predominantly rural states. PAs who started their careers in rural locations were more likely to leave them during the first 4 years of practice than urban PAs, and female rural PAs were slightly more likely to leave than their male counterparts. Those starting in rural practice had high attrition and left for urban areas (41%); however, a significant proportion of the PAs who started in urban practice settings left for rural settings (10%). Because the proportion of urban PAs is so much larger than rural PAs, this kept the total proportion of PAs in rural practice at a steady 20%. Although 21% of the earliest graduates of PA training programs have had exclusively rural careers, only 9% of PAs with 4 to 7 years of experience have worked exclusively in rural settings (Exhibit 5-7). At the state level, generalist PAs were significantly more likely to leave states with practice environments unfavorable to PA practice in terms of prescriptive authority, reimbursement, and insurance (Larson et al., 1999).

Clinical Activities in Rural Family Medicine

A survey of Iowa family practice PAs was undertaken to identify the clinical activities they provide and how these skills and procedures compared with family practice physicians in the same state (Dehn and Hooker, 1999). All reported providing patient education, prescribing and dispensing medication, interpreting radiographs, referring patients, and providing a wide range of services (Exhibit 5-8).

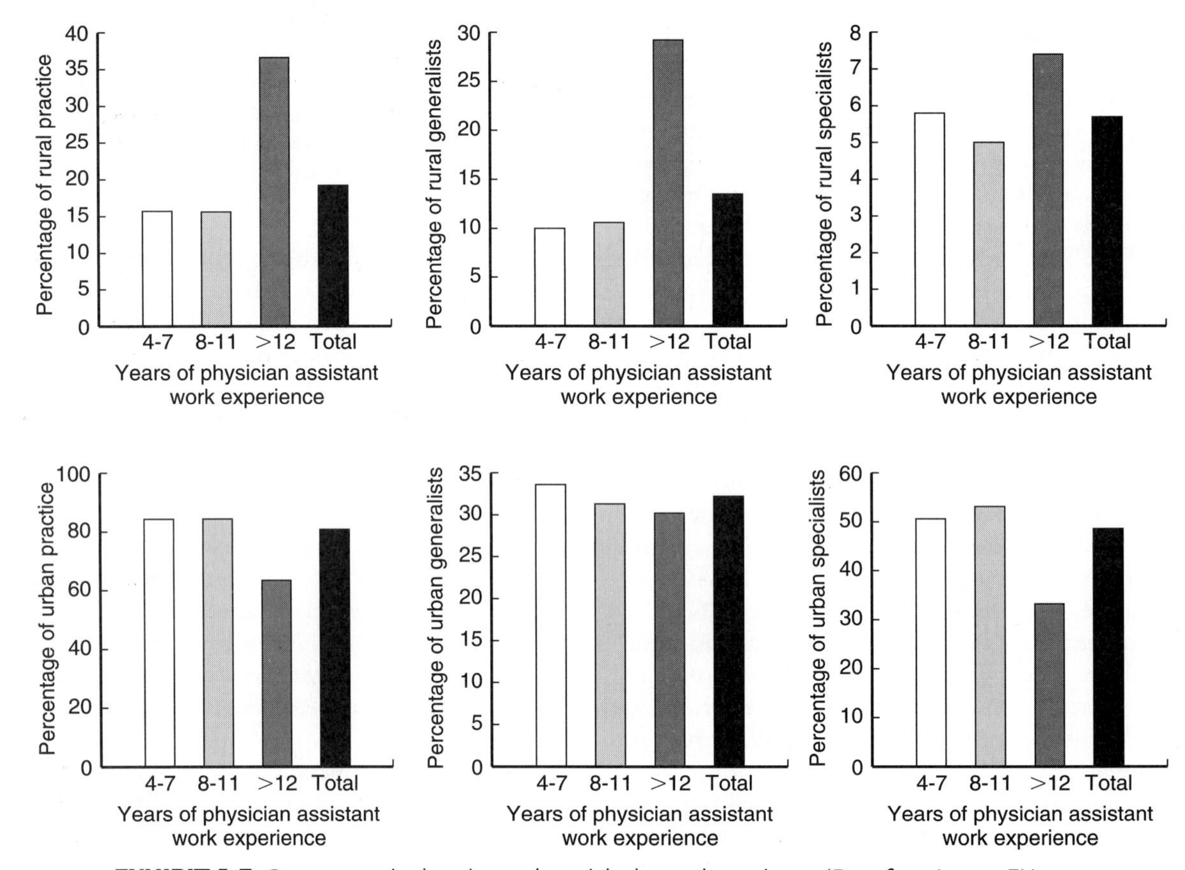

EXHIBIT 5-7 Current practice location and specialty by total experience. (Data from Larson EH, Hart LG, Goodwin MK, et al.: *J Rural Health* 15:391-402, 1999.)

EXHIBIT 5-8

Activities Performed by Iowa Family Practice PAs by Frequency (N = 55)

Clinical skill	Mean	(SD)
Patient education	3.95	(0.30)
Dispense medication	3.44	(1.23)
Make patient referrals directly to specialists	3.39	(0.68)
X-ray film interpretation	3.19	(1.18)
Electrotherapy or cryotherapy of the skin	2.92	(0.81)
Counseling for contraception	2.91	(0.83)
Manage depression by drug therapy	2.82	(0.88)
Counseling for smoking cessation	2.80	(0.88)
Repair and close laceration	2.75	(0.83)
Counseling for stress management	2.61	(0.76)
Electrocardiographic interpretation	2.60	(0.87)
Manage depression by counseling	2.53	(1.03)
Removal of small skin lesions	2.43	(0.82)
Psychologic counseling	2.42	(1.13)
Fluorescein eye examination or foreign body removal from eye	2.36	(0.65)
Perform vision screening	2.33	(1.39)
Use a microscope	2.15	(1.60)
Incision and drainage of abscess	2.09	(0.66)
Counseling for alcohol abuse	1.93	(0.80)
Provide care to patients in nursing homes	1.85	(1.47)
Evaluate wet mounts or potassium hydroxide stains yourself	1.84	(1.50)
Involved in personal management activities	1.81	(1.49)
Splinting and casting	1.78	(0.88)
Skin biopsy	1.73	(0.99)
Removal of ingrown toenail	1.71	(0.99)
Counseling for human immunodeficiency virus testing	1.63	(0.94)
Perform urinalysis yourself	1.56	(1.74)
Regional block with local anesthesia	1.49	(1.20)
Counseling for drug abuse	1.46	(0.88)
Venipuncture	1.25	(1.24)
Neonatal checks	1.19	(1.02)
Primary treatment of psychiatric illness (e.g., bipolar disorder, schizophrenia)	1.16	(1.10)
Nasal packing for epistaxis	1.13	(0.71)
Incise and drain external hemorrhoid	1.07	(0.77)
Provide care to patients in a home setting (house calls)	1.00	(1.03)
Perform audiometry	0.87	(1.18)
Low-risk prenatal care	0.85	(1.15)
Bladder catheterization	0.79	(0.57)
Administer pulmonary function test	0.78	(1.15)
Joint injection	0.68	(0.83)
Perform cardiopulmonary resuscitation	0.65	(0.62)
Perform advanced cardiac life support	0.65	(0.73)
Bartholin cyst drainage	0.64	(0.52)
Reduce fractures and dislocations	0.64	(0.73)
Diaphragm fitting	0.57	(0.64)
Arthrocentesis	0.55	(0.72)
Perform advanced trauma life support	0.55	(0.69)
Nasogastric tube placement	0.33	(0.58)
Endotracheal intubation	0.32	(0.51)
Arterial blood gas draw	0.31	(0.63)
Use a slitlamp	0.30	(0.64)
Perform breast mass aspiration	0.28	(0.49)
Norplant insertion/removal	0.25	(0.43)
Perform Gram stain	0.11	(0.37)
Central venous line placement	0.06	(0.23)
Chest tube placement	0.04	(0.19)

Continued

EXHIBIT 5-8

Activities Performed by Iowa Family Practice PAs by Frequency (N = 55)—*Cont'd*

Clinical skill	Mean	(SD)
Paracentesis or thoracentesis	0.04	(0.19)
Lumbar puncture	0.02	(0.14)
Suprapubic tap on infants	0.02	(0.14)
Colposcopy	0.00	(0.00)
Flexible sigmoidoscopy	0.00	(0.00)
Obstetric ultrasonography	0.00	(0.00)

*Mean frequency of reported activity on a relative scale of 0 to 4. Never = 0; a few times a year = 1; at least once a month = 2; at least once a week = 3; daily = 4.

In a statewide survey of Georgia PAs and NPs, rural providers tended to be older and less educated, to possess fewer specialty credentials, and to be employed longer than urban providers. Again, providers who preferred smaller communities were significantly more likely to mention the importance of community dynamics, while providers who preferred larger communities were significantly more likely to mention professional contact (Strickland, Strickland, and Garretson, 1998).

The future for rural employment of PAs may be bright. Two studies by Shi and others suggest that the demand remains fairly strong in rural areas (Shi et al., 1994; Shi and Samuels, 1997. There seems to be no difference in demand between PAs and NPs, reinforcing other observations that the demand is similar for both regardless of the setting (Shi et al., 1993).

ISSUES AND NEW ROLES OF PHYSICIAN ASSISTANTS IN PRIMARY CARE

House Calls

While the era of house calls by physicians may be remembered by a diminishing number of people who reside in the United States, it still occurs, although in different forms. In Las Vegas two physicians, six PAs, one NP, and three vans are used to visit patients. Two thirds of the patients are seniors, and most of the visits are scheduled. Many of the patients are established with the group and prefer the ambulatory service coming to them instead of them journeying to the medical office. Most services are reimbursed by Medicare (Swann, 2000).

Referrals to Specialists

Referring is an important activity in primary care but is poorly understood. The referral may help bring an episode of care to a conclusion, such as a referral to an ear surgeon to place tubes in the tympanic membrane for chronic recurrent otitis media. It can also represent an alternative to treatment such as a referral to physical therapy for acute shoulder tendinitis when the patient declines a shoulder injection. However, not all insurance carriers want their providers to liberally refer, and not all specialists want referrals from PAs.

To begin understanding referrals by PAs, Enns, Muma, and Lary (2000) surveyed 500 primary care PAs across the United States about their referral practices and perceived barriers to referrals (Exhibit 5-9). They found that 71% of respondents identified barriers to referral of patients to specialists and 86% were satisfied with their level of autonomy in making referrals. The most frequently identified barrier (38%) was the patient's insurance company. This is not an unexpected finding, considering the managed care environment in which medicine is practiced in the United States. In addition the longer the PA was in practice the fewer barriers were perceived by the PA. The high degree of autonomy expressed by the surveyed PAs may reflect the level of confidence that supervising physicians have in the PA's ability to make appropriate decisions regarding referrals.

SUMMARY

PAs have displayed an impressive track record in primary care. This has been accomplished through role delineation studies, the education

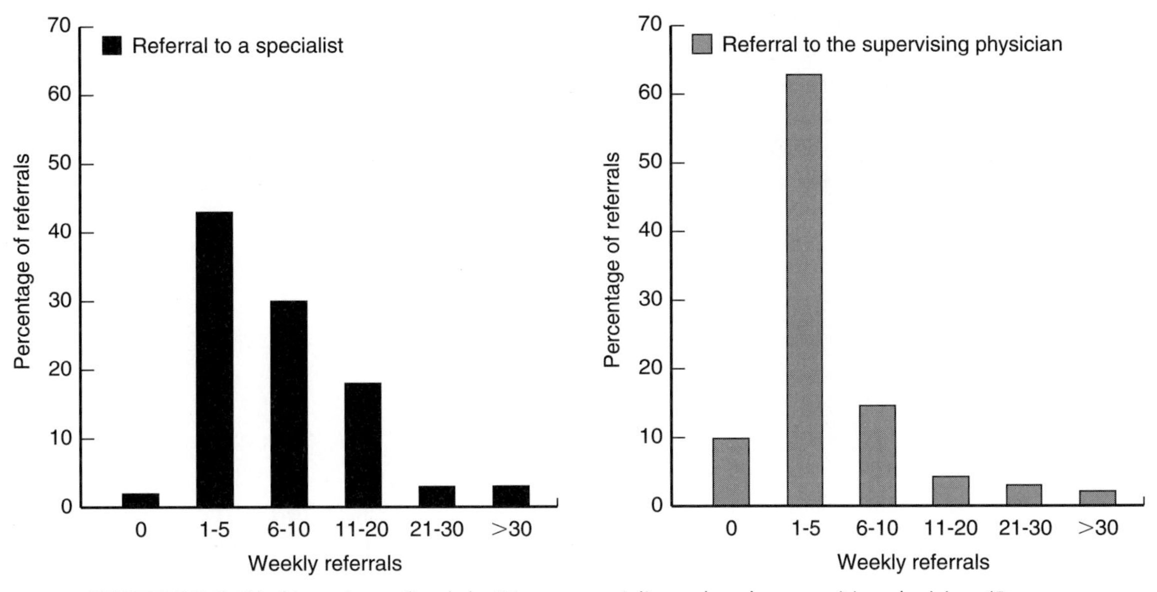

EXHIBIT 5-9 Weekly patient referrals by PAs to a specialist and to the supervising physician. (Data from Enns SM, Muma RD, Lary MJ: *J Am Acad Physician Assist* 13:81-82, 84, 86, 118, 2000.)

process, and physicians who are willing to apprentice assistants in their offices and places of practice. PAs have shown themselves to be safe and capable providers of primary care services. Ironically, despite the success of the PA, it remains a challenge for practices to attract enough of these providers to rural and other needy areas. Where there were once clear barriers to their full practice effectiveness, there is now the recognition by state boards, insurance carriers, and physician groups of the vital roles that PAs play in the delivery of primary care health services.

The PA profession has determined that primary care should remain the cornerstone for PA education. A report published by the AAPA states that

> The PA profession should remain rooted in its primary care foundation, with an emphasis on life-long learning. Although PAs do work in specialty areas, the generalist basis of their education remains critically important to their future. Life-long learning is an important component of PA education. The health care system is rapidly changing; a commitment to continuous life-long learning is a way for PAs to enhance the value they bring to physician practices as well as the health system at large. (Benjamin et al., 1999)

By the end of 2002 there were over 70,000 NPs and over 45,000 PAs in active practice. These providers, along with family physicians, general internists, and general pediatricians, comprise the U.S. primary care workforce, yet there remains little planning or coordination among the professions in terms of meeting health system and societal needs for primary care services. A recent analysis from the AAFP's Robert Graham Center for Policy Studies in Family Practice and Primary Care notes the uncoordinated growth of the U.S. primary care workforce. The AAFP report states that family physicians, NPs, and PAs are distinctly different in their clinical training, yet they function interdependently. Together, they represent a significant portion of the primary care workforce. Training capacity for these professions has increased rapidly over the last decade, but almost no collaborative workforce planning has occurred.

Family physicians, NPs and PAs have complementary and interdependent functions that are important to primary care. PAs always work with physicians, as do most NPs. Despite this functional interdependence, since 1990 there has been tremendous growth in the production capacity of all three professions without joint workforce planning. Like NP and PA education, family practice residency training capacity has expanded significantly in the past decade. Positions in family practice residency programs have increased 34%, from 2393 in 1990 to 3206 in 2000.

Because of the pressing need for primary care clinicians and the potential for increasing access while containing labor costs, the role of the primary care PA is generally believed to be secure for the near term. Health policies determining the future of the health care workforce are dictating that PAs and other nonphysician providers need to be part of the labor force mix.

6

Specialization

INTRODUCTION

The profession of medicine is broadly divided into two disciplines: medicine and surgery. These disciplines then divide into numerous specialties and subspecialties. From the earliest days of the profession, physicians recognized the value of physician assistants (PAs) and employed them into these disciplines. It is these disciplines and the activities within the disciplines that define the specialty of PAs as well. Although one half of all PAs are in primary care, approximately one quarter of PAs are involved in a surgical practice: general surgery, orthopedics, cardiovascular surgery, or some other surgical activity. The other quarter have roles spanning the myriad of medical disciplines such as cardiology, nephrology, oncology, rheumatology, hematology, pulmonology, and gastroenterology. Postgraduate programs have sprung up to accommodate PAs who wish to have additional training in various areas of medical care.

The PA profession was created to provide basic medical services to populations that were underserved or that did not receive any care. Although this is fully recounted in the history of the profession (see Chapter 3), the original intention of Eugene Stead and Richard Smith in creating the profession is not fully appreciated. They envisioned these new practitioners as assistants to doctors in a very general and literal sense and did not confine the activities of PAs to working only with primary care physicians. Stead and Estes intended that PAs would provide a wide number of services for physicians in all types of medical practice. The original Duke curriculum, for example, not only provided training in the performance and interpretation of electrocardiograms, but also gave instructions on how the machine could be repaired if broken. Thus the original design of the Medex and Duke programs was that the PA would perform medical tasks—some involving diagnosis and therapeutic management and some involving technical and routine procedures—that relieved the busy physician and allowed the doctor more time for continuing professional education, dealing with complex patient illnesses, and seeing more patients (Estes, 1968). Both models trained PAs as all-purpose generalist assistants to doctors. This concept became markedly altered as the PA movement gained momentum in the late 1960s. Another movement in specialization that took place in the late 1960s was a surge of new programs to train nonphysician providers in certain specialty areas of medicine. Some of these programs include the orthopedic assistant and the urologic physician's assistant, which were 2-year programs designed to train personnel to work directly for specialists. One experiment was the 4-month "health assistants" training program sponsored by Project Hope in Laredo, Texas. The only requirement was that the student be 18 years of age and be interested in health care. Of the 11 students who entered the first class, 8 lacked high school equivalence but were able to earn their general equivalency diploma certificate on completion of the program (Sadler, 1972). Other programs of various training missions and duration were developed in gastroenterology, allergy, dermatology, and radiology.

None survived past 1975, with the exception of the surgical assistant, the pathologists' assistant, and the child health associate program.

Because PAs are employed by physicians and emulate physician behavior in many ways, it is not surprising that they would move into specialty practices. Most of the trends observed among physicians are also seen in PA specialization, including the trend to work in a non-primary care role and the increase in wages that specialization brings.

As the profession evolved, PAs were attracted to primary care as well as non-primary care roles. Today the profession is evenly divided. Why this has occurred is not clear. Hooker (1992) hypothesized that PAs probably respond to the same forces that shape physician specialty choices: the training process, the specialty that fits the lifestyle and geographic preferences of the physician, and market forces (Exhibit 6-1). Genova (1995) examined the influence of market forces on PA practice settings in Maine and concluded that at least there, the market was weaker for primary care PAs than for the services of specialty care PAs. Studies of new graduate employment show that the specialty distribution of new graduates closely resembles that of the entire profession and the market is strong for graduates (Cawley, Simon, and Blessing et al., 2000).

In approaching the issue of specialization, we divide this chapter on non-primary care PAs into surgical and nonsurgical specialties. PAs who participate in surgery or work in the surgical specialties represent a major component of PA practice. This is a rich history and begins shortly after the formal PA was created. The remainder of the chapter is devoted to many of the non-primary care disciplines. After surgery these are presented in alphabetical order.

PHYSICIAN ASSISTANTS IN SUBSPECIALTIES

PA practice in subspecialty practice areas has expanded considerably since 1980. In this chapter we refer to all areas of medical practice outside of primary care (internal medicine, family practice, and pediatrics) as specialty and subspecialties. Increasing demand for and use of PAs in specialty and subspecialty roles tends to fluctuate as the result of many factors. Specialty practice areas expected to remain strong for PAs in non-primary care roles include emergency medicine, cardiovascular surgery, orthopedic surgery, and a large number of internal medicine subspecialties. The trend of using PAs, sometimes as replacements for residents, raises several policy issues in health care workforce planning. The recent proposed restriction of resident hours to 80 per week could have a significant effect on the use of PAs in hospital settings. Another consideration is that neither PA programs nor teaching hospitals provide many financial incentives to participate in the clinical education of PAs in specialty or inpatient care areas. It may be difficult for some PA programs with curricula focused on primary care to expand numbers and adequately prepare PAs for inpatient care or specialty roles. Exhibit 6-2 is a list of some of the clinical practice specialties and subspecialties in which PAs are used.

What are the factors that influence or lead PAs to choose a particular specialty or practice? Why PAs choose a particular specialty is only partially known. Employment opportunities play a significant role. Studies show that differences between primary care and non-primary care PAs do exist. For PAs in non-primary care roles the most influential factors determining specialty choice are technical orientation and income/ employment. These factors seem to differ from PAs in primary care, who identify prevention, academic environment, debt/scholarship, intellectual content, and peer influence as more important factors (Singer and Hooker, 1996) (Exhibit 6-3).

SURGICAL PHYSICIAN ASSISTANTS

In 1967 John W. Kirklin, MD, chairman of the Department of Surgery at the University of Alabama and an internationally renowned pioneer in cardiac surgery, began the first program to train surgeon's assistants (SAs), or surgical PAs, to assist in the surgical care of patients (Byrnes, 1991). Kirklin's decision to train nonphysician providers to assist in the preoperative, intraoperative, and postoperative care of surgical patients was the culmination of his years of work in medical education and the realization of the value of a trained professional assistant who was not a physician but who could provide a competent continuity of care (Condit, 1992).

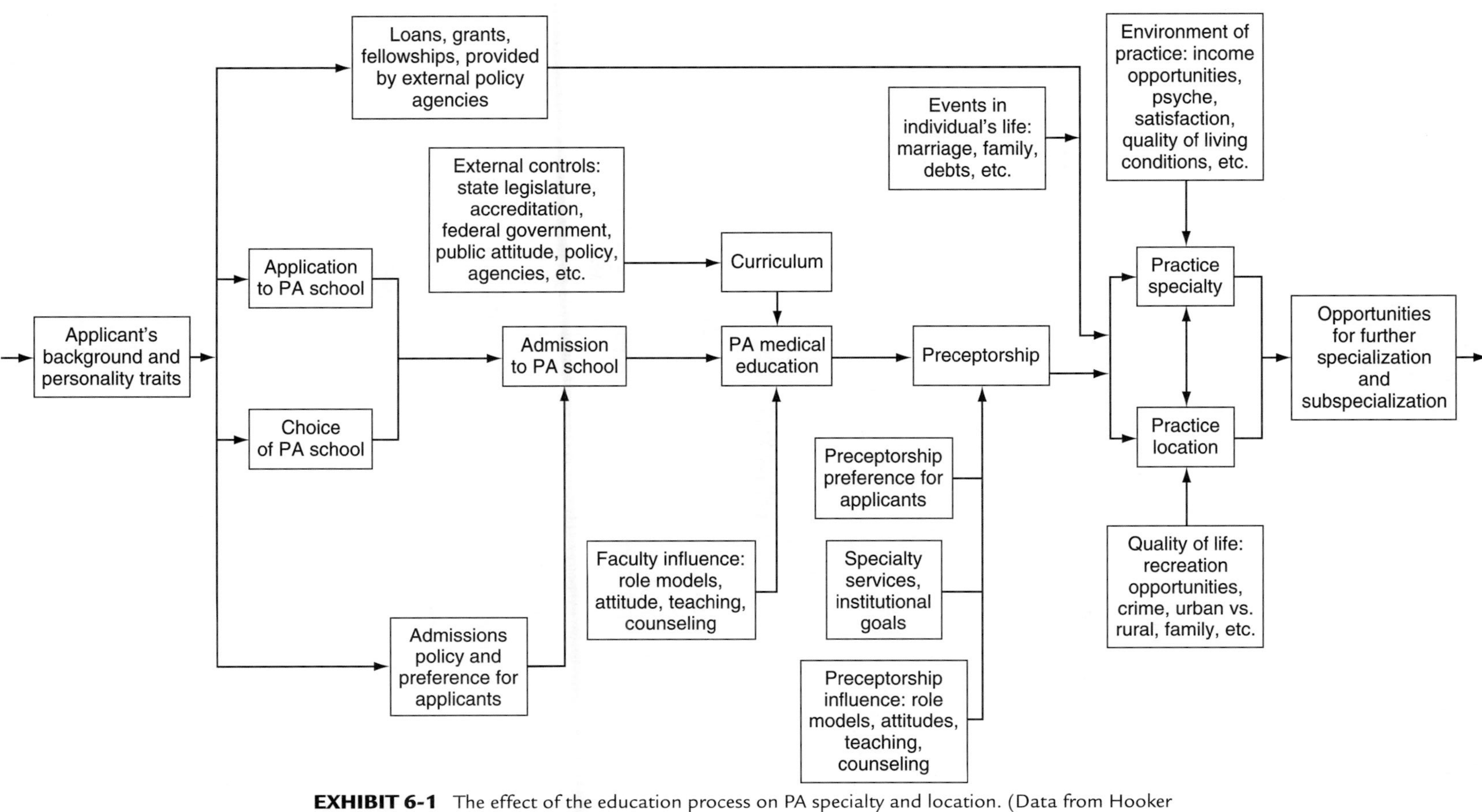

EXHIBIT 6-1 The effect of the education process on PA specialty and location. (Data from Hooker RS: *J Am Acad Physician Assist* 5:695-704, 1992.)

EXHIBIT 6-2

Partial Listing of Non–Primary Care Areas Using PAs	
Allergy	Neonatology
Anesthesiology	Neurosurgery
Cardiothoracic surgery	Obstetrics and gynecology
Clinical research	Occupational health
Critical care units	Oncology and pediatric oncology
Dermatology	Ophthalmology
Emergency medicine	Organ procurement and transplantation
Forensic medicine and pathology	Orthopedics and sports medicine
Gastroenterology and endoscopy	Otorhinolaryngology: head and neck surgery
Gerontology	Physical medicine and rehabilitation
Hematology and oncology	Plastic surgery and burn care
Infectious disease and immune deficiency	Preventive medicine
Interventional radiology	Rheumatology
Invasive cardiology	Substance abuse
Mental health and psychiatry	Urology

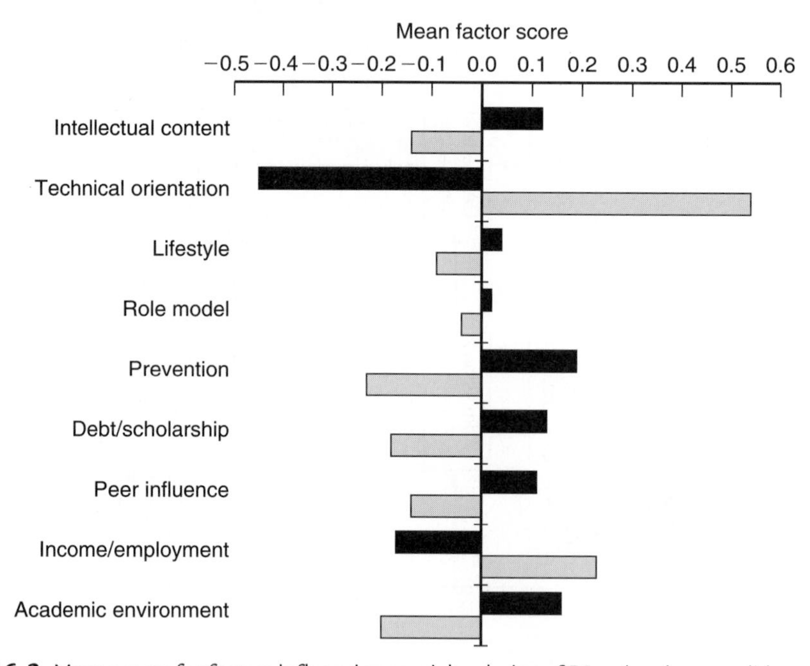

EXHIBIT 6-3 Mean scores for factors influencing specialty choice of PAs who chose or did not choose primary care in their first practice year. (Data from Singer AM, Hooker RS: *Acad Med* 71:917-919, 1996.)

Kirklin's program was typical of a number of programs that tried to develop a type of PA who could assist a physician in either primary care or some specialized service. In 1973 the federal government demonstrated interest in the training of PAs when Congress passed the Comprehensive Health Manpower Training Act, which placed emphasis on primary care programs (Kress, 1971). In 1972 the Bureau of Health Manpower (now known as the Bureau of Health Professions) assumed responsibility for funding 24 of the existing 31 PA training programs. The intent of this act was to relieve problems of geographic and specialty maldistribution of health care delivery. This was interpreted as primary care, so the emphasis of specialty care and surgery programs was left without funding. As a consequence, many of the specialty programs eventually converted to primary care programs or disbanded.

At the same time that policy directives were shaping the PA health care workforce in the early 1970s, there was much debate over the role of the PA in surgery. This debate centered on whether or not surgeons should use nonsurgeons as first assistants. In 1973 the American College of Surgeons (ACS) issued its statement on SAs, in which they supported the concept. This support was published in *Essentials for the Educational Training Programs of Surgeon's Assistants* (ACS Bulletin, 1973).

Surgical PAs can be trained in one of three ways:

- Formally in a structured SA program
- As a graduate PA with on-the-job training
- In a postgraduate training program

The first PA postgraduate training program in any specialty was instituted at Montefiore Medical Center/Albert Einstein College of Medicine in 1971 under the direction of Richard G. Rosen, MD. The Montefiore program began as a means of using PAs as surgical house staff. In 1976 the first class of 12 students was admitted to the Department of Surgery of the Yale University School of Medicine. This program was developed by Yale University and Norwalk Hospital (Beinfield, 1991). These programs became the models of PA postgraduate education.

The American Association of Surgeon Assistants (AASA) was established by a group of surgical PAs in response to opposition from some primary care PAs in 1972. The AASA maintains an active relationship with the ACS and the American Academy of Physician Assistants (AAPA). The Association of Physician Assistants in Cardiovascular Surgery maintains a liaison with the American Association for Thoracic Surgery.

Today surgical PAs are widely employed throughout the United States (Exhibit 6-4). They are distributed in rural and urban areas, in community hospitals and major medical centers, in general surgery, and virtually all surgical subspecialties (Condit, 1992).

Little has been done to compare the skill set of a surgical PA who has been trained in a formal surgical PA program, a postgraduate surgical program, or on-the-job training. Some believe that the on-the-job training takes years to master what a postgraduate-trained PA learns in a relatively short period. Beinfield (1991) maintains that the "... highly structured program offers increasing responsibility under supervision of a knowledgeable and dedicated faculty of senior PAs, physicians, and surgeons in an academic setting.".

EXHIBIT 6-4

Distribution of Surgical PAs

Specialty	**%**
General surgery	35.4
Orthopedics	26.9
Cardiovascular surgery	19.5
Neurologic surgery	4.5
Urologic surgery	4.3
Plastic surgery	2.5
Vascular surgery	1.8
Thoracic surgery	0.8
Traumatic surgery	0.3
Colon and rectal surgery	0.1
Other surgery	3.1
Practice setting	**%**
Hospital	55.4
Group office	21.6
Clinic	15.7
Solo office	8.7
Health maintenance organization	3.0
Inner city	1.9
Rural clinic	0.4
Corrections	0.3
Other setting	4.2

Data from American Academy of Physician Assistants, Census, 1991.

Surgical Physician Assistant Profiles

PAs in surgery command the higher end of salaries in the profession. The mean 1999 salary for all surgical PAs was $70,871; the median income was $74,444. For new PA graduates in 1999 the starting salaries were $55,511 and $55,849, respectively (Exhibit 6-5). The vast majority draws a straight salary or a salary plus bonus, and fewer than 10% have some sort of shared revenue relationship with their employer.

It seems very early in the development of PAs, the attitudes of doctors about surgical PAs have been positive (Legler, 1983). With cost-containment, surgical residencies going unfilled, and advancements in surgical techniques, as well as an increasing acceptance of PAs and SAs, the

EXHIBIT 6-5

Surgical PA Salaries, 1999

Salary type	% of respondents	
Straight salary	53.8	
Salary + % revenue	7.6	
Salary + bonus	37.6	
Partnership	1.0	
Salary distribution	**Overall ($)**	**New graduates ($)**
Mean	70,871	55,511
10th percentile	54,818	42,841
25th percentile	63,523	50,469
50th percentile	74,444	55,849
75th percentile	85,893	61,855
90th percentile	94,500	66,516

Data from American Association of Surgical Assistants, *Surgical Physician Assistants,* 2000. Odyssea Publishing, Inc., Bernardsville, NJ.

field of surgery for PAs is likely to continue to grow at least until 2010 (Exhibit 6-6).

PHYSICIAN ASSISTANT SPECIALTIES

A great deal of experimentation has taken place in developing PA programs. While the greatest area of concentration has been in formally preparing PAs for primary care roles, some of this experimentation has been in creating surgical and medical subspecialty roles. This usually occurs because there is a perceived need for PAs in these roles. Other reasons for PAs shifting into specialty roles include an unfilled niche for a provider in a particular specialty or a physician specifically inviting and directing the PA into this specialty.

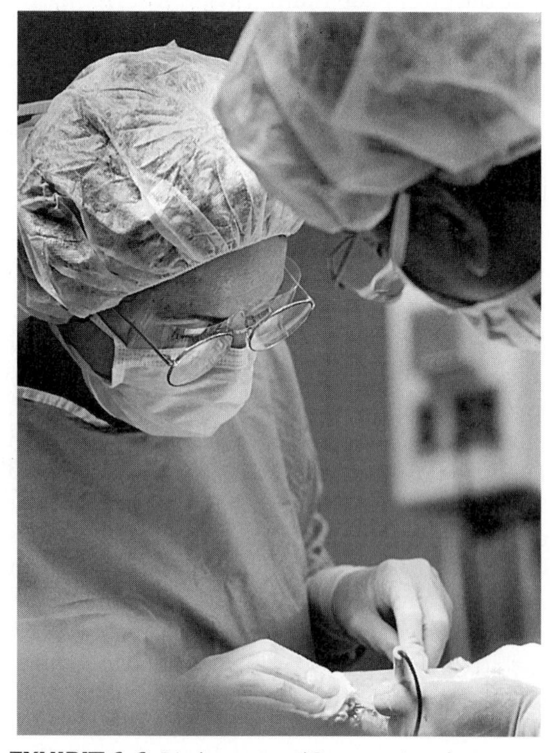

EXHIBIT 6-6 PAs in surgery. (Courtesy American Academy of Physician Assistants.)

The following sections present specializations for PAs identified from the literature or in conversations with PAs in these roles. The list is far from complete.

Administration

Clinical experience as a PA increases their marketability in health care administration, particularly if the PA has credentials in management. Nevertheless, little is known about how many PAs are in administrative roles. Many PAs share both clinical duties and administration in offices, and these roles may even fluctuate depending on the demands in either sector. Various attempts have been made to form special interest groups that involve PAs in administration, but these groups do not endure. Some PAs have used their degrees as steppingstones to administrative roles in hospital and clinic administration, sometimes acquiring administrative degrees along the way (Mayer, 1988).

While the PA profession depends on the physician as employer, this does not preclude the PA from developing a business in health care delivery. Barnes and Hooker (2001) surveyed 56 PAs who administered their own businesses providing health care—oftentimes employing physicians (Exhibit 6-7).

EXHIBIT 6-7

Practice Setting of Self-Employed PAs

Specialty	No. of PAs	Mean
Emergency medicine	7	12%
Family practice	22	39%
Multispecialty	5	7%
Surgery	19	35%
Other	4	7%

Data from Barnes D, Hooker RS: *Physician Assist* 25:36-41, 2001.

Alcohol and Drug Abuse (Substance Abuse)

A small but growing number of PAs provide alcohol and drug abuse management from the clinical side. Also known as substance or addictionology, often their roles include admission and discharge from detoxification units and the provision of medical management of substance abuse patients in outpatient settings (Srba, 1981). Substance abuse and chemical dependency is taught in almost all PA programs (Judd, 2001) (Exhibit 6-8).

Allergy

Although most allergists are pediatricians, many family medicine physicians perform some allergy testing and treatment. This is not an area widely occupied by PAs. A program, which trained PAs in allergy, lasted for 2 years at the University of California, San Diego. Developed in 1969 the program trained PAs to prepare, administer, and evaluate allergens for those with suspected allergic conditions. This was a labor-intensive and technical skill. Because manufacturers prepare almost all allergens, this technical role is no longer needed. Nurses skilled in allergy have largely supplanted the role of the technical PA in allergy.

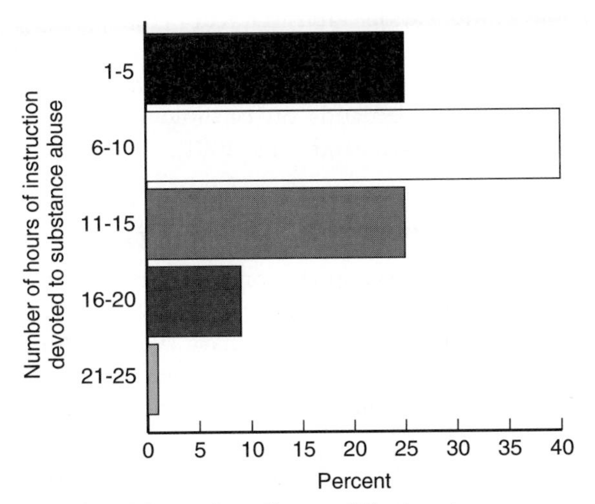

EXHIBIT 6-8 Number of hours of PA education instruction on substance abuse. (Data from Judd CR, Hooker RS: *Perspectives on Physician Assistant Education* 12(3): 172-176. Association of Physician Assistant Programs, Alexandria, Va., 2001.)

Anesthesiology

The concept of an anesthesiologist's assistant (AA) was initiated in 1969 at Case Western Reserve University in Cleveland, Ohio, and at Emory University in Atlanta, Georgia. Having been advised of the programs' purposes and operations, by 1975 the American Society of Anesthesiologists (ASA) was supportive of this emerging occupation. The Emory University curriculum was designed as a master of science degree. Case Western Reserve offered a bachelor of science degree, designed largely as a premedicine curriculum.

In 1976 the ASA petitioned the American Medical Association (AMA) Council on Medical Education (CME) for recognition of the AA as an emerging health profession. The council's recognition followed in 1978. An ad hoc committee within the ASA to worked collaboratively with the AMA's Department of Allied Health Education and Accreditation on the development of educational standards. Because of differences in opinion about the level of the credential and about the need for graduates in this field, in 1981 the ASA withdrew its collaboration with the AMA in the development of accreditation standards and in the accreditation of educational programs.

By 1982 the Association of Anesthesiologist's Assistants Training Programs (AAATP) was created and incorporated. The following year the AAATP and the American Academy of Anesthesia Associates (AAAA) petitioned the AMA CME to recognize them as collaborative sponsors for the program designed to educate AAs. In 1984 the AMA CME reinstated its recognition of the AA profession. *Essentials* for the education and training of AAs were adopted in 1987 by the CME, the AAATP, and the AAAA. In 2000 the AAPA estimated that approximately 40 people in the country were both formally trained PAs and work as anesthesiologists (Legislative Watch, 2000).

The AA functions under the direction of a licensed and qualified anesthesiologist, principally in academic medical centers. The AA assists the anesthesiologist in collecting preoperative data, such as taking an appropriate health history and performing physical examination; in undertaking various preoperative tasks, such as the insertion of intravenous and arterial lines, central venous pressure monitors, and special catheters; in airway management and drug administration for induction and maintenance of anesthesia; in administering supportive therapy, such as intravenous fluids and vasodilators; in providing recovery room care and in performing other functions or tasks relating to care in an intensive care unit or pain clinic; in providing anesthesia monitoring services; and in performing administrative functions and tasks, such as staff education. *Direction* implies the presence of a designated anesthesiologist within the hospital and immediately available to the operating room. AAs are trained in general, epidural, spinal, and peripheral anesthetic nerve blockade.

In addition to the duties described in the occupational description in the preceding discussion, AAs provide technical support according to established protocols. This support includes first-level maintenance of anesthesia equipment; skilled operation of special monitors, including echocardiographs, electroencephalographs, special analyzers, evoked-potential apparatuses, autotransfusion devices, mass spectrometers, and intraaortic balloon pumps; the operation and maintenance of bedside electronic computer-based monitors; supervised laboratory functions associated with anesthesia and operating room care; and cardiopulmonary resuscitation.

AAs are likely to be employed by hospitals with at least 200 beds and with staffs of 15 or more anesthesiologists, nurse anesthetists, and AAs. These settings use a team approach to anesthesia service in facilities for open-heart surgery and have a graduate medical residency training program for anesthesiologists.

There are two anesthesia assistant programs in the United States: Emory University and Case Western. The programs are essentially 2 years, based on a master's degree model. The programs require a baccalaureate degree with a major in cell biology, chemistry, physics, mathematics, computer science, or physiology.

AAs have sought recognition as PAs, using as justification the premise that the term *physician assistant* includes all assistants to physicians. For many years AAs have been recognized as "type B" PAs in Georgia; this designation reaches back to a recommendation by the National Academy of Sciences in 1970 that PAs be classified as types A, B, and C by degree of specialization and level of judgment involved in practice. That designation scheme is now defunct. Another battle is between the AAs and certified registered nurse anesthetists (CRNAs). The lines are drawn between CRNAs who are seeking independence and AAs who are maintaining their physician-dependent role.

Cardiology

The cardiology PA is one member of an organ-specific team that provides comprehensive and quality patient care. Many individuals participate including cardiologists, PAs, nurse practitioners (NPs), pharmacists, nutritionists, physical therapists, behavioral medicine specialists, technologists, and others (Dracup et al., 1994). The cardiology PA role includes ambulatory care, hospital admission and discharge evaluations, early myocardial infarction management, treadmill and stress testing, and other procedures (Mayes, 1991).

DeMots et al. (1987) evaluated the feasibility of PAs performing coronary arteriography. The complication rate and facility in performing the procedure was compared with that of cardiology fellows. The procedure and fluoroscopy times were similar, and more important the mortality rate was zero. Other complications were favorable when compared with published standards (DeMots et al., 1987). Additional experience with this same model and two additional PAs includes more than 1000 patients, with no mortality and low complication rates (Dracup et al., 1994). Other specialized roles for cardiology PAs are emerging as technology becomes increasingly invasive and demands on cardiologists stretch their capacity (Krasuki et al., 2001).

Cardiovascular and Thoracic Surgery

PAs have been working alongside vascular surgeons since the first Duke class (Cooper, 1971; Rothwell, 1993). Their roles have evolved along with the fast moving technologic specialty cardiology is and includes the recognition of early postprocedural complications of surgery, ambulatory care, hospital admission evaluation, and early post-myocardial infarction management. Routines include hospital visits, discharge planning, and follow-up appointments (Mayes, 1988). They improve operating room efficiency and thus free up the surgeon as consultant for other roles (Mauney, 1972; Miller, 1978) . From 1970 to 1974 a program at the Oregon Health Sciences University in Portland trained approximately 15 PAs in cardiovascular surgery among other roles.

One of the more important roles for the cardiovascular surgical assistant is harvesting the saphenous veins for coronary artery bypass grafting (Chaffee, 1988). Some PAs have further specialized as bypass pump technologists.

The Association of Physician Assistants in Cardiovascular Surgery includes PAs who participate in the surgical treatment of cardiovascular disease that encompasses three specialty areas: general thoracic surgery, surgery for congenital heart disease, and surgery for acquired heart disease. Cardiothoracic PAs work for practices involved in heart surgery, chest surgery, and peripheral vascular surgery. Peripheral vascular surgery usually involves surgery of the circulatory system outside of the thorax.

The role of services in cardiovascular and pulmonary surgery ranges from first and second assists in surgery to those who provide preoperative and postoperative care, as well as medical office patient responsibilities. Responsibilities include performing a complete pulmonary and circulatory examination, explaining the surgical procedure to the patient and family members, and answering their questions. Procedures include heart or lung transplantation, liver transplantation, and routine heart procedures. Technical skills involve the intraaortic balloon pump, right and left ventricular assist devices, cardiopulmonary support systems, and extracorporeal membrane oxygenators. At least 10% of cardiovascular surgical PAs are also certified clinical perfusionists operating the heart-lung machines.

Few studies have actually examined the safety of cardiovascular PAs. In one 3-year retrospective examination of 1226 central venous cannulations in 732 patients undertaken by PAs in a vascular surgery section of Geisinger Medical Center, 7 patients experienced a pneumothorax as a complication. Six of the seven procedures were performed by different PAs. Although statistics were not included for physicians the less than 1% incident of pneumothorax for this procedure is considered low compared with 4% overall major complication rate of surgical house officers, anesthesiologists, and other house officers (Marsters, 2000).

A survey of cardiovascular and vascular (CV/V) PAs in early 2000 found that the average surgical practice had three to six (average 5.1) PAs and five to six (average 5.1) surgeons. Sixty-seven percent of the 572 PA respondents were based in private practice; 16% in universities; 7% in hospitals; 3% in health maintenance organizations (HMOs); 3% in clinics; and 2% in the military. In all the practices that employed a PA, other providers were employed as well: registered nurses (RNs) (52%), NPs (26%), certified surgical technicians (CSTs), resident physicians (20%), RN first assistants (RNFAs) (15%), and nonsurgeon physicians (10%). The group most often involved in preoperative care and evaluation consultations was PAs (71%), followed by NPs (15%), RNs (13%), nonsurgeon physicians (7%), CSTs (5%), and RNFAs (4%). Other settings in which PAs were used significantly more than all other nonsurgeon practitioners by CV/V surgeons included postoperative intensive care unit (ICU) care, postoperative care on the ward, and outpatient care (81% vs. 12%; $p < .001$). PAs in these settings report being used at highly skilled and technical levels that differentiate them from other nonsurgeon providers (Exhibit 6-9) (Lee et al., 2000).

Postoperatively cardiovascular PAs manage the patient in the ICU and the hospital wards. Providing optimal patient care includes managing the patient's surgical condition and other disease processes they may have such as hypertension, diabetes, and other conditions. Other roles include overseeing cardiac rehabilitation,

EXHIBIT 6-9

Use of Surgical PAs by Clinical Setting

	All	Preoperative	First assistant	Intensive care unit	Ward	Office
PAs (%)	81	81.1	94.5	70.8	89.9	66.1
Non-PAs (%)	12.3	54.2	54.4	56.6	63.7	57.3
p value	<.001	<.0012	<.001	<.001	<.001	<.003

Data from Lee J, Cooper J, Lopez EC, et al.: *Surg Physician Assist* 6:14-21, 2000.

teaching diet, and discharging the patient. Even then, the involvement with the patients continues by answering telephone calls regarding their concerns after returning home and seeing them in the office for postoperative visits (Gray, 1997).

Correctional Medicine

PAs have been playing a role in correctional medicine since 1973. While often listed as a specialty (as it is here), in reality correctional medicine is a primary care discipline that is practiced under extenuating circumstances, challenging behavior, and ethical considerations, along with certain legal constraints (Lombardo, 1982; Jarmul, 1991; Smith, 1996). PAs often work independently and deliver a number of primary care and specialty services depending on the size of the institution (Salker, 1978; Freeman, 1981). The mission statement of correctional institutions is no different from that of any other organization: provision of essential health care for inmates with professional staff consistent with acceptable community standards.

In one study the employment of a PA in a Baltimore City jail resulted in a decrease in use of prisoner sick call and an increase in duration of encounters. Improvement in prescribing pattern and categories of prisoner complaints was observed as well (Freeman, 1981).

Each county and state, like most large cities, have a prison system with opportunities for PAs. The Department of Justice recruits PAs to staff the Federal Correctional System, better known as the Bureau of Prisons, either as civil service employees or public health service officers. As of 1996 there were 90 federal prisons and 654 PAs working within the federal prison system (Smith, 1996). Anecdotal information suggests that this role of medicine offers a great deal of satisfaction for PAs (Brutsche, 1986). In one federal correctional institution in Georgia with 1750 inmates, responsibilities are shared among 10 full-time PAs, 2 physicians, 3 administrators, a nurse, and numerous ancillary staff (Smith, 1996).

Sometimes the title of PA is not well understood. In 1930, the Federal Bureau of Prisons was established to maintain secure, safe, and humane correctional institutions. In 1974 the bureau created its own PA program at the Federal Medical Center in Springfield, Missouri. The design of the program was similar to that of today: 1 year of academic study and 1 year of clinical work. In 1976 the bureau employed the first trained PAs. The Springfield program operated until 1978 and then discontinued, partly as a result of an inability to provide satisfactory obstetrics and gynecology and pediatric rotations and in large measure because it was not cost-effective.

In 1978 between one half and two thirds of the bureau's medical technical assistants were given the job title PA within the bureau after they passed a written and oral examination. Several graduates of that program went on to pass the Physician Assistant National Certification Examination (PANCE) and are still employed by the bureau in various positions (Vause, Beeler, and Miller-Blanks, 1997). As of 1996 there were 724 authorized positions for PAs in the bureau, approximately 654 of which were filled. Of these employees, 86 are certified PAs and 114 are noncertified PAs. The balance is made up of personnel who qualify under the U.S. Office of Personnel Management standards for PAs (and not always technically a formally trained graduate from an accredited program who is certified by the National Commission on Certification of Physician Assistants [NCCPA]) (Vause, Beeler, and Miller-Blanks, 1997).

For both new and experienced PAs, opportunities abound in the bureau. The great diversity and international complexion of the inmates provides a challenging clinical experience. There are probably no greater opportunities to examine health care staffing while holding a vast number of variables constant than to practice medicine in this the quintessential managed care setting. Prisons allow the PA to follow through with their patients longitudinally while monitoring compliance (Cornell, 2000a).

Critical Care Medicine

After 3 months of rigorous training, two PAs were assigned to the ICU at the Veterans Administration Medical Center in Allen Park, Michigan. Their performance, as well as the operation of the ICU over a 2-year period, was evaluated and compared with 2 proceeding years when house officers operated it. There were no changes in occupancy, mortality, or the rate of complications. Instead there seemed to be evidence for more careful evaluation of patients before admission and discharge, manifesting as slightly fewer admissions and slightly longer duration of hospitalization. The authors concluded there is a role for PAs in providing health care in intensive care settings (Dubaybo, Samson, and Carlson, 1991). Experience in other hospitals is similar (Grabenkort and Ramsay, 1991).

Another comparative study involving 5 PAs, 11 NPs, and 41 resident physicians in two critical care units found similar roles (Rudy, 1998). The tasks and activities performed by these three types of providers are similar and the outcomes of patients tended by these three providers are the same. These tasks and activities are outlined in Exhibit 6-10. Resident physicians tended to treat older and sicker patients and work longer hours than PAs and NPs. The role of the intensive care specialist sometimes involves performing a number of procedures. The procedures listed in Exhibit 6-11 are those recorded over a 14-month period (Rudy, 1998).

EXHIBIT 6-11

Invasive Procedures Performed by Critical Care PAs and NPs

Venipuncture
Arterial or venous cutdowns
Percutaneous placement of arterial catheters
Placement of pulmonary artery catheters
Placement of central venous catheters
Placement of pigtail catheter
Placement of chest tube
Oral or nasal endotracheal intubation
Paracentesis
Thoracentesis
Arthrocentesis
Lumbar puncture
Insertion of drains
Bone marrow aspiration
Liver and other biopsy
Wound closure (superficial and deep)
Wound débridement
Placement or removal of nasogastric or feeding tube
Insertion or removal of nasal packing
Removal of superficial foreign body
Placement of transcutaneous pacemaker
Application of plaster cast

Data from Rudy EB, Davidson LJ, Daly B, et al.: *Am J Crit Care* 7(4): 267-281, 1998.

Global Medicine

Diverse opportunities are available for the PA who wants to work in another country. From the U.S. Peace Corps to *Doctors Without Borders* to missionary programs, these opportunities abound, with most stints ranging from 1 or 2 years. More than 20 agencies recruit volunteer PA, physician, nurse, and allied health personnel to work in underdeveloped countries. Usually transportation and a small stipend are provided for the volunteer. Physician Assistants for Global Health (PAGH) is the network organization for PAs with international experience. Employers of PAs include the government (Peace Corps, U.S. Agency for International Develoment, State Department, and others), nongovernmental organizations, and private corporations.

To practice in Kenya, one PA had to apply for a reciprocal license as a "clinical officer," a designation more or less equivalent to the U.S. designation of PA, but she was allowed to function autonomously 6 miles from the Tanzanian border on the shore of Lake Victoria. In this role she was the highest ranking clinician and oversaw 18 Kenyans who had been trained informally by previous U.S. staff. She supervised the staff, provided most of the administration, and saw patients. The nearest physicians were a 1-day's drive over a difficult road (Chidley, 1997a).

Opportunities for PA students to participate in international experiences are discussed in Chapter 4.

EXHIBIT 6-10

Activities of Acute Care PAs, NPs, and Resident Physicians

Formally present and discuss patient with staff, nursing, and others
Provide hands-on treatment
Serve as preceptor or instructor
Chart, dictate, compute, and write orders
Discuss care and interact with patient, family, and others
Perform formal consultation
Perform hands-on assessment
Arrange, obtain, or review laboratory test results
Review chart notes or records
Transfer patient on or off unit, or discharge
Conference or lecture
Perform administrative or research duties

Data from Rudy EB, Davidson LJ, Daly B, et al.: *Am J Crit Care* 7(4): 267-281, 1998.

Dentistry

In the early 1970s when the role of the PA was less clear, there was an interest in developing dental associates modeled after PAs (Keith, 1974).

Unlike many health problems, dental diseases and the procedures commonly used to resolve them require direct practitioner intervention. Many procedures are routine and well suited for delegation. Unfortunately the dental profession has been generally conservative in employing a dental assistant to assume responsibilities analogous to the contemporary PA, and efforts to promote them have met with strong resistance from organized dentistry (Keith, 1974). However, PAs have been used successfully to teach physical diagnosis in a dental school (Devore, 1978).

Dermatology

In the late 1960s a type C PA program developed briefly at the University of Chicago Pritzker School of Medicine in the Dermatology Department under Stanford I. Lamberg, MD. This was a 12-month program that graduated a certified PA in dermatology. The requirements were high school diploma plus 3 years of health care experience such as an RN or medical corpsman (Sadler, 1972).

Interest in expanding the role of the primary care PA into dermatology has been present for more than two decades (Krasner, 1977; Katterjohn, 1982). In one descriptive study the PA was found to be a useful addition in relieving some of the burden of patient care, but neither patient flow nor income was favorably affected (Laur, 1981). In another dermatology practice, PAs specialize in removal of suspicious moles, acne scars, port-wine stains, and other birthmarks. Lasers are used for hair removal, tattoo removal, and the treatment of hemangiomas (Samsot, 1998). The economics of managed care and current emphasis on cost reduction are making PAs more attractive to dermatologists (Dermatology World, 1996).

An analysis of the 1996 and 1997 National Ambulatory Medical Care Survey (NAMCS) data found that the dermatologic conditions evaluated by PAs accounted for 14% of all primary care visits. Dermatologic symptoms were the primary reason for a visit to all physicians 11% of the time. The NAMCS identified that approximately 2.5% of all patient visits involved a PA as the provider of care (Clark et al., 1999).

In 1999 there were more than 300 formally trained PAs who identified their clinical practice as dermatology and who belong to the Society of Dermatology Physician Assistants (SDPA), which is part of the AAPA Medical Congress. Almost all (97%) worked in private dermatologist's offices and reported seeing or billing for an average of 28 patients a day. The largest concentration of SDPA members is in Texas, California, and Florida (Clark et al., 1999). The procedures they are experienced in are listed in Exhibit 6-12. Postgraduate programs in dermatology are at the University of Texas Southwestern Medical Center in Dallas and at Kirksville College of Osteopathic Medicine. These programs provide 6- to 12-month fellowships and a stipend for PAs interested in dermatology.

Diabetology

The Diabetes Trust Fund in Birmingham, Alabama, established the only known diabetes PA program in the late 1960s. This 2-year program offered a certified diabetes PA degree (Sadler, 1972). Little is known about this program other than that the graduate was a PA in diabetes management.

One book has been written detailing diabetes management in HMOs using primarily PAs (Power, 1973). Diabetes is considered the domain of endocrinologists and primary care; however, the American Diabetes Association has recognized that a diabetologist is anyone who is involved with the diagnosis and management of diabetes and its complications.

Emergency Medicine

Shortly after the first few PA classes were practicing, PAs were occupying roles in hospitals, and

EXHIBIT 6-12

Procedures Frequently Performed by PAs in Dermatology
Cryotherapy of benign lesions
Intralesional injections
Laser surgery
Incisional and excisional biopsies
Wound closure of flaps and grafts
Phototherapy
Patch testing
Hair transplantations
Sclerotherapy
Mohs' surgery
Chemical peels

Modified from Clark AR, Monroe J, Feldman SR, et al.: *Dermatol Clin* 18:297-302, 1999.

before long they were in the emergency departments (EDs). It seemed a natural fit because many had developed trauma expertise in the military, and some had wartime experience that honed their skills further. Others had worked as trauma nurses and technicians. Sometimes they were used to manage the less acute patients such as in a fast-track/urgency care clinic, and other times they were seeing undifferentiated acute medical and trauma patients. There is much consensus that the education process seems to prepare the interested PA for ED services (Gentile, 1976; Friedman, 1978). In 2002 approximately 8% of PAs reported that they were employed in an ED setting.

Only a few studies describe the range of services a PA provides in an ED setting: In a small rural community hospital a PA could competently manage 62% of all presenting conditions (Maxfield, 1975); in an urban setting the roles are quite diverse and help bridge complex cultural gaps in medical surgical services (Goldfrank, Corso, Squillacote, 1980). No study has identified the full range of services that can be provided by an emergency PA or NP, but most believe it is similar to that of physicians. Regarding the concentration of both types of practitioners in some EDs, results of a survey of 111 Veterans Affairs Medical Centers showed that a mean of 1.9 full-time-equivalent (FTE) PAs are employed in 37 EDs and a mean of 2.1 FTE NPs are employed in 29 EDs. They work between 43 and 44 hours per week (Young, 1993).

Hooker and McCaig (1996) analyzed the results of the National Ambulatory Hospital Medical Care Survey that began in 1992. Combining PAs and NPs for statistical purposes, they found that PAs and NPs manage 3.5 million (4%) of the approximately 90 million nonfederal ED visits in the United States. They conclude that there are few differences in the type of patient seen at PA and NP visits compared with physician visits when gender, reason for visit, diagnosis, and medications prescribed are compared (Hooker and McCaig, 1996). In another study, Arnopolin and Smithline (2000) compared patient encounters between PAs and physicians and reached a similar conclusion that the distribution of diagnostic groups between PAs and physicians was similar. Some differences that did emerge were the time for patients and the total charges (Exhibit 6-13). Overall, visits were 8 minutes longer and total charges $8 less when a PA treated a patient. Patients who had headache, otitis, respiratory infection, asthma, gastrointestinal or genitourinary disorder, cellulitis, laceration, or other musculoskeletal disorder had a longer visit when seen by a PA. The difference ranged from 5 minutes to 32 minutes longer (Arnopolin and Smithline, 2000). Innovative programs have included laceration management by PAs, which has been shown to improve care and outcome, decrease cost, and satisfy patients (Katz, 1994).

A few postgraduate programs are available to train the PA in emergency medicine. Active programs include Alderson-Broaddus in West Virginia and Montefiore Hospital in New York. The University of Southern California, in Los Angeles, was the first but closed in 1995. The Army implemented a postgraduate program to train Army PAs in emergency medicine in 1992. These military programs are located at Brooke Army Medical Center in Texas and Madigan Army Medical Center in Washington State (Herrera, 1994).

Patient satisfaction with PAs in the ED seems to be as high as that for physicians. In a study in 1999 patients who were seen in a fast-track ED were surveyed about their experience with the PA who took care of them. A total of 111 survey results were analyzed. The mean response was 93 (on a scale of 0 to 100). This demonstrates a high degree of satisfaction with ED PAs. Only 12% of the patients said they would be willing to wait longer to be seen by a physician (Counselman, Graffeo, and Hill, 2000).

Cutbacks in residency programs of surgical specialties have necessitated substitutions for traditional trauma providers. Miller et al. (1996) examined the use of PAs in a large Flint, Michigan, trauma center. Over the 3 years spanning 1994 through 1996 the use of a trauma surgeon–PA team was introduced in an effort to off-load some of the surgeon's workload. During this period of PA use, the injury severity scores increased 19%, transfer time to the operating room decreased 43%, transfer time to the ICU decreased 51%, and transfer time to the floor decreased 20%. The length of stay for admissions decreased 13%, and the length of stay for neurotrauma ICU patients decreased 33% (Exhibit 6-12). Some of the procedures performed by PAs included chest tube insertion,

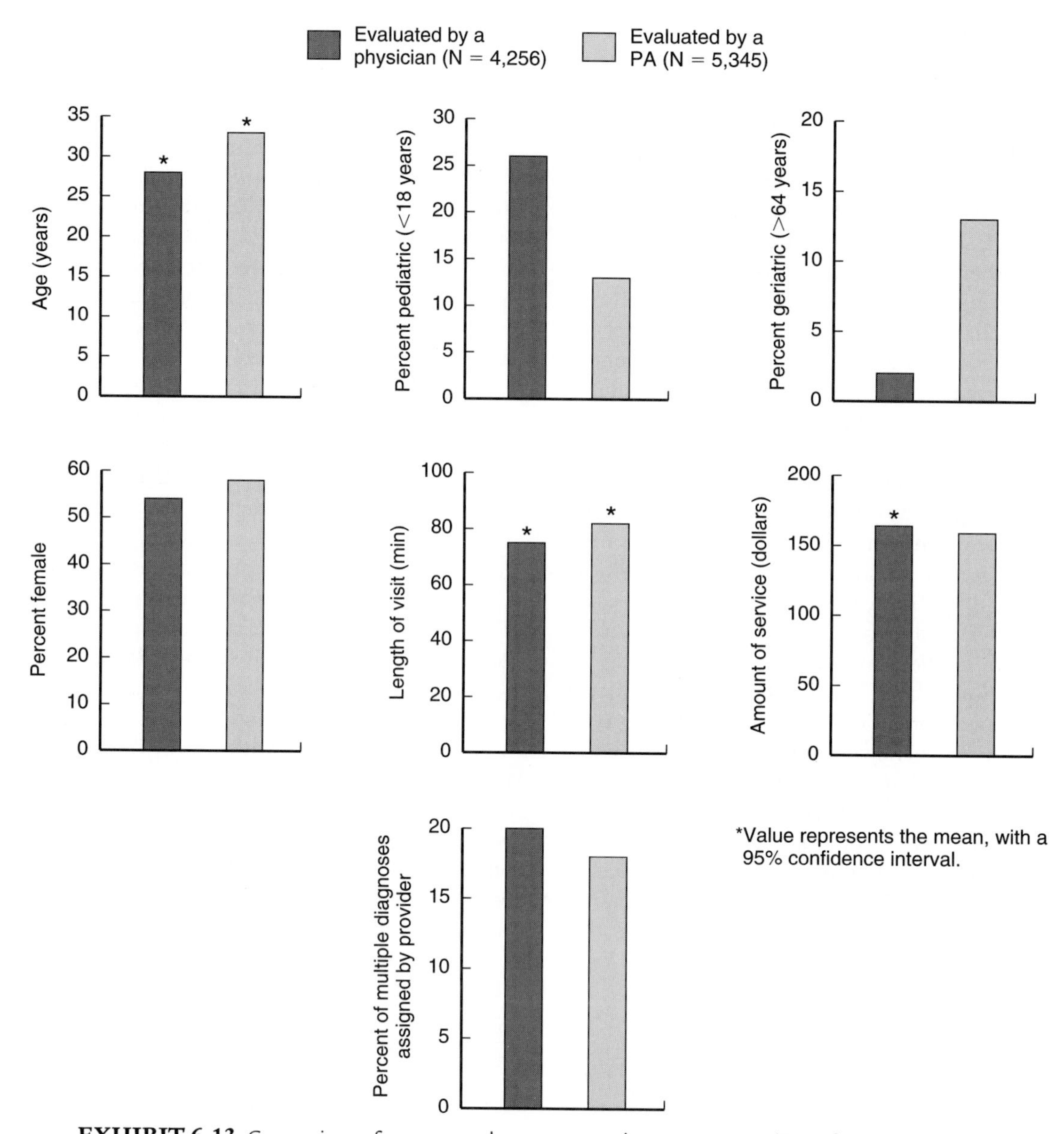

EXHIBIT 6-13 Comparison of emergency department patient encounters. (Data from Arnopolin SL, Smithline HA: *J Am Acad Physician Assist* 13:39-40, 49-50, 53-54, 81, 2000.)

admit and discharge summaries, central venous and pulmonary artery catheter placements, and subclavian catheterizations (Miller et al., 1998). The authors concluded the decreased length of stay in critical care units and in the hospital as a whole resulted in significant savings by the employment of these two trauma PAs.

Few studies on outcomes of care have been undertaken comparing PAs with physicians in the ED. One prospective, nonrandomized descriptive study compared the traumatic wound infection rates in patients based on level of training in ED practitioners. Wounds were evaluated in 1163 patients using a wound registry and a follow-up visit or phone call. Exhibit 6-14 demonstrates the results on wound care. There was no significant difference in level of training and wound care rates between medical students, interns, PAs, resident physicians, and attending physicians (Singer et al., 1995). The conclusion is that the delegation of wound management to PAs is a safe one and that they perform similarly to physicians in the same setting (Exhibit 6-15).

EXHIBIT 6-14

Trauma Service Summary, 1994-1996

	1994	1995	1996
Mechanism of injury			
Blunt (%)	64	64	63
Penetrating (%)	26	23	25
Burn (%)	10	11	10
Injury Severity Score			
All admissions	10.0	12.0	10.8
Critical care	13.4	16.25	16.0
Stepdown	7.3	8.5	8.4
Floor	5.6	7.1	5.1
Transfer to (hours)			
Operating room	2.3	2.0	1.5
Step/intensive care unit	5.9	5.1	2.9
Floor	4.9	4.8	3.9
Length of stay (days)			
All admissions	5.4	5.1	4.7
Critical care	9.3	7.8	6.2
Stepdown	3.1	3.2	2.9
Floor	6.4	3.2	3.8

Modified from Miller W, Riehl E, Napier M, et al.: *J Trauma* 44:372-376, 1998.

Forensic Medicine, Coroner, Medical Examiner

PAs are employed as forensic investigators in a number of jurisdictions. Examples include the Office of the Medical Examiner, Suffolk County, New York (Golden, 1986; Wright and Hirsch, 1987), Pueblo, Colorado (Chidley, 1997b), New Hampshire (Sylvester, 1996), Washington, D.C., and New York City. For some PAs, these jobs are full time, and for others, they are employed in the role part time. Qualifications vary by state, but it is not unusual for a public coroner to be a PA, even though the role of coroner is largely investigative. The coroner examines the crime scene, records what is present at the scene, and then makes determinations as to whether an autopsy, judicial hearing, or coroner's inquest is necessary. While a board-certified pathologist undertakes the autopsy, preferably a forensic pathologist in criminal cases, the medical examiner can be a PA with a good background in pathology.

That PAs would be attracted to medical death investigation is interesting because there seems to be little emphasis on forensic pathology as a potential area of practice in the current PA education curriculum (Cardenas, 1993). As one coroner put it, "Forensic medicine requires many of the same skills looked for in applicants to PA school. It has to be someone who is interested in medicine, someone with the ability to make decisions, someone who can communicate and is compassionate, firm, and fair. And, of course, you have to have the ability to understand scientific data" (Chidley, 1997b). (See the section on pathologist's assistants later in this chapter.)

Gastroenterology and Endoscopy

PAs are trained formally and informally in flexible sigmoidoscopy, colonoscopy, and gastroscopy. The benefit of a PA in one gastroenterology setting included staff efficiency, improved house staff education, and ability to perform an increased number of procedures with existing staff over a 3-year period (Lieberman, 1992) (Exhibit 6-16). It is probably no coincidence that this study was done at a Veterans Administration center because of the historical role they have played in developing the PA concept, and because the large scale of these medical centers allows them to experiment with alternatives to physician-directed services.

Nonphysician endoscopy is not new. From 1972 to 1976 a type C PA program in gastroenterology developed briefly at the University of Washington and the Veterans Administration

EXHIBIT 6-15

Level of Training, Wound Care Practices, and Infection Rates

ED practitioner and wounds per no. of cases sutured	Wound infection rate (%)
Medical student (0/60)	0
All resident physicians (17/547)	3.1
Physician assistants (11/305)	3.6
Attending physicians (14/251)	5.6
Junior practitioners (medical students and interns) (8/262)	3.1
Senior practitioners (PAs, residents, attending physicians) (34/901)	3.8

Modified from Singer AJ, Hollander JE, Cassara G, et al.: *Am Emerg Med* 13:265-268, 1995.
p = .58, not significant for any difference.

EXHIBIT 6-16

Impact of a Gastroenterology PA on Procedure Workload

	PROCEDURES/YR			
	1987 before PA	**1989 after PA**	**1990**	**Percentage change 1987-1990**
Sigmoidoscopy	313	386	442	(+) 41
Panendoscopy	646	810	821	(+) 27
Colonoscopy	373	437	439	(+) 18

Data from Lieberman DA, Ghormley JM: *Am J Gastroenterol* 87: 940-943, 1992.

Hospital in Seattle. This 12-month federally funded program trained about 12 PAs to do rigid sigmoidoscopies, blind biopsies of the esophagus, and manometry; to process tissue; and to assist in other aspects of endoscopy, all of which preceded the development of flexible fiberoptic instruments. Although this program did not survive long, the role of the PA in various endoscopic procedures has persisted. Several screening flexible sigmoidoscopy programs have relied on PAs, NPs, and RNs for more than a decade (Roosevelt, 1984; Weissman, 1987; Schroy, 1988; Cargill, 1991). The question of sanctioning independent endoscopy has been debated in the literature (Palmer, 1990; Smith, 1992).

Other roles in gastroenterology include consultation for liver disease and liver biopsy, managing patients with celiac sprue, inflammatory bowel diseases, irritable bowel syndrome, and other intestinal disorders (Gunneson, 2002). Hospitals with large gastroenterology centers will often use a PA for procedures, monitoring treatment for hepatitis C, and routine maintenance of certain diseases.

Geriatric Medicine

More than 20 studies on the use of PAs in geriatric medicine have been published. The consensus is overwhelming: PAs are very effective in patient management and care in geriatric facilities, contributing to quality care by allowing more patients to be seen and relieving the physician of fewer pressing problems (Isiadinso, 1979; Kraak, 1979; Sorem, 1983; Romeis, 1985). More than one study has demonstrated shorter hospitalization and overall lower medical costs using PAs in geriatric institutional settings (Tideiksaar, 1982, 1984). A study by the Rand Corporation demonstrated improvements in care and outcomes when PAs and NPs were introduced into nursing homes. Both nursing home administrators and directors in the demonstration model expressed higher levels of satisfaction with the process of care (Buchanan, 1989).

In one study on the impact of adding a PA to a large nursing home the hospitalization rate was dramatically altered. A 6-year case series examined hospital events of one nursing home before and after a PA joined a 92-bed teaching

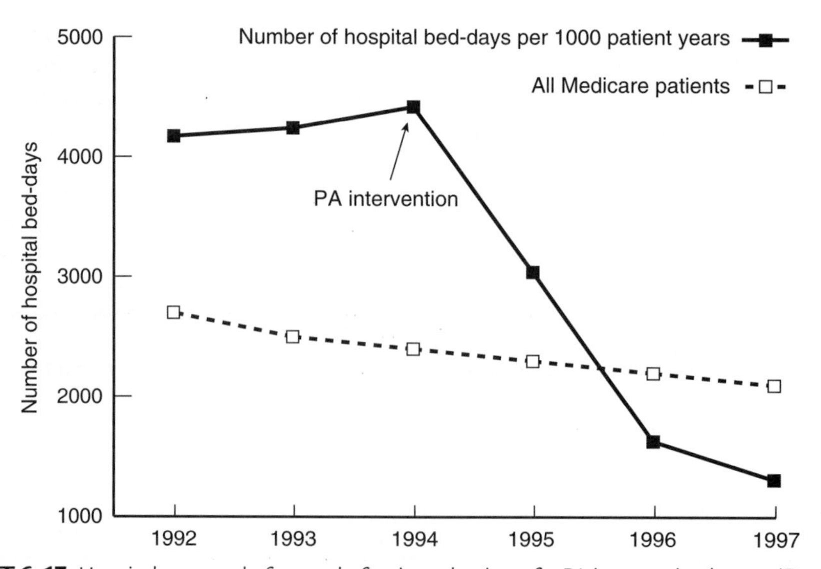

EXHIBIT 6-17 Hospital use rate before and after introduction of a PA in a nursing home. (Data from Ackerman RJ, Kemle KA: *J Am Geriatr Soc* 46(5): 610-614, 1998.)

hospital in central Georgia. After the PA started, the number of annual hospital admissions fell by 38%, and the total number of hospital days per 1000 patient years fell by 69%. The number of nursing home visits increased by 62% (Ackerman, 1998) (Exhibit 6-17).

Historically, neither medical schools nor PA program curriculum has emphasized geriatrics (Yturri-Byrd, 1984; Tideiksaar, 1986). With the revision on Medicare and Medicaid reimbursement for nursing homes, geriatric health care became center stage, and with it came the renewed interest in and the cost-effectiveness of PAs (Fox, 1980; Kane, 1980; May, 1988). The increase in the geriatric population and the growing medical concerns of this population have increased the need for more PAs in this area (Gambert, 1983; Olson 1983; Schafft, 1987; Dychtwald, 1988). Since the late 1980s, most PA programs have tended to include gerontology (Ouslander, 1989; Kane, 1991; Aaronson, 1992).

Although fewer than 2% of all PAs report that geriatrics is their primary clinical responsibility, both students and graduates report a high interest in this area (Bottom, 1988; AAPA, 1995). Virtually all studies on the aging population of both the United States and the world agree that the health care needs of the elderly will continue to increase. The opportunities for PAs in new and expanded roles in geriatric medicine and administration are predicted to increase dramatically in the decades to come (Dieter, 1989).

In 1985 the Bureau of Health Professions joined the AAPA to verify the role of the PA in providing geriatric care (Schafft, 1987). The study developed models of geriatric care provided by PAs and suggested appropriate uses of PAs with increasing demands for elderly medical services. Both inpatient and outpatient settings were outlined.

The Society of Physician Assistants Caring for the Elderly (SPACE) began in 1997 by a group of PAs interested in enhancing the care for the elderly. One of the goals is to promote education and training of all PAs in geriatric health care.

Hospital and Inpatient

PAs are often trained in hospital settings and are used extensively in many inpatient arenas. This role is extensively outlined in Chapter 7.

Infectious Disease, Immunology, Immunodeficiency

Many PAs are infectious disease specialists, both inpatient and outpatient. Some have assumed this role from the communicable disease nurse in hospital settings; others function as a consultant for both traveler's advice and patients with immune deficiencies. In this latter role many PAs are involved with infectious disorders such as acquired immunodeficiency syndrome (AIDS). How these roles are formalized and in what capacities they are performed have not been detailed in the literature.

The Physician Assistant AIDS Network (PAAN) is a national human immunodeficiency virus (HIV)/AIDS clinical interest group for PAs who have substantial involvement in HIV/AIDS direct care, education, or research. The network was developed in association with the AAPA in 1995 and was designed to facilitate access to current information and the exchange of ideas among PAs who serve people with HIV/AIDS.

Maritime Physician Assistant

The U.S. Public Health Service Hospital at Staten Island, New York, developed a 12-month PA program for former military medical corpsmen who wanted to continue their medical career. It was operational briefly in the late 1960s as a type C PA program for the Merchant Marine fleet. The graduates were referred to as marine PAs and were stationed on ships that employed large crews to oversee their health and safety (DeMaria et al., 1971; Sadler, 1972). The duration of this program and why it closed are not known.

We know of one PA who served as a ship's medical officer on a luxury ocean liner. Responsibilities were divided between passengers and crew, and few medical problems came up that the PA was unable to handle. Another PA works for a company that provides medical care to the yachting industry worldwide.

Mental Health (Psychiatry)

Nonphysician therapists who provide psychosocial services dominate the mental health field. Most of these workers are psychologists, social workers, and mental health counselors, but increasingly PAs are becoming visible as psychiatric PAs (Mahon and Batrus, 2000). PAs in the mental health setting are unique because they can see patients who need psychologic services, prescribe psychotropic medication, and provide other medical services. The first documented use of a PA functioning in a psychiatric role was in 1977 (Greenlee, 1977).

A few studies exist on how well PAs perform in the mental health field. One clinical assessment study (Coryell, 1978) found that PA interviews in psychiatric evaluations were comparable to those of physicians for all items including those thought to require the most clinical and medical judgment. Another study (Mathew, 1982) found PAs could successfully identify the medical disorders that accompany psychiatric disorders, which caused the psychiatric symptoms. And in a third study (D'Ercole, 1991) PAs detected nearly three times as many physical illnesses as the psychiatrist. The psychiatrists were significantly more likely to miss diagnoses among older patients and women (D'Ercole, 1991). Sometimes the PA provides a role as the primary care clinician managing most of the medical needs of the patient.

Psychiatry reports critical shortages in the availability of trained specialists like PAs who can be used in state hospitals. One institution's addition of PAs to the mental health staff significantly increased the time that psychiatrists had in which to plan and implement treatment. There was a very high degree of acceptance of the PAs in this setting (Matthews, 1984). Other cost-effective roles include using PAs to provide primary care and nonpsychiatric inpatient care in psychiatric settings (Morreale, 1977).

An Association of Psychiatric Physician Assistants was formed in the late 1990s. The Association of Postgraduate Physician Assistant Programs approved a psychiatric PA program in 1998. This program provides residency-style on-the-job training to PAs who are interested in enhancing their knowledge and therapeutic skills in caring for the mentally ill (Rose, 2001). The successful student who completes the program is eligible to receive a certificate of completion from the University of Texas Medical Branch Managed Care Health Service. Another mental health program for PAs is in Cherokee, Iowa.

Neonatology

One formal postgraduate neonatology program exists for PAs at the physician assistant neonatology residency program in Los Angeles. Two other residency programs in pediatrics also train the pediatric PA to neonatology: Norwalk Hospital and the Wolfson Children's Hospital in Jacksonville, Florida.

Evidence suggests that using neonatal PAs and NPs in the intensive care setting is an effective alternative to using pediatric residents. No significant differences in management, outcome, or charge variables can be demonstrated when comparisons are made between patients cared for by either provider at Wolfson Children's Hospital in Jacksonville, Florida (Carzoli et al., 1994; Schulman, Lucchese, and Sullivan, 1995). At the Bronx Municipal Hospital Center the phasing in of PAs and neonatal NPs overlapped the phasing out of pediatric residents. A study on the survival by birth weight comparing both pediatric residents and neonatal PAs and NPs failed to find any difference (Exhibit 6-18). Additionally after a period of adjustment to the PA/NP staff the authors found work rounds required less time with the PA/NP staff than with the residents. The number of errors in ordering parenteral alimentation solutions (as noted by the hospital pharmacy) had fallen as well (Schulman, Lucchese, and Sullivan, 1995).

The use of nonphysician providers in the neonatal unit has been endorsed in some form since the early 1980s. The Committee on Fetus and Newborn of the American Academy of Pediatrics published a statement on advance practice nurses, which strongly supported its role as members of a

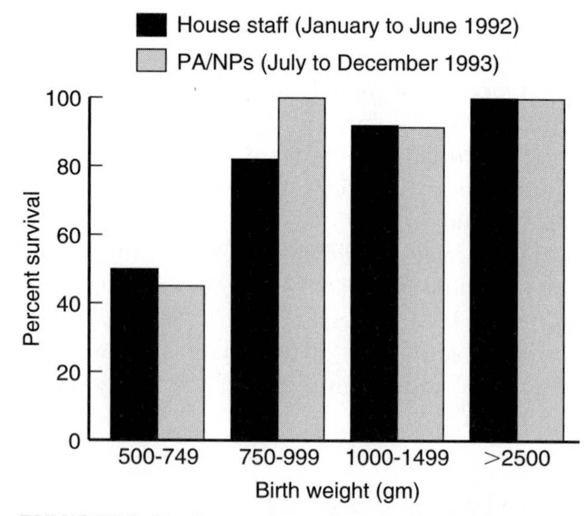

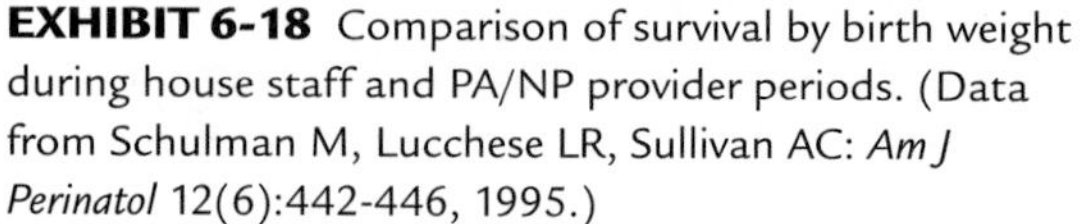
EXHIBIT 6-18 Comparison of survival by birth weight during house staff and PA/NP provider periods. (Data from Schulman M, Lucchese LR, Sullivan AC: *Am J Perinatol* 12(6):442-446, 1995.)

care team in the neonatal ICU (American Academy of Pediatrics, 1982). These studies conclude that the neonatal PA deserves this inclusion as well.

Neurology

PAs are practicing neurology both in primary care and associated with neurologists. A 1987 study of members of the American Academy of Neurology revealed that 29% used PAs and/or nurse clinicians (NCs) in their practice. Institutionally based neurologists were more likely to use PAs and NCs than those in private practice (Gunderson, 1988). At the time of this study many of these physicians were bringing their office PAs and NCs into the hospital. Unfortunately, this study did not define what a PA was, so presumably these were medical assistants and doctor's assistants.

In 1998 there were 60 PAs who identified their primary responsibility as neurology. Some of these PAs were associated with university-based academic programs and either taught or were involved in research (Samsot, 1997). Taft and Hooker (1999) conducted a telephone survey of 46 full-time neurology PAs working in a neurology office, mostly group practices (Exhibit 6-19). They found that the range of conditions seen by neurology PAs was similar to that of neurologists (Exhibit 6-20). Most PAs performed lumbar punctures (63%) and initiated multiple sclerosis therapy (50%). Other procedures that were usually reserved for neurologists were also done by PAs (Exhibit 6-21). Half were involved in clinical research studies. Clearly, PAs in neurology practices are performing a wide range of services that are probably not appreciated by physicians who do not work with PAs.

Neurosurgery

Neurosurgery is a labor-intensive surgical subspecialty. It is not surprising that neurosurgical PAs provide some role in this discipline. This surgical specialty tends to be in a higher range of pay for PAs, particularly when they first assist in lieu of another surgeon. Neurosurgical PAs sometimes perform certain procedures on their own, such as carpal tunnel releases.

A study in which the PA functions in an intern-equivalent capacity in neurosurgery was described in the late 1970s. This study suggests that patient care and patient acceptance were universally improved. The editor of the journal that published the study cited a number of reasons why he personally was opposed to the use of PAs in this area (Sonntag, Steiner, and Stein, 1977).

EXHIBIT 6-19

Practice Setting Characteristics of Neurology PAs (1998)

PRACTICE SETTING	
Group	26
Hospital-based practice	12
Solo practice	6
HMO	2
TOTAL	46

CHARACTERISTICS	Mean	Range	N
No. of years as a PA	13.5	1-25	46
No. of years working in neurology	7.2	1-25	46
No. of years employed in current neurology practice	5.7	2-19	46
No. of neurologists in your practice	4.2	1-20	46
If you see hospitalized patients, how many do you see in a typical week?	26	4-120	36
If you are in an outpatient practice, how many patients do you see in a typical week?	43	12-100	33
Hours employed to see patients	43.8	16-55	46
Do you see patients in a nursing home?	Yes = 7	—	—
Do you "take call?"	Yes = 17	—	—

Data from Taft JM, Hooker RS: *Neurology* 52:1513, 1999.

EXHIBIT 6-20

Neurology PA-Managed Conditions by Order of Frequency
Headaches (all types)
Cerebral vascular accidents
Parkinson's disease and other movement disorders
Seizure disorders
Multiple sclerosis
Low back pain
Peripheral neuropathies
Chronic pain syndromes (fibromyalgia, focal myofascial pain, and others)
Dementia, Alzheimer's disease, and others
Head injuries
Neuromuscular disorders (congenital and acquired)
Neurovascular disorders
Motor neuron disease
Myasthenia gravis
Muscular dystrophies
Hereditary sensory motor neuropathy
Radiculopathies (cervical and lumbar)
Neck pain
Spinal cord injuries
Postpolio syndrome

Data from Taft JM, Hooker RS: *Neurology* 52:1513, 1999.

EXHIBIT 6-21

Procedures Performed by Neurology PAs by Percentage (N = 46)

Procedure	**%**
Lumbar punctures	63
Initiate multiple sclerosis therapy	50
Tender point injection	14
Nerve conduction studies	14
Initiate and monitor tissue plasminogen activator	11
Nerve blocks	11
Evoked potentials	7
Quantitative sensory testing	2
Botulism injections	2
Interpret EEGs	2

Data from Taft JM, Hooker RS: *Neurology* 52:1513, 1999.

Obstetrics and Gynecology (Women's Health)

The shortage of health care personnel in obstetrics and gynecology (OB/GYN) has been cyclical and in the 1970s was significant (Schneider, 1972). The earliest studies of PAs in women's health found that they could care for at least 80% of well patients in family-planning clinics without the need for consultation with a physician (Ostergard, 1975). Two programs, Stanford University and the University of Washington, experimented with postgraduate programs to train PAs and NPs as midwives (Briggs, 1978; Stark, 1984). A third postgraduate program for PAs in OB/GYN existed at Montefiore Medical Center in New York. The 15-month program consisted of advanced training in medicine, surgery, gynecology, preoperative and postoperative care, cardiac and trauma life support, and critical care (McGill et al., 1990).

PAs in female reproductive health perform in various roles including family planning (Mondy, 1986), routine examinations, mammogram interpretation (Hillman, 1987), and termination of pregnancies (Freedman, 1986; O'Hara, 1989; Donovan, 1992). Literature on the advance practice nurse suggests that NPs and CNMs occupy this niche with high levels of employment and that PAs may have trouble entering women's health care provider roles where competition for NPs is high. Anecdotally, we hear many female PAs prefer women's health roles and even when they are in family medicine will often have a large patient load primarily of women.

Occupational and Environmental Medicine (Industrial Medicine)

Occupational and environmental medicine (also known as occupational, industrial medicine, and corporate medicine) has used PAs as early as 1971 and has been an optional rotation within many PA programs (Barnes, 1971; Howard, 1971; Lowe, 1971; Lynch, 1971). One of the early uses of PAs in industrial medicine was on the Alaska Pipeline Project in the 1970s. The delivery of routine physical examinations for industries and insurance companies by PAs can result in substantial savings compared with the cost when this service is performed by a physician, which makes the PA particularly attractive (Medical World News, 1973; Richmond, 1974; Weisenberger, 1974). Industrial health studies conducted primarily by PAs, instead of physicians, have been a trend in certain sectors for the last two decades (Harbert, 1978; Romm, 1979; Elliott, 1984). Occupational medicine is one of the three subspecialties of preventive medicine; the other two are general preventative medicine and aerospace medicine.

The role of the industrial and occupational medical PAs encompasses the delivery of physical, mental, and emotional health care, as well as preventive medicine. While health promotion and disease prevention is stressed, much of the role PAs provide encompasses primary care. Activities include occupational health and safety, stress reduction, smoking cessation, and wellness. Involvement of PAs in this area escalated in 1978 as industry responded to cost-containment pressures; PAs perform annual employee physical examinations, exercise stress testing, occupational health education, drug screening, and treatment of work-related injuries. Work settings initially focused on underserved areas; today they include plant sites, private industrial medicine clinics, and corporate medical administration. Use continues to expand. The American Academy of Physician Assistants in Occupational Medicine, founded in 1981, develops continuing medical education programs and educates industry and the public about PAs in occupational medicine (Ramos, 1989). The trend has been for PAs and NPs to become hospital employee health managers, replacing RNs (Hospital Employee Health, 1991).

Hooker and Mackey undertook an administrative study of the activity of PAs and compared them with physicians in the same industrial medicine setting. The location was a large industrial medicine clinic where 30 physicians and 15 PAs provided care to industrially employed patients in 1999. The results reveal that PAs work more hours and see more patients per year than physicians. The characteristics of patients seen by each provider are similar in age, gender ratio, and severity of injury. Physicians see, on average, 2.8 patients per hour and PAs 2.5. The average charge per patient visit and total charge for an episode of care were similar. Differences between PAs and physicians were on the duration of limited duty prescribed: PAs prescribed, on average, 15 days and physicians 17. PAs were likely to refer a patient to an outside provider 19.7%, while a physician referred 17.4%. The salary of a physician was approximately twice as much as a PA. We conclude that the use of PAs in OEM may represent a cost-effective advantage from an administrative standpoint (Hooker, 2002, unpublished data). See Exhibits 6-22 and 6-23.

The University of Oklahoma physician associate program at one time sponsored a graduate

EXHIBIT 6-22

Comparison of OEM PAs and Physicians by Outcomes of Episodes of Care

	PA average	Physician average	Overall average	p	SD	95% CI
Average no. of days of limited activity assigned	15.6	17.4	16.8	.015	48.2	16.1-17.5
Likely to refer a patient to an outside provider	19.7%	17.4%	18.2%	.0001	38.6%	17.6-18.7
Average no. of patient visits per hour	2.5	2.9	2.8	.008	1.9	2.8-2.8
Average charge per visit	$284.77	$302.53	$296.72	NS	$159.76	294.50-298.93
Average total charges for episode of care	$565.98	$608.13	$594.33	NS	$751.46	583.91-604.75
Average severity score of problems treated (mild, 1; moderate, 2; severe, 3)	1.92	1.93	1.93	NS	.33	1.93-1.94
% of male patients	74.3%	72.5%	73.1%	.007	44.3%	72.5-73.2
Average age of patients (yr)	35.3	35.5	35.5	NS	11.2	35.3-35.7
Probability patients likely to keep their appointment	81%	76%	79%	.0024	1.04	78.0-80.9

EXHIBIT 6-23

Occupational and Environmental Medicine Provider Characteristics

	No.	Age (average) (yr)	Gender	Average salary	Average no. of visits per day
Physicians		50	18 M: 6 F	$143,056	
PAs		45	7 M: 5 F	$74,208	
Average	32.72				23.31

occupational health program that trained and granted a master's degree in public health and industrial medicine.

Oncology

The roles of PAs in oncology encompass pediatric oncology and radiation oncology (Kelvin et al., 1999; Rose, 1999). Major academic centers such as the M.D. Anderson Center in Houston employ more than 75 PAs in oncology, and the Fred Hutchinson Center in Seattle employs more than 50 PAs. The Oncology Center at the Johns Hopkins Hospital in Baltimore employs a large cadre of PAs in multiple roles. A postgraduate program for PAs in oncology started in 2001 at the M.D. Anderson Center.

Orthopedic Physician Assistants

There is a great deal of confusion about PAs who work in orthopedic settings, technicians who call themselves orthopedic PAs (OPAs), and the different organizations of PAs who specialize in orthopedic medicine. Formally trained PAs who work in an orthopedic setting differ from another group of technicians trained to assist the orthopedic surgeon. Both groups have *orthopedic* in the title, and many refer to themselves as *OPAs*. To add to this confusion, there is the American Society of Orthopedic Physician Assistants (ASOPAs), OPAs, and the Physician Assistants in Orthopedic Surgery (PAOS). Approximately 8% of formally trained PAs in 2001 reported they were employed in an orthopedic practice (AAPA, 2001).

The history of OPAs begins with assistants to the orthopedic surgeon. They seem to have been present since at least 1954 in some capacity, whether to assist applying a cast or to hold a retractor. Many developed some expertise while in the military. It is unclear when the first formal orthopedic technical program started; however, the AMA House of Delegates first adopted minimum educational standards for OPA education in 1969 upon a recommendation from the American Academy of Orthopedic Surgeons (AAOS). Eight OPA programs had been accredited by 1973. This proved somewhat controversial, and 1 year later the AAOS announced its intent to withdraw sponsorship from the accreditation program. After substantial consultation with the AAOS, the AMA CME announced a moratorium on the accreditation of any additional orthopedic programs and informed accredited programs that accreditation would be discontinued upon graduation of the classes that would be matriculating in the fall of 1974. It is important to note that the AMA without the involvement of the medical specialty society does not sponsor accreditation efforts in allied health education or societies and the related allied health organizations most closely associated with the occupation.

During this brief period of AMA sanctioning of OPAs in the mid 1970s, eight OPA programs were accredited by the AMA CME (Exhibit 6-24). None of these orthopedic assistant programs remain in existence today. The one at Kirkwood Community College in Cedar Rapids graduated its last class in 1988. The AMA Committee on Allied Health Education and Accreditation never accredited any of the OPA programs as PA programs.

EXHIBIT 6-24

Orthopedic Assistant Technical Programs

Program	Location	Graduates
Bismarck Junior College	Bismarck, N.D.	—
Cerritos College	Norwalk, Calif.	3
Chattanooga Technical Institute	Chattanooga, Tenn.	1
City College of San Francisco	San Francisco, Calif.	2
Highline Community College	Midway, Wis.	12
Foothill College	Los Altos, Calif.	—
Kirkwood Community College	Cedar Rapids, Iowa	36
Marygrove College	Detroit, Mich.	62
Normandale Orthopedic Program		0

Data from various sources including conversations with the admissions departments of some of the schools. Number of graduates may not be accurate because of lack of verification.

The orthopedic assistant programs were confined to training technical orthopedic tasks without the substantial background in the basic medical sciences that the primary care PA programs stress. The educational qualifications of the two groups—OPAs and PAs—differ substantially. Orthopedic assistants were trained as technologists in an 18-month course at a junior college, which was more closely related to other technical programs, such as respiratory therapy, surgical technology, and medical or dental assisting. Anywhere from 500 to 1000 graduates are estimated to have matriculated from these eight programs, along with some similar programs in the Air Force.

Graduates of the orthopedic assistant program are *not* eligible to sit for the PANCE, administered by the NCCPA. A national board handles an examination for OPAs for certifying OPAs (NBCOPA). This NBCOPA is not equivalent to the NCCPA's examination, and the organizations are not affiliated in any way (Kappes, 1992).

Although both PAs and OPAs work for orthopedists, Minnesota is the only state with a law regulating OPAs. In 1978 Michigan included a grandfather title protection for "orthopedic physician's assistants," but OPAs remain an unlicensed occupation in that state. OPAs were also given a finite period to register in Minnesota when regulation of PAs became effective in 1986. In Iowa, home of the Kirkwood Community College program, the 1988 Physician Assistant Practice Act explicitly states that "orthopedic physician's assistant technologists" are not required to qualify as PAs.

The ASOPA represents approximately 400 practicing OPAs and was formed in 1971. Most states do not regulate the practice of OPAs. The exceptions are New York, where OPAs must be registered as specialist assistants, and Minnesota, where for 2 years OPAs were allowed to register as PAs. Medicare does not cover services provided by OPAs (Lindahl, 1994).

Physician Assistants in Orthopedic Surgery, the latest in formation of a special interest group for formally trained PAs, was formed in 1992 at the annual AAPA conference in Nashville. This seems to be the most active organization. It reports working with the Southern Orthopedic Association to develop a membership category for PAs (Wallace, 1995).

NCCPA-certified PAs in orthopedics provide a host of roles that closely juxtapose the orthopedic surgeon. They provide preadmission physical examination, write admitting orders, first assist in surgery, dictate discharge summaries, and conduct fracture clinics (Samsot, 1996).

Broughton's study (1996) examining the range of tasks and the dynamics of practice of orthopedics by PAs helps us to understand the degree of service they perform (Exhibit 6-25). From a survey of 440 PAs in orthopedic practice, all perform history and physical examinations and prescribe medications. Most interpret x-ray films, apply casts, suture wounds, assist in surgery, and reduce fractures. Postgraduate-trained PAs seem to have higher levels of responsibility than the others (Broughton, 1996).

Ophthalmology

There are no formal ophthalmology programs that teach PAs to be clinicians in ophthamology. Two programs developed in the 1960s to train type C PAs in the management of eye diseases: the Georgetown University Hospital in Washington, District of Columbia, and Columbia-Presbyterian Medical Center in New York. Each had a 2-year certification program. Both are defunct. The graduate ophthalmology PA could not only provide refractions but also assist in surgery and manage uncomplicated nonsurgical ophthalmologic problems such as eye infections (Sadler, 1972).

EXHIBIT 6-25

Tasks Performed by Physician Assistants in Orthopedic Surgery

Task	%
History taking	99.0%
Physical examination	99.0
Interpretation of x-ray studies	94.2%
Cast application	94.5
Wound suturing	93.8
Assistance in surgery	92.9
Joint aspiration/injection	80.8
Brace application	76.0
K-wire removal	73.4
Wound incision and drainage	67.5
Fracture reduction	57.1
Dislocation reduction	54.5
Hardware removal	50.3
Compartment pressure measurements	31.2
Administer regional anesthesia	22.1
Tendon repair	22.1
Percutaneous pinning of fractures	21.4

Data from Broughton B: PhD dissertation, 1996, Columbia Pacific University, California.

Approximately 50 PAs who are members of the AAPA report that their primary responsibility is in ophthalmology. Most are employed in large practices that specialize in cataract and radial keratotomy procedures (Wilson, 1990). The role of PAs in ophthalmology is not viewed positively by optometrists who would like to have expanded roles in eye disease care for themselves but are usually prohibited by narrowly defined state laws.

Otolaryngology (Head and Neck Surgery)

The Society of Physician Assistants in Otorhinolayrngology-Head and Neck Surgery was founded in Kansas City during the American Academy of Otorhinolayrngology-Head and Neck Surgery's annual meeting in 1991. The Society was developed to enhance the professional growth development of PAs who worked in the field of otolaryngology. These PAs were seeking an organization that would provide an opportunity to meet and interact with PAs who share a common interest and to obtain continuing medical education specific to their field. At least 75 PAs belong to this organization, which has a liaison with the American Academy of Otorhinolaryngology-Head and Neck Surgery.

The roles of PAs in this specialized field include diagnostic tests and procedures such as fine-needle aspiration biopsies, tympanostomy tubes, and sinus irrigations. Many assist in surgery, coordinate admissions, dictate discharge summaries, and provide follow-up care. Additional office procedures include cleaning of ear canals and mastoid cavities, electrocautery for the control of epistaxis, insertion of nasal packing, and immediate postoperative care of patients in the inpatient and outpatient setting. They may also perform rhinopharyngolaryngoscopy, videostroboscopy, and vocal/voice recordings.

In 1995 approximately 23% of PAs in otolaryngology were employed by a solo otolaryngologist, 57% in a group practice, 4% by hospitals, 7% by the U.S. government, and 7% by HMOs (Poppen, 1996).

Pathology

Pathologist's assistants are often referred to as *PAs.* While they are a type of PA, they are not trained in primary care. They are formally trained in pathology and do not have an association with the AAPA or the Association of Physician Assistant Programs. Formally trained PAs who practice forensic medicine are described in this chapter in the section on forensic medicine.

The role of a pathologist's assistant is to perform specific tasks and duties under the direction and supervision of a licensed pathologist. Pathologist's assistants interact with pathologists in the same manner that formally trained PAs perform their duties under the direction of physicians in medical and surgical specialties (Grzybicki, Galvis, and Raab, 1999; Vollmer, 1999).

Pathologist's assistants programs at the University of Alabama and Quinnipiac College in Connecticut have been active since 1971. Both are 2-years master's degree programs and have seen more than 200 individual graduate. The Quinnipiac College program is affiliated with the Veterans Administration Medical Centers in West Haven and with Yale University School of Medicine. Other programs are at Duke University and the University of Maryland. The master's of science in pathologist's assistant at Finch University of Health Sciences, which began in 2000, is the fourth program. The roles and responsibilities of the pathologist's assistant include histopathology, surgical frozen sections, and general autopsies.

Pediatrics

Pediatrics is considered one of the three specialties that make up primary care. However, many PAs specialize in pediatrics both by formal and on-the-job training. One program specializes in pediatrics and two postgraduate programs are in neonatology. In 2002 there were 2.4% of PAs in clinical practice who reported pediatrics as the specialty practiced for their primary employers. The range of PA practices in the pediatric field mirrors that of pediatricians. Most work in general pediatric settings, while a smaller number choose subspecialties of pediatric care. Of all pediatric PAs, two thirds practice with general pediatricians and one third work with pediatric subspecialists. In addition, an estimated 24,000 (77% of clinically practicing PAs) provide care to patients younger than 18 years in general practice settings (AAPA, 1999).

Most PAs working with pediatricians are graduates of programs that offer a broad general medical education that includes pediatrics. The one program that offers a special focus in pediatrics is the University of Colorado School of Medicine's child health associate/PA (CHA/PA) program. Although this is a primary care PA program, it specializes in the care of infants, children, and adolescents. Students originally fulfilled a 3-year curriculum, with in-depth didactic course work serving as a foundation for a 12-month internship in the third year. Through required rotations in general pediatrics, newborn nursery, adolescent medicine, family medicine, inpatient pediatric medicine, and service in underserved or rural areas, PA students in the CHA/PA program gain generalist medical training with a special pediatric emphasis. This program has since been reduced to 24 months.

Pediatric PAs are specialized as well. They are used on pediatric bone marrow transplant units (Trigg, 1990) and work with the homeless, uninsured, poor, and underserved (Rada-Sidinger, 1992). They are members of social service child protection units (Gray, 1991) and work with inpatients to address the problems associated with resident overwork and educational needs of hospital services (Giardino et al., 1994).

Although most PAs go immediately from PA school to medical practice, opportunities also exist for postgraduate training in pediatric and other specialty fields. Norwalk Hospital and the Yale School of Medicine cosponsor the only PA postgraduate pediatrics residency program.

PAs working in the pediatric inpatient setting typically fit one of two models. Either they are employed outside the hospital and have privileges to provide inpatient care, or they are employed as house staff in the pediatric or neonatal unit. Because pediatric PAs draw on both the generalist and the specialist aspects of their medical training, they can effectively handle routine pediatric issues and can address a range of acute problems. Common responsibilities for PAs in the pediatric hospital setting include taking patient histories and performing physical examinations, working with physicians in diagnosing and treating illnesses ranging from common infections to more complex congenital diagnosing and treating illnesses ranging from common infections to more complex congenital diseases, attending to premature babies, and assisting in surgery. PAs in pediatric hospital practice tend to act as stabilizers within the intense and transient pediatric setting, providing continuity of care to the young patients who need it most. A 1999 report by the American Academy of Pediatrics on the role of PAs and NPs in the care of hospitalized children concluded that they "have a meaningful role in the management of hospitalized children. Having already demonstrated their ability to perform in supervised intensive care settings, they should be effective in the general inpatient unit and can play a valuable role in the care of hospitalized children by contributing specialized skills that improve the quality of patient care" (American Academy of Pediatrics, Committee on Hospital Care, 1999).

Patient satisfaction tends to increase when PAs are on staff for several reasons. PAs facilitate patient flow, shorten waiting periods, and ease staff scheduling. By handling routine pediatric questions and concerns, PAs help patients and parents understand their illnesses and treatment options. A PA on the team can help with patient education and follow-up, which improves compliance.

The AAPA 1999 survey of PAs in pediatrics found single specialty physician groups to be the most prevalent employers of pediatric PAs (30%), followed by hospitals (28%), and solo physician practices (10.5%).

Plastic and Reconstructive Surgery

Plastic and reconstructive surgery encompasses the areas of cosmetic surgery, burn management, and hand surgery. PAs in surgery in general, and plastic surgery in particular, can obtain these skills by formal training (e.g., SA or postgraduate training) or on-the-job training.

The plastic surgeon uses the PA in a variety of ways. In the clinic setting the PA may see patients as postoperative cases. In the hospital the PA may assist in the operation, perform admission histories and physical examinations, order routine laboratory tests, dictate discharge summaries, and monitor patients and change dressings (Toth, 1978; Gittins, 1996). Reconstructive microsurgery has relied on trained SAs in this area to reduce operating time (Gould, 1984).

Public Health and Preventive Medicine

The impact of a nonphysician as a manager on full-time public health coverage was first examined in 1980 (Jekel, 1980). In this setting a PA became the public health director of a region in Connecticut. The experience in Connecticut demonstrates that the public health world does not need to rely solely on physicians. The level of care improved when a nonphysician assumed the role of health director (Atwater, 1980). PAs are employed in public health settings on both the state and national level. They have served as epidemiologists in medical offices at the Centers for Disease Control and Prevention (CDC).

Many PAs are employees of the U.S. Public Health Service, both the uniform and the nonuniform branch. In this capacity they work for a number of agencies such as the Coast Guard, National Oceanic and Atmospheric Administration, CDC, Food and Drug Administration, Federal Aviation Administration, Health and Human Services, Office of Health Promotion/Disease Prevention, Health Services and Resources Administration, and the National Centers for Health Statistics. As uniform officers they wear a Navy uniform and retain a Navy rank. The highest ranking PA is a captain.

Radiology

A program to train highly selected, experienced radiologic technologists to become type C PAs in diagnostic radiology (PA-DR) was initiated at the University of Kentucky Medical Center in 1970 (Kierman, 1977). This 2-year program was underwritten by the federal government and was designed to improve the efficiency of radiologic procedures (Department of Health, Education, and Welfare, 1977). Approximately 30 individuals graduated before the program closed after withdrawal of support by the American College of Radiology.

Despite the small number of graduates, six studies have examined the use of PAs in diagnostic radiology. In one study of work activities a radiologist would have performed including examinations and radiograph screening for disease, the PAs performed these activities "accurately and acceptably." Each PA-DR averaged a savings of 34% of the employing radiologist's time (Kierman, 1977). Duties were wide ranging and included fluoroscopic procedures, excretory urography, and chest radiographic screening (Thompson, 1974). Another study trained primary care PAs to perform competently in screening radiographs, intravenous pyelograms, and brain scans. The authors concluded that the PA-DRs performed as well as radiologists (Thompson, 1971, 1972).

At the Johns Hopkins Hospital PAs on the interventional radiology staff performs history and physical examinations and Doppler pressures, schedules laboratory work and admissions, answers referring physicians' calls, and obtains preliminary patient information (White, 1989). The addition of this person decreased mean length of stay for patients undergoing various procedures and increased the capacity for interventional procedures (White et al., 1988).

Surveys of chiefs of radiology departments were generally favorable when asked if they were willing to delegate traditional radiologist tasks to PAs (Thompson, 1971). When private practice radiologists were surveyed, however, at least 60% showed reluctance to delegate these tasks (Parker, 1972). These studies are in need of repeating.

A study on mammograms interpreted by PAs found that the interpretations were more sensitive and as specific as those made by six HMO radiologists who interpreted the same cases and were as effective as those by radiologists described in the literature. The study concluded that mammogram interpretations by PAs were similar to those made by radiologists, took less time, and cost less than those by performed by radiologists (Hillman, 1987).

Anecdotal reports have circulated about a few PA-DRs who still work after the closure of the Kentucky program in the late 1970s. In 1991 a controversial editorial called for renewed interest in training PAs to work in radiology (Ellis, 1991; McCowan, 1991). In 1996 the subject was reviewed again after describing a few PAs who provide radiology services in some different settings (Hayes, 1996). We know of PAs who are involved in interventional radiology where fine catheters are used to reach and destroy tumors in deep organs.

In an interview with three PAs in radiology, the AAPA found that one group of 20 radiologists hired a PA to help out generally in the group and specifically to assist an interventional radiologist who was setting up new programs. In addition to assisting the neuroradiologist, the PA focused on posttreatment rounds and consults. A positive experience with the first PA led to the hiring of another PA to conduct histories and physical examinations, perform and assist with invasive procedures, and write discharge summaries. The physicians also wanted the PAs to perform fluoroscopies. In that state the radiologists could delegate to the PAs anything within their scope of practice, except final interpretations on scans and x-ray films.

In another state an interventional radiology practice hired a PA who started out doing all the first-assisting duties with one physician. Eventually the practice added three physicians: one fellow and two residents. Because the fellow and residents took over the first-assisting duties, the PA was asked to take on a new role. She took over most of the communicating with referring physicians and performing case evaluations, including such duties as determining whether patients needed antibiotics, intravenous orders for hydration, and insulin management.

Another PA working in interventional radiology at a major teaching hospital said he spent most of his time running the outpatient department. He performed histories and physical examinations and wrote laboratory orders. He assisted on some procedures and followed patients afterward. This particular practice had a high percentage of patients with liver disease with biliary tubes. The PA provided patient education on dealing with the tubes, assisted with placement and maintenance of tubes, and removed 95% of the Hickman catheters. He also did a lot of coordination and consultation by phone with patients who needed help with their tubes and with family physicians who needed to know about caring for the patient's tubes.

Research

Almost as soon as there were more than a handful of PAs, there were researchers to study them. At first, medical sociologists, behaviorists, economists, and health services researchers examined the nascent profession and everything that PAs did (Hooker, 1994). Within a few years PAs became part of investigative teams, as well as the subjects of research. Since the early 1970s the PA research agenda has been shaped not only by health researchers interested in the profession but also by PAs formally or informally trained in the social research disciplines (Jarski, 1988). These medical, social, and health services research efforts to involve PAs have been at five levels of activity:

1. Supplying information about ongoing activities as providers
2. Helping to develop new data
3. Participating in data analysis
4. Assisting in research design
5. Coauthoring papers that result from research

PAs are also clinical investigators who participate in drug trials and biochemical research. They assume roles previously occupied by a physician (Morian, 1986). One of us (R.S.H.) has personally participated as a clinical investigator in 14 clinical trials and has been the principal investigator of two of these trials. This experience is not unique because many other PAs around the country conduct clinical trials in many settings, from private firms to university research clinics.

As PA programs shift to grant master's degrees, many of these programs require a research component to the curriculum. Often a PA will assume the role of research director.

The role of the PA in research is likely to increase as the demand for clinical trials increases and the need for skilled clinicians who can be employed at less cost than a physician also increases. Many PA programs on the master's level have a research component as part of the curriculum, which is likely to stimulate further research.

Rehabilitation Medicine and Physiatry

PAs are found in many rehabilitative roles including employment in hospitals and rehabilitative units. They function essentially as physiatrists, helping to diagnose and treat patients with chronic pain disorders and spine problems, and as directors of rehabilitative care. Some have mastered nerve conduction studies and electromyographic skills. Others provide medical care along with management for paralyzed patients those with spinal cord injuries in specialty units. A few of the PAs we know in this specialty were physical therapists before becoming PAs and a few were formally trained as athletic trainers, naturopathic physicians, or chiropractors.

Rheumatology

Although a small contingent of AAPA members consistently cite their primary medical responsibility as rheumatology, their role has yet to be delineated in any literature. In one study of rheumatology referrals in an HMO a PA and two rheumatologists shared approximately equally all of the consultations for that year (Hooker, 1985). The authors know of rheumatology PAs who provide a broad range of services including new patient evaluations, monitoring drug administration, performing procedures such as joint injections and muscle biopsies, and rounding in the hospital. An HMO rheumatologist identified that the number of patients seen by a rheumatology PA was the same as that of two other rheumatologists (Sloop, 1995).

With the demand for rheumatology service increasing, and the number of training programs for rheumatologists shrinking, it seems that this is an unfilled niche for PAs. Their role seems to be welcomed, and PAs are eligible to be members of the American College of Rheumatology.

Sports Medicine

Many PAs provide care in sports medicine clinics, are team health providers, and function in a variety of roles that transcend orthopedics and rehabilitation medicine. Identifying these PAs is difficult because there is no formal designation for PAs in sports medicine and many list their specialty as family medicine or orthopedics. Some PAs come to this specialty having been athletic trainers and others because they are (or were) athletes.

Tissue Procurement

Cadaver organ retrieval is an ideal role for PAs because of their training and because it can directly replace a physician providing the same service. In one 30-month study involving a PA replacing a physician the total number of kidneys increased threefold, the number of usable kidneys increased dramatically, the number of referral hospitals increased threefold, and the number of kidneys shared with other transplant centers tripled as compared with any period before initiation of the PA approach (Schmittou, 1977). Sometimes the tissue procurement PA will follow the organ back into the operating room to assist the surgeon in the transplantation. Other PAs are involved with monitoring transplant recipients for tissue rejection and other related illnesses. PAs are urged to become more active in procurement and transplant programs (Joyner, 1984).

Urology

A type C PA in urology was developed at a time when a number of emerging technologies were requiring a special person trained to manage the tools and instruments of this specialty. In 1970 a program in Cincinnati trained PAs in urology to administer intravenous pyelograms, obtain detailed voided specimens, assist in methods to snare renal stones, perform cystoscopies, and analyze renal calculi. Although there is plenty of opportunity for PAs to continue in this vein, a new type of urology PA has emerged: the medical urology PA. The urology PA's work tends to be performed in a urology office with one urologist or a group of urologists but sometimes extends into the surgical suite to perform lithotripsy procedures and assist in other roles. This PA often provides the initial consultation, performs a cystoscopy, evaluates and performs biopsies on the prostate, and manages the impotent patient. An expanded role for PAs in this field is in sexology.

Veterinary Medicine

While we know of no study on PAs formally employed in veterinary medicine, anecdotes abound about rural PAs providing care for both large domestic animals and small animals. These services include casting fractures, castrating, immunization, administrating antibiotics, and delivering foals. This service should be viewed as only an occasional and informal tradition of the rural general practitioner and should not be taken too seriously as an erosion of the domain of the professional animal doctor.

POSTGRADUATE RESIDENCY PROGRAMS

In the first comprehensive book discussing the PA profession, Ann Bliss wrote in 1975 a section about the future of PAs and how they might be tempted to subspecialize.

> Immediately upon graduation, the physician's assistant is in considerable danger of being swallowed whole by the whale that is our present entrepreneurial, subspecialty medical practice system. The likely co-option of the newly minted physician's assistant by subspecialty medicine is one of the most serious

issues confronting physician's assistants. (Sadler 1972)

Bliss was alluding to the already emerging trend of PAs working with surgeons and other specialists in acute care medicine and surgery in the hospital setting. Instead of threatening the well-being of the profession, however, these trends marked the beginning of expansion of the ways in which PAs were used and on a very practical level indicated that PAs were seeking out and filling the jobs that were becoming frequently available to them.

The first postgraduate program began at Montefiore Medical Center in the Bronx, New

EXHIBIT 6-26

PA Postgraduate Residency Programs

Specialty	Program	Length	Award
Surgery	Advanced Physician Assistant Studies, Arizona School of Health Sciences	–	–
Surgery	Physician Assistant Surgical Residency Program, Montefiore Medical Center/Einstein College of Medicine, N.Y.	15 mo	Certificate
Surgery	Physician Assistant Surgical Residency Program, Norwalk Hospital/Yale University School of Medicine, Conn.	1 yr	Certificate
Surgery	Cedars-Sinai Medical Center, Los Angeles, Calif.	1 yr	Certificate
Surgery	Geisinger Medical Center, Danville, Pa.	1 yr	Certificate
Surgery	Martin Luther King, Jr./Drew Medical Center, Los Angeles, Calif.	1 yr	Certificate
Surgery	Mayo Foundation, Rochester, Minn.	1 yr	Certificate
Surgery	Butterworth Hospital/Western Michigan University	1 yr	Certificate
Surgery	Physician Assistant Residency in Cardiothoracic Surgery, St. Joseph Mercy Hospital, Ypsilanti, Mich.	–	–
Emergency medicine	Alderson-Broaddus College, Philippi, W.Va.	2 yr	Master's degree
Emergency medicine	U.S. Army, Fort Sam, Houston, Tex., and Madigan Army Medical Center, Tacoma, Wash.	1 yr	Certificate
Emergency medicine	Emergency Medicine Physician Assistant Residency, Los Angeles County/University of Southern California Medical Center	1 yr	Certificate
Family Medicine	Nova Southeastern University Clinics Postgraduate Program in Family Medicine, Fort Lauderdale, Fla.	–	–
Dermatology	University of Texas Southwestern Medical Center, Dallas	–	–
Dermatology	Kirksville College of Osteopathic Medicine, Mo.	–	–
Dermatology	Dermatology Associates of Tallahassee and Nova Southeastern PA Residency Program in Dermatologic Studies	–	–
Gynecology/Obstetrics	Montefiore Medical Center, Bronx, N.Y.	15 mo	Certificate
Geriatrics	University of Southern California School of Medicine, Los Angeles	1 yr	Master's certificate
Orthopedics	Illinois Bone and Joint Institute, North Chicago, Ill.	–	–
Orthopedics	Physician Assistant Orthopaedic Surgery Residency, New York, N.Y.	–	–
Orthopedics	Watauga Orthopaedics Physician Assistant Fellowship	–	–
Oncology	M.D. Anderson Medical Center, Houston, Tex.	1 yr	Certificate
Oncology	Arrowhead Regional Medical Center, San Bernardino, Calif.	–	–
Rural primary care	Alderson-Broaddus College, Philippi, W.Va.	2 yr	Master's degree
Pediatrics	Physician Assistant Postgraduate Residency Program in Pediatrics, Baptist Medical Center, Wolfson Children's Hospital, Jacksonville, Fla.	1 yr	Certificate
Pediatrics	Physician Assistant Pediatric Residency Program, Norwalk Hospital, Conn.	1 yr	Certificate
Pediatrics	Psychiatric Physician Assistant Postgraduate Training Program, The University of Texas Medical Branch, Galveston, Tex.	–	–
Urology	Postgraduate Physician Assistant Urology Residency Program, Northwest Metropolitan Urology Associates, Chicago, Ill.	–	–

York. In 1972 Richard Rosen, MD, a surgeon, was concerned that the large size of the surgical residency training program of that institution was worsening the already apparent overproduction of surgeons. He believed that PAs could be hired to provide the same type of patient care as physician surgical house staff, thereby limiting the production of future surgeons in what was becoming an overcrowded field. The notion that PAs could substitute for house staff was quite different from the existing mainstream philosophy of how PAs were to be used. Rosen recruited PAs to work on inpatient units, first in surgery and later expanding into other departments. He thought that PAs ought to be used in settings where there were many physicians (e.g., in hospitals) and was convinced that PAs should be allowed to provide care that does not have to be given solely by a physician (Rosen, 1986).

This unique use of PAs pioneered by Rosen led to other postgraduate residency programs for PAs (Exhibit 6-26). The Norwalk Hospital affiliated with the Yale University School of Medicine program began in 1976 and instituted a 1-year training experience that consisted of a 4-month didactic training session of the fundamentals of surgical anatomy and physiology, followed by 8 months of clinical rotations through surgical wards at Norwalk. PA surgical residents perform a full range of inpatient surgical duties, including preoperative care, assisting in surgery, and postoperative care (Heinrich et al., 1980) (Exhibit 6-27).

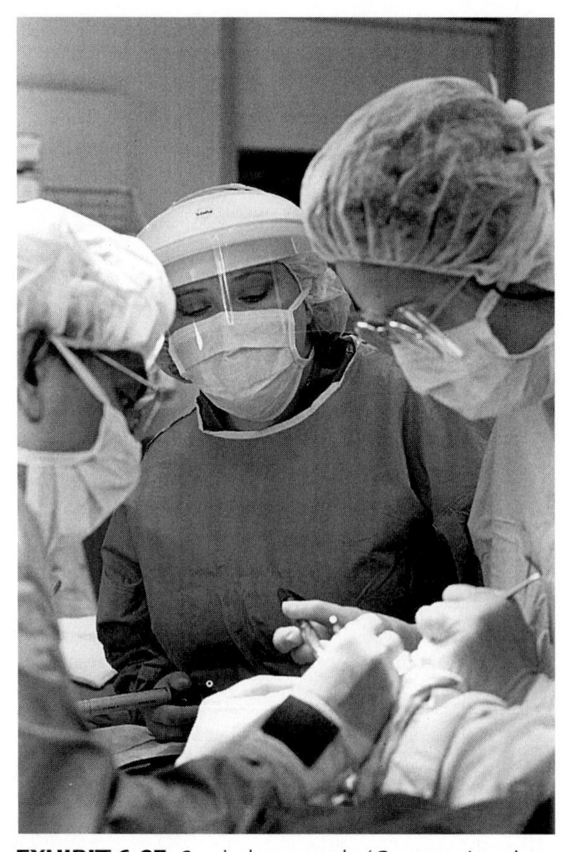

EXHIBIT 6-27 Surgical teamwork. (Courtesy American Academy of Physician Assistants.)

The National Association of Postgraduate PA Programs was established in 1988 to assist in the development and organization of postgraduate educational curricula and programs for PAs. This organization assists in the definition of the role of the PA in the specialties and in the development of evaluation methodologies for postgraduate educational curricula and programs. Other activities include information for the public and profession about postgraduate educational curricula and programs.

Despite the remarkably diverse and growing number of PA postgraduate residency programs, we are unaware of any study that examines where these graduates are dispersed and what they are

EXHIBIT 6-28

AAPA Constituent Organizations

American Academy of Nephrology PAs
American Academy of PAs in Allergy, Asthma, and Immunology
American Academy of PAs in Occupational Medicine
American Association of Plastic and Reconstructive Surgery PAs
American Association of Surgical PAs
Association of Family Practice PAs
Association of Neurosurgical PAs
Association of PAs in Cardiovascular Surgery
Association of PAs in Obstetrics and Gynecology
Association of PAs in Oncology
Association of Psychiatric PAs
PAs in Orthopedic Surgery
Society of Dermatology PAs
Society of Emergency Medicine PAs
Society of PAs in Addiction Medicine
Society of PAs Caring for the Elderly
Society of PAs in Otolaryngology/Head and Neck Surgery
Society of PAs in Pediatrics
Urological Association of PAs

Data from American Academy of Physician Assistants, *AAPA Census Report, 1999.* Other medical specialty PA groups exist in various stages of development but have not attained AAPA constituent organization status at the time of the development of this section.

doing. Whether PAs who are formally trained in surgery, PAs who are informally trained in surgery, or PAs who are postgraduates in surgery perform different duties or see different types of patients is not known. Clearly, research must be conducted to answer the charges that PAs in postgraduate residencies are providing anything more than a ready source of labor for institutions.

CONSTITUENT ORGANIZATIONS

The AAPA maintains a number of constituent organizations for specialty PAs who want a professional society that is more focused on their needs (Exhibit 6-28). These organizations vary in membership size and activity but generally publish a newsletter periodically and meet at the AAPA annual conference. Constituent organizations differ from the AAPA caucuses, which are groups of PAs who have cultural ties that bind them.

SUMMARY

One of the major rationales for the development of the PA profession was to augment the supply of medically trained providers in those specialties in greatest need of assistance. The diversity of employment settings is an indication of the maturity of the profession. While the primary care role of the PA is the root of the profession and remains the basis of PA education, the PA profession has become much more specialized over the last decade, which is primarily the result of economic pressures: This is where the jobs are and the role may be more enhancing. PAs are widely dispersed throughout the spectrum of medical disciplines and seem to have become well integrated. Many PAs enjoy membership status in physician specialty societies or professional specialties of their own making. These specialty pathways involve PA residencies, master's degrees in clinical and nonclinical disciplines, and entry into other fields through experience and formal training. Specialization will remain an important component of the PA program, but with the exception of surgery, no one specialty is likely to dominate.

7

INPATIENT SETTINGS

INTRODUCTION

At the turn of the new century there were a little more than 6000 hospitals in the United States. Physician assistant (PA) use in hospital roles has become commonplace in a wide variety of medical center settings. PAs work in a many types of hospitals including major teaching hospitals, medium-size hospitals, small community and rural hospitals, and other types of inpatient care institutions. As of 2001 approximately 40% of clinically active PAs are employed by a hospital in some capacity (AAPA, 2002).

According to findings from a sample of 1690 PAs employed in hospitals who responded to a national survey, 45% of these PAs were "house officers." More than 90% of responding PAs held formal medical staff privileges and were credentialed under hospital bylaws. A similar percentage of hospital PAs have written job descriptions that permit them to write diagnostic and therapeutic orders within the institution (American Hospital Association [AHA], 1992). Another national study of 116 teaching hospitals reported a 62% use of PAs and/or nurse practitioners (NPs) in at least one of their departments. In these hospitals PAs were used to perform some tasks previously done by physician residents. Of the 178 departments using PAs as substitutes for traditional physician services, 42% were surgical, followed by primary care (25%) and medical specialties (21%). In this study PAs were more likely than NPs to work in surgery and emergency departments (EDs), although NPs were more likely than PAs to work in pediatrics and neonatal care (Riportella-Muller, Libby, and Kindig, 1995).

The role of PAs in inpatient settings tends to be focused in specialty and subspecialty areas. Of the 1600 PAs who work in hospitals, 20% (3200) work in inpatient units and 6% (950) work in critical care units. About 22% (3500) are in outpatient units, and 27% (4300) are in emergency departments. Another 21% (3300) work primarily in the operating room (AAPA, 2001). Hospital employed PAs also work in primary care or ambulatory care departments, in community outreach clinics, in the hospital employee health center, and in the ED at remarkably high levels (Hooker and McCaig, 1996).

Hospital experiences with PAs on inpatient services in many institutions demonstrate they bring a high level of safety, skills, and clinical efficacy. Published reports attest to successful experiences of PA use in inpatient internal medicine (Frick, 1983), surgical and surgical subspecialty (Heinrich et al., 1980), and pediatric services (Silver and McAtee, 1984). In addition, PAs have been found to be effective and are employed in critical care units (Dubaybo, Samson, and Carlson, 1991; Grabenkort and Ramsay, 1991); subspecialty services (e.g., diagnostic radiology) (White et al., 1988), and EDs (Goldfrank, Corso, and Squillacote, 1980; Sturmann, Ehrenberg, and Salzberg, 1990; Hooker and McCaig, 1996). The addition of PAs to inpatient medical staffs reveals high levels of acceptance by employing physicians and patients, a favorable cost-benefit margin to the institution, and maintenance of high levels of patient care quality (McKelvey, Oliver, and Conboy, 1986).

Montefiore Medical Center (Bronx, NY) was among the first hospitals to use PAs as a means to augment inpatient medical and surgical house staff. Beginning in 1971 PAs were hired for house staff roles at Montefiore on surgical wards to offset reductions in resident numbers. Today the institution employs more than 150 PAs not only in surgical areas but also in internal medicine, the medical subspecialties, emergency medicine, obstetrics and gynecology (OB/GYN), on the employee health service, on transplantation services, in burn units, and in a broad range of administrative, education, and research roles.

Another early model of the effectiveness of using PAs on inpatient services was developed and has flourished at Geisinger Medical Center, a 577-bed referral facility located in rural northeastern Pennsylvania. Geisinger began employing PAs in the mid 1970s and now has PAs serving in clinical roles spanning primary care, as well as in specialty and subspecialty roles. The Geisinger, like a number of other institutes, uses both PAs and NPs to staff family medicine clinics and the ED, in general medical internal medicine specialties, in general surgery and surgical subspecialties, in high-technology diagnostic and therapeutic service areas, and in roles in outpatient clinics at satellite settings (Walters, 1986; Harbert, Shipman, and Conrad, 1994). PAs are employed in substantial numbers in many acute care hospitals across the country.

HOUSE OFFICERS

PAs are the primary candidates to substitute for residents because of their skills in physical assessment, medical management, and pharmacology. Many PA programs train students in the hospital setting to work alongside residents or house officers. A small but growing body of literature documents that teaching hospitals have favorable experience using nonphysician providers (NPPs) on the wards, in critical care, and in surgery (Cawley, 1988).

The use of PAs and NPs has been particularly widespread in surgery to fill positions once filled by residents. In fact, some residency programs have lost accreditation because they lacked sufficient cases to provide adequate clinical experience (Foreman, 1993). In other institutions PAs have assumed responsibility for preoperative and postoperative care, obtaining histories, conducting physical examinations, and performing noninvasive procedures. For example, at Butterworth Hospital in Grand Rapids, Michigan, PAs serve as house officers in cardiothoracic surgery, neurosurgery, urology, and orthopedics.

Under certain circumstances PAs may be preferable to residents. Some faculty would rather work with PAs and NPs who have a lower turnover rate, greater familiarity with departmental procedures, and more clinical experience than first- and second-year residents (Silver and McAtee, 1988). Using PAs may also ensure that residents have richer educational experiences. One time-and-motion study of residents at three Minnesota teaching hospitals found that residents spent 12% of their time inserting catheters and drawing blood, procedures that can be done by PAs (Lurie et al., 1989). Because these tasks lose their pedagogic value after a certain number of repetitions, delegating them to PAs would free residents to focus on more complex cases.

Clinical, financial, and practical criticisms have been raised about the use of PAs as substitute residents. Although PAs may work well as substitutes for first- and second-year residents, some suggest they may require additional training to assume responsibility for more complex cases that call for more advanced medical decision making or greater technical skill. In a study by Riportella-Muller, Libby, and Kindig (1995), this was not the case in teaching hospitals. In this national sample, PAs and NPs were filling positions that had been filled by both junior and senior residents (Exhibit 7-1).

Another barrier to using more PAs is the view that they are more expensive to hire than residents and work fewer hours. For example, the 2001 average salary for PAs was $70,000 compared with the average stipend of about $36,000 for second- and third-year residents. Residents are likely to work more than 50 or 60 hours a week while PA house officers tend to work fewer than 45 hours per week.

Another financial issue is that unlike residents who bring graduate medical education (GME) payments (through Medicare) to the institution, hospitals do not always receive an explicit payment for the services of the PA. Currently Medicare pays PAs for hospital services when such services would be covered if furnished by a physician, including assistant-at-surgery services. However, PAs may cost the institution less than salary figures suggest because they may be more efficient than residents, use fewer

EXHIBIT 7-1

Distribution of Departments Where PAs Are Performing Some Tasks Done by Resident Physicians

	PHYSICIAN ASSISTANT ONLY		NURSE PRACTITIONER ONLY		BOTH		TOTAL	
Specialty	**No.**	**%**	**No.**	**%**	**No.**	**%**	**No.**	**%**
General surgery	20	17.2	0	0.0	9	14.5	29	11.4
Surgical specialties	36	31.0	14	19.2	9	14.5	59	23.1
Internal medicine	16	13.8	11	14.3	11	17.7	38	14.9
Pediatrics	1	0.9	13	16.9	4	6.5	18	7.1
Other primary care	5	4.3	8	10.4	7	11.3	20	7.8
Emergency	14	12.1	2	2.6	3	4.8	19	7.5
Neonatal	0	0.0	15	19.5	2	3.2	17	6.7
Other specialty	14	12.1	6	7.8	5	8.1	25	9.8
Unspecified	10	8.6	8	10.4	12	19.4	30	11.8
TOTAL	116	100	77	100	62	100	255	100

Modified from Riportella-Muller R, Libby D, Kindig D: *Health Affairs* 14:181-191, 1995.

resources, and require less faculty supervision. In the long run the cost utility to the institution may be less when the PA house officer, as a permanent employee, does not need to be retrained each year, is knowledgeable about the system, and operates at a higher level of visibility with the staff. An annual transition to new staff and scheduling arrangements takes time and money. In New York, implementation of resident work-hour regulations, coupled with new requirements for continuous supervision of residents and 24-hour availability of intravenous, phlebotomy, and messenger/transport services, has cost approximately $225 million. This is about a 2% increase in total hospital expenditures (Thorpe, 1990). Economists generally regard the services of a resident as neutral or negative because efficiency is less than that provided by a permanent staff house officer and the educational commitment to train and pay the resident is expensive (Kearns et al., 2001; Nasca et al., 2001). On the other hand, hospitals pay salaries to PAs to be house officers with the expectation that greater continuity and coordination of care will contribute to better outcomes, shorter length of stay, and savings. In a study evaluating the effect of replacing residents with PAs and NPs in New York City–area hospitals, it was found that, depending on the replacement strategy used, thousands of PAs and NPs could be hired, costing more than $200 million annually to cover patient care services (Green and Johnson, 1995). One limitation of this study was the assumption that 35% of what a resident physician does is exclusively physician oriented and that it takes three PAs and/or NPs to replace one resident because residents work more than 80 hours per week and PAs and NPs would work only 40 hours. More contemporary views suggest these statistics require revision because of reduced resident hours. The other is that house officer responsibilities assumed by PAs are extensive and vary widely among hospitals. These responsibilities depend on such factors as how many PAs are employed on the service, the extent of attending physician coverage, and supervision of residents. Other issues include the credentialing policies of the institution, the latitude allowed by the hospital PAs and state medical practice laws, and third-party reimbursement policies.

Teaching hospitals have relied heavily on house staff (physicians in training or residency) to provide inpatient care. However, beginning in the early 1990s changes in hospital financing and residency training and the emergence of managed care prompted the development of new cost-effective models of health care delivery. Regulations governing residents' work hours and required shifts in the site of residency from impatient to outpatient settings decreased the availability of residents to staff inpatient wards (Thorpe, 1990; Knickman et al., 1992). These decreases in resident physician labor worsened the house officer/patient ratio. Further cuts in the federal government's support for resident training have been proposed. With these current and proposed limitations imposed on residency programs the roles of hospital-based PAs continue to expand.

Frequently, the roles of house staff PAs encompass a fairly standard list of functions (Exhibit 7-2). Duties may go beyond the basic job description, depending on the PA's experience and training and the approval of the hospital credentials committee. House staff PAs within internal medicine departments have assumed a wide assortment of duties including bone marrow aspiration, thoracentesis, lumbar puncture, coronary angiography, invasive radiologic procedures, and numerous other technical procedures.

House staff PAs are also involved in clinical research activities in which their duties may include collecting specialized data on patients, monitoring therapeutic effects, participating in the analysis of clinical data, and overseeing professional communication. If the hospital is a teaching institution, the house staff PA may participate in teaching rounds, assist in the training of residents, medical students, and PA students, and be involved in other medical educational activities.

The role of the hospital PA as inpatient house staff has become well established in many hospitals. Institutions often employ 6 to 12 PAs, covering with physician residents and attending physicians services of 50 to 150 beds. Sometimes PA house staff duties encompass periods of ED or outpatient clinic duties, depending on service and institutional needs.

Knickman et al. (1992) from New York University addressed the clinical potentials for several types of NPPs to fulfill resident roles While the estimates of PA-specific capacities for resident substitution are not precise, these data offer insight by comparing the proportion of levels of PA capabilities to assume physician resident inpatient clinical duties in teaching hospitals. The exercise is useful in addressing current workforce issues related to PA roles in the downsizing of GME programs (Exhibit 7-3).

In their time-and-motion study examining the clinical activities of two NPs and eight internal medicine residents in two New York City teaching hospitals, researchers documented the time taken by physicians versus other types of health care personnel in performing inpatient medical care tasks traditionally done by physician residents. They compared those times estimated using physicians and nonphysicians under a revised inpatient staffing model. To determine the time per task activity potential for resident substitution, inpatient clinical, educational, personal, and administrative activities were classified by (1) tasks that had to be done by physicians, (2) tasks that were educational only, and (3) tasks that could be done by NPPs or other health care personnel. A total of 1726 specific activities were recorded. Under scenario 1, the traditional model in which the physician serves as the primary medical manager of the patient, about half of a resident's time was spent

EXHIBIT 7-2

Basic Job Description of a House Staff PA

As a member of the health care team the PA will provide medical and/or surgical support to the hospital's attending physicians, nurses, and patients and may perform the following functions:

- Review patient records to aid in determining health status.
- Take patient histories, perform physical examinations, and identify normal and abnormal findings on histories, physicals, and commonly performed laboratory studies.
- Perform developmental screening examinations on children.
- Record pertinent patient data in the medical record.
- Carry out or relay a physician's orders for diagnostic procedures, treatments, and medication in accordance with existing drug laws.
- May transcribe the orders on the patient chart as a verbal or telephone order from the physician and then sign it. Orders written by PAs may be reviewed by the physician.
- Collect specimens for commonly performed blood counts and laboratory procedures.
- Assist in surgery, fulfilling all requirements of a surgical assistant.
- Provide preoperative and postoperative surgical and medical care.
- Provide patient education, health promotion, and disease prevention instructions.
- Screen patients to determine need for medical attention.
- Perform other duties as delegated by the physician and approved by the credentials committee and the bylaws of the institution.

EXHIBIT 7-3

Personnel Who Could Be Substituted/Needed to Perform Physician Resident Activities, Two Staffing Scenarios, by Percent Time

	TRADITIONAL MODEL		PA/NP MODEL	
	No.	**%**	**No.**	**%**
Physician only	6,248	46.7	2,693	20.0
None (education activities)	2,778	20.7	2,778	20.8
None (personal time)	1,800	13.3	1,800	13.4
Nurse	588	4.5	449	3.4
Laboratory technician	160	1.2	160	1.2
Unskilled personnel	822	6.1	822	6.0
PA/NP	988	7.4	4,681	35.0
TOTAL	13,384	100.0	13,383	100.0

Modified from Knickman JR, Lipkin M, Finkler SA, et al: *Acad Med* 67:429-438, 1992.

in activities that must be performed by a physician. Under an alternative model in which a PA or NP assumed an appropriate level of clinical responsibility for day-to-day patient monitoring, only 20% of activities required a physician. The study concluded that there is substantial potential for PAs and NPs to assume inpatient medical tasks, that only 20% of each resident's lost time must be replaced with other physicians' time, and that to achieve this level of clinical efficiency, inpatient hospital staffing models would need to be restructured in which the contributions of nonphysicians can be used to augment physician services (Knickman et al., 1992).

Reducing the number of residency positions in U.S. teaching hospitals poses special problems for many cities, particularly on the East Coast where the per capita number of physician postgraduate training slots is the highest. This is particularly true in New York City–area hospitals, which rely heavily on residents to deliver patient care services. One study analyzed the costs of replacing residents with PAs and NPs under proposals considered in 1994 by Congress to limit the number of first-year training positions and alter the configuration of primary care physicians and specialists produced. The study found that depending on the replacement strategy used the proposals could require New York City–area hospitals to hire thousands of PAs and NPs and other staff, costing a minimum of $242 million annually just to cover patient care services managed by house officers (Green and Johnson, 1995).

HOSPITAL CREDENTIALS

Although the PA is a dependent practitioner, he or she must develop and exercise some degree of independent clinical judgment to be effective. The parameters for the application of PA clinical judgments are usually first defined by existing state statutes on PAs and their scope of practice. Today all states and most territories have laws regulating PAs. Beyond state regulations hospitals develop their own institutional guidelines for employed PAs through amendments to the medical staff bylaws. Bylaws are policies laid out by the hospital board of directors that act as a type of governance for the conduct of the hospital. It spells out important procedures and standards to which members of the hospital must adhere. Physicians must be credentialed by the hospital under the bylaws if they are to have the privilege of entering the hospital for professional purposes.

Hospitals review and approve the qualifications and backgrounds of health care professionals before granting specific privileges. Since 1980 a wide variety of nonphysician health care professionals have been awarded medical staff privileges by hospitals. These include PAs, NPs, certified nurse midwives, optometrists, psychologists, and other members of the health care delivery system. Typically the credentials committee of the medical staff develops guidelines delineating the duties of a PA. These guidelines take into consideration the intended duties, the specific needs and requirements of the medical attending staff, the expected training and qualifications of the PA, and provisions regarding supervision and monitoring of the PA's performance. An important part of these guidelines is the PA job description, which is often developed for each type of service on which PAs work (e.g., medicine, surgery, and pediatrics). The PA's job description must accommodate both the common tasks and the specific duties on a given service.

Some of the basic methods of delineating clinical privileges include the following:

- Job description
- A list of procedures likely to perform
- Categorization according to severity of illness, level of training, or degree of required supervision
- Primary or supervising physician

Most hospitals use the same form or process for PAs that they use for physicians in granting privileges. The system for granting provisional status for physicians is used for PAs as well. Usually this requires proctoring until competence is shown. The American Academy of Physician Assistants' (AAPA) document *Hospital Privileges Summary* includes the major issues that a PA may encounter in seeking hospital privileges and typical hospital responsibilities.

Each state enabling legislation may also contain PA credentialing guidelines that specify which type of educational and professional qualifications a PA must have to receive privileges. Typically a PA candidate is required to be (1) a graduate of an American Medical Association–approved PA training program, (2) eligible for or have passed the national certifying examination administered by the National Commission on Certification of Physician Assistants (NCCPA), and (3) properly registered with the state's medical licensing board.

Credentialing and Privileges

Credentialing is a process of validating the background and assessing the qualifications of professionals to provide health care services in medical institutions (Exhibit 7-4). This involves the evaluation of a person's current licensure, training or experience, competence, and ability to perform the privileges requested. *Privileges* are authorizations granted by the governing body of an institution to provide specific care services within defined limits; granting of privileges is based on a person's licensure, education, compe-

EXHIBIT 7-4

Information Collected for Credentialing and Privileges of PAs

Address (home and work)
Social Security number
License or registration number
NCCPA certification
State prescribing number
DEA number
Degrees and certificates:
  From PA program
  From other education
Additional training (e.g., advanced cardiac life support, advanced trauma life support)
Professional experience, including names of employers
Teaching appointments
Past and current privileges
Legal and administrative actions taken against an individual:
  By employers, hospitals, other institutions
  By government agencies
  By professional societies
  By other monitors of professional conduct
Professional liability:
  Current liability coverage
  Past and current claims and suits
  National Practitioner Databank
Personal health
References
Practice-related information

Modified from Calabrese WJ, Crane SC, Legler CF: *J Am Acad Physician Assist* 10:121-122, 1997.

tence, health status, and judgment (Calabrese, Crane, and Legler, 1997).

The primary purpose of credentialing providers is to protect health care organizations and institutions from the legal liability that could result from the actions of unqualified providers. Evaluation of an organization's credentialing program features prominently in surveys by the Joint Commission on Accreditation of Healthcare Organizations and the National Committee for Quality Assurance. By ensuring that providers are qualified, credentialing also promotes quality care. While the major emphasis of credentialing is to judge the qualifications of physicians, other providers, such as PAs, who participate in the delivery of medical services and who may be legally liable for the quality and safety of the procedures performed are also being credentialed (Calabrese, Crane, and Legler, 1997).

Appointment to the medical staff of a hospital usually lasts 2 years. To be reappointed, staff members must update the information on their original application, provide evidence of continuing education, and document any professional training that may be pertinent to a proposed modification of their privileges. PAs must have the same standards of quality, competence, and patient satisfaction that are expected of a physician. To ensure that credentialing is used most appropriately PAs must become involved in all aspects of the administration of these systems (Condit, 2000).

COSTS AND REIMBURSEMENT OF HOSPITAL PHYSICIAN ASSISTANTS

Although hospitals employ PAs for many reasons, cost-effectiveness is one of the most important factors in many of these hiring decisions. It is no coincidence that the period of rapid growth of employment of PAs, beginning in the early 1980s, closely parallels the time when hospitals were coming under increasing pressure to contain costs. Even before the introduction of diagnosis-related groups (DRGs) in 1982, many hospitals were faced with the problems of inadequate staffing, rising costs of physician and nursing staffing, and loss of physician residency training programs. For many hospital administrators the use of PAs in a restructured staffing pattern was an attractive solution to these problems.

Most PAs who work in hospitals are salaried employees. Their salaries depend on the type of service or department, the type of hospital, and the hours worked. The salary of PA house officers is approximately twice as high as salaries paid to interns and residents; it is far below what a fully licensed physician or a hospitalist commands. Hospitals have found that by adjusting the mix of attending physicians, residents, and PAs, they can reduce overall salary costs for inpatient staffing while preserving adequate levels of medical care. Before 1987 payment for services delivered in inpatient hospital settings by PAs was made either retrospectively on the basis of cost or prospectively on the basis of DRGs. Hospitals paid PAs as salaried employees, and there was no statutory provision under Medicare for or against payment of PA services when they were employed by hospitals.

In late 1986 Congress enacted the Omnibus Budget Reconciliation Act (Public Law [PL] 509), which for the first time permitted Medicare reimbursement to hospitals for services rendered by PAs. The act modifies Medicare reimbursement policies and authorizes coverage of PAs assisting at surgery at a level of 65% of a physician's reasonable charge and 75% for PAs employed by hospitals. Payment is made to the employing hospital, physician, or physician group.

This legislation has made PAs even more attractive to hospitals and hospital-based physicians. Recognition of the value of PA services by the Medicare program had been a long-sought-after goal for the PA profession. This policy not only allows PAs to firmly justify their roles in institutional settings but also has promoted the expanded use of PAs by hospitals that were previously reluctant to employ them. Because most third-party payers emulate the Medicare program in terms of reimbursement policies, they tend to reimburse PA services as well.

Another result of this policy change is the public's expanded access to health care and an improvement in quality of care. PAs are well known for being able to spend more time with patients, pay particular attention to patients' psychosocial needs, and place an increased emphasis on patient education and preventive approaches (Cawley, 1992). These attributes and the PA's proven cost-effectiveness should continue to increase the attractiveness of PAs in many institutional health care institutions.

COST-EFFECTIVENESS OF HOSPITAL-BASED PHYSICIAN ASSISTANTS

With recent changes in the health care environment, hospitals are struggling to meet inpatient needs in a cost-effective manner while maintaining a high level of quality. To meet these changes, hospitals are increasing the use of PAs and NPs.

In spite of the observation that PAs are occupying various niches in hospitals, there is very little written about the economics of their labor. In one randomized trial comparing two inpatient staffing models, a PA was incorporated. The study was undertaken to compare the clinical and financial outcomes for general medicine inpatients assigned to resident (teaching) or staff (nonteaching) services. The staff service used a PA and four physicians. When the unit was fully staffed and operational, patients admitted to the staff service had a 1.7-day lower average length of stay than patients admitted to the resident service, lower average total charges, and significantly lower laboratory and pharmacy charges. No differences emerged in mortality rates or readmission rates were found. While the personnel costs were higher on an attending service the staffing arrangement was financially viable because of the more efficient pattern of care. Shorter length of stay was translated into cost savings and increased revenue that was able to offset the higher salary costs (Simmer et al., 1991).

In a similar but retrospective study, van Rhee (2002) compared the use of resources and length of stay between patients cared for by PAs or residents. This study drew its sample from patients admitted to internal medicine attending physicians who rotate between the PA and resident services over 1½ years. A mixed model analysis was used for each of the five DRGs to test for any significant differences in resources used and length of stay. The results of this study revealed no significant differences in usage of resources except for pneumonia, which was significantly lower in the PA group. There were no significant differences in the length of stay (van Rhee, 2002).

With multiple changes occurring in the staffing and cost arrangements of hospitals in the new century it seems that hospitals, at least teaching hospitals, may want to consider incorporating a PA to serve as an adjunct to both staff services and teaching services.

HOSPITAL SPECIALTY ROLES

PAs may enter more specialized roles in hospital settings. Inpatient PAs are on the staff in many medical and surgical specialties and subspecialties (e.g., cardiology, pulmonary medicine, gastroenterology, nephrology, rheumatology, infectious disease, and oncology), in addition to pediatrics, internal medicine, and geriatrics. In these disciplines, PAs not only assist physicians in routine patient care duties but also perform many technical procedures. PAs who work in cardiology, for example, perform exercise stress tests, coronary angiography, and similar invasive and noninvasive diagnostic evaluations. A PA in Parkland Memorial Hospital in Dallas performed most liver biopsies in 2001 and is a specialist in liver diseases.

Hospital-based PAs are also involved in renal transplant teams, burn units, critical care units, intensive care units (ICUs), cardiac transplant teams, and neurology and neurologic units, as well as many specialty-oriented technical procedures. A number of PAs work in anesthesiology, and some PAs who specialize in cardiothoracic surgery have obtained additional formal training and certification in cardiac bypass pump technology. In a 1987 study PAs performing coronary angiograms had a lower rate of complications than did cardiology fellows (DeMots et al., 1987). A study in 2001 validated these findings (Krasuki et al., 2001). PAs are extensively deployed in neonatology and pediatric ICUs (DeNicola et al., 1994). For such PAs three university centers provide extended specialty training programs.

PA roles in cardiothoracic surgery have grown at particularly rapid rates, and it is estimated that there are more than 1000 PAs in this field alone. Nearly all of these PAs are hospital based (typically in academic medical centers or large community medical centers) and perform a wide range of duties. These duties include preoperative evaluation and preparation of the patient, intraoperative assisting (harvesting the saphenous vein, establishing cardiopulmonary bypass, controlling bleeding, and wound closure), postoperative management of the patient in both the ICU and later on the surgical ward, and a variety of other clinical, teaching, and administrative functions (Willams et al., 1984). Some of the many other specialties that PAs have entered include neurology; neurosurgery; ophthalmology; dermatology; urology and urodynamics; renal dialysis; geriatrics; radiology; pathology; allergy and immunology; ear, nose, and throat; and infectious diseases.

The distribution of hospital-based PAs differs depending on geographic location. In 1995 the AAPA asked members to describe their location of practice. On average 27% answered that they were located in a hospital setting. In the Northeast more than 40% of PAs worked in a hospital setting. In the South and West, fewer than one in six PAs was hospital based (Exhibit 7-5).

The distribution of hospital-based PAs has caught the attention of many health policy analysts, and various explanations for this phenomenon have been advanced. One leading reason for this is the disproportionally high use of international medical graduates as house offices on the East Coast. The increasing difficulty in filling these resident positions has led to replacement by PAs. This trend began in the early 1980s and seems to be increasing.

Another explanation for the difference in geographic distribution is the type of training programs on the East and West Coasts. The Medex model that began in Seattle was strictly outpatient based, both in training and in practice of its early graduates. The Duke model, on the other hand, began in the university hospital setting and continues to expose its students to an inpatient role. Many of the programs that sprang up in the Midwest and on the East Coast have followed the Duke model.

The third hypothesis that explains regional role differences for PAs is that the need for rural providers is far greater in the south central and western part of the United States than in most other regions of the country. The PA seems to be better suited to fill roles in these regions than in inpatient settings. Further research will concentrate on to what extent the PA who identifies a hospital as his or her location of practice actually provides inpatient services.

In an effort to describe the roles of PAs in inpatient specialty roles, McKelvey, Oliver, and Konboy (1986) surveyed 23 PAs employed by the University of Iowa Medical Center. Using both written questionnaires and personal interviews, they found that four PAs were in general medicine, one in general surgery, and the rest in various subspecialties: four in cardiothoracic surgery, two in pediatric cardiology, three in hematology, and one each in radiology, psychiatry, occupational health, gynecologic oncology, urology, burn care, and cardiology. Two other PAs were in urologic oncology. The role activities of these providers and the mean percentage of time spent in each activity covered five areas: technical/procedural (18%), patient care (59.1%), administration (10.7%), research (5.2%), and medical education (6.2%). Patient education was identified as an important component of PA patient care activities, ranging from 25% of all patient care time in surgical specialties to 55% of patient care time in pediatrics. Interestingly when PAs' estimates of their activities were compared with their physician supervisors'

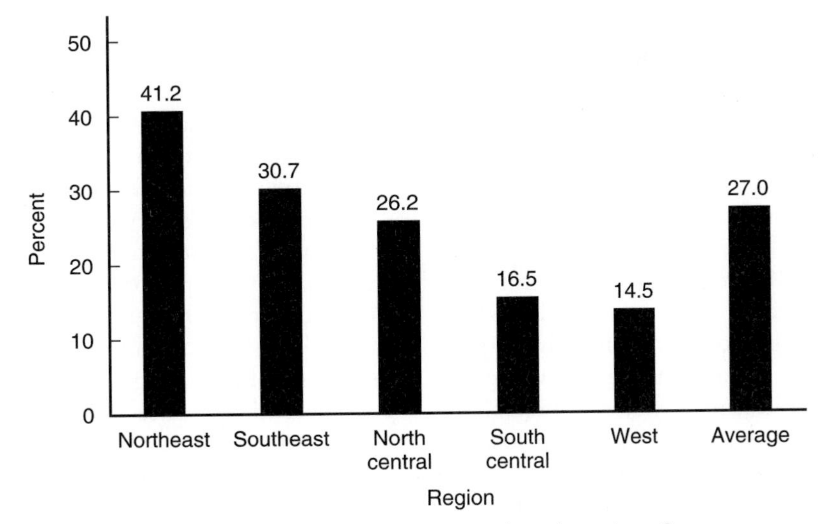

EXHIBIT 7-5 Percentage of hospital-based PAs by region of country.

estimates, more than 75% of the physicians significantly underestimated PA activity in patient education (McKelvey, Oliver, and Conboy, 1986).

The demand on hospitals is already being felt in the medical personnel marketplace. An AHA (1992) survey of 3184 U.S. hospitals found the vacancy rate for PAs rose from 10.1% in 1991 to 12.3% in 1992 and was expected to climb even higher in 1993. The 1992 double-digit vacancy rate for PAs was the second highest ranked profession among the 25 health occupations reported in the AHA survey.

Surgery and Trauma

Surgeons at a hospital in Flint, Michigan, found that when they incorporated PAs in surgery the transfer time to the operating room decreased 43%, the transfer time to the ICU decreased 51%, and the transfer time to the floor decreased 20%. This came at a time when the injury severity scores increased 19% over the previous year's scores. The length of stay for admissions decreased 13% and the length of stay for neurotrauma ICU patients decreased 33%. They concluded that the Hurley Medical Center trauma surgeon–PA model is a viable alternative for verified trauma centers unable to maintain a surgical residency program. Consistency and quality of care indicated by shortened length of stay is a hallmark of such a model providing the highest quality of care (Miller, Craver, and Hatcher, 1978; Miller and Hatcher, 1978).

Neonatal Intensive Care Units

NPPs are increasingly being recruited to fill roles traditionally performed by neonatal residents and fellows (Little, 1996). Downsizing of a pediatric residency program prompted phased replacement of house staff in a 26-bed neonatal ICU (NICU). Subsidized education for neonatal NPs, recruitment of PAs, and NPP leadership took place over 18 months, at which time all house staff functions were assumed by NPPs. The cost to establish this program, the impact on the hospital revenue under New York's prospective reimbursement system, and quality of care were evaluated. The net start-up cost for the NPP program was $441,000 ($722,000 for education, salaries, staff replacement, and recruitment, partially offset by a New York State workforce demonstration project grant). Ongoing costs of the program are $1.2 million per year (including salaries, off-hours medical backup, recruitment, administrative overhead, and loss of indirect and direct medical education reimbursement, partially offset by recaptured house staff salaries and ancillary expense reductions). Access to care was maintained. Quality of care was assessed during the last 6 months of house staff and the first 6 months of full NPP staffing, revealing similar weight-specific survival and an improvement in documentation and compliance with immunization and blood use guidelines during the NPP period. NPPs are expensive in comparison with house staff. Revenue was minimally adversely affected, but access to NICU services and quality of care was preserved and in some cases enhanced with NPP use. The authors concluded that in the context of GME reform, staffing problems such as this hospital experienced will occur increasingly in inpatient subspecialty settings (Schulman, Lucchese, and Sullivan, 1995).

Another study was undertaken to compare patient care delivery by neonatal PAs and NPs with that of pediatric residents in the ICU setting. This study differed from the Schulman, Lucchese, and Sullivan study (1995) in their use of retrospective chart review after developing specific performance criteria, namely, patient management, outcome, and charges. Charts for 244 consecutive admissions to an NICU in Jacksonville, Florida, were reviewed. Patients were cared for by one of two teams: one staffed by residents and the other by neonatal PAs and NPs. The two teams, as determined by patient background characteristics and diagnostic variables, cared for similar patients. Performance of the two teams was assessed by comparison of patient management, outcome, and charges. Management variables included data on length of critical care and hospital stay, ventilator and oxygen use, total parenteral nutrition use, number of transfusions, and the performance of various procedures. Outcome variables included the incidence of air leaks, bronchopulmonary dysplasia, intraventricular hemorrhage, patent ductus arteriosus, necrotizing enterocolitis, retinopathy of prematurity, and number of infants who died. Charge variables included hospital and physician charges. The results demonstrated no significant differences in management, outcome, or charge variables between patients cared for by the two teams. This study underscores other observations that neonatal PAs and NPs are effective alternatives to residents for patient care in the NICU (Carzoli et al., 1994). A survey of neonatal PAs suggests that this is a very satisfying line of work (Otterbourg, 1986).

Intensive Care Units

The use of PAs as providers of care in a medical ICU has also been established. After 3 months of rigorous training, two PAs were assigned to the ICU. Their performance and the operation of the ICU over a 2-year period were evaluated and compared with the preceding 2 years when it was operated by house officers (residents). There were no changes in occupancy, mortality, or the rate of complications. Evidence for more careful evaluation of patients before admission and discharge, manifesting as slightly fewer admissions and slightly longer duration of hospitalization, was also documented. The authors concluded that properly trained PAs may have a role in providing health care in intensive care settings (Dubaybo, Samson, and Carlson, 1991).

Modern ICUs present unique challenges to physician administrators in the current health care environment. Several models of care (e.g., open versus closed ICUs and PAs and NPs in the ICU) are used throughout the country with varying degrees of success. Although all care models may work, the ideal model for a given ICU can be found only through ongoing performance improvement (Stradtman, 1989).

Bone Marrow Transplantation

Bone marrow transplantation is only one of the many subspecialties that are increasingly using PAs. Operating without residents or fellows in continuous attendance, the University of Iowa Hospitals and Clinics Pediatric Bone Marrow Transplant Unit used PAs to assume primary responsibility for patients and to ensure continuity of care. Major tasks assigned to the PAs included evaluation and assessment, writing notes and orders, and clinic follow-up. Basic PA training in pharmacology, physiology, and pathology proved a sufficient background, supplemented by extensive on-the-job training; knowledge of hematology was considered helpful. This PA use model was strongly recommended for other hospitals (Trigg, 1990).

Interventional Radiology

Another emerging area for PAs is the inpatient admitting service. One example that involved interventional radiology demonstrated improved service by developing a clinic and hiring a PA. The service, which began in 1982, was managed by a senior radiologist and fellows. Because of increasing admissions (from a mean of 52 per year from 1982 through 1985 to 110 per year from 1985 through 1987), a 1/2-day, twice-weekly clinic was created in 1985 to evaluate new patients and perform follow-up examinations. In 1986 a PA was hired to assist in the clinic and during patient admissions. Use of the clinic and PA streamlined patient flow and management during hospitalization, resulting in a decrease in mean length of stay for patients undergoing angioplasty (from 3.74 days in 1982 and 1983 to 2.41 days) and a decreased mean cost savings for the hospital under the prospective payment system. Other benefits include improved physician-patient relationships and follow-up, new patients for colleagues (15% of patients had anatomy unsuitable for interventional procedures and were referred to staff surgeons), and increased professional fees.

Psychiatry

Unlike other clinical areas, psychiatry reports critical shortages in the availability of trained specialists. One of the earliest studies on PAs in hospitals was a report on the use of PAs in a state mental hospital. In many state hospitals the number of patients and patient care episodes per psychiatrist is very high, particularly in comparison with the situation at private psychiatric hospitals. In this study the addition of PAs to the staff at this institution significantly increased the time that psychiatrists had to plan and implement treatment, enabling the institution to remain open. The other clinical disciplines showed a high degree of acceptance of the PAs in this setting. The report concluded that psychiatry is a promising area for employment of PAs and PAs are probably underused (Mathews and Yohe, 1984).

Hospitalists

One of the shifts in hospital-based medicine in the United States has been the introduction, or more precisely, the rise of the hospitalist. This is a newly coined term that identifies a physician (usually board certified in internal medicine or one of its subspecialties such as pulmonology) to oversee other physicians' patients. For PAs this has been an emerging opportunity as well (Ottley, Agbontaen, and Wilkow, 2000). Anecdotal information identifies PAs as part of many hospitalist teams (Kessler and Berlin, 1999).

Emergency Departments

To describe current practice regarding the use of PAs and NPs in EDs a telephone survey of 250 health care facilities offering emergency services was conducted by Ellis and Brandt (1997). Of the EDs surveyed, 21.6% were using a PA and/or an NP at the time of the survey, and of those not using PAs and/or NPs, 23.5% intended to do so within the next 2 years. Those using PAs and NPs had been using them for a mean duration of 3.5 years (Exhibits 7-6 and 7-7).

RURAL HOSPITALS

The employment of PAs and NPs by rural hospitals is rising. In 1991 approximately 10% of nonmetropolitan hospitals employed a full-time PA and almost 9% employed an NP. In 1993, 16% employed a full-time PA and nearly 11% a full-time NP (AHA, 1992, 1994). This rise in employment may be because of the need to improve or maintain access to health care services and the inability to recruit or retain primary care physicians (Drozda, 1992).

One study on rural hospital PA employment described and compared 407 sites spread over 8 northwestern states (Minnesota, North Dakota, South Dakota, Iowa, Montana, Idaho, Oregon, and Washington). The results show that rural hospitals are important employers of both PAs and NPs, and there is a greater demand than supply for both providers, in addition to physicians. These hospitals tend to use PAs and NPs to enhance their delivery of outpatient services, and a major factor related to the employment of PAs and NPs is the rural health clinic (RHC) program. The four major reasons for their employment are as follows: (1) to extend care, assist physicians, or increase access to primary care; (2)

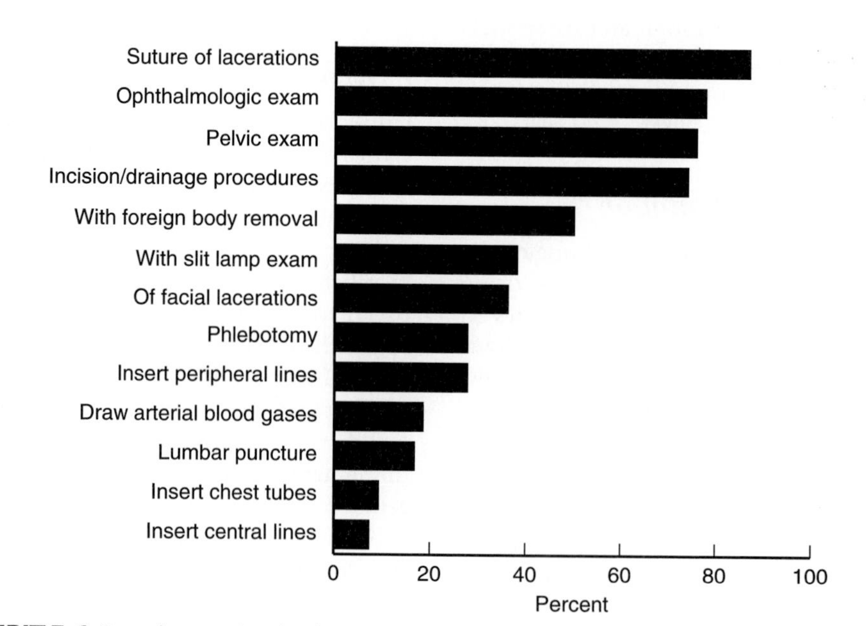

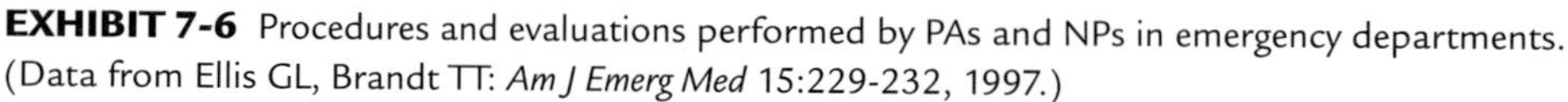
EXHIBIT 7-6 Procedures and evaluations performed by PAs and NPs in emergency departments. (Data from Ellis GL, Brandt TT: *Am J Emerg Med* 15:229-232, 1997.)

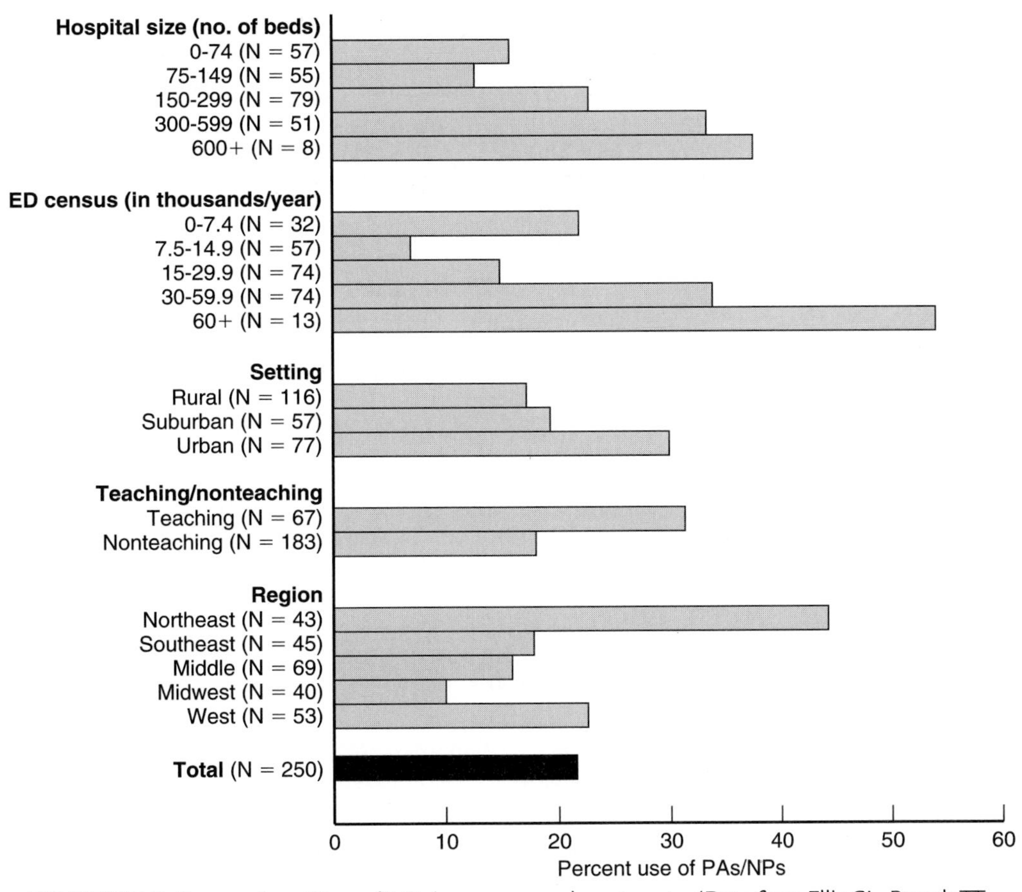

EXHIBIT 7-7 Survey of use PAs and NPs in emergency departments. (Data from Ellis GL, Brandt TT: *Am J Emerg Med* 15:229-232, 1997.)

physicians are unavailable or too difficult to recruit; (3) PAs and NPs are considered cost-effective or more economical for rural areas; and (4) for RHC certification (Krein, 1997a, 1997b) (Exhibit 7-8).

FINANCING ISSUES

As policymakers consider reform measures that would change methods of GME financing and structure, PAs may play an increasingly important role in augmenting medical care services in hospital-based settings. PA use in hospital-based roles, particularly in institutions sponsoring GME programs, has become commonplace. More so than NPs, PAs are employed in teaching hospitals, filling positions in which they essentially substitute for physician residents.

For the training of physicians, financial support through Medicare is provided directly to teaching hospitals sponsoring the clinical specialty training of physicians after medical school. The 3- to 8-year process of GME takes place largely in teaching hospital settings and comprises clinical educational experiences in which physicians complete their medical professional preparation and obtain qualification for state medical licensure and specialty board certification. Medicare finances a large proportion of physician residency training (i.e., GME) by reimbursing hospital charges through a direct cost "pass-through" mechanism and by allowing for an indirect cost educational adjustment for payments to hospitals eligible for reimbursement for educational activities under Medicare Part A DRG payments.

In the 1986 Consolidated Omnibus Budget Reconciliation Act (PL 99-272 Sec 9202), Congress fixed certain limits on the allowable cost per physician resident in an attempt to slow the growth of physician residency programs in

EXHIBIT 7-8

Characteristics of Rural Hospitals That Use PAs and NPs

Hospital and community characteristics	Physician assistants*		Nurse practitioners*	
	Use (N = 216)	Do not use (N = 191)	Use (N = 125)	Do not use (N = 282)
Hospital beds	49 (45)	42 (34)	60[§] (53)	39 (31)
Full-time hospital employees	122[‡] (150)	96 (102)	164[§] (177)	86 (94)
Physicians on active staff	20 (32)	15 (22)	30[§] (39)	12 (19)
No. of specialty types on active staff	4 (4)	4 (4)	6[§] (5)	3 (3)
Primary care physicians on active staff[†]	9 (11)	8 (8)	12[§] (13)	7 (7)
Hospital admissions	1,509[‡] (1,962)	1,183 (1,334)	2,101[‡] (2,362)	1,026 (1,170)
Outpatient visits (emergency and other)	22,621 (25,033)	18,544 (21,566)	31,283[§] (31,655)	16,020 (16,910)
Surgical procedures (inpatient and outpatient)	1,138 (1,739)	867 (1,232)	1,654[§] (2,079)	725 (1,092)
Percent of revenue from Medicare	54% (14.5)	54% (13.4)	51%[‡] (13.9)	55% (13.8)
Owns or manages a rural health clinic	35%[§]	16%	30%	24%
Education site for PA/NP/CNM/CRNAs	28%	14%	22%	21%
Currently recruiting for a physician	66%	68%	74%	64%
Population of the hospital's service area (38,914)	26,731 (33,571)	23,558 (44,993)	35,559[§] (31,056)	20,690
Road miles to a city of 50,000 population	92 (60)	92 (65)	95 (60)	90 (63)

Modified from Krein SL: *J Rural Health* 13:45-58, 1997.
*Mean values with standard deviations in parentheses.
†*Primary care* is defined as general practice, family practice, internal medicine, and pediatrics.
‡$p < .05$ (compared with hospitals that do not use the practitioner).
§$p < .001$ (compared with hospitals that do not use the practitioner).

certain subspecialties perceived to be overcrowded. The act established new incentives for the expansion of primary care residency training and contained mild disincentives for the training of future subspecialists at then current levels.

MEDICARE SUPPORT OF HEALTH PROFESSIONS EDUCATION

Teaching institutions are experiencing cutbacks in Medicare subsidies for medical education. These hospitals are compensated for their GME activities under Medicare payments proportional to the number of Medicare-covered patient days. Medicare's direct medical education (DME) and indirect medical education (IME) adjustment payments are based on hospital eligibility criteria relative to levels of noncompensated care. These payments do not cover PA-delivered clinical services even when augmenting physician residency services in teaching hospital settings. State-imposed legal limitations on the numbers of hours worked by physician residents are also becoming increasingly common and further accentuate hospitals' problems in adequately staffing inpatient services.

In an effort to assess the financial impact of resident cutbacks stemming from the limitation on resident work hours per week in teaching hospitals in New York State, a number of options were examined. Two options for hospitals included enlisting attending physicians to replace residents or hiring licensed physicians to serve as house officers, both expensive options. A staffing mix using PAs with physician residents was determined to be far less costly in providing necessary coverage levels for inpatient services ($160 versus $85 million) than the former option. Yet the adoption of such an approach would require about 1300 additional PAs for New York teaching hospitals alone, when the annual current supply of PAs is 2000 and where many hospitals already have difficulty in attracting sufficient numbers of PAs (Foreman, 1993).

Hospitals employing PAs as general medical house staff and/or in GME substitution roles are believed to be using one of two existing financing methods to obtain reimbursement to cover costs of inpatient PA staffing: (1) by incorporating their costs into per diem charges that are billed and reimbursed under Medicare Part A DRG-based payments or (2) by billing for the clinical services performed by PAs through eligibility under Medicare Part B, which allows payment when PA services are performed in certain settings. Before Part B eligibility (PL 99-509, OBRA, 1986), hospitals employing PAs typically covered their employment costs by building them into the per diem charges hospitals billed under Medicare DRG-based Part A allowances. It is believed that many hospitals continue to finance their use of PAs through this mechanism, rather than by billing for PA services under the Medicare Part B option.

SATISFACTION WITH HOSPITAL PHYSICIAN ASSISTANTS

The speed and efficiency with which PAs can see patients and the quality of the health care they can deliver are often greatly determined by the cooperation of the nursing staff with whom they work. To evaluate nurses' attitudes toward PAs, Erkert (1985) conducted a survey in two hospitals, one of which employed no PAs. The results of the study indicate that nurses who have experience working with PAs or have an understanding of the role of the PA in the health care system have more positive attitudes toward them than those nurses who do not have such knowledge or experience.

Most of the literature on supervising PAs in the hospital is concerned with clinical management. One area of concern that has been overlooked is compliance with quality assurance, continuing education, legal and regulatory requirements, and the normal personnel matters that occur with any employee. The policies and procedures that have evolved along with the use of PAs are an area that has only been superficially touched upon (Synowiez, Fisher, and Royer, 1984).

SUMMARY

Expansion of the roles of PAs into the hospital setting has been the most significant recent trend in health care's use of these professionals (Exhibit 7-9). Initially intended to be primary care providers, PAs have moved into the institutional setting with ease and in large numbers to assume roles as medical and surgical inpatient house staff and as assistants to specialists and subspecialists. In most instances they have adapted to these types of roles without postgraduate training. PAs in hospitals maintain or improve the existing level of quality and access to medical care, are cost-effective in the delivery of inpatient services, and display extensive clinical versatility among the various medical disciplines.

The use of PAs in hospitals emerged from changing forces in the health care personnel supply pool and mandated adjustments in the patterns of GME. Employing PAs has permitted hospitals to cost-effectively maintain the required level of patient care, has allowed residency programs to balance the number of specialty-trained physicians, and thereby has contributed to a more balanced supply of specialists in overcrowded fields. The use of PAs has also contributed to increasing the continuity of care on hospital services and to measures that enrich the quality of residency education for physicians in training.

To accommodate PAs as inpatient providers, amended medical staff bylaws now recognize the education and expertise of PAs and provide the institutional sanction necessary to perform inpatient duties under the supervision of physicians. Accrediting groups, such as the Joint Commission on Accreditation of Health Care Organizations, have acknowledged the roles of PAs as inpatient health care providers and have made recommendations about how hospitals can most appropriately recognize, regulate, and use them.

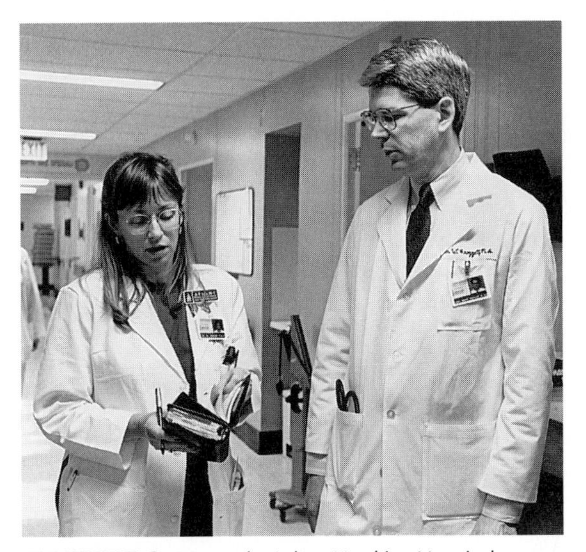

EXHIBIT 7-9 PAs at the Johns Hopkins Hospital. (Courtesy American Academy of Physician Assistants.)

Federal legislation has clarified and established policies whereby employing hospitals are now reimbursed for services provided by PAs. The significance of these actions is the recognition by major third-party payers of the value of PAs in rendering quality clinical services in a variety of settings. Such measures solidify the role of the PA as an important member of the health care team.

Often overlooked by health workforce experts, the demand for PAs in a broad variety of inpatient settings is likely to continue. Employment trends indicate a strong demand for PAs among hospitals and not enough PAs to fill available positions. Most of this is the result of new technology and decreasing availability of residents.

The successful incorporation of PAs in the inpatient hospital setting indicates that these providers are well accepted by physicians, administrators, and patients. This acceptance has been earned by PAs who, working with physicians, have adapted to the demands of the hospital environment. There is every reason to believe that PAs will continue to function successfully in the hospital setting.

8

OTHER PROFESSIONAL ROLES

INTRODUCTION

Physician assistants (PAs) are highly versatile clinicians and professionals, and throughout their careers such mobility leads them in different directions. Surveys suggest about 15% of all individuals who have graduated from PA educational programs are no longer in full-time clinical practice as PAs (Cawley, Combs, and Curry, 1986; AAPA, 2000). With 85% of formally trained PAs in some PA-type role, this level of professional retention is higher than that noted for allied health and nursing occupations. Only physician retention is comparable.

It is not known how many of the 15% of PAs who are not clinically practicing still work within the PA profession or in the health care field but not engaged in patient contact services. Some have obtained additional degrees in medically related fields (e.g., public health, health care administration, education, recruitment, and research) and have developed various careers. A sizeable number are faculty in PA programs and other academic settings. At least 70% of PA faculty members maintain part-time (average of 10 hours per week) clinical practices in addition to their educational duties; 62% of PA program directors remain in clinical practice (Simon, Link, and Miko, 2002). Some PAs have combined their years of clinical experience and expertise with graduate degrees in administration and have evolved into roles in health services management; some have assumed public health positions and roles in research and health policy (Exhibit 8-1). At one time, about 2% of all persons trained as PAs were either allopathic or osteopathic physicians (Jones, 1994).

The PA credential is increasingly recognized in the health care field as a valuable background permitting individuals to move into many types of expanded clinical and nonclinical roles, and attrition from the PA profession does not appear to be a major problem. One can argue that in any

EXHIBIT 8-1

Nonclinical Roles of PAs

Attorney
Academic educator/researcher
Consultant for political candidates
Forensic scientist/legal expert
Hospital administrator
Health facility owner/entrepreneur
Health information management
Health insurance management
Health lobbying
Health planner/regulator
Health services administration
Health services research/health policy
Industrial hygienist
Insurance reviewer
Malpractice reviewer
Medical editor/publisher
Medical epidemiologist
Naturopath
PA service/house staff administrator
PA educational faculty/administration
Pharmaceutical representative
Physician
Politician
Professional recruiter
Public health officer
Researcher, clinical and medical social

profession a predictable number of people will migrate to other related roles or explore new opportunities. Moreover, this is a positive feature that affords individuals in the profession a wide degree of career latitude if they decide to seek expanded or alternative roles. As PAs become increasingly accepted in the health care field, it is likely that more opportunities will surface. As Schneller (1994) writes,

> The fact that some PAs are not satisfied with their level of autonomy and seek career advancement outside of the PA field has not been a concern for the profession. From its origins the PA occupation has been an "accelerator" occupation, allowing members to work to their potential and to aspire to the tasks performed by their supervisor. This is the essence of the occupation's design. A minority will realize that the PA occupation is not their final occupation destination. The one-life, one-career imperative is no longer active. Recall that the PA was designed by physicians and that, in the early years, the occupation was "managed" by medicine. PAs have now come to positions of great respect and power as educators and as members of organizations that represent PAs. These advocates for the PA must not become so attached to the desires of some portion of the membership that they jeopardize the most important features of the occupation.

Although most people who become PAs do so because they want to work with patients, there are PAs who for various reasons have opted to no longer engage in clinical practice (Howard, 2000). This role is similar to physicians becoming administrators, and nurses taking on supervisory roles. While counting these formally trained PAs as part of the census is cumbersome, their work undoubtedly contributes to expanding the understanding of PAs. Many of these PAs remain active in the American Academy of Physician Assistants (AAPA), contributing to development of the profession (Rogers, 2000). Ironically more than a dozen of the past presidents of the AAPA work outside of clinical practice.

We have classified expanding roles for PAs into five categories:

1. Business and management
2. Legal and regulatory
3. Academics, research, and public health
4. Other professional clinicians
5. Journalism, medical writing, and publishing

BUSINESS AND MANAGEMENT

Hospital Administrator

Hospital administration is a natural progression for many health care workers interested in the management side of health care organization. Many PAs start by assuming some of the administrative roles associated with medical office or department management, often balancing clinical activities with organizational roles. These roles include straight administration, health planning, utilization review, and budgeting. Others may pursue a management degree and move full-time into these roles. Various attempts have been made within the AAPA to create a hospital administration coalition of PAs, but most PAs in these roles find their needs are better met by the professional societies devoted to health care organization and management.

For example, there is one hospital administrator who oversees 35 PAs and nurse practitioners (NPs), in addition to numerous other management roles in a modern general acute care hospital. Understanding the needs of employees by sharing a historical background in the same career improves the overall efficiency of management.

Medical Office Administrator

An example of a PA who became a medical office administrator was the result of working in orthopedic surgery for 9 years and then moving into the management side of the organization (Brotherton, 2000). (See Health Facility Owner/Director in this chapter.)

Financial Broker

A background in clinical medicine and pharmacology may be seen as an advantage in certain areas of stock trading and financing. Options are few but exist, as PAs have been able to enter this market as stock analysts. Their ability to assess the market impact of certain drugs and devices under clinical trials and upon release by the Food and Drug Administration make them particularly valuable members of a brokerage house.

Practice Management Consultants

Patient flow and satisfaction of providers are key ingredients to any organization. Numerous PAs have served as practice management consultants for various organizations. Their roles vary: advising senior managers about how to best use PAs and NPs, working with the PAs and advance practice nurses (NPs, certified nurse midwives [CNMs], and certified registered nurse anesthetists [CRNAs]) part of a health maintenance organization (HMO) in negotiations, training support staff in public relations, developing policies and procedures for a new clinic, evaluating staff members, and negotiating salaries for PAs and NPs (Blaser, 1993). PAs have served as consultants to groups to develop and deliver health promotions, provide health-risk analysis reports, and the Center for Medicare and Medicaid Services (CMS) (formerly known as the Health Center Financing Administration [HCFA]) analysis reports. Practice Management Resource Group (PMRG) was developed by an AAPA past president and one of the earliest graduates of the PA profession (Brotherton, 2000). Most of the work is in financial management and Medicare compliance. Having a clinical background is believed to help most consultants in health care management.

Health Facility Owner or Director

PAs have sometimes become owners of health facilities, usually a small medical office. In one scenario two physician owners of a rural clinic hire a PA. After a time one of the partners retires and the partnership half is offered to the PA. With more time the PA may even buy out the second physician or find another physician with whom to partner. In a variation on this theme the PA owner hires a physician as an employee to act as his or her supervising physician.

PAs have been developing or purchasing clinics in small rural towns to run for profit or purchasing part of the business such as the office equipment or the building. Many times these PAs will become the clinic director or manager (Blaser, 1993). Barnes and Hooker (2001) examined these types of practices and found that the PA owners were very satisfied with this type of enterprise (Exhibit 8-2).

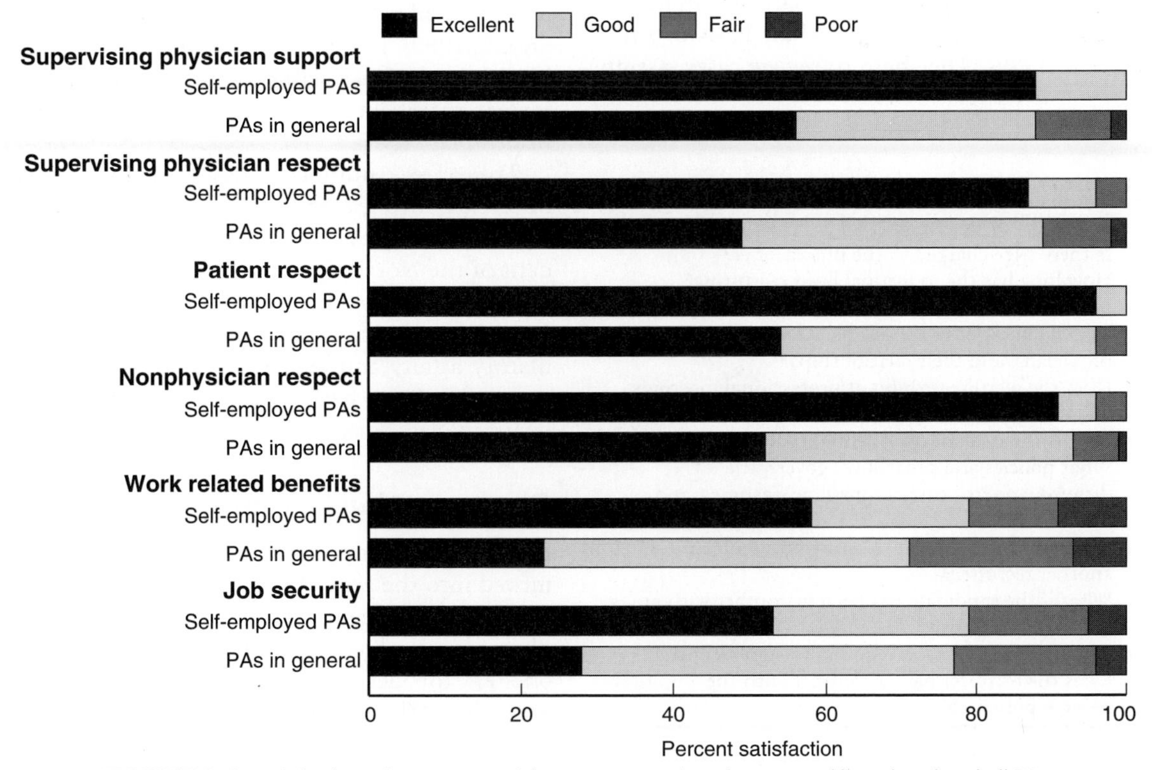

EXHIBIT 8-2 Satisfaction of entrepreneurial PAs: a comparison between self-employed and all PAs.

One enterprise was the development of a company made up of Medex-trained PAs who then purchased small hospitals in rural areas and staffed the senior management with PAs.

Physician Assistant Recruiters

Recruitment of PAs has become a thriving business for placement enterprises and recruitment consultants. Since 1990 the demand for PAs has increased. This is in stark contrast to the late 1970s and early 1980s when PAs had to compete for the few jobs available. PA graduates enjoy a wide choice of employers in most geographic areas (Cawley et al., 2000).

Working with a recruiter can substantially ease, if not completely eliminate, certain out-of-pocket expenses associated with a job search, such as the costs of long-distance phone calls, printing, mailing, and faxing. These can add up, particularly if the PA is willing to relocate and wishes to cast a nationwide net that includes as many potential employers as possible (Exhibits 8-3 and 8-4).

EXHIBIT 8-4

Information a Recruiter Will Need From You

- Curriculum vitae
- Home mailing address
- Phone numbers: home, business, and preference
- PA program attended and year of graduation
- Specialties
- Certifications (NCCPA, ACLS, ATLS, other)
- Work history (to include present and immediate past employers if applicable)
- Motivation for changing positions
- Current salary, benefits, options, and bonuses
- Desired salary
- Relocation availability and requirements
- Important criteria for selection of a new position
- Home ownership
- Family considerations (e.g., spouse's career needs, children's schooling requirements, parents' caretaking needs, and leisure-time interests)
- Interview availability
- Desired start date
- Employers you have previously contacted or positions previously applied for

Modified from Feichter: *AAPA News*. American Academy Physician Assistants, Alexandria, Va., 1997.

Insurance Management

PAs have been employees and managers in health insurance companies (other than HMOs) since the late 1980s. They help to review cases, assign discharge diagnoses (diagnostic-related groups [DRGs]), provide utilization review, analyze reports, summarize the medical literature, and provide advice on policy matters (Webster and Snook, 1990). In one large HMO a PA had a collateral duty of reviewing the medical records of former members who wanted to return to the health plan.

There are a number of PAs who have developed extensive leadership roles in state medical regulatory offices. One PA has served as president of the North Carolina Medical Board and a PA is the executive director of the Arizona Board. Many PAs volunteer part time in state board regulatory affairs and leadership activities. A PA is the chair of the health professions disciplinary board in New York.

EXHIBIT 8-3

Information You May Need From a Recruiter

- Is there a fee charged to the practitioner?
- How long has the individual been recruiting?
- Does the recruiter specialize?
- General knowledge about PAs, NPs, CNMs, physicians, and their relationships?
- Does the recruiter exhibit at professional meetings, and if so, which ones?
- How is the issue of confidentiality handled?
- What policies and procedures govern the dissemination of curriculum vitae, resumes, and references?
- What happens if the applicant finds a job through another recruiter?
- What if the candidate has been in contact with an employer previously?
- Is the PA seeking a job required to sign a contract?
- Does the recruiter have a contract with the employer being represented?

Modified from Feichter: *AAPA News*. American Academy of Physician Assistants, Alexandria, Va., 1997.

Pharmaceutical Representative

Both formally and informally trained PAs have moved into the area of manufacturer representative for pharmaceutical companies. Most major pharmaceutical companies have hired at least one PA for detailing products to prescribers. Sometimes they have remained in the area of sales, but others have found niches within pharmaceutical companies that allow them to specialize as research liaisons to clinical trials, region managers, and administrators.

Clinical Researcher

Some PAs have established clinical research firms and consulting businesses. These entrepreneurial companies contract with pharmaceutical or research companies to conduct part of a clinical trial or recruit participants. They establish a contract with one or more physicians to be principal investigators, using their practice facilities and recruiting their patients into trials (Blaser, 1993). One PA maintains several contracts with pharmaceutical firms in recruiting women interested in trying newer forms of oral contraceptives.

LEGAL AND REGULATORY

Attorney

Pursuit of legal eduction is a career move for some PAs. At times, after experiences or encounters with the legal system, some PAs have become attorneys (Blaser, 1993). Many have retained their identity as PAs and membership in the AAPA, and several PA attorneys have returned to PA education and maintained an interest in medicine and risk management. A few have even returned to medicine after finding the role of a general practice lawyer too competitive. Some PA attorneys have found careers in PA education and PA leadership roles.

Politicians

There have been a few PAs who have attempted to venture into the area of politics. Those who have been successful have been those on the local level. They have functioned as mayors, city council members, and county commissioners; a few have run for state representative in their district (Simmons, 2000). For one PA this came after being a professional lobbyist. Others have done this both as practicing clinical PAs and as politicians (Cornell, 2000b).

Health Lobbyist

Health lobbying attracts health professionals, particularly those who had intense legislative experience working on behalf of their state PA chapters. Most are associated with a health care organization. Some PAs have become part-time professional lobbyists.

Forensic Scientist or Legal Expert

The role of the PA in forensic medicine has been documented on a few occasions (Golden, 1986; Wright and Hirsch, 1987; Cardenas, 1993; Sylvester, 1996). Sometimes these PAs function as city or county medical examiners or coroners; at other times they are called on to act as forensic scientists and experts in homicides. (See the discussion of coroners in Chapter 6.) There are a number of medical examiner offices, including those in New York, Washington, D.C., and other jurisdictions, who employ staffs of PAs.

Disaster Management Expert

A significant number of PAs enter the PA profession with a background, some very accomplished, in emergency medical services. Some of these individuals, following PA graduation, reentered the field of emergency medicine in a combination of clinical and administrative roles; several have attained high-level administrative posts in EMS systems in several jurisdictions and on the national level.

Health Regulator

A good number of PAs participate in health occupations regulatory activities. It is important to distinguish between the hundreds of PAs who serve in part-time roles on state medical regulatory boards. A PA has served in the role of chair of the medical licensing board in one state, and it is now commonplace for PAs (usually practicing clinicians who serve as volunteers) to chair and hold the majority of seats on state regulatory subcommittees overseeing PA practice or chair separate PA boards. One PA is the full-time executive director of a state medical board. PAs have also served as executives of major health professions and health care facility accrediting agencies.

Health Associations/Organizations

A number of PAs have assumed positions in health associations, including the American Academy of Physician Assistants. PAs have also become leaders of health organizations and health-issue advocacy groups.

Consultant for Political Candidates

In the early 1990s most political candidates found that they needed to be particularly informed about health policy and health care reform. As part of a campaign strategy many candidates and political office holders found they understood some of the issues affecting physician, nurse, hospital, and insurance but lacked understanding of other health care workers such as PAs, NPs, podiatrists, psychologists, and nursing home employees. In some instances PAs were involved in campaigns and help shape health policy positions.

ACADEMICS, RESEARCH, AND PUBLIC HEALTH

Academic Educator

The general trend is for PAs to assume the faculty roles in PA programs. Most PA programs have PAs in educational roles such as director, academic coordinator, and clinic coordinator. Because PA programs are set in academic institutions, the program directors and faculty usually have faculty rank from lecturer to full professor. A few PAs have attained the rank of full professor and dean. See Chapter 4 for additional information on PA faculty.

Health Services Researcher

A handful of PAs work in health services research. Although it is difficult to break into this field without significant research background and experience, more and more PA programs are emphasizing this as an area of activity within their mission. With more PA programs expanding into graduate-level studies, undertaking research may become more important for PAs.

Public Health Officer

Several PAs have obtained formal additional training in public health and serve in various roles in that field. One PA works as a state epidemiologist, and another has been chief health officer in several New England jurisdictions. There are a number of roles that PAs have assumed in the U.S. public health service, including posts in the Food and Drug Administration, the Health Services Resources Administration, the National Health Service Corps, and the Bureau of Prisons, among others.

Medical Epidemiologist

The Centers for Disease Control and Prevention (CDC) allows PAs to qualify as health officers through their intensive course medical epidemiologist (Epidemic Intelligence Service). PAs in this role are prepared to respond to disease outbreaks as members of a medical investigation team. There are PAs who serve in the role of medical epidemiologist at the CDC, HRSA, and as state epidemiologists.

Biostatistician

There are number of PAs who have obtained advanced degrees in public health and who have gone on to assume roles as professional-level public health professionals. Typically, this requires a doctoral degree in a public health specialty area such as biostatistics; several former PAs serve in the U.S. public health service as professional biostatisticians or epidemiologists.

Industrial Hygienist

Industrial hygienists are usually employed by industry or large manufacturers to help with the health management of their employees. The petroleum companies were the first to use PAs in occupational health, and since the late 1970s many companies have expanded their corporate goal of reducing worker-related injuries and illnesses by employing PAs in occupational hygienists. These include roles combining aspects of the PA role with administrative duties in which the manager oversees the nurse and clinicians, monitoring the health of the employees.

CLINICAL HEALTH PROFESSIONS

Physician

For a small number of PAs, the desire to become a physician motivates them to seek admission to medical school. About 2 percent of persons who have been trained as PAs have gone on to medical school, both in allopathic and osteopathic schools. Typically, Liaison Committee on Medical Education (LCME)-accredited medical schools do not grant advanced standing to enrollees who are PAs. That only 2% of PAs have gone on to medical school is noteworthy. In the formative years of the PA profession, arguments were put forth about why this new health occupation would fail. Among these arguments was the idea that PAs would become frustrated in their role and leave the field for greener pastures. The sources of frustration envisioned by these critics was the stress and strain of being an "almost doctor," without the intrinsic or extrinsic rewards that society provides for physicians. The intrinsic rewards of professional autonomy in clinical practice would not be available because of the need for close supervision by a physician. The initial view held by some that physician assistants would be frustrated because of a narrow and limited professional role is now untenable. A career as a PA has developed as an attractive alternative to the years of competition, pressure, long hours, and expense required to complete medical school and finish residency training. The PA career is an alternative to the narrower scope of work and lower pay available to the nursing profession.

Chiropractor

There are an unknown number of persons who have been trained as chiropractors who have become PAs. Some of these persons indicate a level of dissatisfaction with chiropractic practice and seek to perform a wider range of patient care services working in a physician's practice.

Naturopath

PAs have formally trained as doctors of naturopathy (NDs). Sometimes they combine their roles to allow for prescription writing, and sometimes NDs have gone on to train as PAs. While these are clinical roles for the most part, many NDs provide education and counseling services.

Podiatrist

Similar to the circumstances with chiropractors, there have been a number of former podiatrists who seek a wider range of patient care duties as a PA.

Summary

Many PAs have expanded their professional positions in health care. Some have used their PA background and experience to branch into related fields, whereas others have acquired further formal education. Employment opportunities and training have led many PAs into more complex and different roles. About 2% of all PAs have moved on to medical/osteopathic school. Employment patterns for PAs are extremely variable, depending on the interests, capabilities, and personalities of the individuals involved. All have used their PA training as a springboard for this change.

9

Economic Basis

INTRODUCTION

Are physician assistants (PAs) cost-effective? Are they productive enough to be considered replacements for physicians? If they are cost-effective, do the benefits of employing PAs accrue to the employer, the patient, or society as a whole?

What happens to the output of a physician's practice, inpatient service, or outpatient clinic when a PA is added to the clinical staff? What are the outcomes in terms of access to patient care services, level of quality of care, practice revenues, and productivity? Although the practice contributions of PAs are determined by multiple influences, many of which are difficult to measure, a number of PA clinical performance characteristics have been well described in health services research. Many of the findings, some of which are from some studies performed years ago, still appear to be valid (Schneider and Foley, 1977; Greenfield et al., 1978).

Numerous studies have shown that within their spheres of practice competency, PAs provide lower cost health care that is comparable and in some instances superior to that provided by physicians (Office of Technology of Assessment [OTA], 1986; Hooker, 2000). While PA cost-effectiveness has not been conclusively demonstrated in all clinical practice settings (McKibbin, 1978), substantial empirical and health services research evidence confirms the findings that they are cost-effective in most of the settings studied (Romm et al., 1979; Record et al., 1980; Cawley, Combs, and Curry, 1986). Probably more significant is that their popularity and use in clinical settings would be unlikely if these health care providers were not cost-effective.

Evidence indicates that the organizational setting is closely related to the productivity and possible cost benefits of PA use. Scheffler (1979) documented that PAs employed in institutional settings are more productive than those in private practice because they see more patients in the same period. Record (1981b) noted correlations among productivity, delegation of tasks, and organizational size and proposed that personnel economies of scale and cost-savings incentives were the likely explanations for the observations on PA cost-effectiveness in the health maintenance organization (HMO) setting.

The performance of PAs in the delivery of medical care services has been studied since the early 1970s. Initially there was an interest in developing a more effective approach to the division of medical labor. Some researchers wanted to document the PA's effectiveness, whereas others thought the stories of PA use were overstated and needed to be refuted. Few professions just beginning have known such scrutiny. Spitzer (1984) notes that "the introduction of physician assistants has been a responsible policy and . . . that many other innovations mediated by medical practitioners have gained widespread acceptance with much less rigorous prior evaluation than was given to . . . physician assistants."

The impact of PAs on access to health care services, quality of care, and physician and patient acceptance continues to be measured with positive results. While the precise degree of productivity and cost-effectiveness of the use of

PAs remains to be determined, the downstream benefits of PA employment are unclear because the vast majority of PA productivity studies have viewed PAs as substitutes rather than members of interdisciplinary health care teams (Scheffler, Waitzman, and Hillman, 1996).

Almost all the economic research on PAs has examined cost-effectiveness of PA employment. Cost-effectiveness analysis is an economic technique designed to compare the positive and negative consequences of a specific resource allocation. It seeks to measure the comparable benefit of a particular investment versus its cost. In health care, this technique is commonly applied to new medical technologies, diagnostic and laboratory tests, health facilities and delivery systems, and drug treatment and immunization programs.

The application of cost-effectiveness analysis in general to the delivery of medical care services and specifically to the provider of such services is a complex endeavor. It is difficult to measure accurately the content of a medical encounter, given variations in such factors as severity of illness, types of treatment, patient preferences, extent of use of diagnostic tests, level of provider training, and the site and mode of care delivery. Add to these factors the differences in the type of provider delivering a similar service and different styles of task delegation, and it becomes obvious that any efforts to determine cost-effectiveness tend to be methodologically difficult and quite expensive.

PAs provide medical care services that overlap to a large extent with those services provided by physicians. Understanding what percentage of overlap exists constitutes the heart of the question for physician employers and health planners. Most studies suggest that PAs can substitute for physicians in various ways. What is not clear is which services are included in these percentages and which are left out. The percentages vary considerably depending on practice setting and specialty, the degree of delegation of tasks by an individual physician to a PA, and the amount of supervision the PA requires or needs.

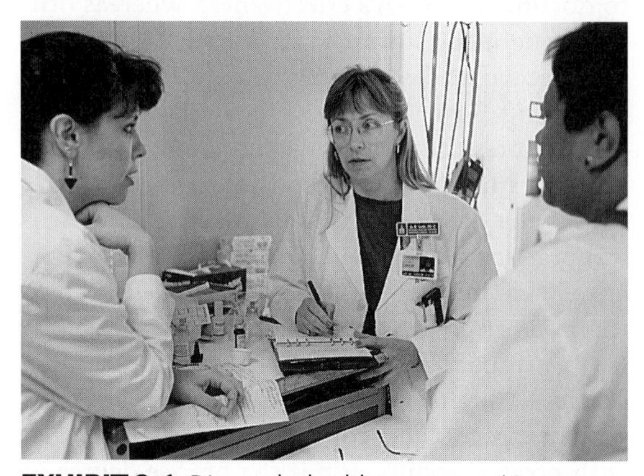

EXHIBIT 9-1 PAs on the health care team. (Courtesy American Academy of Physician Assistants.)

PHYSICIAN ASSISTANTS AS SUBSTITUTES OR COMPLEMENTS

Many studies have examined the role of the PA, and many authors have tried to determine whether PAs substitute for or complement physician services (Exhibit 9-1). In the classic economic definition, a *substitute* replaces a service with something in kind. For example, a kidney machine replaces a donated kidney, so both are substitutes for the real thing. A bicycle substitutes for an automobile (although not a perfect substitute, it is nonetheless a substitute). On the other hand, a *complement* is something that enhances the service being provided. Butter complements a piece of toast.

Feldstein (1988) points out that in medical care it is not always easy to know when an input is a complement or a substitute based just on the task to be performed. A PA may be as competent as a physician to perform certain tasks; if the PA works for the physician, however, and the physician determines the performance or directs the task, then the PA is a complement and will increase the physician's productivity. However, if the PA performs the same task and is operating relatively independently of the physician, then the PA is a substitute for the physician in providing that service. The essential element that determines whether an input is a complement or a substitute is who controls the use of that input (Feldstein, 1988). Substitutability, as the term is used here, implies that quality of care is not threatened. In examining the literature on this question, Sox (1979) concluded that a PA should be able to "provide the average office patient with primary care that compares very favorably with care given by the physician."

Most studies examining cost-effectiveness of PAs have suffered some flaws based on the preceding constraints. For the most part, they have been small sample sizes, analyzed experiences in only one type of ambulatory setting, compared nurse practitioners (NPs) and nurses instead of physicians, focused on primary care functions, and were incomplete in regard to revenue generation and cost data (Lawrence, 1978). Furthermore, most of these studies were performed in the 1970s when the role of the PA was still developing.

Bearing in mind these limitations and recognizing that the published data are suggestive but not conclusive, it is asserted that the cost-effectiveness of PAs can be reasonably confirmed and measured to some extent by the data. Major studies of PA productivity and cost-effectiveness have shown that PAs usually generate practice revenue far beyond the costs of their salaries and overhead (Schneider and Foley, 1977; Mendenhall, Repicky, and Neville, 1980). In addition, an important factor not commonly emphasized in major reviews is the nonmonetary contribution made by PAs to medical practice—a factor even more difficult to quantify than cost-effectiveness. Finally, even though one may never be able to precisely measure the cost-effectiveness in every practice setting and specialty, the fact that more than 45,000 PAs are employed is significant empirical evidence for cost-effectiveness to some degree. Employers—physicians, federal agencies, clinics, and hospitals—would not hire PAs if they were not to some degree cost-effective.

PHYSICIAN ASSISTANT COST-EFFECTIVENESS

Given satisfactory quality and patient acceptance the substitutability of PAs for physicians depends on the volume of services delegated and the degree to which the PA's productivity matches that of the physician in performing the delegated services. The delegation and productivity numbers can be combined to produce a physician/PA substitution ratio. For example, if half of the physician's services are delegated to a PA, and the PA's productivity is half that of the physician, it will take one PA to substitute for half a physician, and the substitution ratio will be .50 physician:1 PA, or .5.

A review of the literature examining the issue of delegation identified 10 studies that used office visits as an output measure. The findings of these studies are summarized in Exhibit 9-2. In the aggregate, the range of delegation is extremely broad, 6% to 99%, with considerable overlap of the delegation level among the settings.

From the bulk of published studies evaluating PA performance, it is clear that most of the services performed by primary care physicians can be provided by PAs without consultation. The most rigorous of all PA economic studies showed that the substitution ratio of traditional primary care medical office visits is .83, suggesting that it takes one PA to substitute for 83% of a physician in primary care ambulatory settings (Record, et al., 1980). Other studies confirm that the clinical productivity of PAs in primary care ranges between 75% and 100% (Page, 1975; Scheffler, 1979; Mendenhall, Repicky, and Neville, 1980; McCaig et al., 1998).

If we accept the fact that PAs are at least three fourths as productive as physicians and are capable of managing at least 83% of all primary care encounters, and if we recognize that the mean salary of a PA is half that of a licensed primary care physician, we can begin to appreciate the considerable cost-effectiveness that PAs bring to clinical practice. These figures tend to become jumbled as a result of misunderstanding of the terms that economists use: practice arrangements, delegation, supervision, consultation, and cost-effectiveness.

Practice Arrangements

Practice arrangement is the organizational structure where the PA is employed. Studies have looked at estimates of PA productivity to try to determine the practice arrangements that best utilize the clinical services of PAs. Past activity analyses used to develop a model of primary care practice organization and productivity consisted of listing the preponderance of tasks that fully describe most typical primary care practices. From this list, a model was developed that estimated that the introduction of a PA could increase medical practice productivity from 49% to 74%; that is, a physician usually producing 150 office visits per week may increase that number to 275 visits per week simply by hiring a PA. Nelson et al. (1975a) also found that when PA providers were actually studied in medical practices, they increased practice productivity as

EXHIBIT 9-2

Delegation of Office Visits to PAs: Summary of the Literature

Reference	Study period	Setting	Patients	Method of triage	Level of delegation
Record (1978)	1971-1973	HMO	200,000 health plan enrollees	By receptionist	79%
Record et al. (1980)	1972	HMO	200,000 health plan enrollees	By receptionist	83%
Pondy (1973)	1972	HMO group, solo (two), institution	Unknown	Not described	81% HMO 36% group 39% solo 24% solo
Miles and Rushing (1976)	1971-1974	Solo	27,000 rural Appalachia	N/A	33%
Henry (1974)	1971-1972	Satellite/ independent	3500 in rural Florida	All patients seen by PA	80%
Riess (1976)	1974	Satellite/ independent	5300 in rural Pacific Northwest	All patients seen by PA	90%
Watkins (unpublished data, 1978)	1977	Emergency department of an institution	200,000 health plan members	Triaged appropriate patients to PA	45%
Ott (1979)	1975	Solo and group	Nine practice settings	By receptionist to CHAs	99%
Ekwo et al. (1979)	1977-1978	Solo, group, and satellite	19 primary care practices in Iowa	By receptionist and independent	87%, 87% (satellite)
Weiner, Steinwachs, and Williamson (1986)	1975	Three HMOs	More than 300,000 health plan members	Varied by health plan	47% 15% 6%

Data from Hooker RS: *Physician Assist* 24:67-85, 2000.
CHA, Child health associate or pediatric PA.

measured by the number of office visits by 12% during the first year after their introduction, and 37% after their first year in the practice.

Reinhardt (1972) found that physicians who practiced in groups could manage more patient care visits than those working in solo practices. He noted that medical care services delivered by physicians exhibited clear *economies of scale,* that is, showed patterns that the mean level of clinical productivity for each health care professional working in the practice serves to increase the total productivity output of the practice as more personnel who can substitute for a portion of the physician are added.

Measures of PA productivity in the HMO setting are consistent with findings observed in studies in rural private practices, urban ambulatory care clinics, and geriatric settings (Frick, 1986; Hansen, 1992). Scheffler (1977) found that PAs spend more of their time in patient care when working closely with three or fewer physicians in general medicine.

Delegation

Delegation is the percentage of primary care medical responsibilities that can be safely handled by a PA under optimal conditions. The term *delegability* was adopted by Record to refer to the maximum level of delegation that can be achieved without threat to quality of care (Record et al., 1980).

In one study at Kaiser Permanente a multidisciplinary panel of health professionals developed a set of medical principles, focusing on the patient's complaint and medical history, for determining the limits of PA substitutability. The team examined an outpatient utilization database for a year of clinical experience to identify the office visits that would have been triaged to PAs had the panel's medical criteria been fully in effect. The team found that the PA-appropriate medical office rate, or delegability, was 83% of the total in adult primary care during the study period (Record, 1980). A number of conservative assumptions were used to conduct this study. Significant illnesses such as cancer, renal failure, congestive heart failure, and similar progressive illnesses were triaged away from PAs; all patients were given a choice of a physician or a PA at the appointment; and no patient was seen more than twice consecutively by a PA for the same diagnosis. PAs and physicians were assigned the same number of appointments each day.

Because of the economy of scale, large practices seem to be more likely to use PAs and nurse practitioners (NPs), and in these settings, physicians tend to delegate a larger percentage of medical services. The positive correlation of size and delegation is further supported by Breslau and Novack (1979), who studied 70 primary care teams and found delegation of technical tasks to be 24% greater and delegation of patient care tasks to be 6% greater in large medical organizations than in small office-based practices.

In a study of the potential for PAs substituting nonphysicians for resident physicians at two New York City hospitals, Knickman et al. (1992) conducted a time-motion study analyzing physicians' clinical tasks under two models: a traditional model in which the physician resident is the primary medical manager and an alternative model in which a PA or an NP performs baseline patient care monitoring. In the traditional model, residents spent almost half their time on tasks they could not delegate. Under the alternative practice model, only 20% of the resident's time was nondelegatable.

The results of the hospital substitution study are applicable to many U.S. teaching hospitals. One survey of 144 teaching hospitals found that 60% of the medical directors reported experience with PA or NP substitution in their hospitals. One third of the hospital departments said they were planning to increase the number of PAs and NPs (Riportella-Muller, Libby, and Kindig, 1995).

Van Rhee (2002) compared a sample of patients admitted to an internal medicine service where cases were compared between PA and teaching services. A total of 16 PAs and 32 postgraduate residents (spread over 1 to 3 years of training) on the internal medicine service were compared with PA service over a 2-year period in the mid 1990s. Resource use was measured using direct costs expressed as relative value units. The results revealed that PAs used fewer ancillary services for pneumonia, stroke, and heart failure. The conclusion is that PAs may be more efficient than residents on some hospital services.

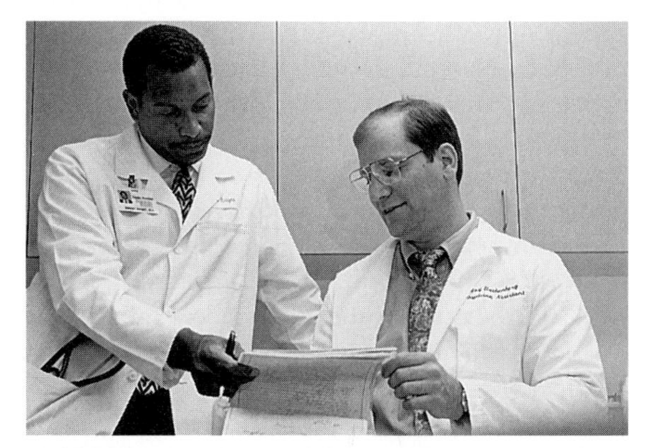

EXHIBIT 9-3 Physician-PA consultation. (Courtesy American Academy of Physician Assistants.)

Consultation

Consultation is the PA's decision to request a physician's assistance in a specific medical office visit. It differs from delegation, which is the physician's decision to assign to the PA some subset of the physician's service. The consultation is some part of the total delegated medical office visits for which the PA is responsible. Many circumstances determine a consultation rate because the consultation can take many forms, with varying time and cost results. Merely signing a prescription, verifying a radiograph finding, or approving a proposed medical management plan may take the PA's supervisory physician only a minute or two, or it may take a prolonged time if a complicated case needs to be reviewed and the physician needs to examine the patient (Exhibit 9-3). The summation of the time consulting with the PA decreases the time the physician has for his or her own tasks and decreases the overall productivity of the PA-physician team. A newly graduated PA will seek more consultations from a physician than a PA who has been practicing primary care for 20 years. In a state that limits PA prescribing or dispensing the PA may have to consult with the physician on every patient who needs a prescription.

The consultation rate is the number of consultations of any kind over the total number of visits assigned to the PA in a given time. It may be closely related to the level of delegation in a certain specialty or if the physician wants to use the

PA as his or her personal assistant. In other circumstances, willingness to delegate a broad range of services to a PA may be based on the assumption that consultation will be frequent or that the PA needs little supervision. It is important therefore to know the consultation rate and the delegation level. Because the consultation is usually informal, little is known about the PA consultation rate. Considered higher for inexperienced PAs and lower for experienced PAs, the rate is undoubtedly controlled by many variables such as relationship with the physician, time, availability, and patient mix. When the PA and physician share an office, the rate is undoubtedly higher than when they are separated by distances and office layouts that inhibit formal and informal consultations. Time-motion studies documenting every minute of a physician-PA relationship would need to be conducted over a prolonged time to understand the importance of this labor assessment.

Supervision

Supervision is a state-legislated term that has both legal and economic implications. (See Chapter 11.) Competent supervision is essential for quality of patient care but can carry with it restriction of delegated tasks and loss of physician productivity because of employer administrative tasks associated with this relationship. How much time is devoted to supervision depends largely on the PA-physician relationship. Little study has been devoted to this important function. In 1992 the Veterans Administration surveyed more than 100 supervising physicians of PAs and NPs (Alexander and Lipscomb, 1992). The average time assigned as the supervisor of a PA or NP in this system ranged from 9.2 to 16.1 hours per week based on a workweek of approximately 30 hours of direct patient care (Exhibit 9-4). Although assigned the role of supervising the PA or NP, the supervising physicians were also engaged in patient care, usually in the same setting.

In one large HMO that employed both PAs and NPs the supervising physician's patient load was decreased by 10% per day. This was assigned as administrative time and was inserted into the schedule to compensate the physician for supervising the PA or NP and reviewing a set of medical records used by the PA and/or NP at the end of the day (Hooker and Freeborn, 1991).

EXHIBIT 9-4

Physician Survey Mean Responses to Questions on Supervision of PAs and NPs

	PHYSICIAN SUPERVISES	
	PAs (N = 75)*	**NPs (N = 34)***
Hr/wk physician spends in direct care	33.0	29.7
Hr/wk physician assigned to supervise the PA/NP	16.1	9.2
Percent time PA/NP takes first call for physician	20.2	26.4
Percent time supervision involves		
Overseeing medical procedures	23.7	27.2
Checking orders with PA/NP	25.7	41.5
Other activities	50.6	31.3

Data from Alexander BJ, Lipscomb J (eds.): *Physician Staffing for the VA*, Washington, DC, 1992, National Academy Press.
*Number of responding physicians.

Clinical Productivity

One of the first economists to study PA labor defined productivity this way:

> In theory, productivity is a simple concept: it measures changes in the total output that occur when small changes are made in one factor of production, with all other factors and circumstances held constant. Because these conditions can be met in the real world only rarely, productivity numbers are almost always rough estimates. Certainly that is the case with respect to [PAs]. (Record et al., 1980)

The findings on PA productivity reflect the changing policy concerns of the U.S. health care system. Initially emphasis relied on documentation of increased access to services, usually within the organizational framework of solo practice in rural areas. Later investigations focused on issues of costs and delegation in organized health care settings. An important contribution of health services research has been the documentation of the multifaceted effects of PAs on clinical productivity, meaning the overall output of a clinic or medical office when a PA is added to the staffing mix. A common measure of productivity, one that can positively affect access to health care, is the number of patient visits performed in a clinical setting. The next question is whether the productivity of PAs compares favorably with that of physicians.

In virtually every study on productivity, PAs compare favorably with physicians (Crandall et al., 1984; Scheffler, Waitzman, and Hillman, 1996). In fact there is evidence in some settings that PAs see more patients per unit time than physicians (Hooker, 1986; McCaig et al., 1998). Generally PA productivity can be compared with physician productivity in two other ways: (1) on the basis of tasks PAs are qualified to perform and (2) on the full range of tasks performed by a physician. The comparison of the range of these tasks is sometimes known as the *functional delegation* (Record, 1981a). For most practices, depending on the degree of task delegation, practice case mix, the health care delivery system, the context in which the PA performs the clinical service, and institutional policy on the use of PAs result in higher clinical productivity rates.

One study looked at nine medical practices that employed PAs. When these practices were compared with control practices, Golladay, Miller, and Smith (1973) found that the physician-PA team practices increased clinical productivity 4.4% (as measured by the number of office visits), whereas the control practices increased only 1.3% during the same time. Another study assessed the impact of a PA in a small practice on the distribution of physician time. After a PA was employed in primary care, a larger proportion of physician time was spent in seeing older patients, more seriously ill, hospitalized patients, and in communicating with patients (Nelson, Johnson, and Jacobs, 1977).

A small-scale study of the cost-effectiveness of nonphysician health care providers including PAs was conducted in another type of ambulatory care setting. This report describes the performance of four nonphysician providers (NPPs) (e.g., PAs and NPs) and five family practice physicians, comparing measures of the practice costs of both types of health care providers working in a student health clinic, a type of prepaid system, and in a fee-for-service family practice clinic. Total hours worked, numbers of patients seen, revenue generated, and provider salaries were collected for the nine primary care providers over 49 weeks. In the student health clinic the average cost for salaries to the clinic for each patient visit was $5.49 for NPP services, whereas it was $8.53 for each visit to the physician. In the family practice clinic, revenue generated per dollar of salary was $2.68 for NPPs and $2.62 for family physicians (Hansen, Stinson, and Herpok, 1980).

Mathematical models have been developed to explore the most efficient contribution of health care personnel in different settings. These settings include private group practices, urban medical centers, military settings, and managed health care settings such as HMOs (Golladay, Miller, and Smith, 1973; Zechauser and Eliastam, 1974; Schneider and Foley, 1977; Cyr, 1985; McCaig et al., 1998; Ortiz et al., 2000) and tertiary care centers (Harbert et al., 1994). These models provide the theoretic documentation for the clinical productivity of PAs, with estimates ranging 50% to 95% of physician productivity (where physician productivity equals 100%). These theoretic and carefully documented empirical approaches are similar in their assessment of PA clinical productivity. Hooker (1993) studied the hourly, daily, and annual productivity of PAs, NPs, and physicians in the primary care departments of internal medicine, family practice, and pediatrics and found that on an annual basis PAs see more patients than physicians in the same amount of time (29%). This difference is due in part to PAs being primarily outpatient based, whereas physicians had hospital responsibilities that took them away from the medical office (Exhibit 9-5). Patient visits to physicians and PAs tended to be similar in 90% of cases (the functional delegation level) but differed in illnesses associated with a hospitalization such as for

EXHIBIT 9-5

PA Clinical Productivity in an HMO Setting

Department	Patients/hr	Patients/day
Family practice		
Physician	2.39	17.4
PAs	2.61	19.0
Internal medicine		
Physician	3.10	22.5
PAs	2.97	21.5
Pediatrics		
Physician	3.14	16.5
PAs	3.07	22.3

Data from Hooker RS: The roles of physician assistants and nurse practitioners in a managed care organization. In Clawson DK, Osterweis M (eds.): *The Roles of Physician Assistants and Nurse Practitioners in Primary Care.* The Association of Academic Health Centers, Washington, DC, 1993, The Association of Academic Health Centers.

acute cardiac illnesses, cerebral accidents, and cancers (Hooker, 1993).

While some practices employ PAs to meet increasing demand, others employ them to relieve physicians of excess workload. Some authors noted that after practices hired PAs, more patients in the practice were seen by appointment and more patients in the practice had specific plans for follow-up visits, suggesting more efficient patient flow (Kane et al., 1978; Kane, Olsen, and Castle, 1978; Olsen et al., 1978). Other researchers reached similar findings, which are displayed in Exhibit 9-6.

PA clinical productivity compares favorably with productivity levels of physicians, particularly in organized ambulatory care practice settings that use team approaches and structured division of medical care staffing. While it seems likely that similar levels of PA clinical productivity exist for PAs working in other types of patient care settings, performance measures in newer practice areas such as inpatient hospital settings have not been performed. Additional studies examining levels of PA clinical performance characteristics are needed because the content of clinical care (the specific medical tasks) delivered by PAs differs within various clinical settings. It would be useful to know the number, content, and patient outcomes of clinical services of PAs compared with those of physicians.

One of the many variables that are difficult to control in comparing productivity of PAs in different settings is the population base. Many significant differences exist between groups of PAs depending on the work setting, type of specialty, or years of experience. However, when some of these data are aggregated, it has some interesting findings. Using data collected on the 1995 American Academy of Physician Assistants (AAPA) membership census, Kraditor (personal communication, 1996) examined the productivity of PAs in terms of number of outpatients seen per day controlling for a number of variables. Exhibits 9-7 through 9-9 present summary statistics on these measures of outpatient produc-

EXHIBIT 9-6

Physician Productivity When a PA Is Added to the Clinic

Study by first author	PA/physician ratio	Productivity (%)*
Hooker (1993)	1:2	110.0
Cyr (1985)	1:1	80.1
Greenfield et al. (1978)	1:1	92.0

**Productivity* is defined as the percentage of patients seen in an outpatient setting compared with a physician's patient load.

EXHIBIT 9-7

Outpatient Visits of PAs per Day by Work Setting, 1995

Setting	No. of respondents	Mean	SD
Clinic	763	21.9	9.6
Group physician practice	517	21.6	7.7
Solo physician practice	190	22.7	9.9
HMO	198	21.3	6.2
Other managed care organization	19	20.1	7.0
University hospital	72	15.0	13.1
Hospital (nonuniversity)	260	23.7	10.7
Inner city clinic	116	19.9	12.2
Military facility	248	24.8	8.3
Corrections facility	51	23.7	12.4
Nursing homes	5	19.4	4.7
Rural clinics	357	20.2	8.9
Self-employed PA	10	35.9	14.5
VA facility	58	16.6	5.5
Industrial facility	44	20.1	9.3
Academic facility	33	22.4	7.9
Public health facility	27	21.0	6.8
Other government facility	14	23.4	20.6
Other clinical setting	109	20.7	10.6
TOTAL	3091	21.7	9.5

Data from American Academy of Physician Assistants, Research Division, 1996.
Based on PAs reporting outpatient visits but no inpatient or nursing home visits. Data collected on the 1995 AAPA member census.

tivity for groups of PAs defined in terms of work setting, years of experience as a PA, and field of practice. All analyses used only data for PAs who reported being in full-time clinical practice and working for a single employer.

Findings from this study include a statistically significant difference observed in the number of outpatients seen per day by work setting, with the largest differences reflected by PAs working in military facilities or correction facilities. When data on years of experience are examined, PAs with more experience see more patients per day than PAs with less experience. Field of experience also seems to make a difference in terms of patients seen per day. The largest differences are found in emergency medicine, in which PAs report seeing 24.6 patients per day on average.

In terms of workweek the vast majority of PAs report working 44 hours a week on average. PAs employed in inner city clinics work fewer hours a week, and those in military facilities work more hours per week than those in all other settings.

The extent of PA productivity cannot be determined without reference to an array of interdependent variables, which assuming that all of them can be identified are difficult to evaluate. The classic conceptualization of how productivity should be measured—by observing what happens to total output when small homogeneous units of one input (in this case the PA) are added while other inputs and the larger context are held constant—is difficult to measure in a big practice and virtually impossible in a small one (Record et al., 1980).

EXHIBIT 9-8

Mean and Standard Deviation of Outpatient Visits per Day by Years of Experience

Yr of experience	No. of respondents	Mean	SD
<1	139	18.6	7.2
1-3	821	20.8	8.8
4-6	505	21.9	10.1
7-9	341	21.2	8.5
10-12	410	21.6	8.6
13-15	371	22.5	10.2
16-18	343	22.8	10.5
>18	296	23.3	10.3
TOTAL	3226	21.7	9.4

Data from American Academy of Physician Assistants, Research Division, 1996.
Based on PAs reporting outpatient visits but no inpatient or nursing home visits. Data collected on the 1995 AAPA member census.

EXHIBIT 9-9

Mean and Standard Deviation of Outpatient Visits per Day by Field of Practice

Field of practice	No. of respondents	Mean	SD
Family/general medicine	1836	22.1	8.2
General internal medicine	255	18.9	8.6
General pediatrics	115	24.4	9.9
Emergency medicine	316	24.6	11.2
General surgery	6	18.3	7.3
Internal medicine specialties	130	16.8	13.6
Pediatric specialties	33	18.7	15.1
Surgical specialties	145	20.0	10.6
Obstetrics and gynecology	88	20.0	10.4
Industrial/occupational medicine	181	21.7	10.3
Other	173	21.4	10.6
TOTAL	3278	21.7	9.6

Data from American Academy of Physician Assistants, Research Division, 1996.
Based on PAs reporting outpatient visits but no inpatient or nursing home visits. Data collected on the 1995 AAPA member census.

THE COSTS OF PHYSICIAN ASSISTANTS

Cost implications of the use of PAs can be viewed from three perspectives. The first is that of the entrepreneurial medical practice concerned with whether the increase in practice revenue resulting from hiring a PA will exceed the additional costs of adding a provider. The second is if market conditions warrant, whether it is more desirable to hire a physician or a PA. The third is the societal concern of how to deliver high-quality care at minimum cost. The societal view is that all costs, no matter where they come from, are ultimately borne by society. This economic approach considers not only employment costs but also training costs.

Employment Costs of Physician Assistants

When a PA is employed a number of direct and indirect costs must be considered. These include salary, benefits, malpractice insurance, office space, equipment, support staff, supplies, and other direct and indirect expenses. Although data on this subject are sparse, there is little to suggest that the costs other than compensation are different from those associated with employing a physician. Only one outcome study has been undertaken demonstrating that a PA uses no more laboratory and imaging orders and drugs for an episode of care than physicians (Exhibit 9-10) (Hooker, 2002). Aside from anecdotal reports suggesting that malpractice insurance may be cheaper for the PA because the litigation rate is less than it is for physicians, there seems to be little to suggest that PAs lose any of their cost-effectiveness by the way they practice medicine.

In contrast to other costs, the income differential for PAs and physicians is clearly quite large. Most PAs are employees and therefore salaried, whereas physicians receive not only a stream of revenue for their own services but also entrepreneurial benefit from employing a revenue-generating provider.

Based on the AAPA data collected in 2002, $7,046 was a reasonable average salary estimate for an experienced primary care PA in that year (AAPA, 2000). The figure for a primary care physician in the same year was approximately $142,000 (Wassenaar and Tran, 2000). This places the PA at .50 of the salary of physician in primary care.

Compensation/Production Ratio

One of the better ways to examine the net value of a PA is the income generated to the employer in private practice. *Compensation,* which includes salary and benefits collectively, is usually examined. The most useful ratio is the amount of compensation the employer forgoes to retain the PA divided by the amount of revenue the PA returns to the employer. Basically the smaller the ratio the more economical the provider is to the practice. The Medical Group Management Association (MGMA) collects these data annually (Exhibit 9-11). In 2000 the compensation/production ratio for PAs was .38. In comparison the compensation/production ratio was .44 for family practice physicians, .40 for pediatricians, .41 for NPs, and .48 for psychologists, suggesting the PA is relatively more economical to employ (MGMA, 2001).

While the number of NPPs used for this study is not large, the relative ratios between providers

EXHIBIT 9-10

Multivariate Regression Cost Model Holding Different Variables Constant While Examining for Differences Between Types of Providers

Provider	N	Total Cost	Visit Cost	Med Cost	Image Cost	Lab Cost
BRONCHITIS EPISODE COSTS						
Physician	1336	$234.74	$133.63*	$96.42**	$3.31	$1.37
Physician assistant	411	$224.13	$92.23*	$125.74**	$4.65	$1.50
TENDINITIS EPISODE COSTS						
Physician	264	$183.33**	$144.77*	$30.14	$7.50	$0.93
Physician assistant	90	$149.80**	$98.77*	$40.65	$9.53	$0.84
OTITIS MEDIA EPISODE COSTS						
Physician	6246	$188.39*	$140.07*	$47.77	$0.0	$0.54
Physician assistant	2008	$136.60*	$83.29*	$52.99	$0.0	$0.32
UTI EPISODE COSTS						
Physician	1633	$262.17*	$142.73*	$83.91	$17.67*	$17.86**
Physician assistant	878	$210.50*	$97.70*	$91.50	$5.80*	15.48**
TOTAL	12,866					

Data from Hooker RS: *JAAPA* 14, 2002.
*Significant at p <0.001.
**Significant at p <0.01.

EXHIBIT 9-11

Compensation/Production Ratio for PAs

Provider type	No. of providers	Medical practices	Mean
Overall for PAs	124	40	.381
Organization type			
Single specialty	19	13	.433
Multispecialty	105	27	.372
Other providers			
Family practice physician	1,117	135	.447
Internal medicine physician	883	134	.447
Pediatric physician	501	107	.409
Nurse practitioner	71	31	.419
Midwife	15	7	.472
Optometrist	57	20	.423
Psychologist	104	32	.477
Podiatrist	31	19	.334

Data from Medical Group Management Association: *Physician Compensation and Production Survey: 2001 Report Based on 2000,* Medical Group Management Association, 2001, Englewood, Colo.

do give an indication of the efficiency a PA brings to a practice. For every $1 in revenue generated, the employer pays $0.38 to employ the PA.

Education Costs of Physician Assistants

The cost of educating and using PA health care professionals and the annual levels of their compensation are far less than comparable costs for physicians (at least for allopathic physicians). Economic analyses of the use of PAs indicate that these and other nonphysician health care providers appear to be underutilized in their roles in health care delivery and are limited in their potential to contribute to health care delivery (Safriet, 1998). Theoretic economic projections of the cost savings that could accrue under optimal conditions of nonphysician use are considerable, perhaps as much as $4 to $5 billion for NPs alone (Nichols, 1980; Salcido et al., 1993).

The education costs of PAs, like those of virtually all other health care professionals, have been borne by tuition of the students and to some extent by society through grants to institutions and tuition subsidies to students and trainees. Typically the medical practice does not share directly in the cost of education. A PA student, judging the return to medical education, perceives "costs" as opportunity costs (tuition, books, and lost income) and is likely to observe a high rate of return on his or her investment in the education because the income as an employed PA is usually substantially higher than that earned from a previous career.

For physicians the three education-cost components are (1) medical school costs, (2) graduate (resident) training costs, and (3) opportunity costs. The value of services to patients provided during the postgraduate years of training is often debated. There is a high cost of supervision and decreased productivity because of this supervision, as well as staffing costs, inefficiencies in care, and overhead. Most economists tend to consider the value to society during the resident years as a net sum of zero in internal medicine and family medicine. More important, the opportunity cost (forgone years of practice) is large during this training period because productivity is delayed until after the period of postgraduate training.

Because virtually no physician begins practice after graduation, we must consider the cost of medical training as 7 years based on 4 years of medical school and at least 3 years of residency. The PA chooses a different career path that is only 2 years long. If the medical student had chosen to be a PA, practice income would have begun after 2 years of professional training. If we use the PA salary rather than the potential income of a 4-year medical school plus 3-year postgraduate-trained physician, we can estimate the cost differential of physicians and PAs.

Both the PA and the medical student start approximately from the same place academically.

The average PA student has a baccalaureate degree, as does the medical student. Most have the same type of background with varying combinations of academic course work in their undergraduate years. Given the overlapping training periods for physicians and PAs the opportunity costs for physicians and PAs can be calculated.

In Exhibit 9-12 the PA and physician students are assumed to begin medical education after completion of 3 to 4 years of undergraduate study (most enter medical school and PA school with a baccalaureate degree acquired after 4 years). The PA becomes fully productive after 2 years of education and the physician becomes a fully productive provider of care 5 years after the PA. Using the assumption that a provider is valued by his or her salary level, and that the PA salary is $65,000, the PA has delivered $325,000 ($65,000 × 5 years) worth of care before the physician begins practice. This figure is defined as the opportunity cost of additional medical education and training. It is also the value of care that would have been delivered to society had the medical student chosen a PA training course.

Exhibit 9-12 also illustrates the opportunity cost of additional medical education and training. If direct training costs are assumed to be approximately $20,000 for a PA and $100,000 for a primary care allopathic physician, the difference between the physician and a PA in total training costs in 2000 may be calculated as $100,000 minus $20,000, plus the protracted training ($100,000 - $20,000 + $325,000). The differential is nearly $405,000 per PA that society gains by having a PA trained instead of a physician. Put another way, the PA produces $405,000 worth of patient care before the physician begins practice.

If salary costs are used as a proxy for employment costs, the physician/PA differential is $74,000 (the differences between the average primary care salaries of $142,000 for physicians and $65,000 for PAs). This means the salary cost of a PA is .45 of a physician. If it requires 10% of a physician's time to supervise a PA, 10% of $142,000 should be added to the cost of employing a PA. The PA/MD cost ratio as viewed by an employer would then become $65,000:$156,000, or .42. When Record et al. (1980) made the original calculations using 1977 data, they found the cost ratio of hiring a PA to be .38 based on a wider disparity between PA and physician salaries. Since that time both physician and PA salaries have steadily climbed, and in 2002 are closer to .50.

	PA student	MD student
Cost/year	$10,000	25,000
Years of training	2	4
Total	$20,000	100,000

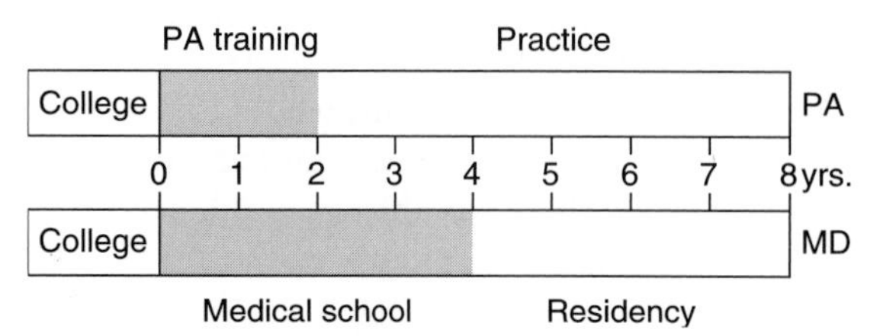

EXHIBIT 9-12 Cost comparisons of PA and MD training programs in 1995 dollars. (Modified from Simon CJ, Born PH: *Health Affairs* 15(3):124–133, 1996.)

Substitution Ratios

Substitution is the degree of labor one worker can assume for another. Primarily the level of delegation and comparative productivity of physicians and PAs for the delegated services determine the physician/PA substitution ratio. A substitution ratio of 1.0 implies unity and is achieved when one PA completely substitutes for one physician. PAs in rural and isolated clinics often function at very high levels, often replacing the physician who was previously occupying that role (DeBarth, 1996). These accounts are largely anecdotal however, and little is known about the types and numbers of patients seen by physicians versus PAs in comparable settings. The best studies occur in large managed care settings where some of the variables can be controlled and physicians and PAs work alongside each other, seeing similar patients at the same time.

Using an urban health care center as a paradigm, one study constructed production functions that would best exploit the possibilities of substituting PAs for physicians. It was estimated that one PA could replace half of a full-time physician. From data developed in a national survey of physicians, Scheffler (1979) estimated that a 10% increase in the medical office visits output of a practice would require, on average, an increase of 3.5% in physician hours or 5.4% in PA hours. These percentages suggest a marginal substitution ratio of .63, as compared with the overall .50 ratio estimated by Zeckhauser and Eliastom (1974). Another mathematic model tested with data from seven HMOs to demonstrate the potential impact of PAs and NPs on physician requirements found that in adult medicine, the addition of 12.72 PAs and/or NPs would permit physician numbers to drop from 16.44 to 9.74. Thus the 12.72 PAs and/or NPs could replace 4.59 physicians (Schneider and Foley, 1977). The respective substitution ratios can be calculated as .53.

Record (1981a) estimated that if enough PAs were hired to perform all of the services for which they were considered competent by physicians in the Department of Internal Medicine at Kaiser Permanente, and if the PA and physician workweeks were equal, the substitution ratio would be .76. Steinwachs et al. (1986) studied ambulatory care in another HMO and found the substitution ratio to be .38 in adult care and .48 in pediatrics. The ratios might have been higher if the base had been primary care, as it was in the Record study (1981a), with outpatient specialty services excluded. Hooker (1993) developed data that suggest the ratio was .90, and Page's work (1975) in the military was close to unity (.99)

Most of the estimates of substitution ratios fall mostly in the range of .65 to .95, suggesting it would take, on average, approximately one PA to substitute for three fourths of a primary care physician. For managers, this suggests that four PAs could replace three physicians.

ISSUES AFFECTING THE EFFECTIVENESS OF PHYSICIAN ASSISTANTS

How cost-effective is a PA? The answer, though not known exactly, is contained in the difference between the physician/PA substitution ratio (.75) and the PA/physician cost ratio (.42). The meaning of these two numbers is that a PA can substitute for at least 75% of primary care physician services at approximately 45% of the physician's direct cost in salary. If the physician's time is reduced because of supervision, then the ratio is 50%. The social cost figures are even more impressive because the PA/physician ratio including training costs is smaller than the employment cost ratio. Finally the employment of a PA is fairly economical because the compensation/production ratio at 38% is more efficient than most other types of providers. Exhibit 9-13 presents a summary of the economic exercises in this chapter. These figures, however, must be viewed with caution. They are based on the "best studies" (those studies considered the most rigorous in investigation), or the average of different studies, using fairly conservative figures.

Prescribing Authority

Almost all states, the District of Columbia, and Guam authorize prescribing privileges for PAs and most of those allow some limited prescribing of controlled substances. The first state

EXHIBIT 9-13

Cost-effectiveness of Primary Care PAs*

Issue examined	Range	Average or best study
Delegation	0.40:1.0	0.83
Supervision	0.10:0.60	0.10
Physician/PA substitution ratio	0.40:1.0	0.75
PA/physician cost ratio (salary)	0.40:0.50	0.43
PA/physician cost ratio (with supervision)		0.52
Compensation/production ratio	0.25:0.52	0.38
Societal cost training a PA (compared with a physician)	0.20	
Average no. of outpatients seen	18:35	21.7
PA/physician cost-benefit ratio	—	—

*Based on a review of the literature up to 1980, using conservative estimates, and extrapolating to 1995 costs.

statute to authorize prescribing privileges for PAs was passed in Colorado in 1969. It stipulated that graduates of the University of Colorado child health associate program (pediatric PAs) could prescribe medications without immediate consultation from supervising physicians provided that the latter subsequently approved the script. New York authorized prescribing privilege to PAs in 1972; Maine, New Mexico, and North Carolina followed in 1973. By 1979, 11 states had passed laws allowing PA prescribing privileges. There was a steady trend among states throughout the 1980s and 1990s to authorize PA prescribing either by statute or by regulation in recognition that prescribing medication is part of the PA's clinical role and the supervising physician has the authority to delegate such tasks to qualified health professionals.

A study in Iowa reported that 95% of physicians and 93% of PAs believed that PAs were qualified to prescribe medications with little or no supervision by the physician (Johnson, Driggers, and Huff, 1983). Similarly, all 29 Montana physicians who responded to a survey expressed confidence in the ability of the PAs they were supervising to prescribe most therapeutic agents, and 40% had no reservations about the PA's ability to prescribe any agent (Rabin and Spector, 1980).

Prescribing authority generally applies to the outpatient or ambulatory setting. Medications for patients in the hospital are considered medical orders and usually fall under the purview of institutional medical staff bylaws. States typically place certain stipulations on PA prescribing activities. These may include (1) requiring physician co-signature for a PA prescription, (2) limitations on the drugs that may be used (e.g., those listed in a specific formulary), (3) excluding selected schedules of drugs (usually schedule II agents (i.e., those defined by the Controlled Substances Act as having the potential for abuse), (4) prescribing using drug treatment protocols, and (5) limiting the quantities of certain drugs that PAs may prescribe.

A 1990 survey administered to PAs working in states having prescribing authority found that 90% of them included prescribing as part of their clinical activities. Sixty percent of PAs reported that they prescribed urinary/vaginal agents, upper respiratory tract medications, gastrointestinal tract agents, antiarthritic/antigout agents, and analgesics. The mean number of prescriptions written per week was 50, and it was estimated that PAs wrote 35.5 million new prescriptions each year; with refill prescriptions, the total approximated 65 million. The most frequently PA-prescribed classes of drugs were nonnarcotic analgesics, antibiotics, antihistamines, antihypertensives, and cough and cold preparations (Willis and Reid, 1990).

Prescribing Behavior

According to a marketing industry that tracks the behavior of physicians and other health care professionals, Scott-Levin Source Prescription Audit estimated that PAs wrote 17.8 million prescriptions in 1999, an increase of 45% from 1998 (Scott-Levin, 2000). This is estimated to account for 6% of the total market for 1999. Unfortunately, these data are probably incorrect and grossly underestimate what is probably the true number, because the data rely on Drug Enforcement Agency (DEA) numbers to be linked to the prescription and not all PAs have DEA numbers (Herrick, 2000a). While there were 37,865 PAs in October 1998 when the original study was undertaken, only 11,322 had a unique DEA number.

One of the shortcomings of tracking PA prescriptions is the method used. The current method involves a prescription written by a physician and given to a pharmacist. The patient has the prescription filled at a local pharmacy. The pharmacist uses the DEA number of the physician who wrote it. Auditing prescriptions allows marketing companies such as Scott-Levine to generate audit reports of what and how many prescriptions are written by individual physicians.

An independent study commissioned by Clinicians Publishing Group, a publishing group that specializes in marketing to PAs and NPs, indicated that the number was closer to 175 million prescriptions written in 1998 and 169 million prescriptions in 1999 (Herrick, 2000a). This estimate is based on a 5-day workweek, 48-week year, and 35,000 practicing PAs. Efforts have been made to improve the accuracy of determining the prescription rates of PAs (Yackeren, 2000).

Another Scott-Levin study (2000) reports that in 2000 physicians wrote the most prescriptions per week, 95, but PAs reported writing a weekly average of 89. NPs averaged 68.

Barriers to Practice Effectiveness

On a public policy level, the phrase *barriers to practice* refers to factors known to have a significant limiting effect on the practice effectiveness of PAs and other nonphysician health care practitioners. Barriers to practice are commonly used within discussions of the utilization of PAs to denote the multiple health system factors that limit the full capabilities of PAs to provide health care services. These factors comprise medical, legal, and economic elements and prevent PAs from discharging the full range of authorized medical tasks for which they are educated and certified to perform (OTA, 1990; Office of Inspector General [OIG], 1993; Emelio, 1994).

PAs are often constrained in their capabilities to augment medical practices because of restrictions imposed by states. Barriers to the full practice effectiveness of PAs may reduce or eliminate the cost benefits that accrue from their use and deter them from serving populations in need of medical care services or from practicing in certain areas. Uneven state medical practice acts, the lack of authorization to prescribe medications in some states, and the absence of private third-party reimbursement that exist in many rural ambulatory practice settings have been shown to have restrictive effects on PA use (Willis, 1993).

While conventionally defined barriers to practice (i.e., state government regulatory policies for supervision requirements and prescribing authority) clearly work to affect levels of PA clinical productivity in a broad sense, on the day-to-day practice level, findings suggest that differences in the delegatory styles of individual employing physicians are also important determinants of PA effectiveness. On a fundamental level, barriers to practice (i.e., practice laws and regulations) represent the parameters drawn for NPPs, usually by physicians. At the margins, because clinical activities between physicians and PAs overlap considerably, scope of practice and professional domain issues arise among these health professionals. Physicians now share a great deal of their medical diagnostic and therapeutic responsibilities with PAs. This willingness to share medical functions is a result of forces affecting the evolution of the division of medical labor in the U.S. health system.

States and their licensing boards have considerable control over the practice activities of PAs and other NPPs through their authority to license and regulate the health care occupations. Restrictions to the full practice effectiveness of PAs and similar health care providers may reduce or eliminate the cost benefits that accrue from the use of these professionals and may prevent them from serving populations in greatest need of medical care services or from practicing at all (OIG, 1993).

Because states exert considerable control over health care practitioner usage patterns through professional licensing and regulation, Sekscenski et al. (1994) from the Bureau of Health Professions analyzed variations in the regulation of PAs (and NPs and certified nurse midwives [CNMs]) and their abilities to practice to full effectiveness in all states and the District of Columbia. In their approach, key factors related to the licensure and legal status, prescriptive authority, and eligibility for reimbursement for PAs were delineated and quantified according to specific criteria across all 51 jurisdictions. Summary scores estimating the favorability of the practice environment for PAs were derived from points assigned to each of three categories—scope of practice, prescribing authority, and reimbursement eligibility—which were then compared with the numbers of individual practitioners, ratios of generalist physicians, and proportions of underserved persons in each jurisdiction. Only nonfederal PAs and physicians were counted in the analysis (Exhibit 9-14). These numbers are expected to change significantly when this study is repeated.

PA practice favorability scores ranged from a high (maximum attainable) of 100 points in three states (Washington, Iowa, and Montana) to a low of 0 (lowest attainable) in Mississippi, with a mean score of 73.1. Twenty-one states had practice favorability scores of 90 or greater, and 14 had scores less than 5. Lower scores generally correlated with the lack of PA prescriptive authority. A significant relationship ($p < .001$) was observed between practice favorability scores and a state's PA/population ratio. States tended to cluster into three groups, reflecting the association between favorability scores and PA/population ratios: states with high favorability

EXHIBIT 9-14

Provider Practice Scores for PAs, NPs, and CNMs by State, 1992

State	PAs	NPs	CNMs
Alabama	39	33	32
Alaska	90	93	84
Arizona	99	86	76
Arkansas	54	48	35
California	58	30	80
Colorado	80	59	50
Connecticut	87	58	93
Delaware	55	60	60
District of Columbia	92	53	60
Florida	48	68	98
Georgia	59	32	70
Hawaii	38	27	42
Idaho	89	46	54
Illinois	59	14	31
Indiana	37	34	25
Iowa	99	73	55
Kansas	87	52	68
Kentucky	42	78	68
Louisiana	37	20	37
Maine	94	42	90
Maryland	49	93	69
Massachusetts	83	68	57
Michigan	89	45	70
Minnesota	83	68	100
Mississippi	0	72	59
Missouri	39	63	27
Montana	98	98	98
Nebraska	93	46	50
Nevada	98	73	30
New Hampshire	95	95	70
New Jersey	37	65	54
New Mexico	94	62	78
New York	98	93	67
North Carolina	92	43	90
North Dakota	87	98	55
Ohio	51	14	60
Oklahoma	46	40	54
Oregon	99	100	80
Pennsylvania	86	66	34
Rhode Island	93	50	84
South Carolina	37	41	59
South Dakota	94	65	70
Tennessee	42	27	56
Texas	77	42	54
Utah	93	91	73
Vermont	86	68	57
Virginia	42	38	47
Washington	100	90	70
West Virginia	96	89	47
Wisconsin	95	67	62
Wyoming	97	94	80
Mean	72.5	60.2	62.1
Median	86	62	60
Standard deviation	25.3	23.8	19.2

Data from Sekscenski ES, Sansom S, Bazell C, et al.: *N Engl J Med* 331:1266-1271, 1994.

scores and high PA/population ratios, states with midrange scores and midrange ratios, and states with low scores and consequently low ratios. These findings confirm the widely held view that scope of practice regulations, the existence of prescribing authority, and eligibility for reimbursement all affect PA use. If these factors are unfavorable, they serve as barriers to PA practice effectiveness. This policy analysis is believed to have played a significant influential role in states improving their enabling legislation for non-physician clinicians in the 1990s.

Prescribing authority has been a particularly troublesome barrier to PA practice effectiveness, and its presence in state law is reflected in the patterns of marketplace demand and utilization of PA providers. State prescribing authority can have a marked influence on the capacity and efficiency of PAs to contribute to health care delivery (Gara, 1989). One example was seen in Texas, where before the passage of PA prescriptive authority, there were only 26 PA rural health clinics. By 1992, only 15 months after the passage of prescriptive authority for PAs in Texas, the number of PAs employed by these clinics had nearly quadrupled to 99. During the same period the percentage of Texas PAs practicing in rural areas tripled, increasing from 5% to 15% (Willis, 1993).

THIRD-PARTY REIMBURSEMENT POLICIES FOR PHYSICIAN ASSISTANTS

Medicare Coverage for Physician Assistants

The first Medicare coverage of physician services provided by physician assistants was authorized by the Rural Health Clinic Services Act in 1977. In the following two decades, Congress incrementally expanded Medicare Part B payment for services provided by PAs authorizing coverage in hospitals, nursing facilities, rural Health Professional Shortage Areas and for first assisting at surgery. In 1997, however, the Balanced Budget Act extended coverage to all practice settings at one uniform rate.

As of January 1, 1998, Medicare pays the PAs' employers for medical services provided by PAs in all settings at 85 percent of the physician's fee schedule (Exhibit 9-15). This includes hospitals (inpatient, outpatient, and emergency departments), nursing facilities, home, offices and clinics, and first assisting at surgery. Assignment is mandatory and state law determines supervision and scope of practice. Hospitals that bill Part B for services provided by PAs may not at the same time include PA salaries in the hospital's cost reports.

Outpatient services provided in offices and clinics may still be billed under Medicare's "incident-to" provisions, if Medicare's restrictive billing guidelines are met. This allows payment at 100 percent of the fee schedule if: (1) the physician is physically on site when the PA provides care; (2) the physician treats all new Medicare patients (PAs may provide the subsequent care); and (3) established Medicare patients with new medical problems are personally treated by the physician (PAs may provide the subsequent care).

According to the Balanced Budget Act, PAs (using the 85 percent benefit) may be either W-2, leased employees, or independent contractors. The employer would still bill Medicare for the services provided by the PA. All PAs who treat Medicare patients must have a provider identification number (PIN).

Effective April 1, 2002, the Centers for Medicare and Medicaid Services issued new instructions that will allow PAs to have an ownership interest in an approved corporate entity (e.g., professional medical corporation) that bills the Medicare program, if that corporation qualifies as a provider or supplier of Medicare services. The new policy also removes a provision that prohibited Ambulatory Surgical Centers from employing PAs.

Medicaid Coverage

Presently, 50 states cover medical services provided by PAs under their Medicaid programs. The rate of reimbursement, which is paid to the employing practice and not directly to the PA, is either same as or slightly lower than that paid to physicians.

Private Insurance

Private insurers generally cover medical services provided by PAs when they are included as part

EXHIBIT 9-15

Medicare Policy for Physician Assistants

Setting	**Supervision requirement**	**Reimbursement rate**	**Services**
Office/clinic when physician is not on site	State law	85% of physician's fee schedule	All services PA is legally authorized to provide that would have been covered if provided personally by a physician
Office/clinic when physician is on site	Physician must be in the suite of offices	100% of physician's fee schedule *	Same as above
Home visit/house call	State law	85% of physician's fee schedule	Same as above
Skilled nursing facility and nursing facility	State law	85% of physician's fee schedule	Same as above
Office or home visit if rural HPSA	State law	85% of physician's fee schedule	Same as above
Hospital	State law	85% of physician's fee schedule	Same as above
First assisting at surgery in all settings	State law	85% of physician's first assist fee schedule†	Same as above
Federally certified rural health clinics	State law	85% of physician's fee schedule	Same as above
HMO‡	State law	85% of physician's fee schedule	Same as above

*Using carrier guidelines for "incident to" services.
†For example, 85% × 16% = 13.6% of surgeon's fee.
‡Some Medicare/HMO risk contracts may exclude nonphysician providers.

of the physician's bill or as part of a global fee for surgery. A long-standing American Medical Association (AMA) policy (April 1978) recommends that:

> . . . reimbursement for services of a physician['s] assistant be made directly to the employing physician. In instances where the PA is providing services in the physician's office and in conjunction with the physician, the cost of such services would appropriately be a part of the physician's charge as is now the case with other personnel he employs. When the PA provides physician-like services to a patient under the direction of, but in a location physically remote from the employing physician, AMA has recommended that the physician bill for such services on the basis of the usual, customary and reasonable charges concept.

TRICARE/CHAMPUS

TRICARE, formerly know as the Civilian Health and Medical Program of the Uniformed Services (CHAMPUS), covers all medically necessary services provided by a physician assistant. The PA must be supervised in accordance with state law. The supervising physician must be an authorized TRICARE provider, and the employer bills for the services provided by the PA.

The allowable charge for all medical services provided by PAs under TRICARE Standard, the fee-for-service program, except assisting at surgery, is 85% of the allowable fee for comparable services rendered by a physician in a similar location. Reimbursement for assisting at surgery is 65% of the physician's allowable fee for comparable services.

PAs are eligible providers of care under TRICARE's two managed care programs, TRICARE Prime and Extra. TRICARE Prime is similar to an HMO. TRICARE Extra is run like a preferred provider organization in which practitioners agree to accept a predetermined discounted fee for their services.

Medicare Reimbursement/"Incident To"

There appears to be some confusion over the basic concept of "incident to" services under Medicare both in terms of which services fall into the "incident to" category, and what set of circumstances need to be present in order for a service to be reimbursed as "incident to" at 100% of the physician's fee schedule. We will attempt to clarify this issue with a brief look at the rationale behind the "incident to" designation, an example of what we feel to be a covered service and language taken from the November 25, 1991, Federal Register. The Federal Register contains regulatory language from the Department of Health and Human Services and the Health Care Financing Administration (HCFA) setting forth the final rules for Medicare fee schedule payments beginning January 1, 1992.

The definition of "incident to" services from the Medicare carriers manual is as follows: "Services furnished as an integral although incidental part of a physician's personal professional services." This idea recognizes the value of the physician assistant (PA)/nonphysician practitioner as a "physician extender" and the important role that they play in the delivery of health care in this country.

There has been some discussion as to whether Medicare intended for PAs to be reimbursed at 100% of the physician's fee schedule when performing medical services when the physician was not directly involved in the treatment of the Medicare beneficiary. Some would argue that the PA should be paid at a (discounted) percentage of the physician's rate.

The Department of Health and Human Services sent Congress a model Medicare Modified Fee Schedule for Physicians' Services in September of 1990. In that publication, the specific question of how nonphysician practitioners should bill a service which was performed in the physician's office/clinic with the physician on the premises was addressed. There was also a question as to whether or not the physician had to actually see the beneficiary or actively participate in each service. The answer to those questions, taken from the report, is as follows: "Visits made to allied health professionals (e.g., nurse practitioners, social workers, physician assistants, etc.) who are employed by a physician may be covered by Medicare as "incident to" the physician's service if the physician is on the premises when the service is provided, even when the beneficiary does not see the physician (see section 2050.1 of the Medicare Part B Carriers Manual)."

It is extremely difficult to make a comprehensive listing of the services that can be considered "incident to" because the scope of medical services PAs perform is so expansive. Generally, for a procedure to be considered an "incident to" service, all of the following criteria must be met:

- The service must be medically necessary.
- The service performed must be one that is typically performed in a physician's office.
- The service performed should be within the scope of practice of the PA.
- The physician should be in the building (on-site) when the service is rendered.
- The physician must personally see the patient on the patient's *first* visit to the practice.

Note: The Health Care Financing Administration allows the carrier(s) in each state a certain degree of latitude in interpreting this "incident to" regulatory language. Check with your carrier for specific information on this issue.

For medical services provided by Physician Assistants that do not fall within the "incident to" category, Medicare pays the PAs' employers for medical services provided by PAs in all settings at 85 percent of the physician's fee schedule. This includes hospitals (inpatient, outpatient, and emergency departments), nursing facilities, home, offices and clinics, and first assisting at surgery.

JOB SATISFACTION OF PHYSICIAN ASSISTANTS

Job satisfaction is not often thought of as an economic issue. However, a high rate of turnover of professional personnel in a clinic is disruptive to patient care and organizational stability, as well as to the individual clinician. When turnover occurs, productivity and the efficiency of the health care service are negatively affected. The major reason PAs, NPs, and physicians leave an organization is usually management (Pantell, Reilly, and Liang, 1980).

Research on PAs and job satisfaction is fairly extensive and PAs seem to be reasonably satisfied with their work experience and practice conditions. PAs express an overall level of satisfaction that compares favorably with that of other professionals such as lawyers, accountants, and engineers (Perry, 1978). PAs report less stress and have lower turnover rates than nurses and many other health care workers (Holmes and Fasser, 1993). PAs also are more satisfied than NPs, who sometimes regard themselves as better-trained and more effective alternative practitioners.

The major determinants of job satisfaction among PAs seem to be the professional and personal support the PA's supervising physician provides, the amount of responsibility for patient care, and opportunities for career advancement (Baker et al., 1989). The strongest correlates of both job performance and job satisfaction are the degree of physician supervisory support and amount of responsibility for patient care (Freeborn, Hooker, and Pope, 2002; Davis et al., 2000). Location in smaller communities is also associated with greater satisfaction (Sells and Herdener, 1975), although a more recent study found that satisfaction levels were equally high for PAs practicing in both urban and rural settings (Larson, Hart, and Hummel, 1994). Lack of opportunities for career advancement has been frequently cited as a major concern and the main cause of attrition from the PA profession (Osterweis and Garfinkel, 1993). Inadequate financial compensation and control over income are other reported sources of dissatisfaction (Willis, 1992). Acceptance by patients and by other health care workers has not been found to be a significant problem (Nelson, Jacobs, and Johnson, 1974; Record et al., 1980; Record, 1981a).

Among PAs, job satisfaction is highly correlated with the level of clinical responsibility and professional autonomy, the extent of professional and personal support provided by the supervising physicians, and the opportunities for career advancement. The majority of studies addressing the job/career satisfaction of PAs reveal that they are largely satisfied in their professional roles and quite happy with their career choice, a set of findings a bit surprising in view of the status of PAs as dependent practitioners.

Holmes and Fasser (1993) reported findings of occupational stress and professional retention in a survey conducted of 1360 randomly selected practicing PAs responding to a mailed questionnaire. The typical respondent was male (53%), white (88%), age 37 years (mean), and devoted most work time to patient care activities. Job satisfaction was high overall, and it was correlated positively with independence, challenge, and job security. Issues of salary, perceived opportunities for advancement, and the management style of the employer were associated with the highest levels of job dissatisfaction and role stress (Holmes and Fasser, 1993).

When Freeborn, Hooker, and Pope (2002) compared perceptions about the practice environment and job satisfaction of PAs, NPs, and physicians in primary care, they identified that autonomy was not a problem and they were satisfied with most aspects of practice in a managed care organization. However, the common areas of dissatisfaction included patient load and the limited amount of time with patients. PAs and NPs were more likely than the physicians to experience stress on a daily basis and indicated they were less likely than physicians to choose the practice setting again (Exhibit 9-16). In the HMO where this study took place, they also were significantly less satisfied than physicians with their incomes and fringe benefits (Freeborn, Hooker, and Pope, 2002).

Researchers at the AAPA identified that by 1999, only 15% of all PAs who have ever graduated from a formal PA program had left the profession. The AAPA surveyed the profession and with a 74% return identified that by all measures PAs were satisfied with their work environment, satisfied with clinical practice, satisfied with their job, and had a favorable outlook on the profession (Marvelle and Kraditor, 1999).

In one of the few career satisfaction studies that compares PAs with other occupations that have similar levels of responsibility, Freeborn and Hooker (1995) examined PAs in an HMO with NPs, optometrists, mental health workers, and chemical dependency counselors. PAs expressed the most satisfaction with the amount of responsibility, support from co-workers, job security, working hours, supervision, and task variety. They were less satisfied with workload, control over the pace of work, and opportunities for advancement. Chemical dependency counselors expressed the highest levels of satisfaction across various dimensions of work, and optometrists the lowest (Exhibit 9-17). NPs also tended to be satisfied with most aspects of practice in this setting. In a number of instances they were more satisfied than the PAs. Most PAs were also satisfied with pay and fringe benefits (Freeborn and Hooker, 1995).

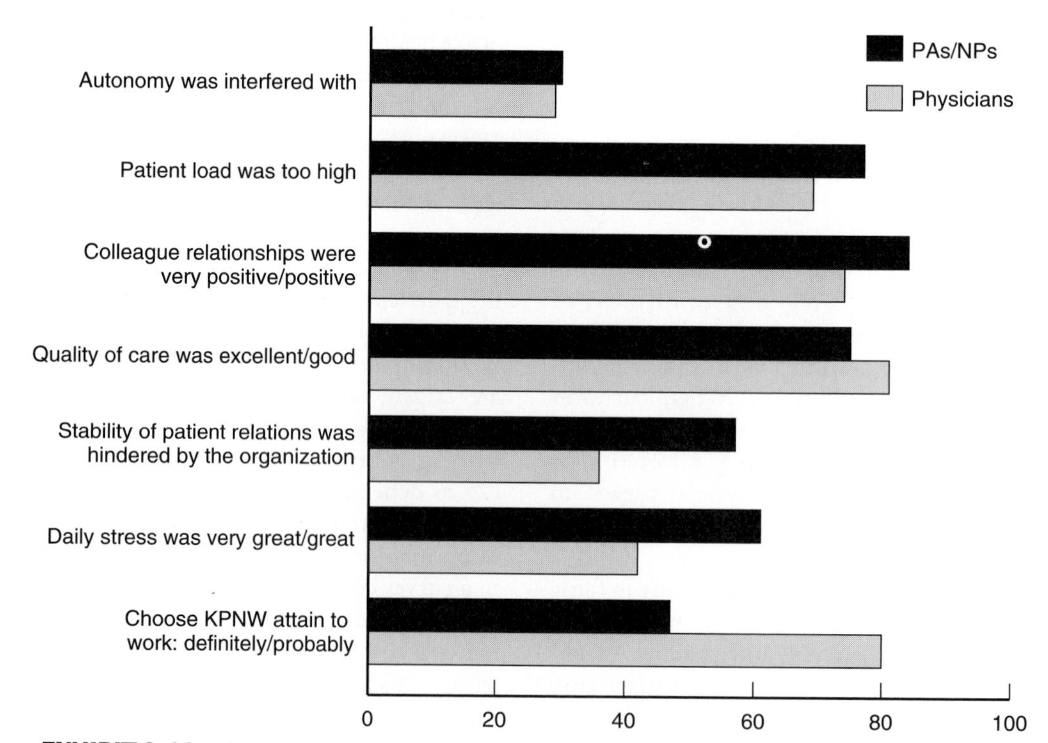

EXHIBIT 9-16 Kaiser Permanente primary care providers' attitudes about selected aspects of practice. (Data from Freeborn DK, Hooker RS, Pope CR: *Eval Health Prof* 25[2], 2002.)

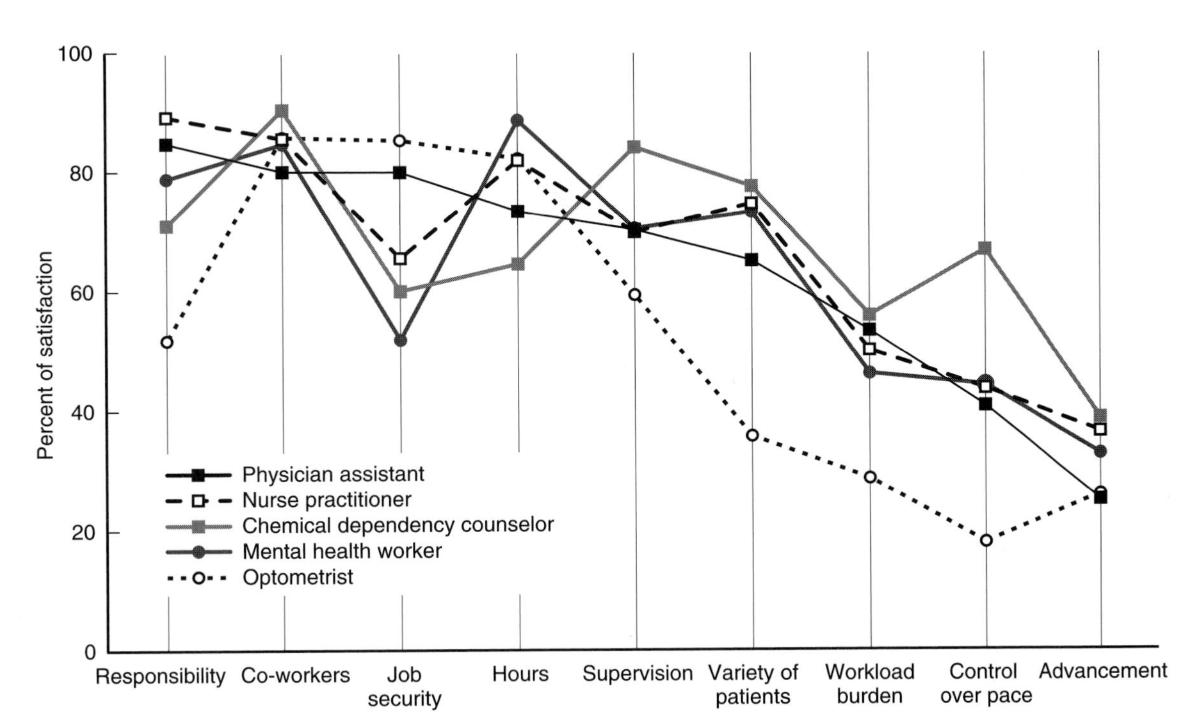

EXHIBIT 9-17 Comparison of job satisfaction between nonphysician providers. (Data from Freeborn DK, Hooker RS: *Public Health Rep* 110:714-719, 1995.)

These findings, along with those of other studies, suggest that institutions, group practices, and HMOs are favorable settings for PAs. The organization of health care in an HMO model may be consistent with how the PA views himself or herself as member of a health care team.

Perry and Redmond (1984) noted the following:

> Little is known about why PAs leave their careers. Clearly some do so to raise families and some may return to resume at least part-time. We estimate that the attrition rate is approximately two percent a year. Background may play a role since men, former military medical corpsmen, and graduates of military PA programs exhibited the lowest attrition in one study.

SUMMARY

Clear evidence exists that PA use results in the production of far more revenue than the costs of their employment in almost all settings. Yet for various reasons, PAs also tend to be underused in some clinical practice settings. Why PAs are not used more in pediatrics and mental health offices bears exploring.

Knowledge about performance and the potential contribution of PAs is significant and continues to mount. The data suggest strongly that a large portion of primary care services can be safely delegated to PAs at levels that exceed 85%. When PAs provide these services, they perform at high levels of productivity that compares favorably with physicians. When the difference between substitution ratios and cost ratios are compared, even when the ratios are conservatively estimated, the differences are so large as to ensure cost savings for employers.

The societal cost savings of PAs in the form of training suggest that a great deal is gained when PAs are trained, because they provide care at substantial savings for 5 years longer than physicians. State barriers in the form of restrictive legislation and reimbursement policies interfere with fuller use of PAs. Research is needed to determine at what level employing PAs in Medicare and Medicaid programs saves tax dollars. However, the cost advantages of employing PAs instead of physicians could diminish if the gap between physician and PA earnings narrows significantly.

Prepaid group practice studies and research from other large institutions suggest that physician comfort levels and practice styles in delegating medical tasks to the PAs with whom they work have a significant influence on PA use and effectiveness in clinical practices. In studies of performance and patterns of utilization of NPPs, scholars have noted a marked difference in the observed versus normative rates of delegation of medical tasks by HMO physicians when working with both PAs and NPs.

Measures of the clinical practice activities and professional characteristics of these health care providers continue to be observed in both inpatient and outpatient settings. Results suggest that NPPs are underused in many health care systems. The factor most critical in determining the effective use of NPPs is the medical task delegation style of the supervising physicians. We offer that staffing efficiency in many organizations could be increased if physicians were more aware of the clinical roles and practice capabilities of these PAs and were better equipped to delegate tasks appropriately.

10

RELATIONSHIPS

INTRODUCTION

This chapter describes the different relationships that physician assistants (PAs) have forged as they have sought recognition. Those relationships include physicians, nurses, nurse practitioners (NPs), managed care, organized medicine, and patients. All are integral members of health care delivery in the United States and a strong relationship is needed with each entity.

The Department of Labor estimates that more than 100 occupations deal with patients in some aspect of the health care workforce. This is in dramatic contrast to the way medicine was originally organized. In the colonial period of America up through the 1930s, all medical services were under the purview of the physician. The patient's family provided assistance informally. Formal nursing arose from a need to assist the physician in treatments, tend to the sick, and develop public health roles. Since the 1860s there has been a constant genesis of new health care occupations. Most health care occupations have taken a common path—an assistant to the physician or nurse. Since the origin of the American PA movement is no different, it is not surprising that the PA profession should try to foster a relationship with medicine and nursing for both support and survival.

PHYSICIAN ATTITUDES TOWARD PHYSICIAN ASSISTANTS

PAs originated from a concept developed by physicians—the need for an assistant who could assume physician-type responsibility and extend their usefulness. As a result of this concept, a close working relationship with physicians has held PAs in good stead. Therefore it is not surprising that PAs and their physician employers agree about the degree of supervision and autonomy, and physicians report that the quality of their lives have improved as a result of hiring a PA.

Theoretic Basis of Physician Dominance

The theoretic basis of the relationship between physicians and PAs is best understood when viewed as part of a larger system of stratification of medical care occupations. With more than 100 health care occupations, physicians have established hierarchical dominance relative to all the other occupations. The physician is considered more powerful in terms of influence and prestige than nurses, aides, and auxiliaries (Goode, 1960; Freidson, 1970; Fuchs, 1974; Shortell, 1974; Larson, 1977).

Autonomy in medicine is typically regarded as possible only when a monopoly exists in that occupation. Yet as Starr (1982) points out, physicians did not set out to gain a "monopoly of competence," rather they wanted to use facilities and work with technical assistants while maintaining control of the division of labor. Thus one might expect that the emergence of relatively new occupations such as PAs and NPs would be generally acceptable and perhaps desirable to physicians as long as their professional autonomy is not jeopardized (Starr, 1982).

Abbott (1981) adds that American physicians are a very heterogeneous social category with varying levels of intraprofessional competition and influence. In other words, although physicians generally enjoy a powerful and prestigious position relative to other medical workers, they vary considerably in how they perceive this power and prestige. The power difference between physicians and other occupations is often described as physician dominance, but this dominance is on a very large continuum. Some physicians seek out PAs as colleagues engaged in a team effort to provide care to the needful of society. Other physicians object to any role that may threaten their position in medicine.

Review of the Literature

The empirical research on physicians' receptiveness to PAs varies by scope, purpose, geographic location, and method. Of the few studies available, several have asked physicians (1) whether PAs should practice independently or with a physician, (2) whether they approve of the concept of a PA, (3) whether they would hire a PA for their practice, and/or (4) what types of tasks PAs might handle. Sometimes these studies were specifically about PAs, and other times they queried physicians about a hypothetical "assistant." For example, a survey of Wisconsin physicians in the 1960s examined physicians' receptivity to hypothetical "doctors' assistants" or "clinical associates." Approximately 40% said they would employ such a person (Coye and Hansen, 1969). In another study undertaken at the same time, mothers of small children were asked whether they would feel comfortable having a PA handle specific tasks. Having a pediatric PA care for their children was acceptable to 94% of the mothers. However, when the same question about specific task delegation was presented to the pediatrician—patients' willingness to accept the patient care services of PAs—the pediatrician's willingness to delegate these tasks fell far below (Patterson, 1969).

Spanning the 1970s and 1980s, several surveys about attitudes of physicians regarding PAs examined both the hypothetical duties and the actual activities of PAs. Physicians who employed PAs and those who had no contact with PAs were surveyed. Some of the questions centered on taking histories, taking blood pressure readings, casting, and suturing. All concluded that routine activities were most appropriate for PAs, and regardless of specialty, type of practice, or community need, most thought it practical to employ a PA (Borland, Williams, and Taylor, 1972; Legler, 1983). Sometimes the surveys concluded that physicians felt PAs could provide appropriate care, but legal and liability questions often arose, suggesting there might be some reluctance to employing a PA (Yanni, Backman, and Potash, 1972). Other times the surveys showed a generally favorable attitude toward PAs, but only a few physicians saw PAs as a solution to the primary care doctor shortage (Haug Associates, 1973). A mail survey of Army physicians stationed worldwide found that a majority (74%) of physicians would welcome a PA to relieve them of seeing routine or minor problems, and 81% believed that the quality of care would be improved or at least was not changed by PA use. Most Army physicians approved of the assignment of PAs to remote locations even when they would have an independent role in the care of active-duty personnel (Stuart and Blair, 1974). In the rural South, a very high percentage of physicians expressed a favorable attitude toward PAs, even though many had never worked with them (Joiner, 1974; Fenn, 1987).

In a study of physicians' attitudes toward the effect PAs have on quality of care, risk of malpractice, role threat, and gender bias in a large health maintenance organization (HMO), internists and pediatricians had favorable attitudes toward both NPs and PAs. Obstetricians and gynecologists had somewhat less favorable attitudes (Exhibit 10-1). Several questions were asked to determine whether these physicians—who at the time of this study in 1977 were predominantly men—might have had gender bias, because most of the PAs were men and the NPs were predominantly women. Physician responses indicated that PAs more than NPs should be awarded certain privileges and participation, suggesting the existence of some gender bias (Johnson and Freeborn, 1986).

Physicians were also asked whether it was a good idea to be on a first-name basis with PAs and NPs. In general, these HMO physicians (almost all men) were less inclined to be on a first-name basis with NPs than with PAs. The doctors were also asked about certain privileges such as (1) wearing the same clinical coats except

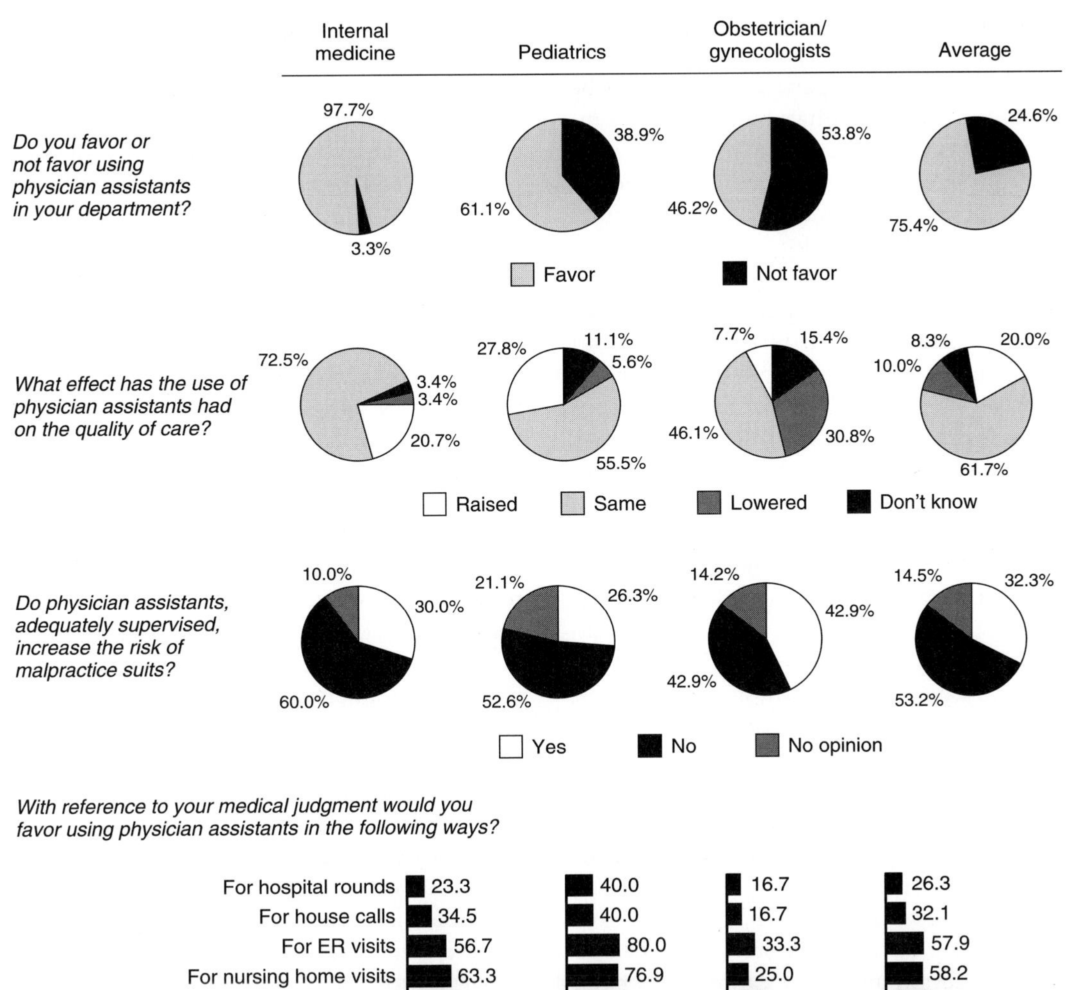

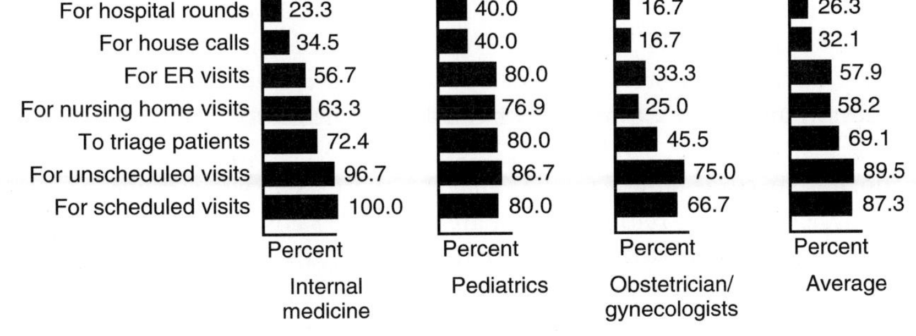

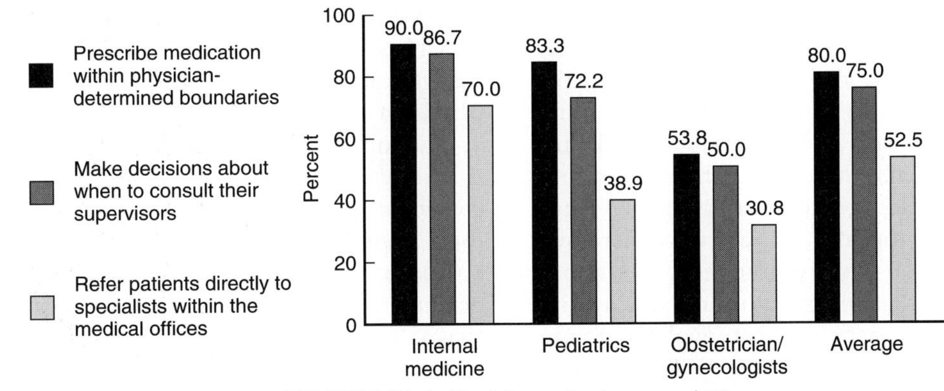

EXHIBIT 10-1 Physician attitudes toward PAs.

for the identification tag, (2) having access to areas reserved for physicians, (3) participating in decisions about how outpatient care was to be delivered, and (4) sitting on various clinical committees. Physicians were generally accepting of PAs. No consistent pattern in their acceptance or attitudes toward PAs emerged in this study (Johnson and Freeborn, 1986).

The ideal relationship between a physician and PA has not been fully articulated in spite of the rhetoric that has taken place coming from the professional societies of physicians. In an interview with a group of physicians on this subject it was expressed that "the role of the PA has to change because integrative models will provide the kind of preventive medicine that managed care demands. The PA is frequently thought of as a substitute, whereas he or she should be complementary to the physician. Physicians will soon begin to lose this. When they do, the relationship between physicians and PAs will be greatly enhanced." Another physician expressed that there is "an abysmal lack of knowledge about PAs." Still another wished that "PAs programs that are tightly integrated with medical school programs should serve as role models and sources of information for 'unintegrated' programs" (Blessing et al., 1998).

Prescribing is considered the last domain of physician autonomy and has been described as "the most common and overt expression of the physician's power" (Pelligrino, 1976). That prescriptive authority has come slowly for PAs may be a result of physicians being reluctant to share this power. The physician's level of confidence in PAs prescribing tends to be more attitudinal than experiential. In Montana, supervising physicians were surveyed about authorizing PAs to prescribe specific agents. Minnesota physicians were asked a similar set of questions. In both instances the physicians strongly supported proposed legislation (Willis and Reid, 1990; Zellmer, 1992). Also in Minnesota, rural family physicians were surveyed about their confidence in the various abilities of PAs. There was a high degree of confidence in the areas of preventive medicine and routine care. Some concern was expressed about the proficiency of PAs taking call, covering the emergency room, and making hospital rounds–activities that involve a broader base of clinical knowledge and diagnostic skills. Other concerns were an increased workload for physicians resulting from their assumed supervisory role; an increased number of complex cases seen by physicians; increased physician liability; job competition among PAs, NPs, and physicians; and supervisory guidelines for physicians regarding collaborative relationships (Bergeson et al., 1997). These attitudes may be different in group and staff model HMOs, in which the role and responsibilities of PAs may be broader and more institutionalized. In many of these HMOs such as Kaiser Permanente, Group Health Cooperative, and Harvard Pilgrim Health Plan the majority of physicians have never known what it was like to not work with PAs (Jacobson, Parker, and Coulter, 1998).

Finally, some physicians offer that the establishment of a collegial role with a PA comes with familiarity. Given time the attitude of physicians toward PAs will improve. The relationship between physicians and PAs should begin with medical students being exposed to PAs and learning more about "how a team approach facilitates good medical care" (Blessing et al., 1998).

Unfortunately, the literature on physician attitudes toward PAs is sparse and may be outdated. Appropriate roles for PAs are not well defined in the minds of most physicians who have responded to surveys and inquiries. PA utilization is dependent on the physician's readiness to hire, work closely with, or otherwise promote the activities of PAs and other nonphysician providers (Glenn and Hofmeister, 1976). Clearly there is a wide range of opinions. As Fottler (1979) concludes, "There is definitely a significant minority of physicians who believe increased delegation of patient-care tasks to properly trained [PAs] is both necessary and desirable.". Since these early studies were undertaken the visibility of PAs in health care systems has steadily improved. Contemporary and well-structured research on their roles may be necessary to adequately address the spectrum of physician attitudes.

The inclination to use PAs is clearly affected by the type of work required. However, there is considerable acceptance of, and even enthusiasm for, PA employment in many quarters. Future attitudes toward acceptance of PAs will depend on the practice patterns of PAs, whether they are viewed as colleagues or competitors and if the economics of PA employment does not infringe on physician income.

Objections to PAs

However overwhelming the acceptance of PAs by physicians may appear, all physicians do not share this view. It would be disingenuous if we did not discuss physician objections to PAs.

For some physicians professional dominance is jeopardized by PAs and other nonphysician clinicians (e.g., NPs, clinical nurse specialists [CNSs], nurse anesthetists, and nurse midwives). One argument advanced by Lichter (1995) is that profit motives and faulty patient satisfaction surveys have contributed to the rise of nonphysician clinician demands for an expanded scope of practice, often achieved legislatively.

Several arguments can be made to counter these views. First is the remarkably opposite view that most policy analysts, economists, and medical sociologists have taken when examining the role of PAs in health care delivery. Their views, endorsed at very high levels, that the use of PAs is an important component in improving health care access and efficiency. Today the U.S. health care delivery system and personnel are perceived by the public to have a number of problems, prompting the need for major reform measures. Many of these problems relate to the composition of its health care workforce and the impact of provider specialty and geographic distribution (White, 1992; Pew Health Professions Commission, 1993). In its Third Report, the Council on Graduate Medical Education (COGME) found the following:

> The rising physician/population ratio will do little to improve the public's health or increase access to services; moreover, it will hinder cost-containment efforts. There is an imbalance of physician specialty distribution, with too few primary care physicians and too many specialist physicians. America's medical educational system is disarticulated between its undergraduate and graduate (GME) components and should be more responsive to regional and national workforce needs. Shortages in the number of primary care physicians contribute to continuing problems in health services access. There continues to be a decline in interest in generalist training among recent medical graduates; only 16% of medical graduates selected residencies in primary care areas and a 57% match rate in internal medicine residency programs in 1993. The preparation of physicians for roles in primary care is often inadequate for future practice responsibilities, particularly in managed care systems. There is a need for better health workforce planning and to restructure financing and reimbursement systems to attain the appropriate specialty mix, racial/ethnic composition, and geographic distribution of physicians. (COGME, 1994)

Strategies aimed at strengthening the ability of the U.S. health care workforce to deliver primary care and improve effectiveness in reducing costs and increasing access will require many years to attain if physicians are the only professionals assumed to deliver medical care services. If overall policy goals for the workforce put forth by the COGME and others are to be achieved, it seems likely that such efforts will require the participation of nonphysicians. It is likely that educational and clinical delivery systems will increasingly use PAs. Future health care delivery systems have been envisioned in which the bulk of primary care services is delivered by PAs and NPs, as physicians assume an increased amount of staff management, administrative, and clinical consulting duties. Such changes in health care professional roles would likely be economically more efficient for medical practices and be a more rational way to use medical training and talent (Meikle, 1992).

Another counterargument is that medicine is being practiced differently and more efficiently now than ever before. This is true throughout all organizational endeavors and is a natural evolution. We have discarded scalpels that need resharpening and needles that need sterilization and have replaced them with disposable and better quality instruments because of the cost-effectiveness of these innovations. Likewise, we have replaced many traditional physician services with alternatives that are more economical than those provided by physicians and in some instances superior to them. History provides us with many examples. Optometrists have taken over the refraction component of ophthalmology care, not because they wanted to, but because physicians were willing to share this role to free their time for other eye services such as surgery. Midwives have been providing birthing services long before there were competent physicians interested enough in assuming this role. A number of studies have shown that contemporary midwifery not only is safe but also may be superior, with the cost of a delivery considerably less than an accouchement assisted by a physician. Other examples abound, such as nurse anesthetists substituting for anesthesiologists, podiatrists for orthopedic surgeons, and psychologists for psychiatrists.

Antiintellectualism

Lichter (1995) also claims that "antiintellectualism has contributed to the rise of PA/NP expanded scope of practice, often achieved legislatively." This may be true because PAs make no claim to be elite providers and instead may be more like nurses that are comfortable allying themselves to the needs of consumers. As Paul Starr (1982) points out, "[Medicine], by its nature, is an inegalitarian institution; it claims to enjoy a dignity not shared by ordinary occupations and a right to set its own rules and standards. These claims go against the democratic grain. They are also exceptionally hard to establish and enforce in a fluid, rapidly expanding society."

The PA role seems more like a blend between the skills of a physician and the patient-oriented role of the nurse. These attributes appear to be attractive to the consumer.

Other arguments contend that the advent of medical boards–guaranteed educational training of practitioners and any movement away from education as the basis of licensure is a step away from medical standards that will have negative long-term consequences (Lichter, 1995). What is not accounted for in this view is the superior educational development that has come out of collaboration between PA training programs and physician training programs. As Dr. Estes (1993) has stated, "The educational system producing physician assistants is more advanced, efficient, and cost-effective than that producing physicians."

Finally, physician attitudes toward an expanded role for the PA in the future are quite favorable (Lapius, 1983; Legler, 1983).

How receptive physicians are to the effective employment of PAs is questionable because the relationship between physicians and PAs is not always well understood, even by physicians who employ them. Ferraro and Southerland (1989) found that physicians are most likely to think that use of PAs should be directed toward caring for the urban poor and is least likely to improve care for obstetrics and pediatrics cases. Physicians may seem more willing to employ and delegate tasks to a PA than an NP (Fottler, 1979), although this view may be reflective of an older concept of both providers.

Remarkably good relationships now exist between PAs and physicians. These relationships are manifested in the types of positions PAs occupy, as well as with organized medicine and physician professional societies.

Are PAs Professionals?

Are PAs professionals? PAs have assumed a number of the characteristics of professionals: They share a body of knowledge with physicians, who are recognized as in the ultimate profession, and are granted a substantial degree of work autonomy within the defined practice scope of the physician. Some would argue that PAs do not qualify as professionals because they do not posses their own body of knowledge and lack total autonomy in their work. Yet the standard of what constitutes a professional appears to be changing. Physician assistants have made great progress in controlling their regulation and legislation, title definition and protection, rules for entry into the profession, accreditation of educational programs, and certification of graduates. While this progress has been incremental, it is based on the increasingly accepted concept of delegated or negotiated autonomy via the supervising physician. There is a need for more research by PAs about physician assistants and health care delivery and a description of the unique aspects that PAs bring to medical practice. PAs have thus far not generated a large body of knowledge about themselves or their practice aspects, but they have resisted the temptation to create an arcane language and "science" in an attempt to bestow professional status on themselves. They remain true to their calling as competency-based providers of health care, with the majority in primary care and many caring for the medically underserved. The PA profession should continue to strive for status as professionals in the altruistic sense, just as physicians ponder returning to their roots in service to society.

ORGANIZED MEDICINE

A relationship between the American Academy of Physician Assistants (AAPA) and the American Medical Association (AMA) has waxed and waned over the years. In 1994 the AMA granted observer status for the AAPA to sit in on the AMA House of Delegates, a signal that this relationship has recently been strengthened.

In 1995 the AMA House of Delegates adopted a set of guidelines for the working relationship between physicians and PAs. The guidelines recognize that PAs practice with physician supervision and the PA and physician together should determine the PA's role in patient care. This recognition came in deference to the practice advocated by NPs. The AMA Board of Trustees wrote:

> [NPs] use terms like "collaboration" and "interdependent" whereas PAs use "delegation" and "supervision." PAs regard themselves as "agents" of the physicians, legally and practically, and view delegated medical acts and understanding the delegatory style of physicians with whom they work as their particular responsibilities. They define "collaboration" as synonymous with physician supervision. In contrast, NPs work towards "independent" practice and decision making under the nurse practice acts. (Gara, 1995)

However, this relationship is not entirely mutual, and in 1995 the AMA developed a set of guidelines that establishes the ideal relationship between a physician and a PA (Exhibit 10-2).

Basically these guidelines reflect the AMA belief that in all settings PAs should recognize physician supervision in the delivery of patient care and that there is no role for PAs either to be in competition with physicians or to practice medicine independently from physicians.

A similar relationship exists with the American Academy of Family Physicians to work on issues affecting continuing medical education. For now the relationship between organized medicine and the PA profession seems secure, providing it remains as physicians want it.

NURSING

In their first decade of existence PAs struggled to distinguish themselves from nurses. When assigned to hospital roles PAs were often placed in nursing departments. In outpatient settings PAs were often linked with a registered nurse (RN), believing this relationship would strengthen the PA's role (Lairson, Record, and James, 1974). Early in the development of the profession, some believed the logical place for PAs was within the nursing profession (Bergman, 1971). PAs are sometimes referred to as *midlevel providers*. This undefined term implies that PAs are somewhere between physicians and nurses. The problem with this term is that nurses feel they are on the same level as physicians as colleagues, not under them; therefore the term *midlevel* seems inappropriate.

EXHIBIT 10-2

AMA Guidelines for Physician-PA Practice

1. The physician is responsible for managing the health care of patients in all practice settings.
2. Health care delivered by physicians and physician assistants must be within the scope of each practitioner's authorized practice as defined by state law.
3. The physician is ultimately responsible for coordinating and managing the care of patients and, with the appropriate input of the physician assistant, ensuring the quality of health care provided to patients.
4. The physician is responsible for the supervision of the physician assistant in all settings.
5. The role of the physician assistant(s) in the delivery of care should be defined through mutually agreed upon guidelines that are developed by the physician and the physician assistant and based on the physician's delegatory style.
6. The physician must be available for consultation with the physician assistant at all times either in person or through telecommunication systems or other means.
7. The extent of the involvement by the physician assistant in the assessment and implementation of treatment will depend on the complexity and acuity of the patient's condition and the training and experience and preparation of the physician assistant as adjudged by the physician.
8. Patients should be made clearly aware at all times whether they are being cared for by a physician or a physician assistant.
9. The physician and physician assistant together should review all delegated patient services on a regular basis, as well as the mutually agreed upon guidelines for practice.
10. The physician is responsible for clarifying and familiarizing the physician assistant with his or her supervising methods and style of delegating patient care.

Data from AMA House of Delegates, June 1995.

Nursing and medicine are occupations that work alongside each other, and although nurses may be employees of physicians, nursing is a profession, complete with a body of theory that assesses the needs of the patient in conjunction with the physician's assessment.

To evaluate nurses' attitudes toward PAs, a survey was conducted in two hospitals. Hospital X employed 19 PAs to work in adult and pediatric ambulatory clinics, the emergency department, the neonatal intensive care unit (NICU), and the newborn nursery. Hospital Y employed no PAs (Exhibit 10-3). The results of this study indicate that nurses who have experience working with PAs or who have an understanding of the role of the PA in the health care system have more positive attitudes toward them than those who do not have such knowledge or experience (Erkert, 1985). Although some tension exists between PAs and nurses on the academic level, the roots of PAs go deeply into the nursing profession. Many PAs had their primary introduction to medicine through nursing. Approximately one fourth of all PAs had some nursing experience. The early military corpsmen were often trained in part by nurses and were often under nursing departments in field and stateside hospitals.

EXHIBIT 10-3

Nurses' Attitudes Toward PAs

1. *In general, do you believe the PAs with whom you have worked to be professionally competent?*

Hospital*	Yes	No
X	91.4%	8.6%
Y	74.2%	25.8%

2. *In general, do you object to performing functions at the request of a PA you believe to be professionally competent?*

Hospital	Yes	No
X	27.9%	72.1%
Y	36.5%	63.5%

3. *In general, are you or would you be comfortable working with a PA?*

Hospital	Yes	No
X	78.4%	21.6%
Y	56.2%	43.8%

4. *Of PAs and NPs, which do you personally prefer?*

Hospital	PA	NP	Both	Neither
X	8.1%	11.1%	58.6%	22.2%
Y	9.6%	35.6%	32.9%	21.9%

5. *How would you describe your overall attitude toward the PA profession?*

Hospital	Positive	Negative	Indifferent
X	52.3%	10.3%	37.4%
Y	35.4%	21.5%	43.1%

6. *I do not clearly understand the need for PAs in the health care system.*

Hospital	True	False
X	37.1%	69.2%
Y	47.9%	52.1%

7. *I do not clearly understand the need for PAs in the hospital.*

Hospital	True	False
X	64.1%	35.9%
Y	74.7%	25.3%

8. *My state Nurse Practice Act:*	Hospital X	Hospital Y
Allows me to legally take orders from a PA	12.3%	6.0%
Legally requires me to take orders from a PA	2.8%	1.5%
Does not allow me to legally take orders from a PA	34.9%	16.4%
I do not know what the Nurse Practice Act says in regard to PAs	50.0%	76.1%

Data from Erkert JD: *Physician Assist* 9:41-44, 1985.
*Hospital X = 19 PAs; hospital Y = no PAs.

Conceptual Models of Nursing

Nurses have formulated a number of conceptual models of nursing that constitute formal explanations of what nursing is. As Fawcett (1994) has noted, four concepts are central to models of nursing: person, environment, health, and nursing. The various nursing models define these concepts differently, link them in diverse ways, and give different emphasis to the relationships among them. Moreover, different models emphasize different processes as being central to nursing. For example, Sister Callista Roy's Adaptation Model identifies adaptation of patients as a critical (Roy and Andrews, 1998). Martha (Rogers, Malinski, and Barrett, 1994), by contrast, emphasizes the centrality of the individual as a unified whole, and her model views nursing as a process in which individuals are aided in achieving maximum well-being within their potential. Nurse researchers increasingly are turning toward these conceptual models for their inspiration in formulating research questions and hypotheses. Other conceptual models of nursing that have been used in nursing studies include King's Open System Model (Johnson, 1998); Neuman's Health Care Systems Model (1989); Orem's Model of Self-Care (1995); and Parse's Theory of Human Becoming (1992). Exhibit 10-4 lists eight conceptual models of nursing, together with a study for each that claimed the model as its framework.

Let us consider one conceptual model of nursing that has received particular attention among nurse researchers—Roy's Adaptation Model (Roy and Andrews, 1998). In this model, human beings are biopsychosocial adaptive systems who cope with environmental change through the process of adaptation. Within the human system, there are four subsystems or response modes: physiologic needs, self-concept, role function, and interdependence. These subsystems constitute adaptive modes that provide mechanisms for coping with environmental stimuli and change. The goal of nursing, according to this model, is to promote patient adaptation during health and illness. Roy's model has been cited as the conceptual framework for adaptation by many researchers.

In addition to conceptual models that describe and characterize the entire nursing process, nurses have developed other models and theories that focus on specific phenomena of interest to nurses. An important example is Nola Pender's Health Promotion Model (Pender and Pender, 1996), a conceptual map. Another example is Mishel's Uncertainty in Illness Theory (1998), which focuses on the concept of uncertainty—the inability of a person to determine the meaning of illness-related events. According to this theory a situation appraised as uncertain will mobilize individuals to use their resources to adapt to the situation. Mishel's conceptualization of uncertainty has been used as a framework for both qualitative and quantitative studies.

These theories, separately and in the aggregate, establishes the theoretical basis of nursing and the contributions they bring to medicine.

EXHIBIT 10-4

Examples of Studies Linked to Conceptual Models of Nursing

Model	Study
King's Open System Model	What is the effect of a nurse-client transactional female adolescents' oral contraceptive intervention on adherence (Hanna, 1993)?
Levine's Conservation Model	What are the dimensions of fatigue as experienced by patients with congestive heart failure (Schaefer and Potylycki, 1993)?
Neuman's Health Care Systems Model	What is the relationship between mood symptoms and daytime ambulatory blood pressure during a 12-hr period in black female caregivers and noncaregivers (Picot et al., 1999)?
Parse's Theory of Human Becoming	What are the factors that influence young women's perceptions of risk for sexually transmitted diseases?
Orem's Model of Self-Care	What is the relationship between self-care agency and abuse on the one hand and physical and emotional health on the other among women in intimate relationships (Campbell and Soeken, 1999)?
Roger's Science of Unitary Human Beings	What is the efficacy of a Rogerian-based intervention of therapeutic touch on anxiety, pain, and plasma T-lymphocyte concentration in burn patients (Turner et al., 1998)?
Roy's Adaptation Model	Do formal cancer support groups help women adapt to the physiologic and psychosocial sequelae of breast cancer (Samarel et al., 1998)?

NURSE PRACTITIONERS

Evolution of patterns in the division of medical labor in U.S. medicine reveals that several types of nonphysician health professionals make important contributions and expand the services available to patients. As part of this evolution of health professional roles, PAs, NPs, and certified nurse midwives (CNMs) have been increasingly incorporated into medical practices and health institutions' staffing.

The NP inception began the same year as the PA inception, in 1965. Most NP programs are affiliated with nursing schools, and almost all are master's degree programs. Like PAs, NPs are well distributed throughout the medical profession, and in many instances PAs and NPs compete for the same jobs, suggesting parity. NP programs tend to be specialty oriented, but the vast majority is primary care based. They do not consider themselves a physician-dependent profession; instead, they believe their care is an extension of the nursing act. This philosophy has been the source of ideological debate and focus of comparison between the two professions.

Despite divergent training (and sometimes acrimonious debate), there is remarkable agreement in how PAs and NPs approach the patient. Because of this attitude, PAs and NPs are often thought of as similar types of health care providers. In a number of clinical settings, such as managed care health systems and ambulatory clinics, the roles of PAs and NPs are regarded as interchangeable, and jobs are often advertised that can be filled by either one. Major research reports and policy analyses that have examined both of these health professions consider PAs and NPs to be equivalent when used in ambulatory practice roles (Office of Technology Assessment, 1986). Even on the clinic level, PAs and NPs have similar views about their roles. When PA and NP attitudes about jobs and roles are surveyed the results are indistinguishable (Freeborn and Hooker, 1995, 2002) (Exhibit 10-5).

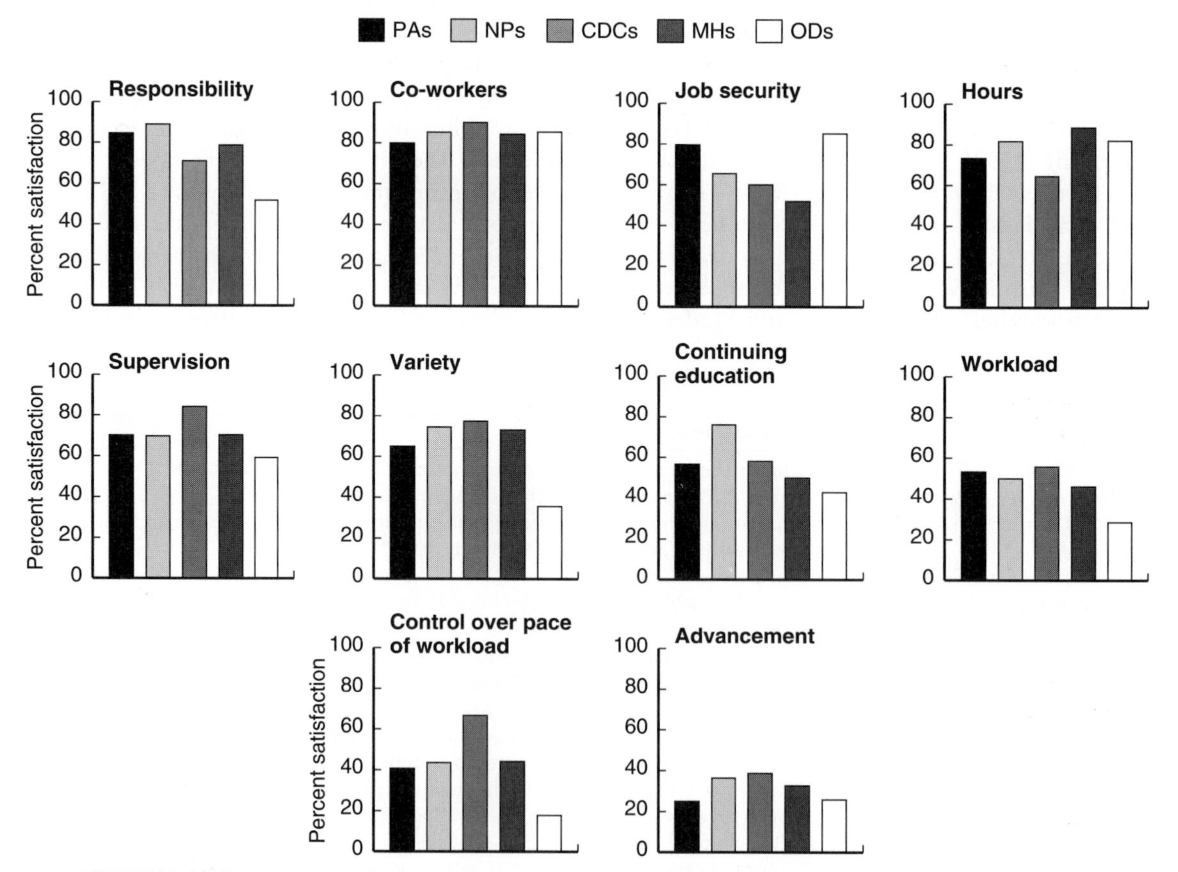

EXHIBIT 10-5 Percentage of Kaiser Permanente providers satisfied or very satisfied with specific aspects of their employment. (Data from Freeborn DK, Hooker RS: *Public Health Rep* 110:714-719, 1995.)

The histories of NPs and PAs have some interesting parallels. In 1965 the first NP demonstration project, funded by the Commonwealth Foundation, was initiated at the University of Colorado Medical Center. Henry Silver, MD, and Loretta Ford, RN, were the developers of this program in pediatrics. The intent was to extend the nurse's role in pediatric medicine. As a 5-year project it was designed to prepare nurses to provide comprehensive well-child care in noninstitutional settings and to study the program outcomes for their applicability for curriculum changes in collegiate nursing programs (Ford, 1979a). This course of study was 4 months, followed by 20 months of field experience with a pediatrician. At completion of this program these nurses were granted a certificate. Graduates of this program were called pediatric NPs.

Despite similarity in origins, important differences between PAs and NPs persist (Exhibit 10-6). As health care professionals, NPs and PAs possess distinctive professional orientations and educational backgrounds, have different state regulatory systems, and show practice characteristics that appear to be moving in different directions. NPs believe that as nurses, they are empowered to act independently, with the authority to prescribe drugs without physician oversight. They want nurse reimbursement rates to be brought up to physician rates for a "like service" (Safriet, 1998). Patients view them differently as well (Conant et al., 1971). These differences have important implications for the future roles of both professions in a reformed health care system. As of 2002, about 100,000 NPs have matriculated from a formal training program and about 70,000 were in active clinical practice (L. Berlin, AANC, personal communication, May 17, 2002). NPs represent 1.3% of the total pool of licensed nurses; of all NPs, about 4500 are CNMs. NPs are distributed mostly in the primary care fields of adult medicine, pediatrics, women's health, student health, and geriatrics. The practice patterns of NPs are largely based in these primary care areas are also expanded geriatrics, nursing homes, home care, and community clinic settings. There are approximately 337 institutions (predominantly schools of nursing), containing approximately 1488 accredited educational programs or separate tracks for NPs (Hooker and Berlin, 2002).

Comparing Nurse Practitioners and Physician Assistants

The origins of PAs and NPs are similar in both time and concept. While their ideologies remain distinct, enough analysis exists to suggest the service to those who reside in the United States is remarkably similar (Hooker and McCaig, 1996; McCaig et al., 1998). The NP data were collected as part of a 1999 survey of U.S.-based NPs (Running et al., 2000). The PA data were collected through an annual census survey of graduates of physician assistant programs (AAPA, 1999). Some information was supplemented by a study comparing PAs and NPs in urban and rural areas undertaken at an earlier time (Pan et al., 1997).

As of January 1999 the number of estimated graduates of all NP programs is almost double the number of PA graduates (Exhibit 10-6). However, the number of practicing PAs is approximately two thirds the number of practicing NPs. Caucasians predominate in the two professions (94.1% for NPs versus 88% for PAs). The vast majority of NPs (72.4%) have a master's degree, versus 50% of PAs. NP programs receive federal support under Title VIII Division of Nursing grants (Hooker, 2001).

The majority of PAs (52.4%) and NPs (67.5%) are in primary care. Primary care in this case is defined as family practice, general internal medicine, pediatrics, and obstetrics and gynecology. NPs are five times more likely to be in pediatrics or women's health than PAs. However, when other subspecialties are included, such as geriatrics, urgent care, corrections medicine, and occupation and environmental medicine, the percent of PAs in primary care is larger.

Almost one fourth of PAs are in surgical roles. The number of NPs in surgical roles was not identified when surveyed. PAs are six times more likely to be in emergency medicine than NPs (9.9% versus 1.5%).

Most PAs and NPs work in urban or suburban settings, although a significant proportion also works in rural areas (PAs, 24.3%; NPs, 20%). The vast majority of PAs report they work full time (87.6%), compared with NPs who report they work full time 58.3% of the time. Some caution is needed in interpreting these figures because each occupation defines the terms full time and part time differently.

EXHIBIT 10-6

Comparison of PAs and NPs

Characteristics	Category	PA	NP
Estimated practicing clinicians (January 1999)		38,112*	60,905†
Total graduates (January 1999)		41,421*	80,000 (estimated)
Gender (%)	Male	46.2*	4.1†
	Female	53.8*	95.9†
Marital status (%)	Married	72.9‡	70.3‡
	Nonmarried	27.1‡	29.7‡
Race/ethnicity	Hispanic/Latino	3.6%*	1.6‡
	Black/African American	3.1*	3.2‡
	Asian/Pacific Islander	2.3*	1.1‡
	Native American/Alaskan	1.2*	0.0‡
	White/European American	88.0*	94.1‡
Education (highest degree)	Associate degree	10.7*	3.0†
	Baccalaureate	62.1*	8.8†
	Master's degree	25.0*	72.4†
	Doctorate degree	3.0*	2.2†
Practice site (primary employment setting)	Metropolitan (urban and inner city)	41.4*	36.2†
	Suburban	32.1*	32.8†
	Rural	24.3*	20.0†
	Other	2.2*	11.0†
Years of practice (mean)		9.5*	9.0†
Specialty practiced	Family practice/general medicine PA or FNP	38.0*	36.0†
	General internal medicine PA or ANP	9.2*	17.8†
	Emergency medicine PA, acute care NP	9.9*	1.5†
	General pediatrics or PNP	2.8*	13.7†
	General surgery	2.8*	—
	Internal medicine subspecialty	4.9*	—
	Pediatric subspecialty	1.4*	—
	Surgical subspecialty	16.8*	—
	OB/GYN PA or WHNP	2.4*	12.2†
	Industrial/occupational medicine	3.4*	—
	Psychiatry/substance abuse PA or mental health NP	1.2*	3.1†
	Geriatrics	0.8*	5.9†
	Other	—	7.0†
Average workweek	Full time	87.6 (32+ hr)*	58.3 (35+ hr)†
	Part time	11.7 (<32 hr)*	32.2 (<35 hr)†
Prescribe medications (%)		88*	82‡
Average no. of outpatient visits per week	Family practice	105‡	75‡
	Adult/internal medicine	90‡	56‡
	Pediatrics	134‡	65‡
	OB/GYN	71‡	67‡

*Data from American Academy of Physician Assistants, 1999.
†Data from Running A, Calder J, Mustain B, Foreschler C: *Nurse Pract* 25(6): 15-16, 110-116, 2000.
‡Data from Pan S, Geller JM, Gullicks JN, Muus KJ, Larson AC: *Nurse Pract* 22(1): 14, 1997.

Even in the absence of far-reaching health care reform, it is anticipated that requirements for the use of NPs are expected to increase in an ever expanding and increasingly demanding health care system. Changes are envisioned for NPs and CNMs, particularly in helping to meet primary care delivery needs under a reformed system providing universal access (Harper, 1996). Projections include requirements for higher numbers of NPs (along with PAs) to fulfill roles as primary care practitioners in private practices, in expanding managed care systems, and in institutional settings.

Unique to NPs are resources that relate to the nursing professional base. Social appeal, political potential through numbers, a different focus on the patient, and substitution opportunities all relate to nursing origins. For PAs the lack of these origins and some of their related phenomena can either benefit from them or hinder them. Unencumbered by "doctor-nurse" conflicts and traditional role perceptions, some analysts believe that PAs have somewhat clearer identities, greater mobility, and willingness—by role, definition, and name—to serve as physician associates than NPs. Their roles are more flexible because of this willing dependence (Salmon, 1985).

Many of the barriers to full use for NPs are common to PAs. These include physician dependence, institutional "job" dependence, limited power when compared with physicians, legal status less than optimal, partial reimbursement, and variance on qualifications and training.

The barriers unique to NPs include time-control needs and a relative lack of professional organization. PAs, on the other hand, may be limited by the social and/or political license afforded NPs because of their lack of a homogeneous professional base. Nursing is the common denominator for all NPs, and the nursing lobby is a powerful voice. Nurses believe they have one foot up the rung of professional acceptance because of their nursing background. PAs, on the other hand, began their profession drawing on their history as former corpsmen but quickly expanded to include applicants with diverse medical backgrounds and now have a wide profession base. The attributes that facilitate or inhibit full expression of a profession are refered to as *enablers* and *barriers* (Exhibit 10-7).

Unlike PAs, who have a single national academy that consolidates all PA efforts (the AAPA), no single organization represents all NPs. The American Academy of Nurse Practitioners, the American College of Nurse Practitioners, the American Nurses Association (ANA), and the National Alliance of Nurse Practitioners all claim some representation and have their advocates and critics. Other organizations represent different specialties of NPs nationally such as the National Association of Pediatric Nurse Associates & Practitioners (NAPNAP), Association

EXHIBIT 10-7

PA and NP Enablers and Barriers to Future Roles in Health Care

Enablers: NPs	**Enablers: PAs**
Professional base	Role flexibility
Independence of physicians	Willingness to assume dependent posture with physicians
Cost-savings potential	Cost-savings potential
Interchangeability with PAs	Interchangeability with NPs
Social appeal	Relatively greater mobility than NPs
Nursing numbers offer wide political potential to influence legislation	Professional organization
Large no. of training programs granting graduate degrees	Relatively clear identity
Barriers: NPs	**Barriers: PAs**
Physician independence	Physician dependence
Limited relative power	Limited relative power
Limited (but growing) reimbursable functions	Limited (but growing) reimbursable functions
Limited power (absolute)	Limited power (absolute)
Limited mobility compared with PAs	Lack of homogeneous professional base such as nursing
Specialized training	Variable qualifications/training
Predominantly women with inherent time-control needs (e.g., part time, day shift, child dependence)	Small number of training programs. Range from junior colleges to graduate programs in academic medical centers
Professional disorganization	

of Women's Health, Obstetrics, and Neonatal Nurses (AWHONN), and the National Association of Nurse Practitioners in Reproductive Health. Four national NP certification boards exist for credentialing NPs, depending on specialty and preference, and many states have certification processes as well. The American Nursing Association, a powerful special-interest group, often acts on behalf of NPs. Because of this splintering of NP factions the likelihood of developing any alliances between NPs and PAs (at least on the national level) remains limited.

NP education is provided in 202 universities and other institutions, with 527 programs or clinical tracks (Exhibits 10-8 and 10-9).

While many people object to the tension between the two nonphysician groups, this tension can also be viewed as healthy, if society is considered best served when there is competition. When both providers strive to improve their image and demonstrate their ability to deliver quality care, patients must surely benefit in the end. Along with the public the respective professions benefit when each is compared alongside the other, as well as with physicians. Delivering quality care at affordable cost and providing choice in types of providers can only enhance the image of U.S. medicine.

EXHIBIT 10-8

Number and Curriculum Focus of NP Programs (Update)*

Nurse practitioner program specialty	No.	%
Family	143	77.7
Pediatric	64	34.8
Gerontologic/geriatric	51	27.7
Adult	49	26.6
Obstetric-gynecologic/women's health	47	25.5
Neonatal	33	17.9
Adult psychiatric/mental health	23	12.5
Acute care (adult)	22	11.9
Oncology	9	4.9
Occupational health	8	4.3
School	6	3.3
Child and adolescent psychiatric/ mental health	5	2.7
Perinatal	5	2.7
Other (includes dual-track options)	18	9.8
TOTAL	483	100.0

Data from American Association of the Colleges of Nursing: *The Essentials of Master's Education for Advanced Nursing*, Washington, DC, 1996, American Association of the Colleges of Nursing.
*Only master's level programs.

The role of the NP in the United States is here to stay. Work on assessing patient outcomes using NPs as the sole providers identifies that the care is identical to physicians' and the cost of

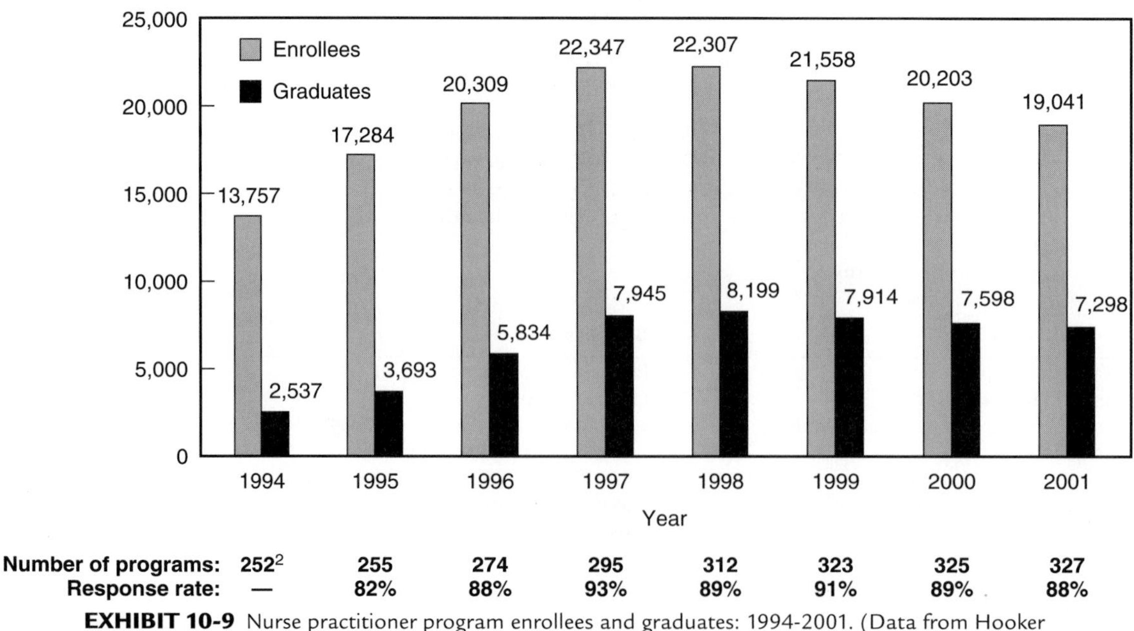

EXHIBIT 10-9 Nurse practitioner program enrollees and graduates: 1994-2001. (Data from Hooker RS, Berlin: *Health Affairs*, 2001.)

care is less than physicians' (Mundinger et al., 2000).

CLINICAL NURSE SPECIALISTS

Little is written on CNSs. The CNS is a nurse in advanced practice who has received advanced education, sometimes at the master's or even doctoral level. The curriculum concentrates heavily on advanced skills in assessment, intervention, health promotion, illness prevention, and critical thinking. In addition, the educational preparation is theoretically grounded in multiple theories of nursing and theories from other disciplines (Huch, 1992). Training and credentials vary considerably. CNSs state that they are prepared to approach the client using a holistic approach, integrating physiologic, psychologic, cultural, spiritual, and sociologic aspects of the patient and family into their care (Lombness, 1994). The CNS is considered both an independent and an interdependent practitioner who functions in a collaborative role with the physician. Educational preparation for the CNS varies considerably. Many demographic studies on NPs and advanced practice nurses include the CNS as an NP.

While the CNS, NP, and PA sometimes perform similar tasks, Lombness (1994) argues that the CNS and PA differ because of the advanced education of the CNS. She believes that CNSs have extended roles that go beyond tasks, require different critical thinking and critical judgment skills, and incorporate case management strategies (Lombness, 1994). To bolster this belief a study was undertaken to examine what differences are seen in length of stay for cardiovascular patients managed by CNSs versus those managed by PAs. A descriptive comparison of two groups was performed. Data were collected using a retrospective chart audit of patients who had coronary artery bypass surgery co-managed by cardiac surgeons and by teams of PAs or teams of cardiac surgeons and CNSs. Complication rates were similar between the two groups. Findings indicated that the CNS-managed group had a statistically significant shorter length of stay (Exhibit 10-10).

Although this retrospective study did show some statistical differences between PAs and CNSs, many variables are not accounted for and need to be adjusted: one hospital's experience, small number of patients, small number of providers, retrospective study, readmission rates, and other factors. However, the study suggests that CNSs may add value to a medical team in outcome of care.

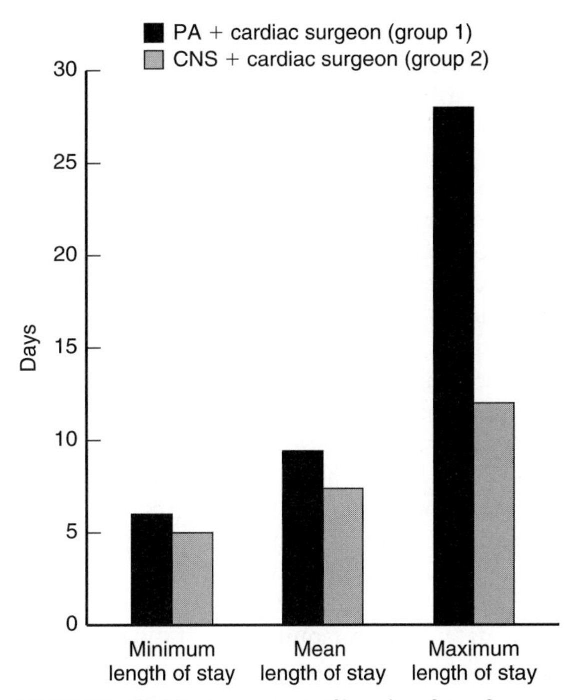

EXHIBIT 10-10 Comparison of lengths of stay for coronary artery bypass graft when managed by certified nurses and PAs.

MANAGED CARE ORGANIZATIONS

PAs have been employees of managed care organizations since the late 1960s. Key health care reform policy goals are to lower medical care access barriers, contain cost, and incorporate largely new organizational structures ("managed competition") in health care services delivery. In effect, this direction likely means a reliance on HMOs and other types of prepaid and managed health care delivery systems. The clinical staffing mix of future HMOs and other managed care organizations will be based in large part on the capabilities and efficiency of employed health care professionals. This means there will likely be both physicians and nonphysicians to provide the required range, access, and quality of medical diagnostic, therapeutic, and preventive care services in a manner acceptable to enrollees.

Many believe these efforts will result in improved levels of health care service access, will promote grater effectiveness in medical care resource allocation, and will place less emphasis on ability to pay as a criterion for people in the United States seeking health care insurance coverage. A likely outcome of any health system reform is the reconfiguration of America's health care delivery system built on HMOs and other managed care plans that have demonstrated success. As these delivery systems become the principal locus of primary care services for many individuals, it is likely that there will be an increased demand for both physician and nonphysician primary care providers (Crane, 1995).

One analysis assessing the requirements for physicians, both primary care and specialty, on a defined population found that managed care systems relied heavily on PAs and NPs (Weiner, Steinwachs, and Williamson, 1986). Projected estimates were developed using clinical performance data, setting requirement standards based on available information obtained from multiple segments of the health care system, and applying these derived standards to the proportion of the U.S. population assumed to be receiving medical care services within each sector. A particular focus was placed on HMO staffing levels under the likelihood that market share will increase with health care reform.

Analysts frequently use HMO staffing patterns to estimate national clinical workforce requirements. This has occurred in some of the military branches and other federal systems. Based on a national survey of group and staff-model HMOs, researchers found that two thirds employ a PA and/or an NP. A correlation analysis also found that HMOs with the lowest ratio of primary care physicians to members also had the highest percentage of PAs and NPs as employees (Dial et al., 1995). The authors concluded that PAs and NPs are being used in high ratios to substitute for physician services in these settings.

GOVERNMENT AND FINANCING ISSUES

The federal government provides substantial amounts in support of health care profession education. Physicians receive a large share of the more than $5 billion Medicare subsidy of GME through direct medical education (DME) and indirect medical education assistance (IMEA) payments. These funds go to teaching hospitals to support the clinical education of physicians and include training assistance for a number of other health care professionals. This Medicare funding does not support PAs or advanced practice nurses (CNSs, NPs, or CNMs). In the past, federal dollars supporting PA and NP training have been administered through grant awards programs, a mechanism that in a number of instances has had positive results. Current incentives and rewards for teaching hospitals sponsoring GME programs are driven more by institutional needs than by societal needs. Changing the structure and financing policies of Medicare to better emphasize the training of generalist physicians has not come to fruition. Making health profession educational programs receiving federal support more accountable to the public in terms of graduate outcomes (e.g., patterns of specialty and practice location) is now an increasingly accepted premise.

Medicare policy has been slow to respond to shifting patterns of physician education and practice. It has long been advocated that generalist physician numbers could be promoted by shifting the locus of GME training experiences to increase residents' time in outpatient and ambulatory care clinics, yet Medicare does not allow funding support in these settings. A policy change in the financing of health profession education is a key part of health care reform. The Clinton administration's proposed bill, the Health Security Act, contained an extensive array of changes affecting GME size and funding. Although this was not enacted, a major reform policy goal remains in place and is aimed to produce a 55% level of primary care physicians in the workforce. To help attain these goals, there has been the development of a new fund to support the cost of academic health center functions beyond the usual provision of patient health care services, establishment of an institute for health care workforce development, a series of initiatives to augment Title VII and VIII funding above the current level, and a GME funding pool of $200 million for advanced practice nursing. This later proposal should be modified to include PAs in the likelihood that they will be used at the same level as or higher than NPs and other advanced practice nurses in reform-restructured inpatient staffing. Incremental changes are anticipated in Congress that may eventually achieve this goal. Until then, PA education will have to rely on limited support through the Bureau of Health Professions.

PHARMACISTS

The last remaining barrier for full use of PAs is in the area of prescribing. On an individual level, where a PA works with a pharmacist, usually within an institution, there is wide acceptance of PAs and the way they prescribe (Hooker, 1993). While historically a few pharmacists opposed the ability of PAs to prescribe, these objections have largely disappeared, perhaps because of the increasing clinical role that pharmacists have been developing since the mid 1990s. For the most part, pharmacists do not seem concerned about PAs from a safety perspective.

One study that examined PA views of drug information sources showed that PAs rate pharmacists the best sources of drug information. Next in descending order of drug information reliability are journal articles, physicians, detail persons, and other PAs. This study also found that PAs view pharmacists with increasing regard the more they come in contact with them (Fincham, 1986).

When PAs were given the authority to prescribe in Wisconsin, a survey of pharmacists indicated that PAs were utilizing the privilege, and that the technical quality of their prescribing was appropriate. However, they were not sure whether it was appropriate for them to prescribe (Huntington and Warnick, 1987). Again, this expressed attitude has disappeared from the literature.

As pharmacists move into the role of limited prescriber in some states, the expansion of the PA role is likely to continue as pharmacists confront the same barriers that PAs once encountered. Alliances are likely to continue in this area.

PATIENTS

The patient's viewpoint is generally considered the most important element in the appraisal of PA acceptance in American society (Exhibit 10-11). While relationships with physicians and nurses are placed high on the list of importance, the PA-patient relationship is the reason PAs have been able to thrive in such a competitive environment. These attitudinal differences are important because if consumers are not satisfied with PAs, no alliance with organized medicine will ensure the PA profession's future. If patient acceptance and satisfaction were low, it is doubtful that PAs would still be in existence. Patient attitudes and satisfaction with their providers is important because satisfied patients are more likely to follow-through on recommendations made by the provider (Janis, 1980).

Literature on Patient Attitudes Toward Physician Assistants

Even before formal PA education had produced more than a few dozen PAs, researchers in the late 1960s were asking mothers of young children if they would feel comfortable with a theoretical "doctor's assistant" who could manage many of the common childhood illnesses. Ninety four percent said such a "PA" would be acceptable (Patterson, 1969).

The first study on patient acceptance of clinically active PAs was conducted within a few years after PAs were beginning to be noticed. This study, anticipating that PAs would be dispersed throughout different socioeconomic classes, sought to determine in which social strata PA acceptance would be highest. The results showed that in 1970 the upper middle class community was more readily accepting of PAs (and NPs) than lower middle class communities (Conant et al., 1971).

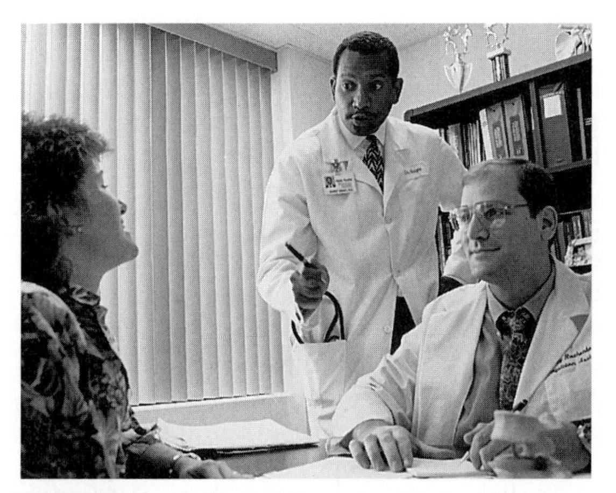

EXHIBIT 10-11 How patients view PAs is critical to their success. (Courtesy American Academy of Physician Assistants.)

In 1972 a study was undertaken in Los Angeles to assess patient acceptance of and attitudes toward the use of PAs in different roles. Acceptance was highest among unmarried middle class respondents who had some exposure to college. As the perceived complexity of procedures a PA might perform was increased, approval decreased; 91% of all respondents approved most procedures, such as injections, administered by PAs. This approval rating diminished to 34% in the case of first examination of a patient with a head injury by a PA (Strunk, 1973). In another 1972 study, patients rated PAs highly in terms of technical competence (89%), professional manner (86%), and access to services (79%), and patients reported improvement in the quality of care (71%) (Nelson, Jacobs, and Johnson, 1974). Other studies helped reinforce findings that PAs were generally well received by the patients they serve regardless of rural or urban setting or social status (Storms and Fox, 1979; Smith, 1981; Oliver et al., 1986).

To address a charge by some that physicians treat patients of higher socioeconomic status and PAs treat those of lower status, Crandall, Haas, and Radelet (1986) undertook a study in three primary care centers in Florida. Data from this study showed no consistent or substantively significant relationships between the patients' social status and the type of provider. In another study using a random survey of all households in Kentucky, Mainous, Bertolino, and Harrell (1992) found that a substantial proportion of households came in contact with PAs and NPs and that satisfaction with PAs and NPs was quite high.

Elizondo and Blessing (1990) examined patient expectations of PAs in dealing with a series of personal, social, psychologic, and health-related items. Results indicated that patients expect the PA to be involved with these problems but do not expect the PA to be an expert (Elizondo and Blessing, 1990). In a follow-up survey a few years later the subject groups were PAs, supervising physicians, and PA educators. The results were compared with those of the previous study, and the findings indicated a higher level of confidence in the abilities of PAs (Elizondo and Blessing, 1990).

Studies of patient satisfaction involving PAs, NPs, and physicians who work alongside each other are few. The impact of provider attitudes affects the outcome of select disorders. The confidence and attitudes of 3 primary care PAs and 18 physicians were assessed 3 weeks after a clinic visit for low back pain in a large HMO. Patients of more confident providers were significantly more satisfied with the information they received than patients of less confident providers. Differences could not be explained by years in practice, length of visit, patient demographics, or the type of providers (Bush, Cherkin, and Barlow, 1993).

In another HMO study by Freeborn and Pope (1994), members in the Pacific Northwest region of Kaiser Permanente rated the "technical competence, skill, and ability" of physicians, PAs, and NPs as "satisfied or very satisfied" more than 75% of the time. Hooker (1993) analyzed the same population spanning an 18-month period in the early 1990s with regard to how members viewed physicians, PAs, and NPs. A 57-item questionnaire specifically asked about satisfaction with a particular medical office visit and a specific provider. Samples were drawn randomly from the automated appointment system and sent within 1 week after a patient's medical office visit. When health plan members were asked how satisfied they were with their latest encounter, adult practice PAs and NPs scored within 1% to 2% of physicians (between 88% and 90% favorable). The technical skill of PAs and NPs rated within 3% to 4% of physicians. As for overall satisfaction, members regarded adult medicine PAs and NPs almost the same and statistically indistinguishable from each other. In this study, pediatricians were viewed approximately 10% more favorably than pediatric PAs and NPs for reasons not clear in this study (Hooker, 1993). In another study using a different instrument, Hooker, Potts, and Ray (1997) compared the attitudes and satisfaction levels of patients with physicians, PAs, and NPs in the same HMO. Analyzing more than 40,000 returned questionnaires, they found neither statistical differences between PAs and NPs nor differences between PAs/NPs and physicians across five different departments (Exhibit 10-12). Even when select variables were examined such as length of experience, gender, and age of the provider, no differences emerged to show any statistical difference (Hooker, Potts, and Ray, 1997).

In a study surveying 1032 patients, Perry (1995) found that nearly one quarter of respon-

EXHIBIT 10-12

Patient Satisfaction as Reported by an 8-item Questionnaire: Comparison of Average Scores for PAs/NPs and Physicians in an Internal Medicine Department, 1997 (N = 41,100)

Question*	PA/NPs	Physicians
How *courteous* and *respectful* was the clinician?	93	94
How well did the clinician *understand* your problem?	90	90
How well did the clinician *explain* to you what he or she was doing and why?	91	90
Did the clinician *use words* that were easy for you to understand?	93.5	94
How well did the clinician *listen* to your concerns and questions?	88	91
Did the clinician spend *enough time* with you?	90	90
How much *confidence* do you have in the clinician's ability or competence?	90	91.5
Overall, how satisfied are you with the service that you received from the clinician?	90	91.5

Data from Hooker RS, Potts R, Ray W: *Permanente J* 1:38-42, 1997.
*Italicized words identify the patient satisfaction characteristic surveyed. No statistical differences were found at $p < .001$

dents said a PA, NP, or CNM sometimes handled their doctor visits. Nearly 9 in 10 said they were very or somewhat satisfied with the care they received, compared with 97% who said they were satisfied with their doctor's medical know-how (Perry, 1995).

Parents

Parents of children are mentioned because of their reaction to the concept of pediatric PAs and child health associates (CHAs). In the mid 1960s, a few years preceding full deployment of CHAs, three separate studies reported favorable parent acceptance of pediatric-trained assistants on alternate pediatrician patient visits at approximately one half the usual pediatric fee (Austin, Foster, and Richards, 1968; Skinner, 1968). In structured interviews in the homes of 145 mothers in the Seattle area, roughly one half of the group had regular pediatric care from private pediatricians, one third from an HMO, and the rest from public health clinics. Approximately 75% of the mothers approved of the pediatric assistant for well-child care, and 94% indicated they would be willing to use the assistant if the physician and assistant were well trained and capable (Patterson, 1969). A third study found that the pediatrician's time could be better spent delegating at least 50% of the workload to PAs (Anderson and Powers, 1970).

Silver and Ott (1973) reported that 94% of the parents expressed satisfaction with the joint services they received from a pediatrician and a CHA team and with their opportunity to maintain adequate communication with the physician. Half the parents of children seen in this setting thought that joint care was better than care they received from a physician alone.

One of the problems with evaluating patient acceptance and satisfaction with health care providers in general is the asymmetry of information. The health care consumer can neither choose the best treatment because of lack of time, nor judge whether the treatment is adequate unless she is a clinician as well. She may perceive the best care for her is the comfort she feels when she is with a certain provider, even though the best care is not being delivered. For many patients the "halo effect" predominates in their thinking, and the clinician (physician, PA, NP, or CNM) is often held above reproach when surveys are conducted.

From the literature, it appears that PAs are held in high regard by patients regardless of socioeconomic status, condition, and setting. These views may reflect confidence in the PA's ability to take care of their medical conditions. The most recent findings suggest patients like the provider as long as the provider is courteous, explains the care, uses terms they can understand, and listens to their complaints. Most likely, *satisfaction* represents the perception of patients whose health care need was largely met. Additional studies are needed to measure and compare both satisfaction and outcome of all types of providers in all types of settings.

Clearly more research must be undertaken in the area of patient satisfaction of PAs. Most of the work is outdated and the few contemporary studies were undertaken in well-defined settings in which PAs and NPs have long been established.

INTERNATIONAL MEDICAL GRADUATES

International medical graduates (IMGs) (formerly known as *foreign medical graduates*) have filled gaps in American medical services during most of the twentieth century. An estimated 100,000 unlicensed IMGs are in the United States, most of whom are foreign born and foreign trained. Unfortunately, not all can meet the requirements for medical licensure. Recognizing this population as a potential source of medical providers, some state medical boards have used various approaches to assist IMGs who have failed to meet requirements for licensure. This includes remedial activities to correct deficiencies in knowledge and skills or limited licensure that allows IMGs to practice as physicians in certain settings and/or under supervision. As barriers to medical licensure have increased, many have sought ways to enter health care in lieu of completing the lengthy and expensive medical licensure process. Some IMGs have sought access to PA licensure as a permanent career change, and others as an interim step toward licensure as physicians. Unlicensed IMGs have organized to promote state laws to make it easier for them to train or practice as PAs. These attempts to recast IMGs as PAs have been criticized as creating a double standard for PA qualification, jeopardizing public safety and creating a regulatory bureaucracy that would be prohibitively expensive (Stanhope, Fasser, and Cawley, 1992; Fowkes et al., 1996).

The AAPA Professional Practice Council maintains that entry to the PA profession should require graduation from an accredited PA educational program and passage of the national certifying examination. The AAPA asserts, "Passage of an examination by itself is inadequate to define the knowledge needed to practice as a PA." Part of the knowledge required is the socialization to the PA role and understanding of the physician-PA relationship, both taught and experienced as a PA student. Having states develop or administer their own examinations as an alternative entry mechanism would compromise the uniformity of a national PA qualifying standard and possibly discourage reciprocity between states. Moreover, there is evidence that IMGs lack the knowledge and skills necessary to practice as PAs or to validate fast-track or abbreviated educational programs as appropriate solutions (Stanhope, Fasser, and Cawley, 1992).

In California, surveys in 1980, 1993, and 1994 collected information about the interest and preparedness among IMGs seeking PA certification. These surveys revealed that few of the IMGs were interested in becoming PAs as a permanent career, and few could show a commitment to primary care of the underserved. Of the 50 IMGs accepted into California's PA programs in recent years, 62% had academic or personal difficulties. Only 34 IMGs became certified. The City University of New York/Harlem Hospital PA program developed an accelerated program for IMGs in 1992. None of the IMGs who took the same clinical competency examination developed for PA students passed (Stanhope, Fasser, and Cawley, 1992).

Some states, including Maryland, Florida, Michigan, and Washington, have used different approaches to alternative pathways to PA licensure for IMGs (Bottom and Evans, 1994; Cawley, 1995). Additional preparatory programs in California that have assessed the readiness of unlicensed IMGs to enter PA programs have shown that the participants did not demonstrate knowledge or clinical skills equivalent to those expected of licensed PAs (Fowkes et al., 1996).

Current thinking is that IMGs are not likely to be granted PA-certified status without attending a formal PA preparatory program. Those who have done so however seem to have adapted to this new career well and do not see conflict with their medical degree and PA certification.

REGISTERED CARE TECHNOLOGISTS

In 1988 the AMA proposed the creation of a registered care technologist (RCT). The proposal called for basic RCT training of 9 months, during which routine patient care duties such as bathing and bedpan and linen changing would be taught. Assisting the nurse in administering bedside medications and more complex nursing duties would require an 18-month training period and would be at a level of an advanced RCT.

The ANA and other nursing groups were vehemently opposed to the creation of the RCT. Nursing leaders expressed their opposition to the proposal as the AMA's desires to strengthen medicine's control over nursing, to weaken their own control of nursing personnel, and to undermine nurses' efforts to standardize their education and credentialing.

In the RCT debate the AMA delegates stressed the essential value of quality bedside patient care and the way in which the RCT would address this immediate need under nursing supervision. The AMA also argued that RCTs could form a new source of nursing applicants and thus be part of the long-term solution to alleviating the nursing shortage.

Six hospitals were recruited to undertake RCT pilot projects, but nursing opposition was so adamant that only one completed a study and no other was started. The official PA position was never condensed. On one hand, the profession espouses the values of quality patient care and the social good of relieving human suffering. On the other hand, there is little interest in weakening nursing's control of their education and credentialing process (Chavez, 1989). In the end the effort died a natural death and the profession was spared taking sides.

REGISTERED NURSE FIRST ASSISTANTS

The Association of periOperative Registered Nurses (AORN) defines an RN first assistant (RNFA) as follows:

> The RN first assistant at surgery collaborates with the surgeon and the health care team in performing a safe operation with optimal outcome for the patient. The RN first assistant practices perioperative nursing and must have acquired the necessary knowledge, skills, and judgement specific to clinical practice. The RN first assistant practices in collaboration with and at the direction of the surgeon during the intraoperative phase of the perioperative experience. The RN first assistant does not concurrently function as a scrub nurse. (www.AORN.org/clinical/rnfaste.htm)

The role of the RNFA has been contentious because of the immediate threat to surgical PAs, who see themselves the natural replacements of the physician first assistant (Larson, 2000). One author believes that PAs are better replacements than RNFAs because they can adjust iontropic and pressor support; insert and remove intraaortic balloon pumps; and perform tube thoracostomies, tracheostomies, and emergent median sternotomies at bedside. Furthermore they can take telephone calls, prescribe and refill medications, and when appropriate, have patients return for follow-up care (Larson, 2000).

Little more has been written other than position statements. To date the literature is silent on what RNFAs can do and what surgical PAs as first assistants can do and how well.

MEDICAL WRITING AND PUBLISHING

Journalism within any profession is a reflection of its maturity. How and what a profession says about itself is an evolving process, and the way it promotes itself in journalism and literature is a measurement of its sophistication. Fortunately this has been a subject of interest to a significant segment of the PA profession, and the increasing numbers of articles authored by PAs have allowed more than one publication to exist at the same time. Cawley (1985) summed it this way: "PAs and health care providers communicate with each other through the pages of the professional journals. These journals reflect the thoughts, direction, and vitality of the profession. It follows then, that our profession is judged in part by the quality and content of the PA literature."

Charles B. Slack, Inc, a publisher in New Jersey, launched the first official journal of the American Academy of Physician Assistants in 1970. Initially, the volumes were titled *Physician's Associate.* This name reflects the few years that the AAPA was the *American Academy of Physician's Associates.* Later, when the name changed to the AAPA, the name *PA Journal* was adopted.

The first PA professional journal listed a number of influential members of the profession: Don Detmer, MD; Ann Bliss, MSW; Carl Emil Fasser, PA; Bill Stanhope, PA; David Lawrence, MD, MPH; Steve Turnipseed, MX; John Ott, MD; and Bill De'Ak, MD. Later known as the "Green Journal" because of its distinctive cover, the *PA Journal* served "as a forum for the discussion and presentation of important issues related to the advancement of the physician's assistant and other health professional auxiliaries . . . " (from the masthead of the *PA Journal,* Volume 4, No. 2, 1974).

While the "Green Journal" was still in publication, a small independent publisher United Business Publications, Inc. launched a magazine in 1976 called *Physician Assistant.* Both journals were competing for essentially the same audience and the same advertising revenue. This competition has remained intense ever since. Ultimately neither journal proved particularly viable financially, and the first version of *Physician Assistant* folded a few years later.

Meanwhile, a new prospective publisher, F & F Publications, entered discussion with the AAPA concerning the possibility of a new journal for the profession. An agreement was reached whereby the AAPA granted a 1-year endorsement to *Health Practitioner* (the initial plan was to distribute it to PAs and NPs). Steve Tiger, longtime PA medical editor and writer, notes in his history of *Physician Assistant,* that potentially a market of PAs plus other "new health practices" the earliest national conferences were designated for "health practitioners," and it was not until a few years later that the annual conference became focused on PAs (Tiger, 1992).

Over the next several years, the name and ownership of the new journal changed. The first issue of *Health Practitioner* was distributed at the May 1977 AAPA conference in Houston. By the end of the year the tag line "Magazine for Physician Assistants" was added to the title. Next, the defunct title *Physician Assistant* was obtained from its publisher, and that title took the place of the tag line for the March 1978 issue, which was called *Health Practitioner and Physician Assistant Magazine.* Starting with the next issue, the name was simplified to *Health Practitioner/Physician Assistant.* In August 1979 the order was reversed, and the name became *Physician Assistant/Health Practitioner* (reflecting the fact that the audience was primarily PAs). Meanwhile PW Communications took over publication from F & F Publications. In 1983 *Health Practitioner* was dropped from the title, and the publication became known by its current name *Physician*

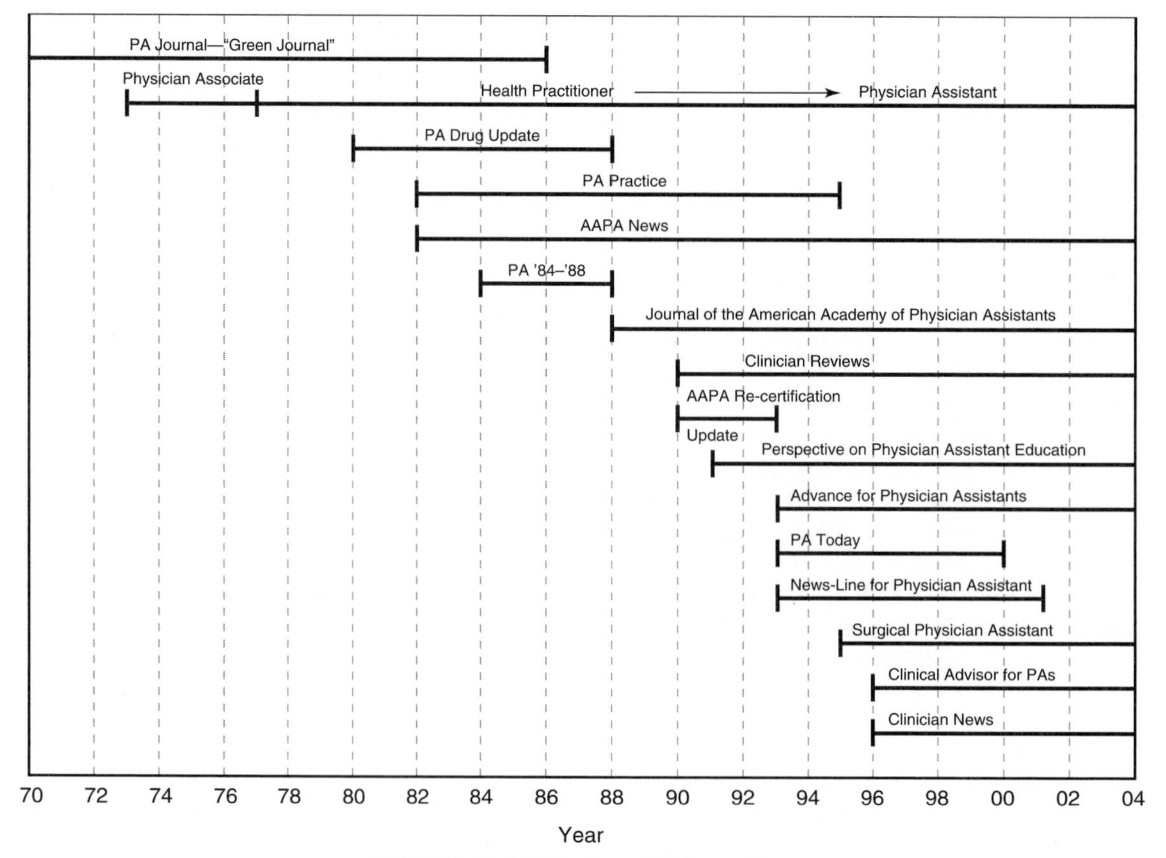

EXHIBIT 10-13 Timeline of PA journalism.

Assistant. Excerpta Medica purchased *Physician Assistant* from PW Communications, which was purchased by Springhouse, and has been listed as the publisher since the October 1989 issue.

The initial endorsement expired after the March 1978 issue. In January 1983, after the green *PA Journal* had finally folded, *Physician Assistant* again became the official publication of the AAPA; that relationship continued through June 1987, when the AAPA was ready to introduce its own new publication, *Journal of the American Academy of Physician Assistants* (Tiger, 1992).

There have been other journals. Peter Frishauf, founder of *Health Practitioner/Physician Assistant,* produced a series of publications that ran for 5 years—*PA 84* through *PA 88. PA Drug Update* began in 1980 as a magazine of "continuing medical education for physician assistants" and went on to found the Internet medical journal *Medscape. AAPA Recertification Update* began in 1990 as a special publication to prepare students and graduates for the recertification process. It ended after 4 years of publication. In 1993 *Advance for Physician Assistants* launched a new publication "to provide timely and useful information about clinical and practice issues." More publications emerged in the 1990s.

That so many journals are published so frequently speaks for the market attraction of the profession (Exhibit 10-13). Some, like *PA Practice, AAPA Recertification,* and *PA Source* were single pharmaceutical manufacturer's publications that may have some endorsement from the AAPA. Single-sponsored monographs have also come and gone. One such example *PA Drug Update* was around from 1982 to 1988. Underwritten by Pfizer Pharmaceuticals, it had a number of topics written by specialists in various fields and was wrapped with a cover and distributed to PAs. Other versions similar to *PA Drug Update* were sent to physicians and medical students under different names but with similar contents.

Advance for PAs is one of the latest publications to seek a niche in the growing PA market. This is just one in a series of 13 "news magazines" by Merion Publications. See Exhibits 10-14 and 10-15.

Clinician Reviews was a breakaway publication of *Physician Assistant.* Formed in 1989 by two PAs (David Mittman and Tom Yakeren), *Clinician Reviews* has done what others have failed to do—appeal to a wider audience than just PAs. This high-quality, glossy monthly journal is marketed to both PAs and NP/CNMs, publishing clinical articles appealing to both providers while occasionally reporting on issues that politically or economically affect both PAs and NPs. *Clinician Reviews* claims a subscription distribution of more than 80,000. *Clinician News* is a newspaper-type publication sent to all NPs and PAs. It

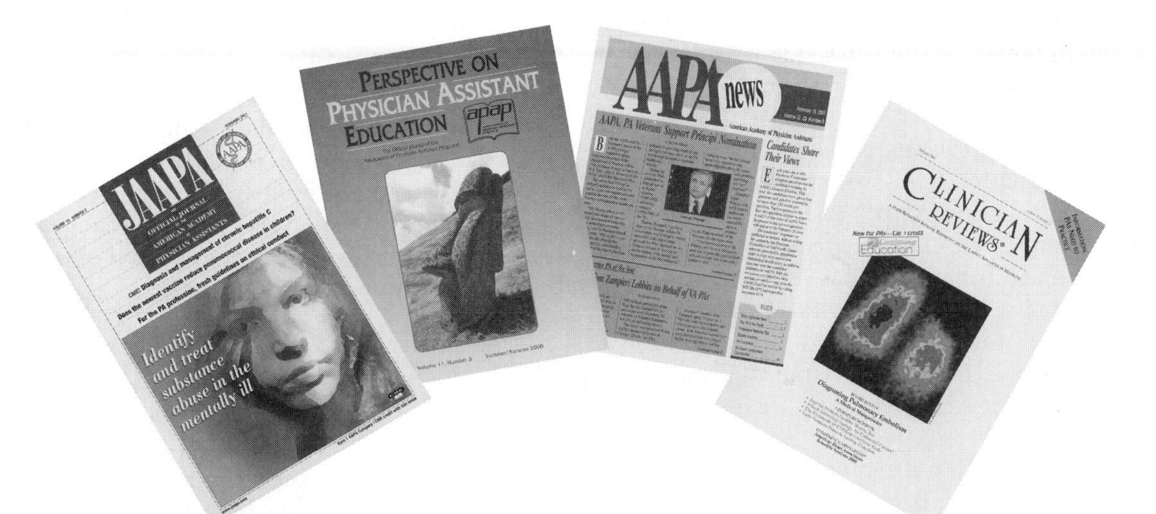

EXHIBIT 10-14 Examples of PA journals. (*JAAPA* journal cover reproduced with the permission of Journal of the Academy of American Physician Assistants and is copyrighted by Medical Economics, Thomson Healthcare, Montvale, NJ; *Perspective on Physician Assistant Education* journal cover courtesy of Association of Physician Assistant Programs, Alexandria, VA, and photo by Kenneth R. Harbert, Ph.D., CHES, PA-C; *AAPA News* journal cover courtesy of American Academy of Physician Assistants, Alexandria, VA; *Clinician Reviews* journal cover courtesy of Clinicians Group, LLC, Clifton, NJ.)

EXHIBIT 10-15

Current National PA-Oriented Journals and News

Journal	Note
AAPA News	Sent to AAPA members only
Journal of the American Academy of Physician Assistants (JAAPA)	Sent to all PAs who have been members of the AAPA
Physician Assistant (PA Journal)	Sent to all PAs who have been members of the AAPA
Advance for Physician Assistants	Sent to all PAs who have been members of the AAPA
Surgical Physician Assistants	Sent to all PAs who have been members of the AAPA and especially surgical PAs
Perspective on Physician Assistant Education	Intended for PA educators; underwritten by the APAP with very little advertising revenue
Clinician Reviews	Intended for PAs and NPs
Clinical Advisor for Physician Assistants	Intended for PAs; a similar journal is marketed to NPs with the same articles
Clinician News	Intended or PAs and NPs

regularly features news that affects PA and NP practices.

In January 1988 for the first time the AAPA published a journal with editorial control in the hands of the academy: The *Journal of the American Academy of Physician Assistants* (*JAAPA*) has its own staff, editorial board, and Leslie Kole, PA, as the editor since its inception (Kole, 1988). Initially published by Mosby, it has been published by Medical Economics since 1994. As of 2000 the *JAAPA* has published more than 8000 pages of clinical articles, policy papers, surveys, scientific studies, editorials, debates, letters, and essays. More than 90% of the contributions have been authored by PAs. It competes side by side with *Physician Assistant* for readership and advertisement revenue.

Perspective on Physician Assistant Education is the official journal of the Association of Physician Assistant Programs (APAP). *Perspectives* is primarily a platform to disseminate research on the education and behavior of PAs. While it was initially started as a newsletter in 1987, since 1998 it has been a formal journal edited by Don Pedersen at the University of Utah. With underwriting from the APAP, its future seems secure in the short run.

Surgical Physician Assistant is published by Odyssea Publishing. Begun in 1995, the journal is distributed to all PAs but reflects the activity of the following surgical PA groups:

- Association of Neurosurgical Physician Assistants
- Physician Assistants in Orthopaedic Surgery
- American Association of Surgical Physician Assistants
- Association of Physician Assistants in Cardiovascular Surgery

Constituent Chapter Newsletters

Since the development of constituent chapters, there has been an attempt to collect and redistribute information on the decentralized and local PA level. Usually this is by and for PAs in state chapters of the AAPA or as affiliations. They ranged the full spectrum in scope and readability. A giant boost in these publications came in the mid 1980s when the Leaderle Corporation made unrestricted grants to all 50 chapters to purchase personal computers (PCs) and other equipment for newsletters. Many of these PCs are currently in use. Today virtually every special interest group stays in touch by paper and increasingly venture into the Internet for better communication.

Books

PAs have authored at least 30 books (Exhibit 10-16). There are several categories, some of which are clinical and others which are on the PA profession. Many PAs have been part of special documents, monographs, and special reports on the profession (e.g., the Pew Commission on Physician Assistants in Managed Care). A few have ventured into fiction and medical history (Currey, 1992).

EXHIBIT 10-16

Books Targeted for PAs

1972	*The Physician's Assistant: Today and Tomorrow*, by Alfred M. Sadler, Blair Sadler, and Ann Bliss; first book on the PA profession
1975	*The Physician Assistant: A National and Local Analysis*, by Ann Suter Ford
1977	*The New Health Professionals: Nurse Practitioners and Physician's Assistants*, by Ann Bliss and Eva Cohen
	The Physician's Assistant: A Baccalaureate Curriculum, by Hu Myers
1978	*The Physician's Assistant: Innovation in the Medical Division of Labor*, by Eugene Schneller
1980	*Physician's Assistant Examination Review*, by Thomas D. Aschenbrener
1981	*Staffing Primary Care in 1990: Physician Replacement and Cost Savings*, by Jane Cassels Record
	The Art of Teaching Primary Care, by Hagen, Carlson, and Golden (Eds.)
	The Role of the Physician Assistants in Primary Care, by Judith Greenwood
1982	*Physician Assistants: Their Contribution to Health Care*, by Henry Perry and Bena Breitner
1984	*Alternatives in Health Care Delivery: Emerging Roles of Physician Assistants*, by Reginal D. Carter
1986	*Physician Assistants: Present and Future Models of Utilization*, edited by Sarah F. Zarbock and Kenneth Harbert
1987	*The Physician Assistant in a Changing Health Care Environment*, by Gretchen E. Schafft and James F. Cawley
1991	*Appleton & Lange's Review for the Physician Assistant*, by P.J. Cafferty and L.J. Stillson
1993	*The Role of the Physician Assistant and Nurse Practitioner in Primary Care*, edited by D. Kay Clawson and Marian Osterweis
	Selected Annotated Bibliography of the Physician Assistant Profession: Fourth Edition, 1993, by Susan M. Anderson
1994	*Physician Assistant: A Guide to Clinical Practice*, edited by Ruth M. Ballweg, S. Stolberg, and E. Sullivan
	Managing Risk Through Quality PA Practice: A Guide For Health Care Providers, by the American Academy of Physician Assistants
1995	*The Physician Assistant Medical Handbook*, by James B. Labus
	Opportunities in Physician Assistant Careers, by Terence J. Sacks
	Physician Assistant Career Planning Guide, by Julie A. Edin
1996	*Physician Assistant: 925 Questions & Answers*, by Richard R. Rahr and Bruce R. Niebuhr
	The Physician Assistant Emergency Medicine Handbook,by Steven W. Salyer
1997	*Physician Assistants in American Medicine*, by Roderick S. Hooker and James F. Cawley
	Don't Call Me Doctor, by G.B. Randall
1998	*The Physician Assistant Surgical Handbook*, by James B. Labus
	Physician Assistant Legal Handbook, by Patricia A. Younger
	Getting Into The PA School of Your Choice, by Andrew J. Rodican
1999	*Appleton & Lange's Review for the Physician Assistant*, by Anthony A. Miller
	National Certifying Examination for Physician Assistant, by Jack Rudman
	Physician Assistant: A Guide to Clinical Practice, 2nd edition, by Ruth Ballweg, Sherry Stolberg, and Edward M. Sullivan
	A Comprehensive Review for the Certification and Recertification Examinations, by Sarah Zarbock Goltzer and Rebecca Lovell Scott
2000	*Physician Assistant: Pretest Self-Assessment and Review*, by Rodney L. Moser
	Appleton & Lange's Outline Review for the Physician Assistant Examination, by Albert Simon and Anthony Miller
	Physician Assistant's Clinical Companion, Anonymous.
2001	*Physician Assistant's Guide to Research and Medical Literature*, by J.D. Blessing
	Physician Assistant's Drug Handbook, by J. Dennis Blessing
	Appleton & Lange's Quick Review: Physician Assistant, by Richard R. Rhar, Salah Ayachi, and Bruce R. Niebuhr
	Physician Assistant Review (Book with CD-ROM), by Patrick C. Auth and Morris D. Kerstein
2002	*Physician Assistant Secrets*, by David A. Tecchio and Donna Hall
	A Kernel in the Pod, by J. Michael Jones.
	Clinical Procedures for Physician Assistants, by Richard W. Dehn and David P. Asprey
	Physician Assistants in American Medicine, by Roderick. S. Hooker and James. F. Cawley

Modified from Hooker RS, Cawley JF: *Perspect Physician Assist Educ* 9:87-90, 1998.

Electronic Formats

Through support by Duke University the Internet is available for PAs in a number of forums: the PA Forum, Student PA Forum, PA Faculty Forum, and PAs in Primary Care Forum. Known as lists, these forums are usually lively exchanges of opinions by PAs and include a wide range of subjects.

As an extension of the Internet, the academy operates a PA page on the World Wide Web (www.aapa.org). The AAPA web site provides

EXHIBIT 10-17

Sources of Information via the Internet

Source of information	Web site address	Comment
Bureau of Labor Statistics, U.S. Department of Labor	stats.bls.gov/oco/ocos081.htm	Projects PA growth
American Academy of Physician Assistants home page	www.aapa.org/	Continuously updated
American Academy of Physician Assistants list of PA programs	www.aapa.org/pgmlist.php3	–
Association of Physician Assistant Programs	www.apap.org/	Official organization of PA programs
Surgical Physician Assistant	www.surgicalpa.com/	Journal web site
Physician Assistant Newsletter	neuropa.hypermart.net/	Private web site offering information on PAs
National Commission on Certification of Physician Assistants	www.nccpa.net/	Credentialing body for graduate PAs
Journal of the American Academy of Physician Assistants	jaapa.pdr.net/	Official journal of the AAPA
Physician Assistant Journal	www.pajournal.com/	Journal for PAs
Clinician Reviews	primarycare.medscape.com/CPG/ClinReviews/public/about.ClinReviews.html	Journal for both PAs and NPs
Physician Assistant Jobs	www.physicianassistantjobs.com/	Job locator
Veteran Affairs Physician Assistant Association	www.vapaa.org/	–
Internet Journal of Academic Physician Assistants	www.ispub.com/journals/ijapa.htm	–
U.S. News and World Report ranking of graduate PA programs as of 2000	www.usnews.com/usnews/edu/beyond/gradrank/gbphysas.htm	–
Accreditation Review Commission on Education for the Physician Assistant	www.arc-pa.org/	The accreditation body all PA programs must pass

basic information about the PA profession that PAs can use to educate others and to answer commonly asked questions about PAs and the academy. Additional information directed to someone in the academy can be obtained via the Internet at aapa@aapa.org. Other Internet sources of information about PAs are available in Exhibit 10-17. This is a partial list of more than 150 web sites on some aspect of PAs. Most of the web sites are individual programs.

SUMMARY

No profession stands alone; all are built on relationships with other players in the same arena. The physician-PA relationship began as a strong one and continues today. The evidence is overwhelming that physicians accept PAs in their many and varied roles, and this is not likely to change as long as PAs avoid seeking independent practice. The relationships with other populations such as nurses, NPs, pharmacists, organized medicine, and patients are stronger today than they have ever been.

PA journalism involves both writing and publishing. A number of ventures have been launched with PAs as the target audience. These enterprises have expanded as the profession has grown and will likely continue, an acknowledgment that this profession has come of age and is an important audience to observe.

11

LEGAL, POLITICAL, AND PROFESSIONAL ASPECTS

INTRODUCTION

Similar to the historical, sociologic, and economic basis of the physician assistant (PA) profession, there is a legal, political, and professional basis as well. The legal basis is found in both the laws and the regulations enacted at first for physicians and subsequently for nurses and other health personnel. These laws were largely developed in the late 1800s and early 1900s and have evolved to their highly codified form today. There are now over 36 regulated health professions in the United States.

Laws authorizing prescribing have been met with a fair amount of resistance. From a patchwork of laws among various jurisdictions, today PA practice regulations are more similar than different. The evidence to date is that PAs handle the delegated role assuming a great deal of responsibility. The evidence that these laws have had their desired effect is in the improved access for U.S. society.

Professional issues often influence the behavior of PAs because many PAs are judged by how they appear in a professional context. These issues include impairment, abortion, unions, detailing by pharmaceutical manufacturers' representatives, and others.

LEGAL BASIS OF THE PHYSICIAN ASSISTANT PROFESSION

Medical licensure laws to regulate physicians were enacted in the United States in approximately their present form during the late nineteenth and early twentieth centuries as a matter of public necessity. Protection of the public against quackery, commercial exploitation, deception, and professional incompetence required legally enforceable standards for entrance into and continuation in the medical profession. The state medical practice acts therefore specify both ethical and educational requirements for physicians relating to personal character, scientific education, and practical training or experience.

Unlike medical licensure laws, state licensure statutes for PAs, allied and auxiliary health personnel, and nurses were not enacted to correct such abuses of independent entrepreneurial practice. Instead, the latter statutes have usually been "friendly" regulations enacted with the cooperation of the professions and occupations and designed to protect both the regulated personnel and the public from unqualified and unethical practitioners. The forms of licensure, however, are generally similar to medical practice acts, except that in some states for PAs licensure is permissive rather than mandatory. Accordingly the statutes define the practice of the various professions and occupations and prescribe the personal, educational, and certification of professional competence qualifications required for such practice.

The most significant and contemporary issues regarding licensure of PAs concern the effect of licensure provisions on the distribution of tasks and duties. For physicians, with unlimited licenses to perform all functions, the critical questions are what functions they may delegate and under what conditions such delegations may be made. For PAs the problems are more numerous and complex. Because their licenses may be limited to a particular segment of health service, it is sometimes necessary to determine those functions that they may not legally perform under ordinary circumstances. These determinations require interpretation of the scope of permissible practice as defined by the relevant licensure statute and the scope of exclusive practice as defined by licensure statutes. Thus, for example, a PA in a urology practice may be violating his or her scope of practice if a patient has a wart removed from his or her foot. In Missouri an early licensure stipulated that PAs could not refract and fit patients with prescription lenses. Countless examples abound.

Functions within the scope of practice for a PA may be either "independent" of, or "dependent" on, receiving orders, direction, or supervision from a physician. Obviously, many variables are involved in determining whether a given function is dependent, and if so, the nature and degree of supervision required for its performance. The same complexity characterizes another problem related to the scope of practice, the delegability of functions. Unlike some allied health personnel such as physical therapists and occupational therapists who have unique skills not likely to be duplicated by a physician, the PA has the same skills more or less than those of a physician. Therefore delegation is not one of authorizing personnel to use their exclusive professional skills, but one of dividing what the physician would normally have to do.

In general, scope-of-practice issues are the most clouded areas in the legal regulation of PAs, because the licensure statutes or related court decisions have not adequately addressed how they should be viewed—as providers with their own set of jurisdictions or as employees of physicians. After more than three decades of experience with delegation of physician tasks to PAs, that so few cases have come under the legal spotlight reflects some confidence that PAs are practicing within their legal jurisdiction.

History

The early licensure statutes reflected the recommendations of the Flexner report on medical education, published in 1910, which initiated efforts to raise standards of medical school admission, instruction, and curriculum to place these schools under the jurisdiction of universities and to provide full-time faculty and adequate facilities for teaching and clinical experience (Starr, 1982). The incorporation in medical licensure laws of requirements that proprietary schools could not meet resulted in the closing of medical doctor diploma mills, as the inadequate medical schools of the time were called. Standards of ethics and competency provided in the early licensure laws were derived from the view of leaders of the medical profession that medicine should be based on an educational system that was responsive to the needs and the social and scientific status of the country at that time.

Although vast changes have taken place in the social and scientific status of the country since the original enactment of the medical practice acts, no fundamental changes have been made in the statutory standards of professional competence and ethical behavior. In investigating the adequacy of current licensure laws to meet modern scientific and social conditions, we turn to the important question of authority for delegation of functions.

Licensing, Certification, and Registration

More than thirty-five years after graduation of the first PA the legal status of the PA still lacks geographic uniformity. Different states provide specific requirements for licensing, certification, and registration. Generally physicians and attorneys are licensed. These are licenses to act independently and without supervision other than peers. This mosaic of enabling legislation by state is displayed in Exhibit 11-1. Requirements in most states include graduation from an accredited PA program, national certification, and some sort of screening questionnaire about involvement with the law for any sort of felony or malpractice.

EXHIBIT 11-1

Physician Assistant State Credentials, 2002

State	Credentials
Alabama	Licensure
Alaska	Licensure
Arizona	Licensure
Arkansas	Certification
California	Licensure
Colorado	Certification
Connecticut	Licensure
Delaware	Licensure
District of Columbia	Licensure
Florida	Licensure
Georgia	Licensure
Hawaii	Certification
Idaho	Licensure
Illinois	Licensure
Indiana	Certification
Iowa	Licensure
Kansas	Registration
Kentucky	Certification
Louisiana	Licensure
Maine	Licensure
Maryland	Certification
Massachusetts	Registration
Michigan	Licensure
Minnesota	Registration
Mississippi	Licensure
Missouri	Licensure
Montana	Licensure
Nebraska	Licensure
Nevada	Licensure
New Hampshire	Licensure
New Jersey	Licensure
New Mexico	Licensure
New York	Registration
North Carolina	Licensure
North Dakota	Licensure
Ohio	Licensure
Oklahoma	Licensure
Oregon	Certification
Pennsylvania	Certification
Rhode Island	Licensure
South Carolina	Certification
South Dakota	Certification
Tennessee	Licensure
Texas	Licensure
Utah	Licensure
Vermont	Certification
Virginia	Licensure
Washington	Licensure
West Virginia	Licensure
Wisconsin	Licensure
Wyoming	Licensure

Data from American Academy of Physician Assistants, 2002.
Summary: Licensure, 36 states; certification, 11; registration, 4.

Most state laws specifically prohibit physicians from delegating professional responsibilities to an individual the physician knows or has reason to know is not qualified by training, experience, or licensure to perform the delegated duties. Physician employers have a responsibility to check regularly to ensure that supervised personnel have kept their licenses, certification, and registrations current and have met all requirements of continuing education necessary for renewal. Establishing an annual review of records is one method to ensure that nothing is overlooked by either the PA, the employer, or the supervising physician.

When a state requires certification the PA must document that he or she has a certificate from the National Commission on Certification of Physician Assistants (NCCPA) that has not expired. The laws generally do not refer to "recertified," they merely require "current certification." The specific language varies by state.

Supervision

Various state statutes require that a physician supervise a PA. *Supervision,* as defined by law, is considered "responsible control." *Control* implies both the establishment of overall limits and the policies to be met by the supervised professional and the day-to-day supervision of care. Direct supervision requires the physician be in the facility and occasionally in the same room as the individual performing the duty. Direct supervision further implies that the physician will be immediately available if the need arises. A typical way this is stated is provided in a New York state statute:

> Supervision shall be continuous but shall not be construed as necessarily requiring the physical presence of the supervising physician at the time and place where such services are performed. (N.Y. [Educ.] Law 6542[3])

More often, supervision is indirect and may be implied or explicitly stated but usually requires the availability of the physician for consultation. This is often interpreted to be by telephone or some other electronic means in a timely or consistent manner.

Availability need not necessarily be the physical presence of the doctor. Carrying a beeper or a cellular telephone for voice availability may be appropriate, depending on the circumstances of the practice site and the rules imposed by the state boards responsible for licensure. The degree of availability usually depends on the complexity of the task, risk to the patient, training of the PA, setting in which care is rendered, necessity for immediate medical attention, and the number of other professionals the physician supervises. Generally the more complex the task and the greater the potential risk to the patient, the more direct and explicit the supervision. Backup should be made available if for some reason the usual methods of contact fail or the supervising physician is out of town.

Review implies the physician will regularly examine the notes and examine the work the PA is doing. This process may consist of a review of medical record progress notes made by the PA or some other predetermined means of ensuring supervision. Generally the physician should be able to demonstrate that the supervised PA is performing at the expected skill level and is compliant with any protocols and procedures that may be in place to ensure quality of care. This should be done with some regularity (Harty-Golder, 1995). How this is done and with what frequency is generally left up to the supervising physician and the PA.

Delegation of Functions

The most significant contemporary questions arising from mandatory licensure for the practice of medicine concern the delegation of functions by physicians to PAs. As previously noted the statutory definitions of medical practice give physicians an unlimited license to perform all functions of health service, even those for which other health care personnel may also be licensed (or even better suited). However, the concomitant licensing of other health care personnel indicates that the statutes do not contemplate all health care service to be conducted by physicians. Rational policy in the division of labor can only be attained by allocating certain tasks to PAs, nurse practitioners (NPs), and other specialized personnel. The need for such expansion of the professional productivity of physicians seems certain to continue and even increase over time.

What is the legal basis for the expansion of PA activity? For example, does the medical practice act and the PA practice act permit a PA to insert a pacemaker in a patient suffering severe bradycardia? For most jurisdictions there can be no certain answers to such questions because legal authorities have not had to deal with the underlying issues. In a few states, however, the answers have begun to emerge from court decisions, attorney general opinions, or legislative enactment. As a practical matter, delegation of health service functions is predominantly governed by prevailing custom and practice. In the few relevant court decisions, however, it has been held that professional custom is no defense for a contravention of licensure laws.

One case in particular is important to illustrate, not only because of the court's handling of elements of licensure, custom, and supervision in deciding the delegation question, but because of its influence on the development of the PA profession. The case *People v. Whittaker* (No. 35307, Justice Court of Redding Judicial District, Shasta County, Calif. [December 1966]), involved the right of a neurosurgeon to use a trained surgical assistant to assist in brain surgery. The assistant was charged with practicing medicine without a license, although he was always within sight and under direct supervision of the surgeon, because he operated a cranial drill and Giegle saw, positioned by the surgeon, to bore holes and excise skull flaps during neurosurgical operations. The surgeon was charged with aiding and abetting an unlicensed person to practice medicine. The jury of a Justice of the Peace Court found both parties guilty of the charges in one instance in which the surgeon had sufficient time to call another physician to assist him but did not try to do so. As a standard for judging the physician's use of an unlicensed trained assistant, working under direct supervision, the following instruction was given to the jury:

> In determining whether acts in this case, if any, performed under the direct supervision and control of a duly licensed physician, were legal or illegal, you may consider evidence of custom and usage of the medical practice in California as shown by the evidence in this case.

The *Whittaker* judgment has since been appealed because of its importance as a test of the right of a physician or surgeon to use an extra pair of hands under conditions not constituting a medical emergency. The case is significant for its allowance of prevailing "custom and usage of the medical practice" in the state to determine the propriety of a physician's delegation and supervision of patently medical, but essentially mechanical, functions.

The interesting footnote to this case is that Roger Whittaker, the defendant, was a Vietnam veteran, a Navy trained corpsman, and a first assistant to the neurosurgeon for more than 125 similar cases. Eugene Stead, MD, the founder of the PA program at Duke University was called to serve as an expert witness in this case. In the course of the legal proceedings, Dr. Stead had the opportunity to meet with Whitaker and told him about the new educational program that had been inaugurated at Duke. Whitaker became a member of the third PA class at Duke and later, president of the AAPA (Condit, 1993).

The key issue in the licensure of PAs is the scope of functions that may be delegated to them and the educational and certification qualifications to permit such delegation safely. The shortage of PAs and other skilled health care personnel, new scientific and technologic developments, and new methods of organizing health services have made the question of delegation all the more important. It appears that licensure laws are in the process of being amended to authorize broader scope of functions for qualified PAs. It also appears that PAs have used their delegated role without much malpractice or criminal judgments against them.

Scope of Employment

In traditional legal theory, an employer is responsible for the acts of the "servant" while the servant performs on behalf of the employer. The thinking is that the employer derives benefit (generally profit) from having the servant (employee) and therefore should pay for any damages the servant might cause (Grumbach et al., 1999).

In an early English case the court held that a master is not responsible for the acts of a servant when the servant is "going on a frolic of his own." In *Joel v. Morrsion* (1834, 6C & P, 501, 172 Eng. Rep. 1338) the court held if the servant steps beyond the bounds of "his master's business," then the master should not be held liable.

In health care, as in many other businesses, what generally determines the "scope of employment" is the employment contract (job description) and the written guidelines or policies. These documents are the basis determining whether the employee has truly been doing the "master's work" or has been off "frolicking on his own."

If a hospital emergency department for a specific emergency medicine role has hired a PA and the PA begins administering cancer therapy without checking with the supervising physician, and the PA has no prior experience in providing cancer therapy, then the PA is clearly going beyond the "scope of employment" from what the emergency department had hired the PA.

Scope-of-employment "violations" can subject the employee to dismissal or can make the PA responsible for all damages in a negligence action. In the case of a negligence claim, if the hospital can prove that it did not know about the employee's activities and had no reasonable way of obtaining that information, it can escape liability and place the entire burden on the "frolicking" employee's shoulders.

Scope of Practice

Scope of practice is the specific regulations of practice set down by the separate state licensing boards. When revising practice regulations the boards generally consider what constitutes the "usual and customary" practice in the area.

The PA practice act in each state outlines what a PA is authorized to do or not do, called *scope of practice.* This "authorized practice" within category also differs widely from state to state. In one state a PA may have prescriptive privileges and in another he or she may not. In some instances the prescriptive privileges may be limited to a certain category of drugs, such as excluding controlled substances, while in other states, certain exceptions may allow PAs to administer certain scheduled drugs in rural and underserved areas. This can become quite confusing when practicing in more than one state. Scope-of-practice regulations tend to be more global than scope-of-employment regulations.

State Practice Acts

State practice acts vary widely, both in regulatory approach and in the scope of practice they authorize. They may influence the formal prescriptive authority and the administrative protocols organizations develop. Within each organization, however, PAs often have wide latitude for prescribing and carrying out protocols. Although practice acts are intended to ensure quality of care, these organizations, from small physician offices to large medical centers and institutions, often provide their own controls on quality in addition to or over and above state practice acts.

Although state practice acts may provide a weak mechanism for guiding actual practices within a state, they play an important role in defining professions and restricting what PAs can do. In some instances they can even define the amount of care a physician can delegate. For example, in Virginia the regulations about PA management state that the supervising physician shall see and evaluate any patient who presents with the same complaint twice in a single episode of care and has failed to improve significantly.

Because these acts may present a threat of litigation for PAs and physicians when practicing within a state, they cannot be simply ignored. The development of model PA state practice acts, as outlined in Appendix 3, can give states an alternative that if developed with input from all affected groups would represent a national consensus (Physician Payment Review Commission, 1994).

Liability of Physicians Who Supervise Physician Assistants

Three legal theories are commonly used to impute liability to the physician from the PA: *respondeat superior, negligent supervision,* and *negligent hiring*. To assess a physician's liability for mistakes of a PA, it is important to understand and distinguish the typical claims from the legal theories on which most actions are based. Two important issues for physicians who supervise PAs focus on supervision and actual control. These are often cited as (1) the "Borrowed Servant Rule" and (2) the "Captain of the Ship Doctrine." Physicians striving to reduce liability from PAs working under them should focus on three main areas: (1) selection, (2) supervision, and (3) standard of conduct. It is important to remember that PAs learn most from the habits of the physicians who supervise them, irrespective of whether those habits are good or bad.

Since about the mid 1980s there have emerged statutory regulations from various states suggesting a legislative trend to reduce and limit the liability for physicians who supervise PAs. Generally the standard of care applicable to PAs is the same as the standard of care for a physician. The tendency is for the elements of each cause of action to reflect the mistakes of PAs and not to hold supervising physicians liable (Gore, 2000).

PHYSICIAN ASSISTANT MALPRACTICE LIABILITY AND LITIGATION

Although there have been malpractice lawsuits involving allegations of negligence by PAs, very few have resulted in reported cases that can be cited as precedent. Nevertheless, a study of select suits filed reveals certain patterns of liability (Zimmerly and Norman, 1985).

Negligence

A claimant who brings a medical negligence action against any health care provider must prove that four elements exist: duty, breach of duty, proximate cause, and damages.

Duty

The claimant first must show that the health care provider had a duty to provide medical care. For example, in all states but Vermont, health care providers are not required to stop and render care in a roadside emergency (Vt. Stat. Ann. tit. 12 519). Therefore they could not be found negligent for failure to provide care. On the other hand, some courts have ruled that a physician on call in an emergency department has a duty to render medical assistance to any emergency patient whether or not the person is eligible for treatment at that facility (*Guerrero v. Copper Queen Hospital,* 537 P2d 1329). In most circumstances the duty to treat is activated when medical treatment is begun and continues until the patient has recovered from the condition or has released the health care provider from the continuing duty to treat.

Breach of Duty

Breach of duty is predicated on provision of the standard of care of a reasonably prudent physician practicing under the same or similar circumstances. This is an objective standard, and an expert witness in a medical negligence trial is not asked what he or she personally would have done in the situation, but what an average reasonably prudent health care provider in the community would have done. This standard of care was spelled out in a case heard in 1988 (*Pike v. Honsinger*, 155 NYS2d 201, 49 NE2d 760 [1988]).

A physician and a surgeon, by taking charge of the case, implied possessing that reasonable degree of learning and skill that is ordinarily possessed by physicians and surgeons in the locality in which he practices, and which is ordinarily regarded by those conversant with the employment as necessary to qualify him to engage in the business of practicing medicine and surgery. Upon consenting to treat a patient, it becomes his duty to use reasonable care and diligence in the exercise of his skill and the application of his learning to accomplish the purpose for which he was employed . . . there must be a want of ordinary and reasonable care, leading to a bad result.

So, breach of duty necessitates a lack of reasonable care under the circumstances.

Proximate Cause

In addition to the duty to treat and a breach of that duty, negligence involves proof that the breach was the actual cause of the claimant's injury. For example, a health care provider may have been negligent, even grossly negligent, in a case of wrongful death. But if the health care provider can show that the patient would have died regardless of the treatment rendered, the negligence cannot be held to be the proximate cause of death.

Damages

A claimant also must have sustained some damage to prosecute a medical negligence suit successfully. For example, medication errors frequently are made in hospitals; too much, too little, or the wrong type of medication is given, or it is administered via the wrong route. Many of these errors can be blamed on negligence, but the vast majority results in little or no damage. Medical negligence suits routinely cost more than $20,000 to prosecute, and it is unlikely that an experienced malpractice attorney would accept a case with estimated damages less than $50,000.

Standard of Care

Of the four requisite elements in negligence cases the most difficult to prove is breach of duty. As previously mentioned, in a medical negligence action involving a physician, the duty is breached only when the physician has not performed as a reasonable and prudent physician would have performed under the same or similar circumstances. But to what standard of care should a PA or other health care extender be held: to that of a reasonably prudent PA or that of a reasonably prudent physician? Two federal court opinions involving a technician and a PA illustrate the confusion in this area.

In the case of *Haire v. United States* (No. 75-55-ORL-CIV-R, 1976), the mother of a 23-month-old girl took her to the pediatric clinic at a military medical center in Florida, where a medical technician saw her. This technician had worked as a medic in Vietnam for 2 years and had received in-service training, primarily observation of the supervising pediatrician, before being assigned to the clinic. The medical technician examined the child and recorded that she had a runny nose as a result of an upper respiratory infection. He prescribed a decongestant and discharged her. Over the next 10 days, the child's appetite diminished and her runny nose persisted. On the tenth day, her temperature was noticeably elevated. The next day, her mother brought her back to the clinic, where the medical technician again saw her. He examined the child's ears and throat and listened to her chest. He told the mother that the patient's tonsils were causing her distress and then discharged the child without referring her to a physician. The next day the patient's mother noted "twitching" of her daughter's hands and a temperature of 103' F. She rushed the child to a local emergency department, where a physician performed a lumbar puncture and diagnosed *Haemophilus influenzae* meningitis. Despite the rapid institution of appropriate treatment the child died 3 days later.

The child's family sued the medical center, claiming that the "physician extender" failed to diagnose or test for meningitis and that the child should have been referred to a physician on her second clinic visit. At the trial a board-certified pediatrician testified on behalf of the family that if a pediatrician had seen the child on the second visit, the physician would have suspected meningitis and conducted ophthalmic and neurologic examinations to confirm the diagnosis. The court held the technician to the standard of care of a board-certified pediatrician, and because he had not performed the neurologic and ophthalmic examinations that a board-certified pediatrician would have performed, the court found him negligent. In 1976 the parents were awarded $15,000 each for emotional suffering.

In the case of *Polischeck v. United States* (535 F Supp 1261 [ED Pa. 1982]), another federal court took a different approach. A 44-year-old woman experienced a headache associated with nausea, vomiting, and fever. She complained to her husband of pressure behind her eyes and the feeling that the "top of her head was blowing off." The next day, she went to the emergency department of a government medical center and was evaluated by a PA. Her temperature was 100.4' F and her blood pressure was 144/90 mm Hg. The PA questioned the patient about her illness and recorded that she had experienced "sudden onset of headache 4 days ago with malaise, nausea, and ocular myalgia." A brief neurologic examination revealed photophobia but no nuchal rigidity. A complete blood count demonstrated a slightly elevated white blood cell count. The PA diagnosed flu syndrome, prescribed an analgesic/anxiolytic/muscle relaxant, and instructed the patient to return to the emergency department if her symptoms became worse. This medical center allowed PAs to use their discretion in deciding whether to consult a physician and did not require supervising physicians to review the charts of patients seen by PAs, so the patient was not seen by a physician and her chart was not reviewed or countersigned by a physician.

Two days later, on a Friday, the patient returned to the emergency department when her condition had not improved. The PA, who referred her to the emergency department physician, again saw her. The physician examined the patient, diagnosed "headaches, etiology unknown" and advised the patient to go to the internal medicine clinic the following Monday if her headaches persisted, or sooner if they became worse. That evening the patient's husband could not rouse her. He took her back to the emergency department, where the same physician examined her and diagnosed intracerebral hemorrhage. Because the medical center was not equipped to handle this type of patient, she was transferred to another hospital, where an arteriogram demonstrated a large subdural hematoma and a right posterior communicating artery aneurysm. A frontoparietal craniotomy was performed. However, the patient never regained consciousness and she died 3 days later.

The patient's husband filed suit in federal court, claiming that the medical center was negligent in not having his wife seen by a physician on her first visit. He also claimed that the physician was negligent in treating the patient on her second visit. At the trial the plaintiff's expert medical witnesses testified that the standard of care in the community required that patients not be discharged from emergency departments until they had been seen or at least their charts had been reviewed by a licensed physician. The court reasoned that the PA himself was not negligent in failing to diagnose the patient's subarachnoid hemorrhage on her first visit.

Indeed, it hardly seems reasonable to expect a person with only 2 years of general medical training to be able to recognize a medical condition when it is presented in a patient possessing only some of the condition's textbook symptoms.

Therefore the court held the PA to the same standard of care as other PAs in the community with similar training; compared with these peers, he was not negligent. However, the court did find the medical center negligent for failure either to have the patient seen or to have her records reviewed by a physician on her first visit, as was standard in the community.

These two decisions disagree about the standard of practice that a PA must meet. Decisions in other cases involving health care extenders may be helpful in clarifying this issue.

Thompson v. Brent (245 S2d 751 [La. 1971]): In removing a cast from a patient's leg with a Stryker saw, a nurse accidentally cut the patient's leg, leaving a scar. The court held her to the standard of care of a physician and ruled that she had been negligent.

Barber v. Reinking (411 P2d 861 [Wash. 1966]): A practical nurse administered an injection that caused injury to a patient. In that state only registered nurses were authorized by law to administer injections. The court held the practical nurse to the standard of care of a registered nurse and ruled that she had been negligent.

Thompson v. United States (368 F Supp 466 [WD La. 1973]): A practical nurse in a Veterans Administration hospital told a drugged disoriented patient to go to the laboratory by himself. On the way the patient fell and injured his finger, which ultimately had to be amputated. The nurse was held to the standard of care of a nurse, not a physician.

Whitney v. Day (300 NW2d 380 [1980]): A nurse anesthetist working in a hospital was held to the same standard of care as other nurse anesthetists in the community, not to the standard of an anesthesiologist.

It would appear from these cases that PAs who are practicing in a state where they are recognized and allowed to practice and who are performing procedures that they legally or traditionally can perform in the community should be held to the standard of a PA. However, PAs who are practicing in a state that does not recognize them and who are performing procedures that only physicians or nurses are licensed to perform in that community probably should be held to the standard of a physician or a nurse.

Evidence of Standard of Care

How is the standard of care proved in a medical negligence suit? In addition to hiring an expert witness the plaintiff's attorneys most likely will subpoena all hospital or clinic manuals, regulations, and protocols referring to PAs. These usually are admissible evidence of the applicable standard of care. If a PA has failed to follow a hospital's protocol or other applicable regulation, there will be strong, though not necessarily conclusive, evidence that the standard of care was not met. Violation of a state law regarding the duties of PAs also is strong evidence of a breach of the standard of care (Exhibit 11-2).

EXHIBIT 11-2

PA Legal References

Vt. Stat. Ann. tit. 12 519
Guerrero v. Copper Queen Hospital, 537 P2d 1329
Pike v. Honsinger, 155 NYS2d 201, 49 NE2d 760 (1988)
Haire v. United States, No. 75-55-ORL-CIV-R, 1976
Polischeck v. United States, 535 F Supp 1261 (ED Pa. 1982)
Thompson v. Brent, 245 S2d 751 (La. 1971)
Barber v. Reinking, 411 P2d 861 (Wash. 1966)
Thompson v. United States, 368 F Supp 466 (WD La. 1973)
Whitney v. Day, 300 NW2d 380 (1980)

This is an incomplete list and does not represent the range of legal cases or literature on litigation involving PAs. The reader is referred to the legal literature for recent cases.

In addition to hospital or clinic protocols and regulations the courts may consult guidelines issued by professional organizations, including standards used by the Joint Commission on the Accreditation of Healthcare Organizations. Therefore it is important that PAs also be aware of the guidelines issued by these organizations.

Although data are limited, current evidence indicates that the increase in the number of malpractice claims, size of awards, and rate increases physicians have been undergoing in the 1980s has not been the PA experience.

PRESCRIBING

As a result of legal statutes PAs are sanctioned to perform a wide variety of services in all the states, the District of Columbia, Guam, and in various federal agencies (Army, Navy, Air Force, Coast Guard, Public Health Service, federal and state correction systems). These statutes allow physicians to delegate authority to PAs to diagnose, test, treat, and follow-up the patients they manage. A substantial amount of evidence indicates that physicians have successfully delegated a great deal of such authority.

One major aspect of treatment that has had limited sanction is drug prescribing. When legally authorized, the privilege of prescribing is usually restricted. Because the use of medication is the most frequently performed treatment in medical care, the absence of this privilege limits the scope of medical practice. It restricts where and how PAs can practice. Consequently the issue of prescribing privilege is a significant concern of the PA profession. It is also an issue among managers, administrators, and policymakers in the larger health care community because PAs appear to be less costly substitutes for physicians in a variety of clinical situations.

Legal Status of Physician Assistant Prescribing

PAs were first authorized limited prescribing privileges in Colorado in 1969. Child health associates (pediatric PAs and NPs) could order drug treatments without consulting their supervising physicians as long as the latter reviewed and approved the order. New York authorized prescribing privilege to PAs in 1972; Maine, New Mexico, and North Carolina followed in 1973. By 1979 PAs had prescribing privileges in 11 states. As of 2002 PAs are authorized by statute or regulation to prescribe in 47 states, the District of Columbia, Guam, and federal facilities including the military and the Veterans Administration.

The underlying principle in these jurisdictions is one of dependent prescribing by PAs to whom supervising physicians have delegated this authority. With few exceptions—such as dentists and veterinarians, and in some states podiatrists, optometrists, and NPs—the legal right to prescribe is a domain of the physician that has not been transferred lightly.

The authorization to prescribe applies to the outpatient setting. Inpatient medications are generally considered orders and usually come under a different review process. Most states in which PAs are legally authorized to prescribe have constraints on their prescribing. Such constraints may include the following:

- Requiring the supervising physician to cosign each prescription order written by a PA
- Prescribing from a drug formulary, and/or limiting prescribing to select classes or schedules of drugs defined by the Controlled Substances Act of 1970 as having the potential of abuse
- Prescribing by drug treatment protocols
- Limiting the quantities of certain drugs that PAs may prescribe

The Controlled Substances Act defines five schedules of drugs, each with drug preparations that have differing potential for abuse by users. Schedule I drugs have the greatest potential for abuse and schedule V the least. Not included in the act are drug preparations that have no potential for abuse by users but whose use requires a written order from a licensed prescriber. These drug preparations, referred to as *prescription legend drugs,* can be prescribed by PAs with prescribing privilege. PAs may also prescribe over-the-counter medications, drug preparations that do not, by law, require the written order of a licensed prescriber.

Among the states with prescribing regulations in place, approximately one third grant PAs prescribing privileges for schedule II through schedule V drugs in addition to "prescription legend" drug preparations. Schedule I drugs are not relevant to this discussion, as it is illegal for licensed practitioners in the United States to prescribe these drugs. In the other states the prescribing privilege applies to schedule III through schedule V drugs including prescription legend drugs, with some restrictions by various states on prescribing schedule III drugs.

Current Extent of Physician Assistant Prescribing

Although PAs prescribe in a wide variety of settings, few empirical data are available about how and when PAs prescribe. The restrictions on prescribing privileges have undoubtedly limited the interest of researchers in examining PA prescribing. Some market surveys and a few published research studies have shown interest with PAs who prescribe. A 1990 survey, administered in the states that had some form of prescribing authority for PAs at that time, found that 90% of a selected sample of PAs prescribe when provided the authority. Sixty percent or more of the PAs reported prescribing urinary/vaginal agents, upper respiratory medications, gastrointestinal agents, antiarthritic/antigout agents, and analgesics (Willis and Reid, 1990). Among these PAs the mean number of prescriptions written per week was 50. It was estimated from the survey that PAs write 35.5 million new prescriptions each year (Willis and Reid, 1990). When extrapolated to 1996, and when refill prescriptions are included, the total is about 75 million. In 1996 the 40 states with prescribing privileges for PAs have more than three fourths of all the PAs in the United States and contain approximately 75% of the total U.S. population.

In 1984 a survey of 170 randomly selected PAs in New York State returned questions on prescribing, with a 67% response rate (Mittman and Mirotznik, 1984). New York permits physicians to delegate prescribing privileges to the PAs they supervise; outpatient prescribing is restricted to nonscheduled drugs. All respondents reported that the most frequently prescribed types of drugs, in order of frequency, were oral antibiotics, antihistamine/decongestants, topical antibiotics, pain/fever medications, and otic/ophthalmic preparations. They also reported recommending over-the-counter preparations an average of nine times a day. Aspirin and other pain medications, cold and allergy products, cough preparations, and antacids were the most frequently recommended. Those in non-hospital-based settings, about one half of the respondents, reported writing an average of 17 outpatient prescriptions per day (Mittman and Mirotznik, 1984). They also attempted to provide some insight into attitudes that could affect PA prescribing. Eighty-eight percent of PAs agreed with the statement that "the average patient does not feel treated without getting a prescription." Seventy-one percent agreed with the statement that "the pharmaceutical companies that regularly call on PAs are the ones whose products the PA will tend to prescribe." Pharmaceutical sales representatives were mentioned by PAs as one of the five factors that most influenced their selection of drug products (Mittman and Mirotznik, 1984).

The findings of these studies begin to show the extent and nature of PA prescribing when delegated but come from small market surveys and nonrepresentative samples of PAs that signal caution in interpreting the findings. The reports consistently show that PA prescribing fits the types of drugs commonly associated with primary care.

Reasons for Restrictions

Several reasons have been advanced as to why state regulatory agencies have limited the prescribing privilege to PAs. One early reason is that PAs are not sufficiently trained to be competent prescribers. Further, because the agencies regulating PA practice have historically been largely composed of physicians, a second reason, related to the first, is the potential of increased legal liability of supervising physicians because of PAs' perceived lack of prescribing competence. Physician reluctance can also come from cultural and economic reasons.

Concerns about patient safety and physician liability have had some historical validity given the substantial amount of variation that has characterized the evolution of PA training and educational programs. The pharmacology and therapeutics component of the PAs' educational experience had been singled out as a major area of concern (Camp, 1984). At one time, the pharmacology preparation varied widely among PA programs and ranged from one semester (covering such topics as basic mechanisms of drug action, enzyme induction, drug absorption, distribution, metabolism, excretions, and various families of drugs) to minimal exposure in practical therapeutics. Not mentioned in these observations was that students gained instruction in pharmacology during clinical rotations as part of their patient management experience under physician supervision. Moreover, during this time no clear definition existed across programs of what drug families the student should know and what specific disease problems the student should learn to manage (Heller and Fasser, 1978). Pharmacology and medical therapeutics are a part of the core requirements of every PA program. Of 55 PA programs surveyed in 1990, 49 averaged 66 hours of instruction in pharmacology, with a range of from 28 to 128 hours (Oliver, 1993). A model clinical therapeutics curriculum was developed in 1996, but how many programs use it is unknown (Wilson et al., 1995).

Another potentially powerful reason is that the medical profession may not wish to share the act of prescribing. The act of prescribing has been described as "the most common and overt expression of the physicians' power" (Pelligrino, 1976). Much of this power is ascribed to the symbolism associated with prescribing. Throughout history the ingestion of substances has been associated with magical, mystical, and religious elements that transcend any pharmacologic effects. When coupled with the ingrained urge to "take something" for an illness, this historical association gives extraordinary power to the person who has the exclusive right to provide the "something" (Pelligrino, 1976).

The act of prescribing manifests the physician's power in a variety of ways. It gives the physician the authority to define the clinical situation as medical, it establishes that the patient is "truly ill," and it implicitly reinforces the physician's ability to handle the illness. The act of prescribing maintains the physician's power by providing the physician time for the illness to unfold when a diagnosis is uncertain or a condition is obscure. The act of prescribing maintains the physician's control of the situation even though scientific observation may indicate no medication is needed. Sharing prescribing privileges with PAs removes physicians as the only source of such power.

The symbolic weight of prescribing has other practical implications for the physician. For one thing, prescribing a drug indicates to the patient that the physician is concerned and is trying to help. Prescribing a drug can take the place of communicating with the patient. Finally, prescribing can be used to both guide and end the office visit, as well as to provide a link with the patient for continuing visits (Pelligrino, 1976). Thus delegating prescribing authority to PAs also empowers them in their relationships with patients and may be perceived as reducing the power of the physician.

Another possible reason to limit the prescribing privilege is an economic one. The initial purpose of the creation of PAs was to alleviate a shortage of physician services. More recently, however, given the more abundant supply of physician services, the distinction of whether PAs complement physician services or are alternatives for physician services is less clear. The latter situation implies that PAs are currently in competition with physicians for patients.

Opposition to prescribing privileges for PAs from other health care professions, such as pharmacists, is another possible reason. The opposition, however, is basically confined to attempting to influence regulatory agencies and state legislatures through testimony and lobbying efforts. Such efforts may delay the granting of prescribing privileges in some states but have not been sufficient to prevent them.

Medical Justification for Physician Assistant Prescribing

Although the data to assess the safety and effectiveness of PA prescribing are sparse, there is ample empirical evidence that PAs prescribe effectively and safely. *Safety,* in this context, refers to the prescribing that minimizes the risk of an adverse consequence from the drug prescribed, and *effectiveness* refers to the contribution of the drug to the outcome of treatment. Such data from outpatient primary care settings would be of particular importance because the largest share of PAs are employed in these settings. Some data are available that compare physician and PA patterns of practice including prescribing as one of the criteria to assess the quality or appropriateness of the diagnostic and treatment processes or the outcomes of care.

Goldberg and colleagues (1981) evaluated the quality of care provided by 23 PAs in Air Force primary medicine clinics, where PAs assumed a considerable portion of the care formerly provided by physicians. Quality-of-care judgments were based on diagnostic, therapeutic, and disposition criteria. Therapeutic criteria included desirable actions (e.g., prescribing the appropriate class of antibiotic for infectious otitis media at the first visit) and undesirable actions (e.g., prescribing an antibiotic for a viral syndrome with gastroenteritis). On five of six such criteria identifying desirable therapeutic action, PAs performed as well as physicians. For all eight criteria identifying undesirable action, PAs performed as well as or better than physicians (Goldberg et al., 1981).

Kane and colleagues (1976) compared the quality-of-care performance of PAs with that of their supervising physicians, one criterion being whether medication was ordered for specific diagnoses. They found that PAs were less likely than physicians to use antibiotics for fevers of undetermined origin and for upper respiratory tract infections, and somewhat less likely to use systemic steroids for contact dermatitis and asthma. These data indicated that PA prescribing decisions for these morbidities were as good as or better than those of physicians (Kane et al., 1976).

Duttera and Harlan (1978) evaluated the appropriateness of care provided by PAs in 14 rural primary care settings. They concluded that PAs were competent both in diagnostic and in therapeutic skills in the three following practice patterns: (1) when all patients were initially seen by the PA and then by the physician, (2) when patients (not preselected) were managed concurrently by physicians and PAs, and (3) when patients with specific problems were assigned to PAs.

Kane et al. (1978) also compared functional outcomes, patient satisfaction with care and outcome, and mean costs per acute episode of care for family practice residents, faculty, and Medex-trained PAs at two family practice centers associated with a university family practice training program. The performance of PAs was as good as or better than the physicians' in each of the measures.

Record and Greenlick (1975) compared the performance of PAs and physicians in a large health maintenance organization (HMO) in handling episodes of four specific morbidities: strep throat, upper respiratory infection, bursitis, and bronchitis. One outcome criterion was safety, in terms of the rate of adverse effects from antibiotics and other drugs provided in the treatment of upper respiratory infection. They found no differences in the rates between PAs and physicians.

Tompkins et al. (1977) investigated how physicians and PAs at two different clinics medically managed patients with acute respiratory illnesses. The PAs used clinical algorithms to guide their choices of diagnostic tests and treatment. The findings showed that the PAs did not prescribe antibiotics needlessly or more than internists for conditions not generally requiring an antibiotic and PAs prescribed antibiotics similarly for treatment of bacterial conditions. Internists had the highest medical care costs per patient. The authors concluded that the care provided by the PAs was as effective as and less costly than the care provided by physicians.

A study in Iowa reported that 95% of physicians and 93% of PAs believed that PAs were qualified to prescribe medication with little or no supervision by the physician (Ekwo et al., 1979). Similarly, all 29 Montana physicians who responded to a survey expressed confidence in the ability of the PAs they were supervising to prescribe most therapeutic agents, and 40% had no reservations about PAs prescribing any agent (Willis and Reid, 1990).

In another study, a stratified sample of 19.6% of Wisconsin pharmacists was surveyed about their attitudes toward PA prescribing (Huntington and Warnick, 1987). The survey was conducted 8 months after PAs were authorized to prescribe nonscheduled prescription drugs with the physician supervisor required to cosign the patient's medical record. Slightly more than one half of the 329 pharmacist respondents (47% response rate) reported dispensing prescriptions written by PAs. At the time of the survey, Wisconsin PAs were prescribing an average of 27 prescriptions per month, or about 1 per day. The findings indicated that pharmacists found PAs' prescriptions "completed appropriately and legibly prepared." They were confident in "filling a prescription from a PA." Nevertheless, Wisconsin pharmacists expressed little support for expanded prescribing authority for PAs (Huntington and Warnick, 1987). Reasons for this conclusion were not mentioned in the analysis.

Hooker (1993) examined prescribing by quantity and found that adult primary care PAs and NPs prescribed 15% of the prescriptions in the department of internal medicine and family practice while staffing the departments at 20% full-time equivalent personnel.

The findings from reports that describe prescribing by PAs and that medically justify prescribing privileges for PAs are limited in number and in rigor. Much of the information about what and how much PAs prescribe has come from market surveys and various reports that have used convenience or otherwise unrepresentative samples of PAs. The findings applicable to medically justify PA prescribing have been compiled from studies that have one or more common methodologic problems. One problem has been the small sample sizes of physicians and PAs in comparative studies. Another problem has been the types of sites of comparative studies, such as military installations, rural practices, university teaching hospitals, and clinics. These settings are not representative of the mainstream of primary care and where most PAs practice (Kane et al., 1976; Duttera and Harlan, 1978; Kane, Olsen, and Castle, 1978; Goldberg et al., 1981). In addition, patient populations have been nonrandomized and measures of quality and appropriateness have been process measures. Finally, medical care record data have not been standardized and in some instances have been incomplete (Sox, 1979; Office of Technology Assessment, 1986). Nevertheless, a consistent finding appears to be that when PAs are delegated the prescribing decision or provided protocols to guide them in specified clinical situations, they do at least as well as physicians in writing prescriptions, ordering drug treatment, and producing "good" processes of care. Although the evidence is not sufficient to generalize to all PA prescribing, it does appear sufficient to predict adequate performance of PAs when they are delegated the handling, including the drug treatment, of acute episodes of illness in office-based primary care. Liability insurance premiums have not increased appreciably, and the remarkably few malpractice claims have not centered on prescribing as an issue of safety.

Although progress has been made and continues to be made in achieving prescribing authority for PAs, it has taken more than 30 years to gain such privilege, albeit generally limited, in most states (Exhibit 11-3).

While the body of evidence is limited, there is good reason to believe that PAs prescribe safely and effectively. If they were not doing so, an abundance of reports would be available to identify the problem. However, it would be useful for health planners, managers, and policymakers to know more definitively how cost-effective PAs are as alternatives to physicians when delegated the

EXHIBIT 11-3

Prescriptive Privileges for PA by State

States	Prescriptive authority	Restrictions	Controlled substances
Ala.	X	Noncontrolled from board formulary	–
Alaska	X	Physician name and DEA number required on prescription	Schedules III through V
Ariz.	X	–	Schedules II and III limited to 72-hr supply
Ark.	X	–	Schedules III through V
Calif.	X	PA may write "drug orders," which, for purposes of DEA registration, meet the definition of a prescription	–
Colo.	X	Written protocol on case-by-case and per-patient-visit basis required: physician countersign on charts required within 3 days	Controlled II through V
Conn.	X	–	Schedules IV and V; schedules II and III hospitals; long-term care II through V
Del.	X	Therapeutics approved by physician and board	–
D.C.	X	Noncontrolled only	–
Fla.	X	Formulary of prohibitive drugs	–
Ga.	X	Formulary	Schedules III through V
Guam	X	–	Schedules III through V
Hawaii	X	–	Schedules III though V
Idaho	X	Board formulary	Schedules II through V
Ill.	X	–	Schedules III through V
Ind.		–	–
Iowa	X	Must be ordered by physician in written protocol or in an emergency	Schedules III through V; schedule II except stimulants and depressants
Ky.	X	–	–
La.		–	–
Me.	X	DEA registration	Schedules III through V (Board may approve schedule for individual practices)
Md.	X	–	Schedules II through V
Mass.	X	–	Schedules II through V
Mich.	X	Noncontrolled only	Schedules III through V; schedule II (30-day supply as discharge med)
Minn.	X	Formulary	Schedules II through V
Miss.	X	–	–
Mo.	X	–	–
Mont.	X	Delegation by physician	Schedules II through V; limited schedule II to 34-day supply
Neb.	X	Physician authorization required	Medications including 72-hr supply of schedule II
Nev.	X	Board approval and pharmacy registration required	Controlled; limited to supervising physician's prescriptive authority
N.H.	X	Pharmacy law examination required	Controlled
N.J.		–	–
N.M.	X	Formulary	Schedules II through V
N.Y.	X	Noncontrolled only	Schedules III through V

EXHIBIT 11-3

Prescriptive Privileges for PA by State—*Cont'd*

States	Prescriptive authority	Restrictions	Controlled substances
N.C.	X	Pharmacy board approval required	Schedules II through V; schedules II and III limited to 7-day supply
N.D.	X	—	Schedules III through V
Ohio		—	—
Okla.	X	Formulary	Schedules III through V
Ore.	X	Physician and board approval and DEA registration required	Schedules III through V
Pa.	X	—	Formulary drugs schedules III through V (limited to 30-day supply)
R.I.	X	State drug control office and DEA registration required	Schedules II through V
S.C.	X	Formulary	Schedule V
S.D.	X	—	Schedules II through V; schedule II limited to 48-hr supply
Tenn.	X	Noncontrolled only	Schedule II through V
Tex.	X	Limited to underserved areas, practices with high rates of indigent patients, physician's primary practice site, hospital, or other site	
Utah	X	—	Schedules II through V
Vt.	X	Physician authorization required	Schedules II through V
Va.	X	Noncontrolled on board formulary	Schedules IV and V
Wash.	X	DEA number required	Schedules II through V
W.Va.	X	2 years of experience, board-approved pharmacology course, and NCCPA. Board formulary. DEA number required	Schedules III through V (schedule III limited to 72-hr supply)
Wis.	X	With written protocols and consultation with physician	Schedules II through V
Wyo.	X	DEA number required	Schedules II through V

Data from American Academy of Physician Assistants, 2002.

handling, including the drug treatment, of conditions common to primary care and in different settings. Because many PAs are specialized, it would be useful to know whether PAs are more cost-effective than the physicians with whom they work.

Rigorous research is indicated to show if PAs with prescribing privilege are as effective; that is, can they provide the same or better outcomes of treatment for the same or less costs than physicians in conditions where drug treatment is indicated. *Effectiveness* refers to expected favorable health- and psychosocial-related outcomes of treatment, whereas *cost-effectiveness* refers to lesser total costs generated to produce similar health- and psychosocial-related outcomes. Favorable health-related outcomes, for example, would be the absence of therapeutic failures (drug re-treatment or refills), complications from undertreatment or overtreatment including the adverse effects of drugs. Favorable psychosocial outcomes include, for example, maintenance of functioning and social roles and satisfaction with the treatment provided. A summary of controlled substances is presented in Exhibit 11-4.

DRUG ENFORCEMENT ADMINISTRATION

Every provider who administers, prescribes, or dispenses any controlled substance, other than as a direct agent of another registrant, must be registered with the Drug Enforcement Administration (DEA). A PA who is required to register must submit a completed Form DEA-224 to the DEA. Before 1994, PAs, NPs, and certified nurse midwives (CNMs) were registered similar to physicians with a registration number beginning with the letter A or B, followed by a letter corresponding to the first letter of their last name. In 1994 the DEA chose to reclassify nonphysician providers under the term *midlevel practitioners* and require new registration numbers

EXHIBIT 11-4

Controlled Substance Act

Schedule I are drugs with no accepted medical use in the United States and have a high abuse potential. Some examples are heroin, marijuana, LSD, peyote, mescaline, and psilocybin.

Schedule II are drugs with a high abuse potential with severe psychic or physical dependence liability. Controlled substances consist of certain narcotic, stimulant, and depressant drugs. Examples of narcotics are opium, morphine, codeine, methadone, and meperidine. Examples of the stimulants are amphetamine and methamphetamine. Examples of the depressants are amobarbital, pentobarbital, secobarbital, and methaqualone.

Schedule III drugs have an abuse potential less than those in schedules I and II and include compounds containing limited quantities of certain narcotic drugs and nonnarcotic drugs such as paregoric and barbituric acid derivatives not included in another schedule.

Schedule IV drugs have an abuse potential less than those listed in schedule II and include such drugs as phenobarbital, chloral hydrate, meprobamate, chlordiazepoxide, diazepam, and dextropropoxyphene.

Schedule V drugs have an abuse potential less than those listed in schedule IV and consist of preparations containing limited amounts of certain narcotic drugs generally for antitussive and antidiarrheal purposes.

beginning with the *M* (for *midlevel*) and the first letter of the last name, followed by a computer-generated sequence of seven numbers.

The registration must be renewed every 3 years. The certificate of registration must be maintained at the registered location and kept available for official inspection. Every prescriber registered with the DEA receives a re-registration application approximately 60 days before the expiration date of his or her registration. If more than one practice location is used from which he or she dispenses controlled substances from personal supplies, then each location must be independently registered. A move to a new location requires a request for modification of registration in writing to the DEA office.

There are some exceptions to this process, such as being in the Armed Forces or other government agencies such as the Public Health Service and the Veterans Administration. Other administrative details such as record-keeping requirements, inventory, prescription orders, control and reporting of substance theft or loss, and guidelines for prescribers of controlled substances can be found in the *1993 Mid-Level Practitioner's Manual: An Informational Outline of the Controlled Substances Act of 1970.*

POLITICS

No chapter on legal aspects of PAs is complete without a discussion of the political ramifications of an expanding workforce that includes PAs. David Mechanic (1974) writes,

> It is becoming fashionable to think of health politics as the process of federal policy making. But the character of health care is molded, equally, by the clash of interests at the community level, the organization and promotion of particular structures of professional organization, and the continuing decisions made at the level of operating agencies of all sorts. Many individuals at many points make decisions about the character of health care. This characteristic, particularly, gives the health context its complex diversity and uneven response to change.

In the article "The Politics of Ambulatory Care," Bellin (1982) has approached this subject by discussing the players who deliver ambulatory care.

> It is logical first to consider the politics of health care practitioners themselves. Government refers to them generically as "providers."
>
> In delivering ambulatory care, not only physicians but also a variety of health professionals and allied health professionals strive for legitimacy. Functional lines of demarcation are increasingly blurred. Territories once the exclusive domain of the [physician] have been challenged, sometimes *de jure* by legal and legislative means, often *de facto* by gradual changes in customary practice. A partial list of combatants includes:
>
> - Orthopedists vs. podiatrist
> - Ophthalmologist vs. optometrist
> - Psychiatrist vs. clinical psychologist vs. psychiatric social worker

- Primary care physician vs. nurse practitioner vs. physician assistant

The medical professional lays historic claim to the entire human body, including the feet, the eyes, the psyche, and the right to make preliminary assessment of a patient's health status. Nevertheless, there appears to be an inexorable and irreversible process at work, periodically made manifest in quarrels among professionals over [anatomy and physiology]. Although the physician possesses extraordinary prestige, there has been, during the past few decades, a progressive demystification of the [physician's] knowledge and skills, in part as a result of the increasing formal education and sophistication of the lay public. Demystification has facilitated the trickling down of certain functions and procedures of [physicians] to the "limited-licensed" health care practitioners, such as the podiatrist, the optometrist, the clinical psychologist, and now those primary care professionals called nurse practitioners and physician assistants. [Doctors] have been disinclined to do certain tasks deemed routine or disagreeable or of low status and have allowed some of these tasks to go by default to others eager to fill the functional vacuum, provide needed service, and enhance their professional status. The podiatrist has been less loathe than the orthopedist to operate on corns and calluses. The ophthalmologist has preferred to perform eye surgery rather than fit glasses, so the optometrist has prescribed and fitted lenses. Local [doctor] shortages have provided further encouragement to the limited licensed practitioner to enlarge his professional territory. Cost has been another factor. Customarily, the limited-licensed practitioner has been less expensive than the [physician] specialist in the same functional domain.

The limited-licensed practitioner has legitimized the acquisition of once [doctor]-specific tasks by legislatively expanding the legal scope of licensure and by adding pertinent courses in the curriculum of the professional school. To the orthopedist's annoyance, the modern podiatrist now performs vascular and bone surgery on the feet and prescribes medications with systemic effects. Despite opposition by ophthalmologists, the optometrist has sought and has won the right in an increasing number of states, albeit with curricular safeguards, to prescribe eye drops for diagnostic purposes. Once the limited-licensed practitioners have secured the right to do certain things once hitherto performed only by MDs, they never give up that right. [Physician] hostility has retarded but failed to halt this process.

In ambulatory care delivery the latest political controversy relates to what is to be the ultimate role of physician assistant (PA) and nurse practitioner (NP), each having come into being originally to alleviate the impact of the critical shortage of primary care physicians. The NP resents ever being placed in a hierarchical or reimbursement position lower than or subordinate to the nonnurse PA. To avoid friction between the PA and the NP, it is sometimes prudent to assign them to different departments or agencies. Yet they have certain political goals in common. Both the PA and NP prefer to attenuate if not eliminate altogether the supervisory role of the [physician] vis-à-vis their own work. Both would like to prescribe, being independent of the [physician's] overview. Although not unanimously held, these views reflect PA and NP expansionist tendencies that characterize all limited-licensed professionals today in ambulatory care delivery. In contrast, the [physician] champions the principle of [physician] supervision of PA and NP, who would remain, of course, nonautonomous. In the [physician]-approved model, the PA and NP would handle routinizable situations according to an unambiguous protocol. There are also pecuniary considerations. Subordinate to the [physician], the PA or NP would cost the [physician] less than another [physician] as employee or partner but could generate income to supplement the physician's.

The contemporary PA is striving for legitimacy in an era of political change. While this is being played out on a number of fronts, the political/policymaking arena is probably the most important. Because the physician no longer has control of this process, it is likely that policymakers will continue to recognize the attributes of PAs based on outcome and economic data, and not the soft social values exhorted by some that all health care should be controlled by the physician.

NATIONAL PRACTITIONER DATA BANK

The National Practitioner Data Bank (NPDB) is a federal repository for any state board actions or malpractice actions against physicians, dentists, PAs, NPs, and other licensed health care professionals. It was established to restrict the ability of incompetent practitioners to move from state to state without discovery of previous substandard performance or unprofessional conduct. All PAs applying for privileges to a hospital or medical center must submit information that is then forwarded to the NPDB.

From 1990 to 1998 the NPDB produced information on more than 176,000 reported actions, malpractice payments, and Medicare/Medicaid exclusions involving 118,142 individual practitioners. A study of data from the NPDB spanning 1990 through 1998 revealed that 252 medical malpractice payments were made by reason for payment regarding PAs (Exhibit 11-5). PAs were responsible for only four payments, representing 0.03% of the total for 1997. The most frequently cited reason for all malpractice payments was diagnosis related, followed by surgery- and treatment-related reasons (Exhibit 11-6). Physicians totaled 104,353 medical malpractice payments spanning September 1990 through December 1997. PAs had 252 payments during the same reporting period. The leading category of reason for medical practice payment for both physicians (34,021 of 104,353) and PAs (129 of 252) was diagnosis error.

Medication-related malpractice payments represented 6.35% of physician reports and 9.5% of PA malpractice reports. Exhibit 11-7 shows the number of medication-related medial malpractice payments by reason for payment (Cawley, Rohrs, and Hooker, 1998).

The NPDB data suggest the rate and amount of malpractice payments for PAs is relatively low compared with that for physicians. In fact the NPDB data reveal one claim per eight practicing physicians versus one claim per 107 PAs over the same time. These findings support perceptions that PAs pose a low risk of malpractice liability to the public in general and to employing practices in particular. One reason postulated for this observed low risk is the communication skills that PAs may provide in patient encounters (Brock, 1998). Whether PAs have communication skills that limit liability remains to be researched.

Important work is needed to further understand the rate of litigation and malpractice by number of visits and types of visits that are managed by physicians, PAs, NPs, CNMs, and other types of providers. While the NPDB has some flaws in its collection methodology, these flaws should not be discounted completely because the

EXHIBIT 11-5

Number, Mean, and Median Medical Practice Payment Reports by Practitioner (1990-1998)

Provider	Payment amount
Physicians	
Mean payment	$139,581
No.	8,619
Median payment	$40,000
Total MD/DOs in 1997	637,186*
Payment ratio: MD/DO	2.4%
Physician assistants	
Mean payment	$55,241
No.	24
Median payment	$12,500
Total PAs in 1997	33,500†
Payment ration: PA	0.76%

*The number of physicians in 1997 is the number of "total physicians" less the number of physicians listed as "inactive" or "address unknown" as of December 31, 1997. Modified from American Medical Association, *The American Medical Association's Physician Characteristics and Distribution in the U.S.*, 1996-1997, Chicago.
†The number of PAs in 1997 is the number of total practicing PAs as of October 1997. From the *AAPA Physician Assistant Census Report*, American Academy of Physician Assistants, Alexandria, Va.

EXHIBIT 11-6

Medical Malpractice Payments by Reason for Payment and Practitioner Type (1991-1998)

Malpractice type	Physician assistant	Physician
Diagnosis	129	34,021
Anesthesia	1	3,455
Surgery	13	28,556
Medication	24	6,622
Intravenous and blood products	0	483
Obstetrics	0	9,279
Treatment	76	18,478
Monitoring	4	1,223
Equipment/product	0	400
Miscellaneous	5	1,825
TOTAL	252	104,353

EXHIBIT 11-7

Medication-Related Medical Malpractice Payments by Reason for Payment and Practitioner Type (1991-1998)

Malpractice type	Physician assistant	Physician
Failure to order appropriate medication	1	416
Wrong medication ordered	3	519
Wrong dosage ordered of correct medication	1	417
Failure to instruct on medication	1	202
Improper management of medication regimen	4	1797
Consent issues	2	99
Error (not otherwise coded)	4	378
Failure to medicate	1	103
Wrong medication administered	2	241
Wrong dosage administered	0	166
Wrong patient	0	1
Wrong route	0	30
Improper technique	0	159
Administration (not otherwise coded)	5	2094
TOTAL	24	6622

MEDICATION-RELATED CLAIMS PER PRACTITIONER

	1997	1996	1995
Physicians	**1:836**	**1:726**	**1:808**
No. of claims	762	878	789
Physician assistants	**1:7000**	**1:4500**	**1:3571**
No. of claims	4	6	7

criteria for databank entry affect both physicians and PAs equally. The work here should offer some reassurance that the delegated responsibility of patient care from the physician to the PA is a relatively safe one.

PROFESSIONAL ISSUES

Professional issues influence the behavior of PAs. They are often political in nature and many issues draw lines as to which side of the health care environment PAs are placed when viewed by physicians. The issues under discussion represent contemporary changes in health care delivery and reconceptualize traditional views of caregivers and services. As new patterns of service delivery evolve, the boundaries between professions and even within some professions will blur.

Physician Assistant Unions

Efforts to organize PAs have met with both acceptance and resistance since the first PAs were incorporated into a health care worker's union in approximately 1975 with Kaiser Permanente in Colorado. In 2000 New York led the nation in the number of unionized PAs through their affiliation with the Service Employees International Union (SEIU), Local 1199, in New York City. The union began incorporating PAs in 1988, and in 1997 the local union created a PA Division, an organizing entity within the local union that represents PAs exclusively. Local 1199 is the first and closest thing to a PA-only union in the country. As of 2000 it had unionized more than 500 PAs, including 75 at the Catholic Medical Center in New York City and 157 at the Riker's Island correctional facility. About half are located in hospitals within New York State (Herrick, 2000b).

The AAPA 1999 census found nationwide that 3.9% of all PAs were in a union. These figures may not reflect part-time and per diem PAs, who are also covered by union contracts but may only have a quasi-membership status within the union (AAPA 2000). While the New York unionization rate is almost triple that of any other state, the vast majority of PAs are not in unions. Not all efforts to unionize PAs have been successful. Although little is known about union successes, much less failures, the authors know of unionization efforts within Kaiser Permanente in Portland, Oregon. In 1988 and 1999 a movement to organize PAs and APNs, 230 full-time employees, into a collective bargaining union met with defeat. A Kaiser Permanente strike of 1000 PAs, nurses, pharmacists, optometrists, physical therapists, and other health care workers in Colorado lasted 20 days in 2000. All but a few PAs joined the strike (Hughes, 2000).

Unionized PAs report that collective bargaining has allowed them to influence how care is delivered and to increase stipends in continuing medical education, work ratios, shift times, and the formation of professional practice committees that decide work and care issues (Herrick, 2000b). Job security is probably the main reason for developing a union.

Pharmaceutical Manufacturer Representatives Detailing Physician Assistants

PAs with prescribing rights are a new audience when pharmaceutical company sales representatives visit doctors' offices. Traditionally physicians were the targets of visits from pharmaceutical sales representatives. Beginning in the 1990s pharmaceutical representatives' attentions increasingly shifted to PAs and NPs who have at least limited prescribing authority. Like physicians, "nonphysician prescribers" receive drug presentations from sales representatives as one way they obtain new pharmaceutical information. Like doctors, PAs read clinical journals, take continuing medical education courses, and discuss prescription effectiveness with colleagues. Surveys by Scott-Levin Associates show drug sales representatives are increasingly targeting nonphysicians who have prescribing rights. Some 52% of PAs polled said they saw drug representatives more often than their supervising physicians did, and 41% of NPs said drug representatives "detailed" them more often than doctors (Scott-Levin Associates, 2000).

Although studies by Scott-Levin Associates and the AAPA indicate PAs are prescribing from 30% to 50% more medications than 5 years ago, the prescribing rate per patient has remained the same at 0.8 prescriptions per patient visit (Scott-Levin Associates, 2000). In a different survey the AAPA said PA prescribing has been slowly increasing over the past 3 years and as of 2000 is at 1.1 per patient visit (Nelson, 2000).

Undoubtedly PAs are increasing total prescriptions because their numbers are growing. In the survey Expanding the Prescriber Base: Nurse Practitioners and Physician Assistants, Scott-Levin Associates found drug representative visits to PAs in 1999 averaged 4.4 per week and 5.2 for NPs. These numbers are expected to rise each year. Visits to doctors' offices increased 10%, to 36 million in 1999 from 33 million in 1995, and 30% of those visits include discussions with nonphysicians. Some 2000 physicians surveyed said they saw from four to five drug representatives per week.

The Scott-Levin survey found that PAs and NPs received 16% of the industry's details in the first quarter of 2000. In comparison, hospital-based doctors received 10%. Pfizer, Bristol-Myers Squibb, and Johnson & Johnson were the top companies calling on PAs and NPs in the first quarter of 2000 (Exhibit 11-8). The bulk of activity focused on the largest group of prescribers, office-based physicians, who accounted for 74% of all details. The study also found a majority of nonphysicians makes recommendations to physicians to either expand use rates or try new drugs (Exhibit 11-9). Some 80% of PAs and 69% of NPs said they make recommendations to physicians.

Another issue that comes into play are the free gifts given to physicians, PAs, and NPs by drug representatives, which can influence prescribing habits. More than half of the $11 billion spent in

EXHIBIT 11-8

Physician Assistant and Nurse Practitioner Calls by Pharmaceutical Representatives*

Corporation	PA calls	NP calls	PA/NP calls
Total market	501,000	728,000	1,229,000
Pfizer	51,000	81,000	132,000
Bristol-Myers Squibb	34,000	53,000	86,000
Johnson & Johnson	30,000	50,000	80,000
Glaxo Wellcome	26,000	41,000	67,000
Schering-Plough	29,000	36,000	65,000
American Home Products	21,000	41,000	62,000
Aventis	29,000	33,000	61,000
Merck	27,000	31,000	58,000
Pharmacia Corporation	25,000	25,000	51,000
All others	202,000	300,000	502,000

Modified from Scott-Levin: Nurse practitioners and physician assistants: all about promotion, patients, and prescribing, 2000. Available at: http://www.quintiles.com/products_and_ services/informatics/scott_levin/1,1261,0,00.html
*First quarter, 2000.

EXHIBIT 11-9

Five Most Esteemed Pharmaceutical Companies by PA or NP, 2000

Physician assistants	Nurse practitioners
1. Pfizer	1. Pfizer
2. Merck	2. Johnson & Johnson
3. Glaxo Wellcome	2. Merck (tie for no. 2)
4. Johnson & Johnson	4. Glaxo Wellcome
5. GlaxoSmithKline	5. American Home Products

Modified from Scott-Levin: Nurse practitioners and physician assistants: all about promotion, patients, and prescribing, 2000. Available at: http://www.quintiles.com/products_and_ services/informatics/scott_levin/1,1261,0,00.html

promotions in 1996 was funneled through company sales representatives. Although this is a concern, there are ethical guidelines on gifts that physicians may accept only from drug representatives that benefit patients or their practice. Similar guidelines have been developed for PAs and NPs.

Assisted Suicide

Assisted suicide has been a topic of debate among health care professionals for decades, and PAs are no exception. In a Michigan survey conducted in 1994, 48% of responding PAs tended to support provider-assisted suicide and 40% were opposed (Hayden et al., 1995).

In 1997 Oregon became the first and only state to legalize physician-assisted suicide. In 1998 provider-assisted suicide was used by 16 patients, and 27 patients did the same the following year. This represents nine provider-assisted suicide deaths per 10,000 total Oregon deaths. As of 2002 there have been over 80 assisted suicides reported, none involving PAs. While the executive director of the Death with Dignity advocacy group, which helped create the Oregon law, is an attorney and former PA—Barbara Coombs Lee—no known case of assisted suicide involving a PA has been reported. Attitudes about this act are likely to change with time and along with it will be the more open involvement of patients, their caregivers, physicians, nurses, pharmacists, and PAs.

Impairment

Impairment of professional performance by alcohol, other drugs, or mental illness is common. An estimated 12% to 14% of physicians experience such problems at some time during their lives, mostly due to chemical dependence.

In 1985 the North Carolina Academy of Physician Assistants created a standing committee to address impaired PAs, modeled after a similar program for physicians in the state. Over the first 11 years 29 PAs were referred for assessment and treatment by the impaired physician program in the state (Exhibits 11-10 and 11-11) (Mattingly and Curtis, 1996). Other states have modeled their PA impairment programs after either the North Carolina model or the existing one for physicians. A support program within the AAPA, called the Caduceus Caucus, assists AAPA members with alcohol and drug addiction.

Liability Insurance

Along with the expanding role of the PA the need for professional liability insurance developed. No matter how careful and competent PAs are, mistakes are made and sometimes judgments on those mistakes are rendered. The future of PA practice can be dependent on whether PAs are properly protected in the event they are sued.

EXHIBIT 11-10

Problems/Diagnoses of Impaired PAs (North Carolina)

Diagnosis	No. of PAs (N = 29)	%
Opioids	7	24
Alcohol	5	17
Polysubstances	5	17
Dual diagnosis	3	10
Psychiatric disorder	3	10
Sexual misconduct	2	7
Other	2	7
Marijuana	1	3
Unsubstantiated	1	3

EXHIBIT 11-11

Status of PA Impairment Cases in North Carolina

	No. of PAs	%
Contract agreements	13	45
Assessed and released	9	31
Not currently licensed in N.C.	—	10
Not currently in N.C.	3	10
Other	1	3

Usually a PA is the employee of a physician, group, or institution, in which case there may be adequate coverage under the employer's plan or a group rate.

Professional liability insurance coverage generally depends on the duties that are performed, the geographic area of practice, and the limits of liability chosen (Exhibit 11-12). The American Continental Insurance Company has classified PAs by the type of activities in which they participate. Class I PAs tend to be in the cognitive disciplines while class III PAs are in the surgical specialties. Generally speaking class II PAs carry twice as much liability as class I insurance, and class III PAs carry three times as much liability insurance as class I PAs. PA students (class IV) are approximately one tenth as much as a class I PA for liability purposes.

These rates vary considerably depending on where the PA practices geographically. Urban locations carry more liability risk than rural areas and the Northeast more than the Southwest (Exhibit 11-13).

Abortion

Legislation on PAs involved with abortions varies by state. As a result of the shortage of qualified providers, much attention has been paid in recent years to the idea that PAs, NPs, and CNMs

EXHIBIT 11-12

Classification of Physician Assistants for Liability Insurance

Class I: A physician assistant who performs tasks ordinarily reserved for a physician and who works under the direction and supervision of a qualified licensed physician to assist the physician in the diagnosis and management of patients.

Class II: A physician assistant who is involved in any of the following:

A. Assisting in surgery: any exposure to an operating room other than for observation
B. Any exposure to trauma/emergency room procedures or responsibilities thereof (10 hr or less a week)
C. Obstetric exposure limited to prenatal or postnatal care
D. Assisting in anesthesiology

Class III: A physician assistant who is involved in any of the following:

A. Assisting in surgery: any exposure to operating room other than for observation with orthopedic surgeon, obstetric/gynecologic surgery, cardiovascular surgeon, thoracic surgeon, and neurovascular and/or plastic surgeon
B. Any exposure to trauma/emergency room procedures or responsibilities (more than 10 hr/wk)
C. Exposure to obstetric/gynecology including delivery room responsibilities
D. Exposure to cardiac catheterization laboratory

Class IV: Students currently attending an AAPA-approved physician assistant program

Data from Maginnis and Associates, Inc., Chicago, 1997.

EXHIBIT 11-13

Examples of Full-Time PA Annual Liability Insurance Rates for Different Classes of PA Activities by Geographic Regions (1998)*

	PHYSICIAN ASSISTANT TYPE			
Location	**Class I ($)**	**Class II ($)**	**Class III ($)**	**Class IV ($)**
New York City	1723	3445	4134	138
New York State	1016	2032	2438	85
Houston, Texas	2050	4100	4919	164
Texas (most areas)	1209	2418	2901	101
Tennessee	1209	2418	2901	101
Oregon	1209	2418	2901	101
California	2050	4100	4919	164
District of Columbia	1209	2418	2901	101
Florida, Dade County	2091	4182	5017	167
Florida State	1233	2466	2959	103
Louisiana	1016	2032	2438	85

Data from Maginnis and Associates, Inc., Chicago, 1997.
*Values are based on $1,000,000 professional liability protection for a single occurrence.

can expand access to abortion services, which in 1999 were unavailable in 86% of U.S. counties. After the U.S. Supreme Court declared in *Roe v. Wade* that women had a fundamental right to terminate a pregnancy, most states enacted laws decriminalizing abortion when performed by a physician. Six states (Arizona, Kansas, New Hampshire, Oregon, Vermont, and West Virginia) do not specify that a physician must perform this procedure. At the same time most states define the scope of practice of PAs as the practice of medicine by trained and licensed professionals under the supervision of physicians. Inconsistencies between physician-only abortion laws and PA statutes have generated some confusion in the medical community over whether PAs working under the supervision of physicians can legally perform abortions. Three attorneys examined some of the case studies surrounding abortions and wrote that "any perceived conflict between physicians-only and PA statutes should not preclude PAs from performing this common surgical procedure" (Lieberman and Lalwani, 1994).

With the introduction of mifepristone, an abortifacient that is distributed directly from the manufacturer to medical practitioners, rather than pharmacies, a number of laws came into effect. Missouri and Michigan law prohibits PAs from performing abortions, and a regulation in Tennessee says that PAs may not accept the delegated authority to issue a prescription or dispense any drug or medication whose sole purpose is to cause or perform abortion. The California attorney general in 1991 ruled that the state's physicians-only law precludes PAs from performing abortions, but in New York the health department reached the opposite conclusion. The Rhode Island Department of Health lifted the physicians-only restriction on medical, but not surgical, abortion. The Montana State Supreme Court overturned a law prohibiting PAs from performing abortions in Montana.

In 1997, 3 years before the Food and Drug Administration (FDA) had approved mifepristone, a survey of a nationally representative telephone survey of U.S. obstetricians and gynecologists (OB/GYNs), family practice physicians (FPs), NPs, and PAs. The results were that most health care professionals surveyed considered themselves at least "somewhat familiar" with mifepristone or methotrexate, but few reported being "very familiar" with the methods. OB/GYNs were most familiar with mifepristone (79%), followed by NPs and PAs (73%), and FPs (62%). FPs and NPs and PAs reported being less familiar with methotrexate than with mifepristone. If the FDA approved mifepristone, 54% of OB/GYNs said they would be "very" or "somewhat" likely to prescribe the drug for abortion, including 35% of OB/GYNs who do not perform surgical abortions currently. About half of FPs and NPs and PAs were interested in offering mifepristone if approved by the FDA. Few health professionals reported ever having prescribed methotrexate for abortion (Koenig et al., 2000).

Pitfalls in Physician Assistant Careers

For the PA the opportunity to practice medicine is a limited license (in most states) and governed by a set of rules. The state board of medical examiners usually oversees these rules. While a fair amount is known about the activity and conduct of PAs in certain states, little has been aggregated and compared across states. Some of these issues involve misrepresentation as someone other than a PA (usually a physician), inappropriate prescribing, improper supervision, and other issues.

Through discussion with representatives of state boards of medical examiners or attorneys who either work for the boards or defend PAs, a list of common errors has emerged (Exhibit 11-14). These are offered as the accumulation of wisdom of many people who regulate the activity of PAs and not scientific fact.

Signing a Death Certificate

In Washington State a funeral director or other person in charge of internment may accept a PA signature on a death certificate if the PA was the last person in attendance of the deceased. Washington State law has long allowed PAs to sign death certificates, but the laws governing coroners had not recognized PA signatures as being acceptable.

1998 Medicare Changes

The law allows PAs to see Medicare patients in the office or clinic without the onsite presence of a physician, with reimbursement at 85% of the

EXHIBIT 11-14

Issues That Are Likely to Jeopardize a PA's Career

1. Failure to pay attention to the whole person
   a. Complaint A was addressed, but B was ignored.
   b. The appropriate questions were not asked of the patient.
   c. The patient and the PA each understood the relationship to be different than it was.
   d. The PA terminated the relationship, but the patient did not have any alternative for care.
   e. A romantic or inappropriate relationship was developed between the PA and the patient.
2. Inappropriate or inadequate supervision
   a. A formal relationship with the physician was not maintained.
   b. The physician supervised more PAs than the law allows.
   c. The change of supervising physicians was not formally made or documented.
   d. The board of medical examiners was not informed that the previous supervising physician relationship was terminated.
3. Inappropriate prescribing
   a. Appropriate forms were not completed allowing authorization for the prescriptive privilege.
   b. The PA prescribed a drug that is not considered appropriate for the scope of practice or the clinical basis of the practice.
   c. The PA prescribed for self or for family.
   d. The medical record entry was not made or did not reflect the prescription that was written.
4. Failure to adequately and accurately document in the medical record
   a. The medical record fails to document the care that was given.
   b. The sloppiness of handwriting suggests an indifference to organization and care of the patient to some reviewers (and juries).
   c. The medical record entry is subject to a loose interpretation.
5. Failure to communicate
   a. The perception of the patient or the patient's family was that the provider was rude, impertinent, arrogant, indifferent, or callous.
   b. The PA lies to the patient or family, and it is then discovered that he or she lied intentionally.
   c. The patient or patient's family's concerns or complaints were not acknowledged and documented.
6. Misrepresenting self
   a. The PA does not disclose that he or she is a PA and/or explain what a PA is, if asked.
   b. The PA fails to wear a name tag that distinguishes him or her as a PA.
   c. The PA misrepresents himself or herself as a physician (by calling himself or herself a doctor even if he or she has a doctorate degree).
7. Becoming visible to the board of medical examiners
   a. The PA fails to register an address change or name change.
   b. The PA fails to renew his or her license.
   c. The PA misrepresents (lies) on a state or federal government form.
   d. The PA fails to file paperwork in the required time frame.
8. Failing to stay current with administrative or legislative changes
   a. Legislation can change the law.
   b. The board of medical examiners can change the rules.
   c. The standards of care can change in the community, the state, or even nationally.
9. Failure to know the state laws and rules
   a. The PA must understand the physician assistant licensing act in his or her state.
   b. The PA must understand the physician assistant rules that the board of medical examiners oversees.
   c. The PA must understand the letter and intent of the pharmacy laws, rules, and policies for both prescribers and pharmacists.
10. Boundary violations
   a. The PA mishandles prescriptions, samples, and medication dispensing.
   b. The PA makes careful documentation of interactions with patients that seem seductive or solicitous.
   c. The PA commits alcohol or substance abuse violations.

physician fee schedule, took effect in January 1998. A number of changes affect PAs:

The "incident to" provision is used for office or clinic services delivered by PAs when the physician is onsite. Payment is 100% of the fee schedule. The previous rules that required the physician to personally treat new patients to the practice and established patients with new conditions remain in effect when billing under the "incident to" provision.

EXHIBIT 11-15

Medicare Policy for Physician Assistants

Setting	Supervision requirement	Reimbursement rate	Services
Office/clinic when physician is not onsite	State law	85% of physician's fee schedule	All services PA is legally authorized to provide that would have been covered if provided by a physician
Office/clinic when physician is onsite	Physician must be in the suite or offices	100% of physician's fee schedule	Same as above
Home visit/house call	State law	85% of physician's fee schedule	Same as above
Skilled nursing facility and nursing facility	State law	85% of physician's fee schedule	Same as above
Office or home visit if rural HPSA	State law	85% of physician's fee schedule	Same as above
Hospital	State law	85% of physician's fee schedule	Same as above
First assisting at surgery in all settings	State law	85% of physician's first-assist fee schedule	Same as above
Federal rural health clinic	State law	Cost-based reimbursement	Same as above
HMO	State law	Reimbursement is on capitation basis	All services contracted for as part of an HMO contract

There is no change in the method of billing for services delivered in hospitals, nursing homes, or for first assisting at surgery. The modifier codes that were in place in 1997 remain in effect. The services should be reimbursed at 85%.

Medicare policy affecting PAs are outlined in Exhibit 11-15.

SUMMARY

Statutory changes permitting physicians to use PAs in an innovative manner have been difficult to achieve, and there is a fair amount of discrepancy in state laws among the states. These laws usually indicate the educational qualifications and the dependent nature of the practice. All states indicate the number of PAs who can work at one time under supervision with a physician.

Registration of PAs also varies widely. Some use a registration process while others use a credentialing or licensing process. In some states the process is flexible and general, and in other states the description must be rigidly inclusive of the activities the PA will perform.

Prescribing is a contentious area for some states despite the limited data on safety. Most states now authorize PAs to prescribe in some form, and others are considering improving prescribing laws. In states that allow prescribing by PAs, reports of prescribing violations or problems are almost nonexistent. The empirical evidence suggests that PAs do it frequently and do it well.

The myriad policies and practices related to the services that PAs deliver in American medicine make this a complex and exacting role. However, the profession is attracting more applicants than ever before and attitudes about PAs continue to favor them. Health reform debate in the new millennium continues to discuss the need for primary care providers and inevitably includes PAs and NPs in the formula. Professional issues will continue to arise and then with time settle as PAs prove their worth.

12

PHYSICIAN ASSISTANT ORGANIZATIONS

INTRODUCTION

How physician assistants (PAs) are represented and remain a viable part of the complex U.S. health care environment lies within the organizations that represent the profession. There are four major organizations within the PA profession that have emerged and been established to assume vital functions:

- The American Academy of Physician Assistants (AAPA)
- The Association of Physician Assistant Programs (APAP)
- The National Commission on the Certification of Physician Assistants (NCCPA)
- The Accreditation Review Commission on Education for the Physician Assistant (ARC-PA)

These organizations are influential bodies of members, officers, and full-time staff devoted to the specific mission of each agency. For example, the AAPA looks after members' interests in federal and state legislative activities. The APAP speaks for PA educators and sponsoring institutions to ensure there is dialog between educators, government agencies, and practicing PAs. The NCCPA ensures to the public and health regulatory agencies that PAs meet a standard level of knowledge and have skills necessary for safe and effective clinical practice. Finally, The ARC-PA ensures that PA educational programs meet established standards for accreditation.

THE AMERICAN ACADEMY OF PHYSICIAN ASSISTANTS

Shortly after the second PA class graduated, it became apparent that some form of communication among all PAs was needed and that it was necessary for the fledgling profession to have some form of representation on the national level. The early graduates of Duke decided that an organization was necessary to reach out to all PAs, both students and graduates (Stanhope, 1992). Out of this effort, the AAPA was born in April 1968, and the first newsletter representing the nascent profession was sent to all graduates in 1969. The Medex program was developing in Seattle, Alderson-Broaddus was launching its program, and the Colorado child health associate program was producing graduates. From a group of 15 PAs (founded in a rented trailer in North Carolina) the AAPA organization has grown to a membership that represents more than two thirds of PAs who have ever graduated from a formal educational program (Exhibit 12-1).

The effort to found the first professional organization was not a direct lineage, and there was competition for an institution that could represent all PAs. Sometime after the founding of the AAPA other organizations emerged, aiming to represent and/or provide services to the new profession. These were proprietary membership associations (Ballweg and Wick, 1999):

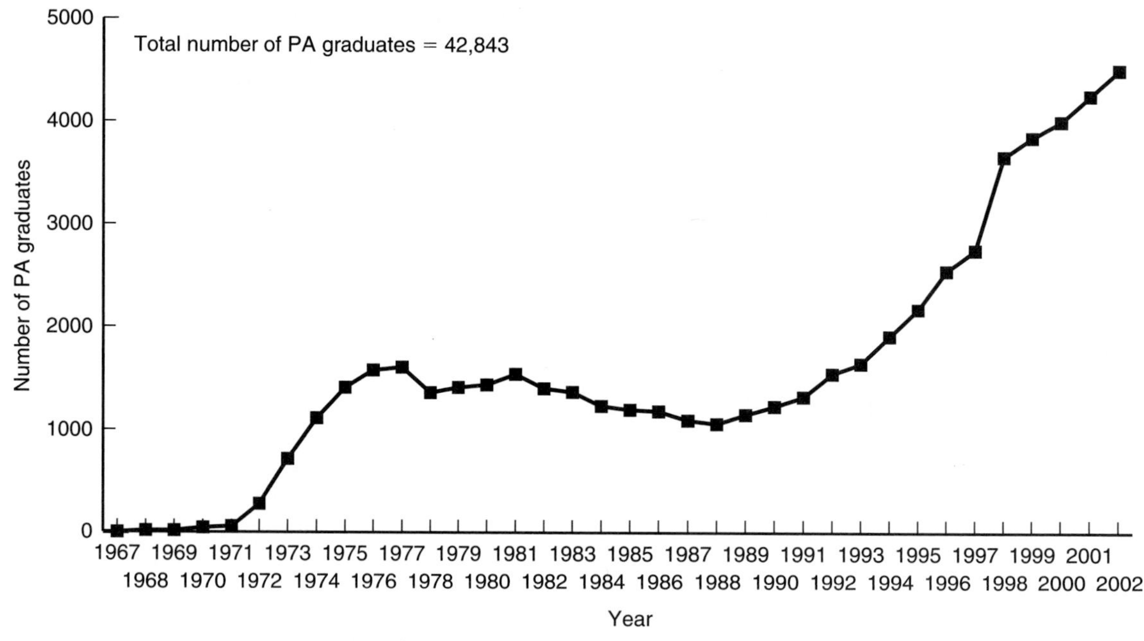

EXHIBIT 12-1 Annual cohort of PA graduates.

- The American Association of Physician Assistants (a group of U.S. Public Health Service PAs at Staten Island Public Health Hospital)
- The National Association of Physician Assistants
- The American College of Physician Assistants (which originated from the Cincinnati Technical College PA program)

In the early 1970s the AAPA and those now-defunct organizations vied for the opportunity to represent all PAs. Newly graduated PAs were asked to join or support one or another organization. Eventually most PAs selected the AAPA, and today it is the only national professional society representing all PAs. The AAPA survived this initial period and prospered in part because of the strong leadership of the newly hired Executive Director, Donald Fisher, PhD, and the support of a number of prominent physicians (Alfred Sadler, Tom Pimme, Joseph Hamberg, and Hu Myers) and the national prominence of its early presidents including Thomas R. Godkins, PA, Carl E. Fasser, PA, and Paul Moson, PA.

Headquartered in Alexandria, Virginia, today the AAPA has grown into a prominent national health professions organization (Exhibits 12-2 and 12-3). The AAPA exists to enhance the role and utilization of PAs; to promote the PA profession to the public; to ensure the competency of PAs through active involvement in continuing education and certification processes; and to promote and conduct research on the PA profession. The academy's mission, reaffirmed by the 1992 House of Delegates, is to promote quality, cost-effective, and accessible health care and to promote the professional and personal development of PAs.

Chapter Structure

The academy is a federated structure of 57 chartered constituent chapters representing the interests of PAs in 50 states, the District of Columbia, Guam, the Air Force, Navy, Army, Public Health Service/Coast Guard, and Veterans Affairs Department. PA educational programs have formed student societies that make up the Student Academy of the American Academy of Physician Assistants (SAAPA).

Purposes and Objectives

Since its founding the AAPA has defined its purposes to include the following:

- Encourage its membership to render quality service to the public

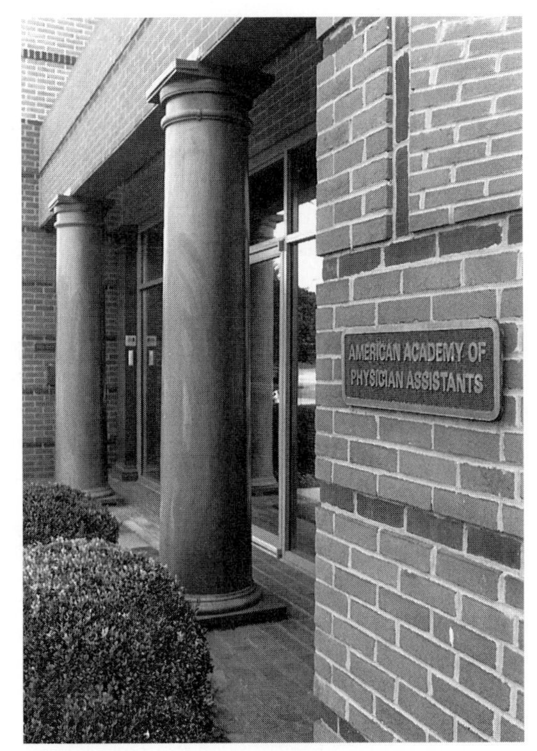

EXHIBIT 12-2 National headquarters. (Courtesy American Academy of Physician Assistants.)

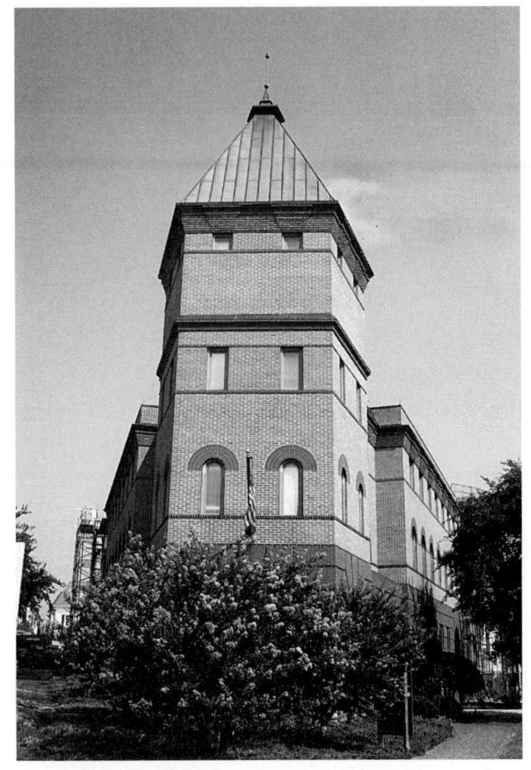

EXHIBIT 12-3 AAPA Building in Alexandria, Virginia. (Courtesy American Academy of Physician Assistants.)

- Develop, sponsor, and evaluate continuing medical education (CME) or medical-related educational programs for the PA
- Assist in the role definition for the PA
- Participate in the development of criteria leading to certification
- Develop, coordinate, and participate in studies having an impact directly or indirectly on the PA profession
- Serve as a public information center to membership, health professions, and the public
- Participate in certification of PAs

The objectives of the Academy include:

- Establishing moral and ethical guidelines for the assurance of continuity in the quality of health care delivery by its members
- Developing CME
- Providing services for members

Governing Bodies

The AAPA House of Delegates meets annually to adopt legislation and policy. The house considers resolutions put forth by its eight standing committees, three councils, the constituent chapters, the Board of Directors, the SAAPA, the APAP, the Surgical Congress, and the Medical Congress. Other affiliates of the AAPA include the Physician Assistant Foundation, which grants scholarships to deserving PA students, and a Political Action Committee, which supports federal candidates supportive of the PA profession, and the SAAPA. The Academy's fellow members and the House of Delegates elect the Board of Directors.

The development of the PA profession and the AAPA were virtually synonymous for the first two decades. PAs are elected as leaders and serve in various roles. The leadership of the AAPA consists of a president, vice president who is also speaker of the House of Delegates, secretary, treasurer, and a Board of Directors. The president and speaker of the house are the most visible of the elected executive board (Exhibit 12-4). The immediate past president serves as chair of the Board of Directors, another visible leader.

The permanent staff is organized under an executive vice president, a chief operating officer, a vice president for member programs, a vice president for governmental and professional affairs, a vice president for information and research services, a vice president for clinical affairs and education, and a vice president for finance and administrative services. Within this framework are a wide variety of technical and professional staff members who deliver an assortment of services for the membership and inquiries (Exhibit 12-5).

Governmental and Professional Assistance

The AAPA is the primary voice in Washington working on behalf of the PA profession. Representing the interests of PAs to public and private policymakers is a vital function of the academy. Consequently it acts as the profession's advocate before federal regulators, policy makers, including the U.S. Congress. The staff of the AAPA provides assistance for policymakers about professional affairs, interprets and comments on proposed or enacted laws or regulations, such as Medicare and Medicaid.

The academy has worked aggressively to improve the regulations of PAs at the state level as well. Through the academy's State Government Affairs Program and its resources, it assists chapters that need help with projects that seek to improve PAs' scope of practice through changes in laws or regulations. This requires a constant monitoring of state legislative activities, the

EXHIBIT 12-4

Leadership of the AAPA

Years	President	Speaker of the house
2003-2004	Pam Scott	
2002-2003	Ina Cushman	Steve Hansen
2001-2002	Edward Friedman	Thomas Lemley
2000-2001	Glen E. Combs	Thomas Lemley
1999-2000	William Kohlhepp	Ina Cushman
1998-1999	Ron L. Nelson	Ina Cushman
1997-1998	Elizabeth Coyte	William C. Kolhepp
1996-1997	Sherrie L. Borden	William C. Kolhepp
1995-1996	Lynn E. Caton	William C. Kolhepp
1994-1995	Debi Atherton Gerbert	M. Randolph Bundschu
1993-1994	Ann L. Elderkin	M. Randolph Bundschu
1992-1993	William H. Marquardt	Debi Atherton Gerbert
1991-1992	Sherri L. Stuart	Debi Atherton Gerbert
1990-1991	Bruce C. Fichandler	Suzanne Reich
1989-1990	Paul Lombardo	Sherri L. Stuart
1988-1989	Marshall R. Sinback, Jr.	Sherri L. Stuart
1987-1988	Ron L. Nelson	Bruce C. Fichandler
1986-1987	R. Scott Chavez	Bruce C. Fichandler
1985-1986	Glen E. Combs	Bruce C. Fichandler
1984-1985	Judith B. Willis	Bruce C. Fichandler
1983-1984	Charles G. Huntington	Burdeen M. Camp
1982-1983	Ron L. Fisher	R. Scott Chavez
1981-1982	Jarrett M. Wise	Charles G. Huntington
1980-1981	C. Emil Fasser	Charles G. Huntington
1979-1980	Ron Rosenberg	John Weed
1978-1979	James E. Konopa	Elaine E. Grant
1977-1978	Dan P. Fox	William Hughes
1976-1977	Roger G. Whittaker	*
1975-1976	Thomas R. Godkins	*
1974-1975	C. Emil Fasser	*
1973-1974	Paul F. Moson	*
1972-1973	John A. Braun	*
1971-1972	Thomas R. Godkins	*
1970-1971	John J. McQueary	*
1969-1970	William D. Stanhope	*
1968-1969	William D. Stanhope	*

Data from American Academy of Physician Assistants, 2002.
*House of Delegates not established until 1977.

EXHIBIT 12-5

Executive Vice President and Staff: AAPA

Name	Tenure	No. of employees
Stephen Crane, PhD	1993-present	86
Harry A. Bradley	1992-1993	46
F. Lynn May	1984-1992	19
Peter D. Rosenstein	1981-1984	5
Donald W. Fisher, PhD	1973-1981	3

Data from American Academy of Physician Assistants.

District of Columbia, and half a dozen territories.

Although it is impossible to list all of the accomplishments of the AAPA, one example may suffice. As the health care reform debate was in the spotlight for much of 1993, the AAPA played an important role in providing timely information to committees about the role PAs play on the health care team. The AAPA provided information to policy makers involved in the health care reform debate. Members of the AAPA were invited to the White House for briefings on health care, and then First Lady Hillary Rodham Clinton confirmed the rising importance of PAs in her address to the AAPA's national convention that year.

Under the academy's Government and Professional Affairs Department the AAPA continues to lobby for Medicare and Medicaid regulations involving PA services in all practice settings. In response to the AAPA's prodding, the *Medicare Carriers Manual* was revised to expand the scope of medical services that PAs can provide. In 1994 a significant advance was gained when the Senate Finance Committee voted for an amendment expanding Medicare coverage for PA services to all outpatient settings at 85% of the physician's reimbursement rate. The 1997 Balanced Budget Act finalized the terms of reimbursement for PA services at 85% of the physician rate in all practice settings.

State activity has always been at the heart of enabling legislation for PAs, and this activity has increased as state legislatures tackle health care reform. To ensure that the PA point of view is heard and understood the AAPA has staff members who work exclusively on state issues. One result of this effort is that PAs can prescribe in almost all states, the District of Columbia, and Guam. In addition, California PAs may write transmittal orders for prescription drugs. A model legislative act for states to enable PAs to function as effectively as possible is contained in Appendix 3. Other services the academy provides include consultation and grants for chapters struggling with improving legislation. Reference materials include *Physician Assistants: State Laws and Regulations,* and the monthly *Legislative Watch.* Other services are a handbook on reimbursement policies and rationales of both private insurers and Medicare.

Constituent Chapter Officers Workshop

The Constituent Chapter Officers Workshop is organized by the AAPA and held in Washington, District of Columbia, every fall. This event helps chapter leaders develop leadership skills, chapter organization, and programming. Leaders also get a chance to meet with their U.S. representatives and senators and national health leaders.

Five regional meetings are held nationwide throughout the year to provide chapter leaders opportunities to network and to meet with leaders of the AAPA.

Publications

A large set of publications is produced by the academy. Many of these are available electronically.

The *Journal of the American Academy of Physician Assistants* is the official clinical journal of the academy. Published monthly by Medical Economics publishing house, it provides news reports, clinical review articles, research reports, a review of research on the PA profession, and other subjects of general interest for the profession. It is sent to all PA graduates, regardless of membership.

AAPA News is published biweekly. It is intended to keep members up-to-date on issues affecting PAs. Information includes updates on legislative and professional affairs, listings of employment, educational programs, data and survey results, and job opportunities.

Research Division

The Research Division performs a number of functions, from internally initiated data collection and analyses to sponsored projects (Exhibit

12-6). The demand for data from the members, leaders, vendors, and government policy analysts is keen because of the highly reliable and remarkably complete databases.

Some of the more important annual surveys conducted by the Research Division are the annual PA census, membership census, the student census, and the conference survey. Individual salary profiles are available to show the compensation range and average salaries of PAs in different areas and different specialties. Outcomes from these studies have improved management capability for the academy, improved revenue, helped promote the profession, helped form strategic alliances, and improved benefit negotiations for PAs.

Education

The annual PA conference is held in late spring in a major city and is attended by more than 9000 PAs. While the main focus is CME, other events include workshops, technical exhibits, interactive computers, and general sessions featuring nationally renowned speakers and academy leaders. Professional exchange draws most participants. Since 2000 research has become a subject of increasing interests to attendees. In 2002 there were over 80 research posters on display.

The first conference was held in 1973 at Sheppard Air Force Base in San Antonio, Texas. A small number of PAs attended, but since then, the annual attendance has continued to climb (Exhibit 12-7). For many PAs this is the one major conference they attend each year. Traditionally the conference spans Memorial Day to honor those serving and have served in the uniformed services.

EXHIBIT 12-6

AAPA Research Division Activity

Internally sponsored or initiated data collection, analysis, and reporting projects
Member census
Census of PA students
Survey of conference preregistrants
Survey of PA programs about applicants
Annual conference evaluation
Market research
Breast and cervical cancer study
Prospective survey of PA students' specialty decision
Survey of demand for advance trauma life support
Pathway II evaluation
Survey to determine no. of practicing PAs
Survey of employment benefits
Surveys regarding member wants, needs, and preferences
Activities to promote and facilitate research by PAs
Data book (historical data on AAPA members)

Data from American Academy of Physician Assistants, Research Division.

Clinical and Scientific Affairs

The academy recognizes the importance of the scientific basis for the clinical practice of PAs and the need to provide more emphasis in activities in this area. To accomplish this goal the academy utilizes the Department of Clinical Affairs and Education, a staff-driven unit, and a Clinical and Scientific Affairs Council. The council identifies and monitors clinical practice and scientific developments related to the practice of medicine as it concerns PAs. Responsibilities include developing reports, issuing papers, and selecting educational documents for the academy.

Continuing Medical Education

The AAPA's Education Council monitors trends in medical education, assesses PA continuing education needs, develops methods to address those needs, develops reports and issues papers regarding educational concerns, and works with the APAP on educational issues.

The AAPA's CME Logging and Reporting Service helps members track CME hours. AAPA members may report their CME hours to the AAPA to log such credits. Beginning in 2004 the NCCPA will exclusively log the required 100 hours of CME.

Public Education

The Public Education Program helps spread information about PAs. Articles about PAs have appeared in major papers and on national television networks. On National PA Day, celebrated each year on October 6, public education activities are spotlighted. Some of these activities include blood drives, food collection and medical education for the homeless, helping people living with acquired immunodeficiency syndrome or human immunodeficiency virus (HIV) infection, and fund-raising for local charities.

EXHIBIT 12-7

List of AAPA National Conferences and Attendance

Yr	Place	Attendance	AAPA CME lectures	Exhibits
2010	–	–	–	–
2009	San Diego, Calif.	–	–	–
2008	San Antonio, Tex.	–	–	–
2007	Philadelphia, Pa.	–	–	–
2006	San Francisco, Calif.	–	–	–
2005	Orlando, Fla.	–	–	–
2004	Las Vegas, Nev.	–	–	–
2003	New Orleans, La.	–	–	–
2002	Boston, Mass.	9120	400	656
2001	Anaheim, Calif.	7346	380	678
2000	Chicago, Ill.	8238	303	673
1999	Atlanta, Ga.	8193	257	652
1998	Salt Lake City, Utah	6200	202	547
1997	Minneapolis, Minn.	6676	304	504
1996	New York, N.Y.	6471	309	342
1995	Las Vegas, Nev.	6817	269	442
1994	San Antonio, Tex.	5349	212	396
1993	Miami, Fla.	4346	201	349
1992	Nashville, Tenn.	4086	219	308
1991	San Francisco, Calif.	3881	187	294
1990	New Orleans, La.	4447	172	248
1989	Washington, D.C.	4513	161	226
1988	Los Angeles, Calif.	3490	159	158
1987	Cincinnati, Ohio	2814	155	208
1986	Boston, Mass.	3813	110	184
1985	San Antonio, Tex.	2864	105	176
1984	Denver, Colo.	2680	115	176
1983	St. Louis, Mo.	2179	75	122
1982	Washington, D.C.	2802	32	145
1981	San Diego, Calif.	1877	29	96
1980	New Orleans, La.	2205	28	103
1979	Hollywood, Fla.	1955	32	88
1978	Las Vegas, Nev.	1940	13	72
1977	Houston, Tex.	1525	21	42
1976	Atlanta, Ga.	1465	5	24
1975	St. Louis, Mo.	765	12	18
1974	New Orleans, La.	525	6	5
1973	Sheppard Air Force Base, Tex.	235	8	1

Data from American Academy of Physician Assistants.

For chapter activities, the academy produces *Fitting in the Pieces,* a public education how-to handbook, distributed to all constituent chapters.

Professional Recognition

The AAPA Academy Awards are the profession's top honors. Awards are given annually to PAs in recognition of the following categories:

- National humanitarian
- International humanitarian
- Rural PA of the year
- Inner city PA of the year
- Outstanding PA of the year
- Public education achievement award
- Educator of the year

Other awards recognize excellence in publishing, public education, and a special honorary membership for those who have made important contributions to the profession.

Professional Practice Council

The Professional Practice Council (PPC) monitors health policy developments in the public and private sectors and writes papers on issues that affect the PA professional practice. The PPC has evaluated and written about the following:

- Stem cell research
- Needle/syringe exchange programs for the prevention of HIV transmission
- Immunization in children and adults
- Hospital privileges and credentialing
- Unlicensed medical graduates
- End-of-life decision making
- Rural health care
- Telemedicine
- Substance abuse disorders
- PAs as Medicaid managed care providers

Generally there is wide agreement among PAs that the AAPA has done a credible job of facilitating and promoting the profession. The PA profession enjoys a relationship with other professional medical organizations that is envied and continues to grow. It has succeeded in winning commission status in all the uniformed services. Medicare reimbursement for PAs has been achieved and continues to improve. The PA profession now enjoys Medicaid reimbursement as fairly standardized in most states. Legislation improving prescribing in most states continues to improve. These efforts have been driven by a sense of what is good for the public and what is good for the profession.

Some believe that with these accomplishments the academy should place more emphasis on the first part of the mission statement, " . . . to promote quality, cost-effective, and accessible health care . . . . " The AAPA has been in the forefront of many public health initiatives including the promotion of Healthy People 2010 (www.health.gov/healthypeople/), promulgated by the surgeon general. At the heart of this document is the goal of access for all people. As the Academy expands its role, it may need to reassess its mission from time to time.

International Affairs

As a result of the increase in interest of PAs to work internationally and the interest among other countries in the PA profession, the AAPA has begun to devote more organizational resources to this area. In 2000 the AAPA formed the International Affairs Committee to serve as a clearinghouse for information on international PA matters. In May 2001 the committee issued a policy statement, *Guidelines for PAs Working Internationally,* which provides guidance for PAs in the international arena:

1. PAs should establish and maintain the appropriate physician-PA team.
2. PAs should accurately represent their skills, training, professional credentials, and identity or service both directly and indirectly.
3. PAs should provide only those services for which they are qualified via their education and/or experiences, and in accordance with all pertinent legal and regulatory processes.
4. PAs should respect the culture, values, beliefs, and expectations of the patients, local health care providers, and the local health care systems.
5. PAs should take responsibility for being familiar with and adhering to the customs, laws, and regulations of the country where they will be providing services.
6. When applicable, PAs should identify and train local personnel who can assume the role of providing care and continuing the education process.

The Physician Assistant Foundation

The PA Foundation seeks to foster the goals and objectives of the academy by supporting the educational and research needs of the profession (Exhibit 12-8). Founded in 1980 as the Education and Research Foundation and later changed to its present name, it is the philanthropic arm of the AAPA. Although most of its activity is focused on scholarships, the foundation does help to support public health services where PAs are involved. Some of this includes free clinics and homeless shelters where PAs provide some of the support staff. The Breitman-Dorn Endowment is an unrestricted grant to assist doctoral students studying the activity of PAs.

ASSOCIATION OF PHYSICIAN ASSISTANT PROGRAMS

The APAP is the national organization representing PA educational programs. The APAP was formed in 1972 for facilitating communication and cooperation among PA programs. The mission of the APAP is to assist PA educational

EXHIBIT 12-8

PA Foundation Presidents

2002-2003	John Byrnes
2001-2002	John Byrnes
2000-2001	Robin Hunter Busky
1999-2000	Robin Hunter Busky
1998-1999	Ann L. Elderkin
1997-1998	Ann L. Elderkin
1996-1997	Paul Lombardo
1995-1996	Paul Lombardo
1994-1995	Lorraine S. Atkinson
1993-1994	Lorraine S. Atkinson
1992-1993	Lorraine S. Atkinson
1991-1992	Lorraine S. Atkinson
1990-1991	J. Jeffrey Heinrich
1989-1990	J. Jeffrey Heinrich
1988-1989	J. Jeffrey Heinrich
1987-1988	James F. Cawley
1986-1987	James F. Cawley
1985-1986	James E. Konopa
1984-1985	Jarrett M. Wise
1983-1984	Jarrett M. Wise
1982-1983	James E. Konopa
1981-1982	James E. Konopa
1980-1981	Noel McFarlane
1979-1980	Donald W. Fisher

Data from American Academy of Physician Assistants.

programs in the instruction of highly educated PAs in numbers adequate to meet society's needs. Specifically the goals of APAP are to do the following:

- Foster faculty development
- Promote excellence within PA programs
- Facilitate research and scholarly activities
- Advocate for PA education
- Maintain and advance the organization

The APAP serves as a resource for individuals and organizations from various professional sectors that are interested in the educational aspects of the PA profession. Critical activities have included the collecting, publishing, and disseminating of information on member programs and their trends and characteristics. The *Annual Report on Physician Assistant Educational Programs in the United States* surveys the activity of PA programs annually. Another activity is to provide effective representation to affiliated organizations involved in health education, health care policy, and the national certification of PA graduates.

Origins

The APAP was founded in 1972 by a group of physicians and concerned PA program faculty who saw a need to address a number of important issues regarding PA education. This consists of accreditation of educational programs, certification, and CME requirements of PAs, and the role delineation of PAs. The overall goal of the APAP is to improve the quality and accessibility of health care through the selection, education, and deployment of PAs. The association shares office space and contracts with the AAPA for management services.

Services

APAP services include two national meetings of PA programs each year: the semiannual meeting in May and the education forum in the fall. It also provides publications, newsletters, consultation services, faculty development and leadership education programs, the systematic collection of pertinent PA program data, and the development of tools to assess and improve the quality of PA education for individuals as well as for programs. The APAP Faculty Development Institute is the umbrella entity that oversees all of the APAP's faculty development initiatives and workshops. A Research Institute oversees all of the APAPs research activities, including the research grant programs and the production of the peer-reviewed journal *Perspective on Physician Assistant Education*.

Governance

The governance of the APAP is a Board of Directors elected by the membership. This consists of a president, president elect, past president, secretary treasurer, director-at-large (two of them), and student president (Exhibit 12-9).

Responsibility for all APAP activities lies with the APAP Board of Directors. The board administers the APAP's financial affairs, appoints standing and ad hoc committees, and conducts all association business between membership meetings. Board members are elected by the APAP member programs. The APAP's day-to-day activities are handled by the APAP staff.

Member Programs

As of 2002 the APAP has 132 member PA educational programs located at various institutions across the United States. All currently accredited programs have elected to join the association.

EXHIBIT 12-9

Presidents of the Association of Physician Assistant Programs	
2003-2004	James F. Cawley, PA, MPH
2002-2003	David Asprey, PA, PhD
2001-2002	Gloria Stewart, PA, EdD
2000-2001	P. Eugene Jones, PA, PhD
1999-2000	Donald Pedersen, PA, PhD
1998-1999	Walter Stein, PA, MHCA
1997-1998	Donald Pedersen, PA, PhD
1996-1997	Dennis Blessing, PA, PhD
1995-1996	James Hammond, MA, PA
1994-1995	Ronald D. Garcia, PhD
1993-1994	Richard R. Rahr, EdD, PA
1992-1993	Anthony A. Miller, MEd, PA
1991-1992	Albert Simon, MEd, PA
1990-1991	Ruth Ballweg, PA, MPA
1989-1990	Steven Shelton, MBA, PA
1988-1989	Suzanne Greenberg, MS
1987-1988	Jesse Edwards, MS
1986-1987	Jack Liskin, MA, PA
1985-1986	Carl Fasser, PA, MS
1984-1985	Denis Oliver, PhD
1983-1984	Robert Curry, MD, MPH
1982-1983	Stephen Gladhart, EdD
1981-1982	Reginald Carter, PhD, PA
1980-1981	David Lewis, EdD
1979-1980	Thomas Godkins, PA, MPH
1978-1979	Archie Golden, MD, MPH
1977-1978	Frances Horvath, MD
1976-1977	C. Hilmon Castle, MD
1975-1976	Robert Jewett, MD
1974-1975	Thomas Piemme, MD
1973-1974	Alfred Sadler, Jr., MD

Data from Association of Physician Assistant Programs.

Only PA programs accredited by the ARC-PA, or its predecessor or successor organizations, are eligible for full program membership. Several yet to be accredited programs have also chosen to affiliate with the association as "colleagues of APAP."

Activities

The APAP aims to promote communication among PA educational programs and faculty. The organization has formed special institutes to support activities particularly vital to the typical activities of PA program faculty. Some of these activities include:

- The Research Institute was established in 1996 as an organizational means to promote and fund research proposals that aim to explore topics pertaining to the conduct and process of PA education.
- The Faculty Development Institute, which was founded in 1997, presents and promotes educational sessions to expand and enrich the skills of PA educators.
- The Centralized Application Service for PA Applicants (CASPA) was instituted in 2001 by the APAP. This service, developed in partnership with the Association of Colleges of Osteopathic Medicine, offers applicants a convenient web-based application service that allows applicants to apply to any number of participating PA educational programs by completing a single application.

Postgraduate Physician Assistant Programs

While not one of the four major organizations of the PA profession, an important component of PA education involves postgraduate PA educational programs. In 1988 a small group of postgraduate PA programs met to formalize a national postgraduate PA program organization. The Association of Postgraduate Physician Assistant Programs (APPAP) was formed to further specialty education for PAs. Since its founding the APPAP has gained the support of the AAPA and the APAP. A liaison representative of the APPAP now sits on the APAP Board of Directors, and APPAP members work with the AAPA and APAP on mutual goals designed to expand the PA profession. Member programs of the APPAP include those formal postgraduate PA programs that offer structured curricula, including didactic and clinical components, designed to educate NCCPA eligible/certified PAs for a defined period (usually 12 months) in a medical specialty. APPAP member programs follow several models including fellowships, master's degree programs, and residency programs. All APPAP member programs must award a certificate or degree or provide graduate academic credit. The APPAP's educational, professional, and informational purposes include the following:

- Assisting in the development and organization of postgraduate educational curricula and programs for PAs
- Assisting in defining the role of the PA, particularly in the specialties

- Assisting in the development of evaluation methodologies for postgraduate educational curricula and programs
- Serving as an information center for PAs, programs training PAs at the entry level, other medical and health care disciplines, and to the public with respect to postgraduate educational curricula and programs for PAs

THE NATIONAL COMMISSION ON CERTIFICATION OF PHYSICIAN ASSISTANTS

After a formal education and training in an accredited program the final stage in the professional preparation of a PA involves the national certification process. The PA credentialing process represents a distinct aspect of the evolution of PA profession systems and represents one different from most patterns observed in other nonphysician health professions. The development of a single respected system of national certification and recertification for PAs is considered an asset of the profession.

The NCCPA, founded in 1975, is the public organization that exists as the only credentialing organization for PAs in the United States. As of 2002, the NCCPA has certified more than 43,000 PAs. The mission of the NCCPA is to ensure the public and others that PAs credentialed by the NCCPA meet established standards of knowledge and clinical skills upon entry into practice and throughout their careers.

The NCCPA administers two national examinations used by state medical licensing boards. Both the Physician Assistant National Certification Examination (PANCE) and the Physician Assistant National Recertification Examination (PANRE) are developed under contract from the NCCPA to the National Board of Medical Examiners (NBME).

Other NCCPA functions include the following:

- Establishing eligibility requirements for the PANCE and PANRE
- Establishing standards for the examinations
- Issuing and verifying certificates
- Reregistering and recertifying PAs who meet CME and reexamination requirements
- Initial certification through the PANCE is required for PA licensure in all states and U.S. medical jurisdictions including the District of Columbia and U.S. territories

Most states require an NCCPA certificate to be licensed or to prescribe; at least half of the states require a current NCCPA certificate for license renewal.

History

The NCCPA arose as a result of the need for an independent agency to certify the level of preparation of the PA graduate for clinical practice. It was acknowledged that because program accreditation is not an infallible science, an additional mechanism to ensure a minimal level of clinical competence should be established. In 1971 the Division of Associated Health Professions of the U.S. Department of Health, Education, and Welfare (DAHP/DHEW), along with the Kellogg Foundation, set out to develop a certifying examination. This activity was later funded through the NBME and was first known as the National Certifying Examination for the Assistant to the Primary Care Physician.

Almost in parallel fashion with developing a national examination for PAs, key physicians within the American Medical Association (AMA) led the effort to develop an independent certifying agency. Thus with the participation and support of the professions then young representative organizations (the AAPA and APAP), with the backing of the federal government and funding from the Kellogg Foundation, the NCCPA was founded.

The Certifying Examination for Assistants to the Primary Care Physician, developed by the NBME, was first administered in December 1973. A number of new health practitioner programs, such as certain nurse practitioner, nurse clinician, and child health associate programs, were gaining momentum, as were Medex, physician associate, and PA programs. Graduates of most of these programs were eligible to take the initial PA certifying examination. Eligibility to those who had not graduated from a formal program was extended to these PAs to allow qualifying as PAs under a grandfather clause. From 1974 through 1985 the NCCPA entry-level certifying examination was open to informally trained PAs who met certain eligibility criteria such as prior clinical experience working in a PA-like role.

Only a few hundred took the examination. With this in mind the AMA and the NBME worked to bring together representatives of a number of medical organizations to form a freestanding independent commission. By 1973 they established the commission as an organization to ensure employers, state boards, and patients that a standard related to the competency of PAs was in place. In 1975 the NCCPA was chartered with headquarters in Atlanta, Georgia. The first executive director of the NCCPA, David Glazer (1973 to 1996), and Thomas Piemme, MD, the first president of the NCCPA (1974), played pivotal roles in establishing the legitimacy of the NCCPA and its certifying examinations among state medical licensing boards. The Board of Directors of the NCCPA comprises representatives from the PA professional organizations (the AAPA and APAP) and major medical organizations. Organizations include the American College of Physicians-American Society of Internal Medicine, American Academy of Family Physicians, the AMA, the American Academy of Pediatrics, the American College of Emergency Medicine, the American College of Surgeons, and the American Osteopathic Association. Additional organizations such as the Federation of State Medical Boards, major employers of PAs such as the Department of Defense, the Veterans Administration, and the American Hospital Association, and the public are included as representatives.

Physician Assistant National Certification Examination

The PANCE, the PANRE, and the Pathway II examination are administered by the NCCPA. These examinations assess essential knowledge and skills of PAs in conducting a variety of health care functions normally encountered in practice. The PANCE consists of 300 standardized questions developed by the NBME and is taken by nearly all PA educational program graduates. Since 2000 it has been administered on computer, and in 2002 over 5000 sat for the PANCE.

Content specifications for NCCPA examinations were developed and validated, in part through use of role delineation studies. The first study was conducted by the NBME in the early 1970s. Subsequently these studies were by the AAPA in 1979 and 1985. Several test-writing committees generate test questions for the PANCE, Pathway II, and the PANRE; test-writing committee members are appointed by the NCCPA and staffed by the NBME. Committee makeup includes physicians and PAs, employed in both academic and clinical settings, including the primary care and clinical specialties. Test committees meet regularly to develop the content for each examination. Committees review the previous year's examination performance, finalize the current examination blueprint, and make assignments for and prepare new test items. In 1995 the number of certifying examinations administered totaled 2913, with 2272 attaining certification. The failure rate was 22%, with 641 candidates unsuccessful in reaching the pass/fail score level. In 2001 there were 4267 first-time PANCE takers who had a 91.5% pass rate (Exhibit 12-10).

The NCCPA content blueprint list is a primary reference for identifying the clinical problems the PA should be prepared to encounter in a typical primary care practice and is reflected in the PANCE, Pathway II, and PANRE. This outline of the organ systems/medical specialties was compiled using various sources including data from the National Ambulatory Medical Care Survey and the National Hospital Discharge Survey (Exhibit 12-11).

To further establish the validity of the three NCCPA examinations the organization periodically conducts an occupational analysis. The 1998 PA Practice Analysis project provided the fundamental basis of the content blueprint used in current NCCPA certifying and recertifying examinations (Cawley et al., 2001). This analysis lists the tasks and essential knowledge and skills that are representative of the actual clinical practice roles, specific tasks and knowledge, skills, and abilities required of PAs. The results of this study identified that the knowledge and skills rated most highly by practicing PAs were as follows:

- Skill in identifying pertinent physical findings
- Knowledge of signs and symptoms of medical conditions
- Skill in recognizing conditions that constitute medical emergencies
- Skill in performing physical examinations
- Skill in conducting a patient interview

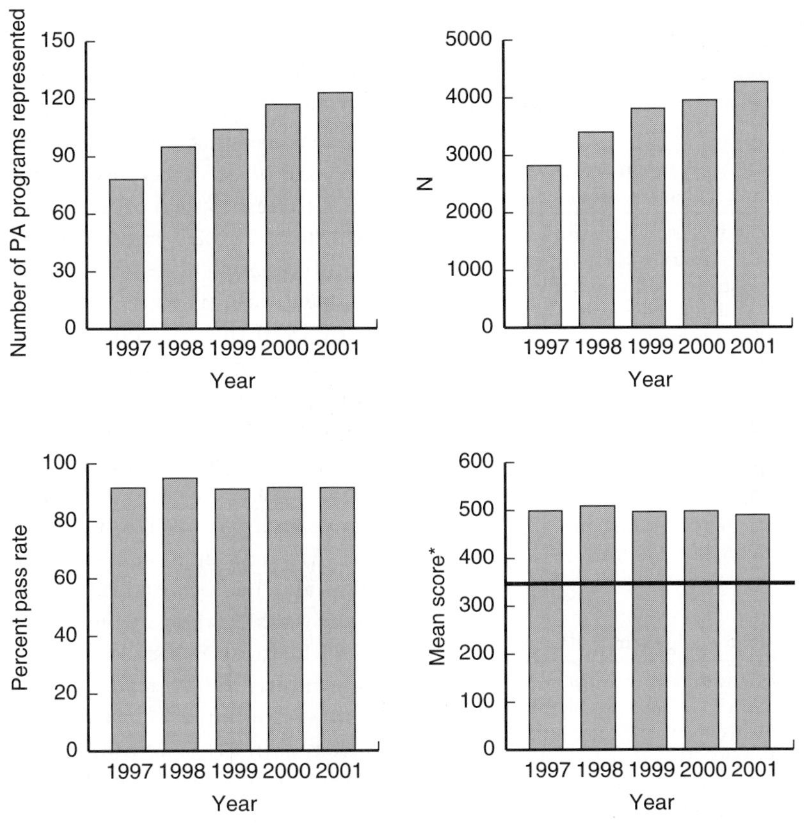

EXHIBIT 12-10 Physician Assistant National Certification Examination annual scores. (Data from Hooker RS, Hess B, Cipher D: *Perspectives on Physician Assistant Education,* 2002.)

- Skill in associating current complaints with presenting history and identifying pertinent factors
- Knowledge of physical examination directed to a specific condition
- Skill in effective communication

The practice analysis study by Cawley and colleagues (2001) found few differences in the tasks performed by PAs based on the length of time worked in the profession. Some response patterns differed across specialties, particularly in the areas of cardiovascular/thoracic surgery, general surgery, and orthopedic surgery. However, and perhaps more importantly, PAs engage in tasks essential for clinical practice. Consistently high ratings were observed in the domains considered being the essential functions of PA clinicians: history taking and physical diagnosis. PAs place great value on additional skills required in the practice of clinical medicine: diagnostic acumen and judgment and knowledge in the development of an effective management plan. The consistency and high ratings of these findings suggest that there are central cores of medical knowledge, tasks and skills valued that are performed often and consistently by practicing PAs. This core of knowledge and skills appears to apply to virtually all specialties and settings (Exhibit 12-12).

Despite that nearly half of all PAs work in primary care specialties, PAs engage in a wide variety of specialized practice activities, and the data suggest individual differences in the specific clinical interventions and procedures performed by PAs in different practice settings. PAs across the country perform procedures in widely varied practice domains, but it is clear that not all PAs perform the same procedures in all areas. PAs rated the knowledge and skills required for clinical procedures and interventions as important in effective clinical practice (Cawley et al., 2001).

EXHIBIT 12-11

Examination Content, PANCE and PANRE, by Percentage of Organ System Diseases, Disorders, and Medical Assessment Areas, and by Knowledge and Skill Areas

% of examination content	Diseases, disorders, and medical assessment
16	Cardiovascular system
12	Pulmonary system
10	Gastrointestinal/nutritional system
10	Musculoskeletal system
9	Eye, ear, nose, and throat
8	Reproductive system
6	Endocrine system
6	Neurologic system
6	Psychiatric/behavioral system
6	Renal/urinary system
5	Dermatologic
3	Hematologic system
3	Infectious diseases
100%	

% of examination content	Knowledge and skill areas
18	Clinical therapeutics
18	Formulating most likely diagnosis
16	History taking and performing physical examinations
14	Clinical intervention
14	Using laboratory and diagnostic studies
10	Applying scientific concepts
10	Health maintenance
100%	

Modified from National Commission on Certification of Physician Assistants: *NCCPA Examination Content Blueprint*, Atlanta, Ga., 2002.

EXHIBIT 12-12

Domains of Knowledge Deemed Most Important by PAs, Rank Ordered

1. Subjective data gathering
2. Assessment
3. Objective data gathering
4. Formulate and implement a plan
5. Clinical intervention procedures
6. Health promotion and disease prevention
7. Ancillary professional responsibilities

Modified from Cawley JF, Andrews MD, Barnhill GC, et al.: *J Am Acad Physician Assist* 14:41-42, 44, 47-50, 55-56, 2001.

PANRE and Recertification

In an effort to ensure career-long accountability the NCCPA developed a two-part program, consisting of certificate reregistration every 2 years, based on the acquisition of appropriate hours of CME, and the policy of recertification using the PANRE by examination every 6 years. To maintain NCCPA certification and retain the right to use the designation PA-certified (PA-C) beyond the date of certificate expiration, PAs must follow a three-pronged process, involving documentation of CME, submission of registration materials, and successful completion of a recertification examination.

In 1980 the NCCPA administered the entry-level examination for the purposes of recertification. This recertification was in part designed to identify any content areas that penalize people working in specialty practices to help identify the "core" area to be tested by a separate recertification examination. The recertification examination was developed as a separate examination in 1984 and has been administered ever since. For many years there was a high rate of passage of the PANRE; most PAs passed the examination and were recertified on that basis. Based on NCCPA policy adopted in 1998, failure of the PANRE once requires that an individual retake the examination; only 50 persons have failed the PANRE twice.

The NCCPA established a policy that every 2 years all certified PAs must submit documentation logging 100 hours of CME. The concept of certificate maintenance is based on the ongoing acquisition of new medical knowledge obtained through attendance at formal CME sessions and periodic recertification examinations. A noted feature of the PA profession is the recertification process. It was determined in 1980 that every 6 years was an appropriate time to retest individuals on their basic medical knowledge. The intent was to ensure the public that PAs are keeping abreast of the core knowledge to practice medicine.

The PANRE comprises 300 multiple-choice questions. In 2001 more than 4500 examinees took the PANRE, and 96% of examinees passed the examination. Fulfilling requirements for NCCPA certification must be accomplished within 6 years after passing the most recent NCCPA examination.

Pathway II

An alternative mechanism for meeting NCCPA recertification requirements grew out of an

AAPA-NCCPA partnership begun in 1992. Pathway II is another recertification process administered by the NCCPA since 1997. As an alternative to the traditional PANRE, Pathway II consists of a take-home examination plus an elective component and was developed in response to the needs of PAs who specialize in a particular medical field. The elective component is divided into nine categories of educational and experiential activities.

Controversies

The NCCPA, and in particular the NCCPA recertification examination, has been the subject of substantial criticism from the PA profession during the late 1980s and early 1990s expressed in statements and resolutions of the AAPA House of Delegates. In particular, the NCCPA policy related to those PAs who fail the PANRE twice has been a topic of intense debate within the profession. The implications of this policy for those PAs practicing in the states requiring valid certification as a condition of licensure are significant. This NCCPA policy was known as "endpointing" because it defined the final consequences for those PAs who failed PANRE twice. Under endpointing, such PAs lose their certification and must take and pass one of the three NCCPA examinations to regain certification status. There have been questions raised on the uses and predictors of success on the PANCE. PA educators are curious regarding candidate performance on the NCCPA examinations and the implications of these findings on adult learners for the recertification process. For example, is there a correlation between the academic degree received in PA education and the likelihood of passing the PANCE?

One older study suggested that the NCCPA examination may need reevaluation because students without academic degrees and those with associate degrees who complete the PA program pass the NCCPA examination at a higher percentage than those with baccalaureate and graduate degrees. The study sample was nonrepresentative; it was suggested that the discrepancy observed could indicate a cultural bias in the NCCPA examination (Carter, 2000). Hooker, Hess, and Cipher (2002) looked at the correlation between PA training at the graduate level and performance on the PANCE and found that students who have graduated from a master's degree program on average do slightly better on the PANCE than those in a certificate or baccalaureate degree program. Nor could they find any other characteristics of programs (size, private, medical school association, duration) or characteristics of students (age, gender) that correlated with pass rates.

Specialty testing is a broad issue facing the profession, its representative organizations, and the NCCPA. Because specialization is a natural evolution in most health care professions, greater numbers of PAs are working in specialty practices. PAs representing specialty and subspecialty groups have spoken openly of the desire to have some form of recognition. Thus far, other than the NCCPA examination in surgery, there are no examinations in specialties for PAs. Some regard the NCCPA requirements regarding certificate maintenance using periodic recertification as a frustrating and time-consuming requirement. Yet PAs must be mindful of the legitimacy derived from the profession's willingness to have a recertification by examination system.

In 2001 a clash between the NCCPA and the AAPA occurred over the matter of who should be given the authority to log CME credits required for certificate maintenance. For many years the NCCPA extended to the AAPA the opportunity to log CME credits for its members. The NCCPA determined that it should be the sole agency to log CME credits, because the NCCPA defines the requirements for certificate maintenance.

THE ACCREDITATION REVIEW COMMISSION ON EDUCATION FOR THE PHYSICIAN ASSISTANT

The ARC-PA is the recognized accrediting agency that protects the interests of the public and the PA profession by defining the standards for PA education and evaluating PA educational programs within the territorial United States to ensure their compliance with those standards. It was initially formed as a component of the AMA's Committee on Allied Health Education and Accreditation (CAHEA), a national allied health professions accrediting entity. Later the CAHEA was transformed into a more independent agency, the Commission on Accreditation of

EXHIBIT 12-13

Accreditation Committee/Commission History Time Line

Date	Action
May 28, 1971	The development of the *Essentials of an Accredited Educational Program for the Assistant to the Primary Care Physician* was undertaken by the American Medical Association (AMA) Subcommittee of the Council on Medical Education's Advisory Committee on Education for Allied Health Professions and Services. The subcommittee included representatives from the American Academy of Family Physicians (AAFP), American Academy of Pediatrics (AAP), American College of Physicians (ACP), American Society of Internal Medicine (ASIM), American Medical Association (AMA), and Association of American Medical Colleges (AAMC). The *Essentials* prepared by the subcommittee were approved by those organizations.
1971	The AMA House of Delegates Committee on Medical Education adopted the *Essentials*, clearing the way for the approval of educational programs that met or exceeded these requirements.
1971	Organizational meeting of the then-titled Joint Review Committee for Educational Programs for the Assistant to Primary Care Physician (JRC-PA) was held.
1972	The first formal meeting of the JRC-PA was convened.
	The JRC-PA made its first accreditation recommendations to the AMA.
1973	The American College of Surgeons (ACS) adopted *Essentials for an Educational Program for the Surgeon's Assistant.* Originally the ACS Committee on Allied Health Personnel reviewed applicant programs' compliance with the *Essentials.*
	The JRC-PA added three graduate PAs as members-at-large for 1-yr terms.
1974	The sponsors of the JRC-PA and the AMA recognized the American Academy of Physician Assistants (AAPA) as the fifth sponsor of the JRC-PA.
1975	The ACS became a sponsor of the JRC-PA.
1976	The review committees for primary care PAs and for surgeon's assistants were merged into the Joint Review Committee on Educational Programs for Physician Assistants.
	The AMA House of Delegates voted to delegate its responsibility for adoption of proposed educational standards (also known as *Essentials*) to the AMA Council on Medical Education and authorized the transfer of responsibility for accreditation from the AMA Council on Medical Education to its Committee on Allied Health Education and Accreditation (CAHEA).
	This new committee was a modification of the council's former Advisory Committee on Allied Health Education. These changes were instituted to achieve complete compliance with the U.S. Office of Education criteria for national accrediting agencies. The CAHEA was designed to represent communities of interest for which accreditation actions were taken. The CAHEA was composed of representatives of allied health professions, medicine, the Council on Medical Education, and the public.
1978	The JRC-PA sponsors recognized the Association of Physician Assistant Programs (APAP) as the seventh sponsor of the JRC-PA.
1981	The ASIM withdrew its sponsorship of the JRC-PA.
1982	The sponsoring organizations reduced their representation from three to two members each, except for the AAPA, which continued to have three representatives.
1988	The JRC-PA was renamed the Accreditation Review Commission on Education for the Physician Assistant (ARC-PA).
1991	The AMA requested that administrative responsibility for the ARC-PA be undertaken by another sponsoring organization.
	The AAPA accepted administrative responsibility for the ARC-PA. The corporate offices of the ARC-PA were established in Marshfield, Wisconsin.
1994	The CAHEA was dissolved, and accreditation activities were transferred to a new, independent agency, the Commission on Accreditation of Allied Health Education Programs (CAAHEP).
	The AMA became the seventh sponsoring organization of the ARC-PA.
1995	The ARC-PA approved the addition of a third representative from the APAP.
	The ARC-PA was incorporated.
1996	A study was initiated to determine the feasibility of the ARC-PA withdrawing from the CAAHEP system and establishing itself as a freestanding accrediting agency.
1998	The ASIM returned as a sponsor of the ARC-PA when the association merged with the ACP.
2000	The members of the ARC-PA voted to become a freestanding accrediting agency.
January 1, 2001	The Accreditation Review Commission on Education for the Physician Assistant (ARC-PA) began operation.
	Commission awards accreditation under the new agency.

Modified from J. McCarty, ARC-PA, Personal communication, February 19, 2002.

Allied Health Education Programs (CAAHEP), which was separate from the AMA. In 2001 the ARC-PA became a freestanding accrediting agency (www.arc-pa.org).

In accomplishing its mission to set standards for PA educational programs, the ARC-PA is composed of a number of representatives. These representatives include the American Academy of Family Physicians, the AAPA, the American College of Physicians–the American Society of Internal Medicine, the American College of Surgeons, the AMA, the APAP, and a member of the public. The ARC-PA appoints site visitors, reviews applications for accreditation, and determines accreditation actions. As an agency to ensure public trust, the ARC-PA encourages excellence in PA education through its accreditation process by establishing and maintaining minimum standards of quality for educational programs. It awards accreditation to programs through a peer-review process that includes documentation and periodic site visit evaluation to substantiate compliance with the Accreditation Standards for Physician Assistant Education. The accreditation process is designed to encourage sound educational experimentation and innovation and to stimulate continuous self-study and improvement.

In addition to establishing educational standards and fostering excellence in PA programs, the ARC-PA provides information and guidance to individuals and organizations regarding PA program accreditation and makes public its accreditation actions (Exhibit 12-13).

SUMMARY

As the PA profession grew and matured, a number of organizations arose to represent the various components of the profession. Each of these organizations, in turn, underwent their own maturation process. As of the new millennium, each organization is well established, has a defined domain, and a relationship with the other three organizations, as well as a constituency to which it reports. Each organization in turn contributes to the organizational efficiency of the profession as a whole.

13

FEDERAL EMPLOYEES

INTRODUCTION

The federal government is the largest employer of physician assistants (PAs). As of 2002 approximately 12% of all employed PAs have a professional relationship with the U.S. government. They serve in the U.S. Armed Forces, Veterans Affairs, Bureau of Prisons (BOP), U.S. Public Health Service (e.g., National Institutes of Health, Indian Health Service), and other federal agencies. The vast majority of federally employed PAs are in primary care services, and most work in positions previously occupied by a physician. Exact numbers are difficult to determine because many agencies and branches of the federal government, including the military, are constantly undergoing staffing changes. Today approximately 1150 uniformed PAs are on active duty and 1200 are in the Veterans Administration (VA) (Exhibit 13-1). Because a federal registry of health care workers is not available, these figures are based on communication with employees in different departments and branches of the federal government.

MILITARY

As of 2002 approximately 1150 PAs are on active duty in the military worldwide. They are on land and sea or in the air, with many in special hardship situations. In addition, approximately 500 or so PAs are employed in civilian practices who also serve in the Ready Reserves and National Guard in 50 states and four territories (Salyer, 2002). Outside these figures are the many nonuniform (civilian) PAs on contract with military branches and federal agencies.

Unlike most civilian PAs the majority of military PAs have been medical corpsmen, and most received their training in the military. PAs in the military also tend to be men, train at an older age than their civilian counterparts, and remain in primary care. Job characteristics tend to differ as well: Level of responsibility is slightly higher and closeness of supervision is lower for the military PA than for the civilian PA.

The history of the PA movement is anchored with the medic and corpsman. Many of the first PAs were the returned veteran who attended the early PA programs in the 1960s and 1970s (Hooker, 1991a). While most remained in civilian attire a few donned the uniform again and returned to the military. All PAs in the uniformed services are commissioned officers.

The PA as a form of medical officer was introduced in the Army, Navy, and Air Force in 1971 and in the Coast Guard in 1975 (Stuart, Robinson, and Reed, 1973; Hooker, 1991b; Gwinn and Keller, 1999). Initially, all were noncommissioned officers, usually with senior enlisted rank. Throughout the 1970s their ranks swelled. The primary reason PAs took hold in the military was largely in response to the termination of the draft for physicians (Gaudry and Nicholas, 1977). Once obligated service was removed for physicians (after the abolishment of the draft for military duty for men), those with little time invested in the military as a career tended to leave. In fact this was largely a wholesale departure of junior physicians from the

EXHIBIT 13-1

Federally Employed PAs, 2002*

Branch	Active duty	Billets†
Department of Defense		
U.S. Navy (including Marines)	235	275
U.S. Army	600	517
U.S. Air Force	330	320
Department of Transportation		
U.S. Coast Guard	30	30
Federal Aviation Administration	1	2
National Oceanic and Atmospheric Administration	3	3
Department of Justice		
Bureau of Prisons	654	724
Immigration and Naturalization Service	30	40
Department of Health and Human Services		
U.S. Public Health Service	88	100
Indian Health Service	30	60
Food and Drug Administration	2	—
Centers for Disease Control and Prevention	4	—
National Institutes of Health	6	—
Health Service Resource Administration	2	—
National Health Service Corps	36	40
Department of Veterans Affairs	**1200**	**1200**

*Data derived from various personal sources in the different agencies and branches, 2002. The numbers are likely to be different at the time of printing.
†A billet means an available position. These are fluid positions subject to change.

military and a medical staffing vacuum was created. Not surprisingly the services found it difficult to recruit physicians. With peacetime military and a need for medical officers the military turned to PAs as a logical alternative (Hooker, 1989). PAs filled the medical officer gap then and remain at high levels of visibility today.

One of the more interesting footnotes in the evolution of the military PA is the commissioning of PAs. While almost all hold a commissioned officer status, this was not always so. The first PAs were from the enlisted ranks. PAs were the medics, the corpsmen, or allied health personnel who matriculated through a formal PA training program (Amann, 1973). In the early 1970s their rank status was changed from *enlisted* to *warrant officer* to reflect their more technical skills and to avoid conflicts when directing services that involved officers (Hooker, 1989). In April 1978 the U.S. Air Force (USAF) promoted enlisted PAs to commissioned officer status. This accession was considered consistent with the skill and responsibility of an officer. It also took place because the Air Force warrant officer program was discontinued (in 1958) and this warrant officer structure was not an option. This left the Army, Navy, and Coast Guard PAs as warrant officers, in contrast to the commissioned officers in the Air Force. As a consequence, a discrepancy in rank, status, and career earnings for military pay emerged that was in stark contrast to the uniformity of rank, pay, and hierarchy of physicians, nurses, dentists, pharmacists, and physical therapists in the military. For a 20-year career the USAF PA was making 25% more than his or her professional peer was in the Army (Hooker, 1989). This disparity became more apparent after economic research revealed the significant differences commissioning could mean for recruitment and retention. After some intense lobbying by the American Academy of Physician Assistants (AAPA) legislative representatives, work by the PA leaders in the different services in the AAPA, PAs in and out of uniform, and some congressional help, the surgeon generals of the different services eventually commissioned for all military PAs (those in the Navy and the Coast Guard in 1990 and those in the Army in 1992). With the commissioning of the Coast Guard Reserve as the final step achieved in 1992, the AAPA could move on to other professional issues.

There is a strong kinship between the military and PAs. As Assistant Surgeon General Moritsugu said to a group of Army PAs in 1994, "You are the germ plasm of all PAs." The first PA student class at Duke University was made up of four Navy veterans, all hospital corpsmen (Condit, 1993). Subsequent classes at Duke and other programs were made up primarily of military veterans, many with Vietnam experience (Hooker, 1991a). For the first 10 years, most PA graduates were veterans.

With the exception of medics, technicians, and corpsmen coming up through the ranks, the number of civilian-trained PAs entering the military is not very large. At one time, all of the services used their own military schools. To meet demand at different times, some military branches contracted with civilian schools to train military PAs. This took place with the Army at the St. Francis University Master of Medical Science PA program, the Coast Guard at Duke University, and the Navy at The George Washington University in Washington, D.C. In 1996 federal budget cuts forced the Department of Defense to consolidate its military training programs. Mixed classes of PA students from the Army, Navy, Air Force, Coast Guard (and at one time the Federal BOP) now train at the interservice PA training program at Fort Sam Houston in San Antonio, Texas, the site of the former Army PA program. The student selection process is the responsibility of each individual service.

The role of the PA in the military has been enhanced in a number of ways, beginning with deployment during international engagements since Vietnam, Panama, the Gulf War, Somalia, Haiti, Bosnia, Afghanistan, and many other places (Exhibit 13-2). PAs have been an integral part of combat-ready troops in the Army, Navy, Air Force, Marines, and Coast Guard. They also serve in the White House, the Pentagon, the office of the Surgeon General, and in a number of policy development positions. Currently the highest-ranking military PA is a colonel. A flag rank for a PA is now considered attainable.

The military has a number of domestic roles for PAs including Reserve and National Guard units. Sometimes these units are called up in times of disasters such as floods, tornadoes, hurricanes, and wild fires. Many reservists including PAs were called up after the September 2001 terrorist attack on the World Trade Center in New York City. Sometimes PAs serve in reserve units that have special missions such as medical units, prisoner of war units, and harbor defense.

EXHIBIT 13-2

Major Military Campaigns That Deployed PAs
Grenada (Operation Urgent Fury)
Panama (Operation Just Cause)
Gulf War: Iraq and Kuwait (Operation Desert Storm/Shield)
Northern Iraq, relief to Kurdish refugees (Operation Provide Comfort)
Balkans: Bosnia, Kosovo (Operation Joint Guard)
Somalia
Macedonia
Afghanistan
Other

Historically the military has always provided an opportunity for enlisted members to expand their medical training and skills while moving up a career ladder. At the turn of the new century the military needs for PAs may be greater than before. Broad-based missions on different fronts require more medical services than when they are concentrated stateside. To expand the applicant pool the services allow officers enlisted from other career tracks to apply.

Air Force

The Air Force has approximately 330 PAs on active duty, serving principally in primary care and family practice clinics (Exhibit 13-3). The PAs in the Air Force enjoy strong support from the highest levels of the Air Force medical command. They are part of the Biological Sciences Corps. A small number of Air Force PAs also have opportunities in orthopedics, head and neck surgery, emergency medicine, bone marrow transplant/oncology, and cardiac perfusion.

At one time the Air Force had its own PA program located at Sheppard Air Force Base in Wichita Falls, Texas, which has now been integrated in the interservice PA program at Fort Sam Houston, San Antonio, Texas. Air Force PAs derive from the interservice program and direct civilian recruitment.

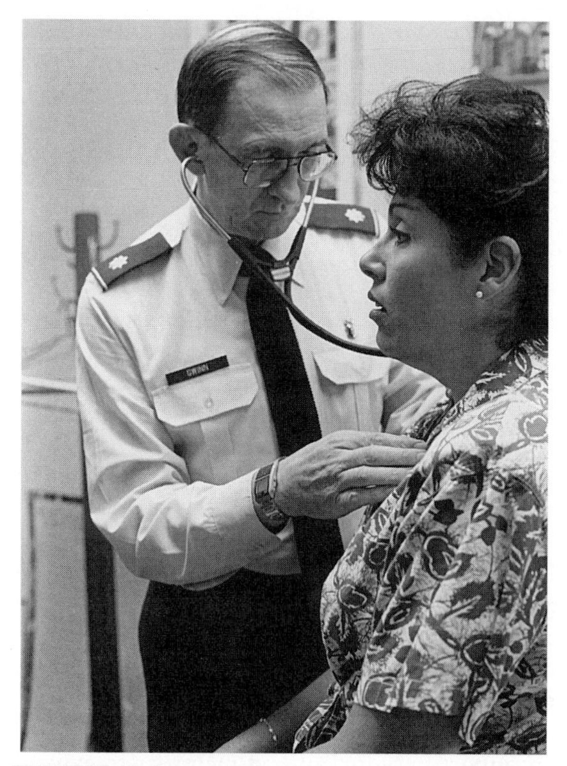
EXHIBIT 13-3 A physician assistant in the Air Force. (Courtesy American Academy of Physician Assistants.)

Army

The Army, with approximately 600 PAs, has the largest contingent in the military. Army PAs are part of the Medical Specialist Corps and work in the field with operational forces, as well as in the primary care setting (O'Hearn, 1991). In addition, Army PAs have opportunities to specialize in occupational medicine, aviation medicine, orthopedic surgery, emergency medicine (Herrera, 1994), cardio perfusion training and other specialties. In the field, advanced trauma teams are often overseen by a PA (Henson, 1999). Frequently the forward team of a battalion aid station includes a PA, a staff sergeant medic, and two junior medics. When sent with units on a mission PAs are often in the "muddy boots" Army (combat units). These units are often at the point of the sword when it comes to first engagement. When these units are deployed, PAs are with them. Eighty percent of Army PAs are in maneuver units at the division level. There are a large number of Army PAs in Korea near the demilitarized zone between North Korea and South Korea, where they are somewhat isolated and live in austere conditions. Because the Army does not have enough PAs to satisfy the demand, Army PAs tend to move a lot. When Army medical units are detached to war-torn areas they are there to not only care for their own troops, but to provide medical assistance in villages and set up clinics to assist the people.

An example of an advanced trauma managed team in the Army is described in a brief paper by Henson (1999). There the forward team of a battalion aid station includes a PA, a staff sergeant medic, and two junior medics. As a team they are dispatched to the Serbian villages to set up clinics and to provide care to the people who remain. Humanitarian endeavors such as this will likely be the mission in the new century for the military.

Army PAs have opportunities to specialize in a number of areas. The Army has four PA residency programs: emergency medicine, occupational health, cardiovascular perfusion, and orthopedics. All are located at large Army medical centers.

The Army's PA service arose from a desperate need for more doctors during the Vietnam War and remains the largest such program in the U.S. military service. Beause of their diverse missions Army PAs may have the most diverse skills of any group of PAs.

Navy

The approximately 235 active-duty Navy PAs are part of the Medical Services Corps. They are used almost exclusively in primary care. A number of operational billets are available for deep-water vessels such as carriers and cruisers, but most are attached to medical centers and shore stations. Navy PAs can be deployed with Marine Corps units; a few serve on independent duty. The Navy PA School was in San Diego but has now consolidated with the interservice program in San Antonio in the mid 1990s. Navy PAs derive from the interservice program and direct civilian procurement, as well as from outside scholarship programs. PAs assigned to the Marines undergo additional training in field medicine.

Coast Guard

Often overlooked as a military branch, the Coast Guard is part of the Department of

Transportation, instead of the Department of Defense. As such the Coast Guard tends to serve domestically rather than overseas. There are 30 PAs on active duty and 10 in the reserves. Many of these PAs are at independent-duty stations (Hooker, 1987). For example, when icebreakers are underway a PA is assigned as the sole medical officer. PAs from the enlisted ranks were trained at the Air Force PA training program in Wichita Falls, Texas, but are now trained at the combined military program in San Antonio. The U.S. Public Health Service (USPHS) supplies some PAs to the Coast Guard (and those PAs wear the USPHS emblem on their uniform), but the majority are both recruited and trained by the Coast Guard. Approximately one third of the medical officers in the Coast Guard are PAs, and the other two thirds are physicians and nurse practitioners (NPs) (Hooker, 1991b).

Because there is no specialty corps in the Coast Guard, PAs are line officers and must compete with other line officers for advancement (Hooker, 1991a). This is in contrast to Coast Guard physicians, who are USPHS commissioned medical officers.

NONMILITARY FEDERAL AGENCIES

Within the federal government are numerous agencies that use medical personnel. The following sections provide a list of some of those agencies.

Public Health Service Corps

The USPHS is of one of eight Public Health Service agencies in the U.S. Department of Health and Human Services. As USPHS officers, PAs serve in the Food and Drug Administration, the Centers for Disease Control and Prevention, the Indian Health Service, the National Oceanic and Atmospheric Administration (NOAA), the Coast Guard, the National Center for Health Statistics, and other agencies. Some of these PAs are commissioned officers; others are civilian or contract workers. All are recruited, and none are trained at the Uniform Services Medical University.

The National Health Service Corps (NHSC) is one program that has health care professionals in more than 500 areas (neighborhoods to rural areas) that are suffering from critical shortages of primary health care providers. The Health Resources and Services Administration (HRSA) Bureau of Primary Health Care administers the NHSC.

A number of recruitment funds support programs that offer financial help for PAs and other medical care professionals in exchange for professional services. These include scholarships, the Federal Loan Repayment Program, the NHSC State Loan Repayment Program, and the Commissioned Officer Student Extern Program (COSTEP).

National Oceanic and Atmospheric Administration

Only a few PAs are assigned to the NOAA. These PAs are part of the USPHS Corps and tend to rotate in the NOAA for only a few years before moving on to another branch of the USPHS.

Bureau of Prisons

The BOP is part of the Justice Department and has numerous PAs serving in various federal prisons. The BOP is the fastest growing federal department and is constantly recruiting PAs for correctional medicine (Vause, Beeler, and Miller-Blanks, 1997). At one time the BOP contracted with the interservice PA program at Fort Sam Houston in San Antonio, Texas, to train PAs for service in the BOP.

Bureau of Indian Affairs

The Bureau of Indian Affairs has employed PAs for work on Indian reservations since 1975. More than 60 positions are available, some of which are filled by NHSC and public health officers.

Peace Corps

The Peace Corps has a rich tradition of using PAs in many roles. The Peace Corps is a branch within the State Department and actively recruits PAs, along with physicians and NPs to be either volunteers or Peace Corps medical officers. Applicants must have and maintain a current license to practice medicine. The Office of Medical Services at the Peace Corps determines the level of provider required at each post before contractor selection. The Peace Corps places people in more than 50 countries, and at least one medical officer is deployed to each country.

The first use of a PA as a Peace Corps medical officer was in the Kingdom of Tonga (South Pacific) in 1975, and a PA has been there ever since (Goddard, 1980).

Immigration and Naturalization Service

The Immigration and Naturalization Service (INS) actively recruits PAs along with many other types of health care employees to look after both INS workers and detainees.

VETERANS AFFAIRS

One of the principal institutional employers of PAs nationwide is the VA. From the very beginning of the PA profession the VA has played a vital supporting role in the education and use of PAs. For example, the VA Medical Center in Durham, North Carolina, has continuously provided clinical education sites, going back to the first PA students at Duke University. The St. Louis University PA program was initiated by the VA in St. Louis in 1971. The VA first began employing PAs in 1968 (Fox, 1983).

Initially, each VA facility largely determined for itself the role of the PAs it employed. In 1972, however, the VA central office issued Circular 10-7-252, entitled "Utilization Guidelines of Physician Assistants." This document, which represented an effort to standardize the role of the PA within the VA system, defined the areas of the hospital in which the PA could be used and specified the type and level of tasks to which they could be assigned (Fox, 1983). This seems to have opened the door for PAs. More than 1100 PAs are working in more than 130 VA locations. However, the VA system is quite large and includes 172 hospitals, 68 satellite outpatient units, and 127 nursing homes. This large system seems to have a constant effort to recruit more PAs.

Several research projects on PAs in the VA have provided a profile on roles and utilization patterns. These evaluations have enhanced the ability of the VA to establish appropriate PA/NP policies. In 1992 a study by Alexander and Lipscomb (1992) identified the allocation of time for PAs and NPs (Kraft, Alexander, and Rowlands, 1992).

The Veterans Health Administration (VHA) is divided into 22 geographic regions designated as Veterans Integrated Service Networks. Not all facilities hire PAs, so the PA presence is larger in some regions than others. In a survey that was undertaken in 1998 in the VHA, 1131 PAs were employed (Lyman, Elli, and Gebhart, 1999). Approximately two thirds (68%) were men, the mean age was 47 years, and the mean length of experience was 16 years. Most of the PAs worked in the outpatient setting (58%), but a surprisingly large group also worked inpatient (40%) (Exhibit 13-4). A majority had clinical roles, but in addition to that, 54% reported some administrative activities (Exhibit 13-5). Almost one third (31%) indicated they would like their administrative duties increased. At the time of this survey (1998), 81% had a salary between \$50,000 and \$70,000. Since then the salaries of PAs within the VHA has been adjusted upward.

OTHER FEDERAL AGENCIES

A number of other federal agencies employ PAs. These include the Central Intelligence Agency, the Federal Bureau of Investigation, the Centers for Disease Control and Prevention, the State Department, the National Institutes of Health, and the Food and Drug Administration.

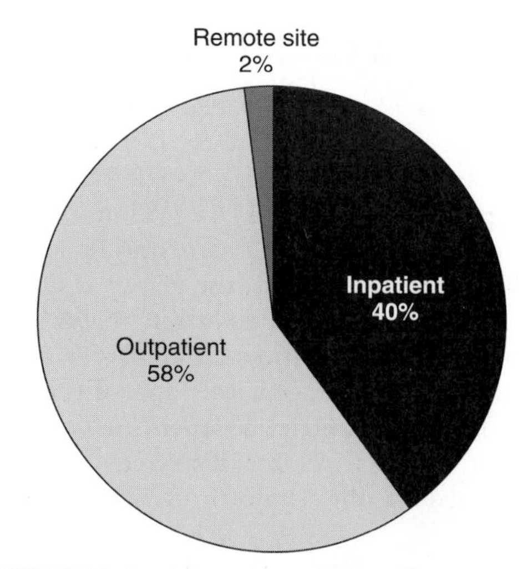

EXHIBIT 13-4 Work settings of PAs in the Veterans Health Administration. (Data from Lyman P, Elli L, Gebhart R: *Veterans Health Sys J* 4:25-29, 1999.)

EXHIBIT 13-5

Work Assignments for PAs in the Veterans Health Administration

Work assignment	No. of responses	%*
Primary care	287	26.9
Medicine and subspecialties	234	21.9
Surgery, anesthesia, and subspecialties	162	15.2
Mental hygiene/psychiatry/substance abuse	118	11.1
Long-term care/geriatrics/hospice/domiciliary	59	5.5
Employee health	46	4.3
Administration	36	3.4
Spinal cord injury	28	2.6
Rehabilitation	27	2.5
Community-based clinic/home care/mobile clinic	25	2.3
Emergency medicine	13	1.2
Compensation and pension examinations	9	0.8
Critical care/urgent care/transitional care	8	0.75
Women's health	4	0.4
Other (research, specialized laboratory, blind rehabilitation, medical informatics, Persian Gulf coordinator)	11	1.0
TOTAL	1067	100

Modified from Lyman P, Elli L, Gebhart R: *Veterans Health Sys J:* 4:25-29, 1999.
*Because of rounding, total percentage does not equal exactly 100%.

SUMMARY

While the federal government remains the largest single employer of PAs, there is no cohesive body that directly recruits PAs for federal service. Each of the military branches of the Department of Defense has devised a strategy for ensuring it has enough PAs for its members and the other federal agencies have similar strategies. Collectively the PAs employed by the federal government represent more than 15 agencies. The fact that more are employed each year suggests their use is valued in large part because of their adaptability to changing roles.

14

FUTURE DIRECTIONS

INTRODUCTION

The physician assistant (PA) in American medicine continues to enjoy an unparalleled success among the health professions. The establishment of the PA concept that began in the 1970s has grown into a widely accepted and highly respected health occupation and is becoming internationally recognized. In the late 1980s PA growth reached a plateau but then expanded during the mid 1990s and continues to grow. Various explanations have been advanced as to why the PA concept has been so successful in the American medical care system. Clearly the PA fits well in the United States, a system different from that of other countries. The key question that arises is what does the future hold for the profession? Will the demand for PA services continue to increase or will it plateau or decrease? Will the brisk demand seen in the past several years continue or will it reach a saturation level? Will patterns of supply and demand for PAs result in the cyclic fluctuations seen in other professions or will a steady and comfortable equilibrium be reached?

This chapter begins by examining why PAs have succeeded so effectively in the U.S. health care system. From this backdrop the next step is to determine where the PA profession is headed. Does the past predict the future? How will the changing face of the U.S. health care system have an impact on the PA profession?

Why have PAs succeeded in becoming an integral part of American health care when they could have failed? The answer to this question is important because if PAs are to understand what the future holds for them, they need to understand their past. A number of experts have analyzed the evolution and success of the PA profession in American medicine and offer what they believe are the major social forces thought to have influenced the PA movement. These include the following:

- The changing lifestyles and practice preferences of physicians who grew out of the 1960s. Physicians, along with others, realized they did not want to work as hard as their predecessors and needed help.
- Women entered the workforce in a major way, with many seeking a return to a new career in health care. Many women were trying out careers that had been traditionally occupied by men.
- The commitment to be a dependent profession closely associated with physicians allowed for widespread acceptance by physicians.
- The early establishment of specific skills and competencies expected of PAs through program accreditation and a national board allowed for state enabling legislation.
- There was a national emphasis on training primary care generalists, with PAs assuming diverse roles after obtaining a set of core competencies (Carter, 1992).

Reflecting on why PAs have succeeded, Fowkes et al. (1983) provides the following summary:

> In the early part of [the twentieth century] the Flexner report changed the emphasis in our medical schools from a practical approach to a biomedical emphasis as the priority in education. This made medical schools slow to

respond to the changing social environment, and less responsive to health care needs. In the 1960s primary care was a new concept. There was a recognized need for these services, a maldistribution of physicians and types of services, and questions about who should do it. A discipline of family medicine was emerging but was not large enough to have much influence. It takes medical schools (and nursing schools for that matter) an enormous amount of time to make critical changes. One of the critical features of the physician assistant movement has been its flexibility and resourcefulness. One only has to look to the way the training programs responded to the early awareness of AIDS, homelessness, drug abuse, and domestic violence by incorporating these conditions in their curriculum. The physician assistant is the only flexible category of health professionals. Both PA programs and PA practitioners have demonstrated their abilities to quickly modify elements of education and practice in response to social need.

The PA profession has also succeeded in part because of the personal and career characteristics and attributes of PAs. It has been and continues to be one of the most exciting careers that have developed in the twentieth century.

THE FUTURE OF HEALTH CARE

Many experts believe that innovation in every aspect of patient care will be nothing less than astonishing as the new century unfolds. The accelerating pace of technology will bring together a remarkable group of health care providers who have the ability to adapt to health care delivery change quickly and adroitly. Futurists have identified and analyzed some of the trends and technologic advances that will likely shape and inform the next generation of medicine. They range from fundamental advances in computing and administration, research, nursing, and patient care delivery to minimally invasive surgery, biomolecular therapies, bionics, and beyond. Other advances in technology will emerge in the next decade that until recently existed only in the realm of science fiction.

Some of the changes that will shape how health care is delivered, and with it the fate of the PA, will take place in the next decade. Each of these is detailed here.

Health Care Finance

Forecasting the changing picture of health care financing necessitates understanding policy changes at federal and state levels, movements in the employer and consumer markets, and tracking long-term shifts in demographics and technology. Changes have been underway for some time and government priorities will continue to expand medical coverage for more and more Americans. These policy changes will increase the number of demands on a health care system that is struggling with labor costs. PAs offer an opportunity to provide this care at less expensive salaries. The substitutability of PAs for traditional physician services means they are likely to be used in increasing ways to help fill the gaps of more demand for health care access.

The New Health Care Consumer

Telecommunications via the Internet is only one example of how the new consumer has fundamentally changed many industries. Is health care next? Newly empowered patients are demanding more accountability of their health care dollar. This is not well balanced in the United States with its tiered health insurance system: Those with good paying jobs have excellent health care coverage compared with those without the benefit of a generous employer. The heavy users of health care services are on average older, poorer, and less sophisticated than the mainstream baby boomers, and their care often has to be cost shifted to make room for those with better coverage. So it is unclear exactly who the new health care consumer will be and how quickly the health care marketplace will change. Increasingly those staffing health care systems are turning to PAs as a temporary solution to meeting the demands of shifting health care consumers.

Health Care Delivery Systems

For many consumers and physicians, managed care was not the panacea that was predicted. New organizations and relationships in health care delivery systems will be built. At the core of each new experiment will be health care providers. Increasingly health care systems realize that diversity of the health care workforce means not only gender and ethnic diversity but also various types of providers such as PAs, nurse practitioners (NPs), midwives, and others. Americans want and demand choices, and this transcends to nonphysician providers.

Technology

The area of information and medical technologies is where the greatest changes will take place. The impact of emerging technologies and new media on patients, delivery networks, insurers, and physicians is difficult to predict, although it will drive up the cost of health care. The role of new medical technologies will be dramatic in the next 10 years. To use these technologies will require a mix of physicians and nonphysician providers such as PAs and allied health personnel. The growth of physicians is fairly flat, so increasingly technology will call on PAs to be part of the technology delivery.

Sociodemographic Trends and Health Status

There is a growing realization that medical care does not alone equal health status, and new definitions of health are emerging. They include consumer demands for new types of health services such as "complementary and alternative" medicine. In 2000 there was more than $14 billion in expenditures in the United States. On top of this will emerge different philosophies about health spending and what contributes to health outcomes. The areas that are likely to dominate U.S. health policy and health care delivery are:

- Human genomics and all the proteins that genes produce
- The empowered consumer
- Internet and telemedicine
- Complementary and alternative medicine
- Technology developments in electronic information and communication
- Impact on patient access and quality

Like technology, each one of the areas that will open up will require increasingly better trained individuals to apply the information.

THE FUTURE FOR PHYSICIAN ASSISTANTS

What does the future hold for PAs? How blue are the skies for the next generation of PAs? Is this a profession that encourages young, bright, and capable people to pursue it? Although these questions are usually replied in the affirmative, the evidence to predict a rosy scenario is mostly conjecture. To make predictions we need to know something of the past and what trends are underway. The most solid evidence we have is that the profession is growing and the demographics are changing.

Economics is one of the tools available to help with prediction modeling. At its most basic level, it is the science of understanding supply and demand largely based on human behavior. If supply exceeds demand, then price goes down. Conversely, if demand exceeds supply, the price increases. The following is an examination of these two fundamental principles as they apply to PAs.

Supply Side

As of 2002 there were 132 accredited PA programs and a few more in various stages of development (Exhibit 14-1). At year's end of 2002, approximately 5000 new PAs had entered the workforce and approximately two thirds of these new graduates are women. Since the new century the PA workforce in the aggregate has been largely composed of women, because there are fewer men applying to PA school and the men in the workforce are older by at least 5 years than their female counterparts. The trend of female PA expansion is calculated to extend to at least 2010. By 2005 there will be 57,500 PAs in the workforce, and by 2010 there will be at least 85,000 PAs clinically employed (Exhibit 14-2). These numbers take into account retirements of both male and female PAs, who are being replaced by more younger women than men. The fairly steady 1.5% attrition of the PA corps up until 2000 will gradually increase to 2.5% by 2006 as more women leave the workforce to pursue families and other careers.

These shifts in gender may create new and different work habits. The length of the workweek is one area in which this is apparent. The workweek is gradually shrinking for physicians, down from

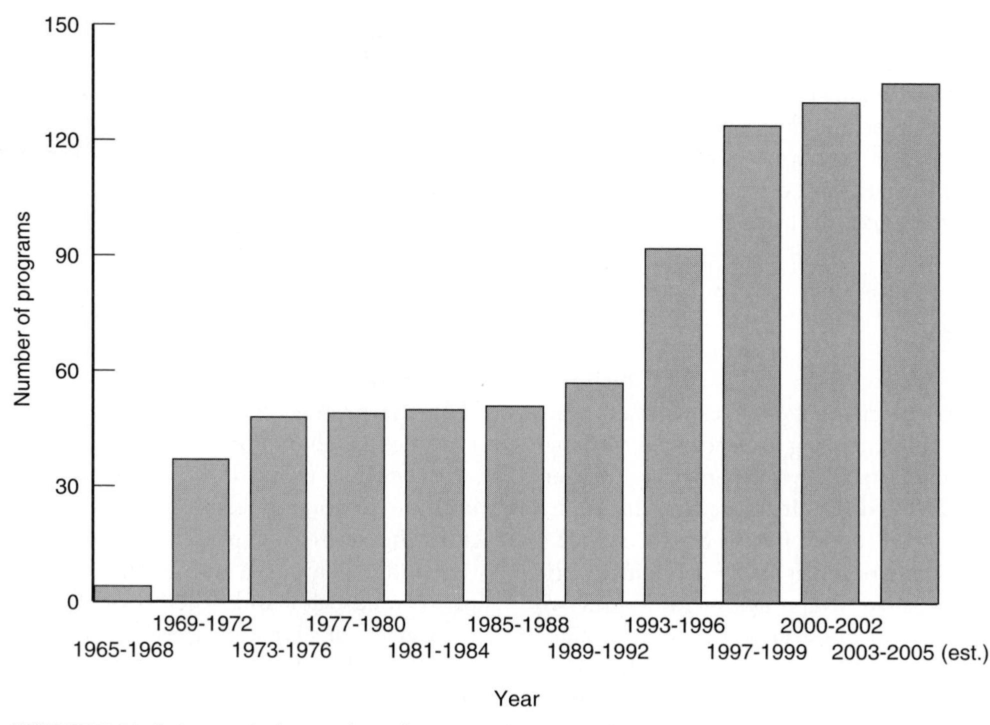

EXHIBIT 14-1 Accumulative number of programs by year of first entering class. (Data from Association of Physician Assistant Programs, Alexandria, Va., 2002.)

55 hours in 1990 to 50 hours in 2000. The 45-hour workweek for PAs has remained fairly steady since 1995.

The obverse side of the PA supply coin is that health care continues to be a labor-intensive enterprise. Because the cost of this labor is expensive, the outcomes of different types of labor will be scrutinized and compared. This bodes well for the profession in the short run. Managers will increasingly recognize the value of PAs as a skilled labor force, able to shift from one area of demand to another. Demand will continue for a while, a slow but steady rise in programs will continue, and from 2000 to 2010 the supply of PAs will double (Hecker, 2001). Many will welcome this expansion, but the greatest threat to the PA profession is the fickle marketplace. As salaries increase the cost-effectiveness of PAs will diminish under this invisible hand–pricing oneself out of the market. "If PA income continues to increase at the levels we have seen recently, then cost, value, and productivity differentials will influence hiring decisions" (Jones and Cawley, 1994). Eventually there will be more PAs than opportunities, and relationships with physicians may suffer.

Until then the dependence of PAs on physicians will probably continue to serve the profession for a while as it continues to reach out to organized medicine for professional guardianship. By demonstrating competence to the physician, the PA's clinical role in practice is ultimately established through a process of ongoing negotiation. Professional autonomy is determined through performance of delegated and negotiated tasks and exists within the practice limits of the supervising physician.

Significant increases in the role of PA and NP use in health maintenance organizations (HMOs) will be augmented by the degree to which physicians can be persuaded to hire them, but whether physicians will use them once hired is less predictable. This uncertainty suggests the need to expand PA program output should be gradual and perhaps underlines the necessity for an administrative structure able to fine-tune and monitor this development.

Because the shape of the U.S. health care workforce is so uncertain, the fundamental question of how many PAs will be enough remains unanswered.

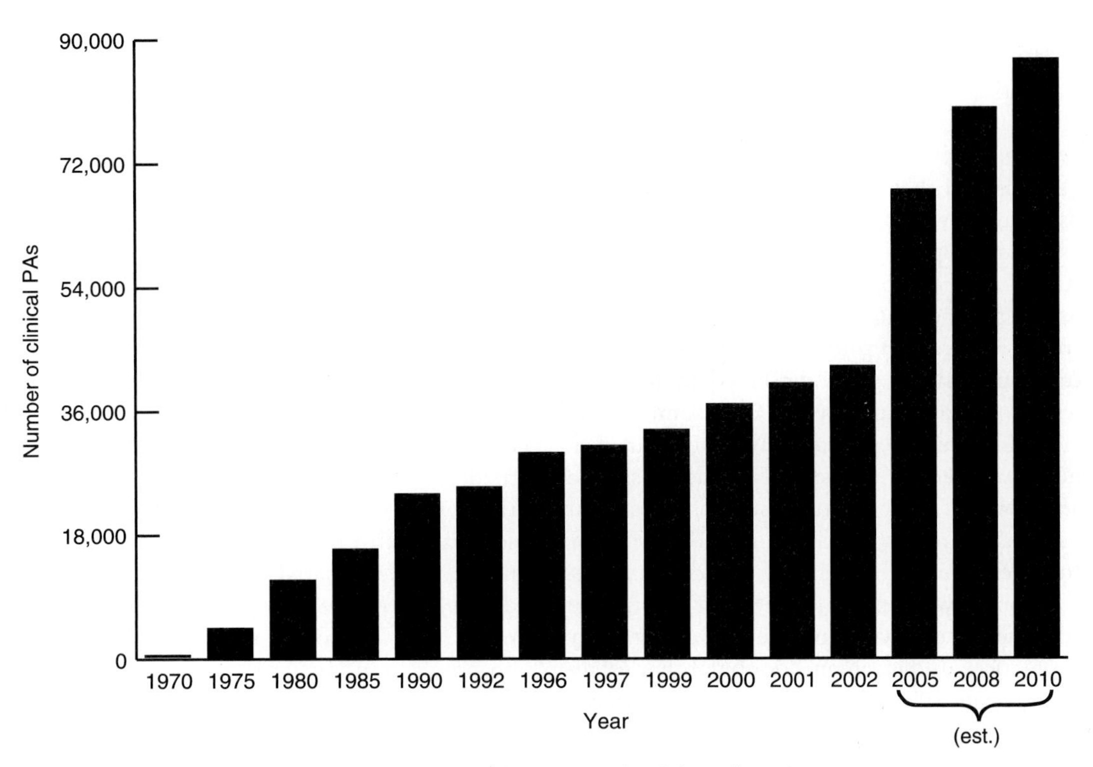

EXHIBIT 14-2 Present and future supply of clinically active PAs.

Demand Side

The demand side of the equation is more difficult to predict and relies on data from other sectors of the health care field. In the short run hospitals will increasingly employ PAs (or NPs) as more intensive services demand that a permanent salaried house staff be present 24 hours. Teams of hospitalists (physicians and PAs) will manage large inpatient populations that require highly skilled personnel because only the very ill will be hospitalized for any period. Ambulatory care, where most PAs reside, will continue to employ more and more PAs as physicians become more and more familiar with their skills and services. These outpatient services will experience many more demands for both primary care and non-primary care PAs. The primary care demand will decrease because there continues to be limited interest in medical students selecting a primary care role. In the non-primary care area, technology will create more and more need for skilled providers such as PAs to aid in the application of the technology. This will occur in areas such as neurology, nephrology, and cardiothoracic surgery. PAs are already frequently present as first assistants in many surgeries.

A gloomier side of the demand curve is that PAs will produce too many clinicians. For example, PAs are in direct competition with NPs and to a lesser extent with nurse midwives. The vast majority of NPs are in primary care and the number of clinically active NPs is almost 50 percent more than the number of PAs (Hooker and Berlin, 2002). Their activity may prevent a firmer foothold in the primary care arena for PAs.

One of the nagging issues facing the profession is the appropriate number of PAs to train. How many PAs should there be in American? Unlike some countries that have developed prescribed physicians/population ratios (e.g., Canada, England, Australia, and the Netherlands), the United States has largely allowed the markets to dictate how many physicians there should be. The only governor of physician supply is the number of medical and osteopathic schools and their ability to turn out graduates. As of 2002 the number of graduates is approximately 16,500 annually. Part of this equation is how many primary care physicians should be available to the population and in what ratio? Should PAs and NPs (and midwives) be considered part of the equation?

There are two sides to the question of how much is enough. Some believe there is a surplus of physicians and that PAs and NPs are redundant. This argument is based on counting physician heads and comparing ratios of physicians to populations and comparing these numbers with those of other countries. However, others believe there are not enough primary care physicians and many communities go underserved in terms of access to primary care services. Still, some believe we should mandate primary care quotas in residencies and reduce specialized residencies. And others believe that it is unrealistic to expect that physicians in any appreciable numbers will by themselves reverse the trend of professional specialization (Cawley and Jones, 1997). If this notion holds true, doctors will continue to avoid primary care practices, and it remains doubtful that established specialist physicians will convert to generalist roles in any appreciable numbers. The continuing decline in interest among young physicians in primary care careers and generalist practices has not yet been reversed, and it will take decades, even if the number of medical graduates choosing primary care significantly increases before adjustments in graduate medical education (GME) outcomes will have an impact on service delivery. This prospect raises the question of which type of health care personnel will provide primary care now and in the future. As physicians become increasingly specialized, moving further away from primary care, PAs are likely to assume a greater profile in delivering primary care services. This is particularly true in settings such as HMOs, other types of managed care systems, and organized health care systems such as the Veterans Affairs (VA) hospitals, state and federal correctional systems, and the military. One veteran workforce observer believes that physicians are really no longer in the primary care business and that PAs and NPs, working with physician "managers," may be the best providers to meet future primary care needs. Meikle (1992) recommends increasing PA educational output and use in primary care roles. Finally, some free market economists believe that as many PAs should be trained as the market will bear because in the end competition produces a public good in distributing products and driving down costs (Hooker, 1997).

In the future the supply of PAs and other nonphysician health professions is likely to be determined by political, economic, and legal factors that affect the evolution of their roles in relation to those of physicians (Jones and Cawley, 1994). As the U.S. health care system changes from one encompassing a disease-oriented and economically open-ended structure to one stressing a more preventive, patient-centered, and cost-conscious direction, nonphysician clinicians (NPCs [i.e., PAs, CNMs, and NPs]) will assume a higher profile. The further evolution of the professional roles of NPCs in U.S. health care will be determined by changing trends in the division of medical labor, more accountable public perceptions of levels of physician responsiveness to societal health care problems, population-based needs, patient satisfaction, and outcome evidence. The future may produce the interdisciplinary team approach to health care that will become a standard at the same time Americans are demanding increasing accountability from its health professionals. This new accountability will require adjustments in the educational preparation of medical and health care providers, approaches extending the biomedical model to encompass both the population-based and behavioral sciences. The PA concept in American medicine has emerged as a creative and effective health workforce approach to augment clinical service gaps in multiple areas. PAs are well integrated into medical practices and have demonstrated clinical competency and versatility. Expansion of PA use will likely continue in several sectors of the health care system.

Trends in primary care practices are likely to evolve. As of 2002 approximately one fourth of all solo practitioners employ an NPC. When we examine just those practices incorporating a PA and/or NP (both solo and group practices), approximately 11% of patients are seen by an NPC (either as the sole provider of record or with the physician). Again, looking just at the population of patients seen by PAs and NPs, approximately one third of all patients are younger than 18 years, suggesting the physician is delegating a great deal of health care to the NPC (Hooker and McCaig, 2001).

The growth of the profession is likely to continue to at least 2010. A swelling of the ranks is expected until at least 2005 when the current level of PA programs (132 PA programs as of

2002) will reach its maximum output. This maximum output is estimated at 6000 PA graduates per year. Under the current scenario, using regression analysis and factoring in an aging profession, more women than men, younger women than men, we predict a PA population of 85,000 active clinicians by 2010.

Medical marketplace demand for primary care PAs is anticipated to grow. One estimate of primary care needs suggests that a primary care physician can cover the needs of 1600 to 1800 persons annually in a managed care practice setting (Hummel and Pirzada, 1994). Given these figures the United States will need 150,000 primary care physicians for a population of approximately 330 million in 2005. However, only 88,000 primary care physicians younger than 55 years are in active practice. With the addition of a PA to the practice, the patient panel for a PA-physician primary care team could increase to at least 2400 (a conservative one-third increase in practice productivity). "This increase in total practice productivity suggests that work force requirements for primary care physicians could be reduced if more physicians were able to utilize PAs" (Cawley, 1995).

The demand for PAs in hospitals is expected to increase as well. In most institutions, residency program directors are already using PAs and NPs, and there is no reason to believe they will not continue to employ them. A survey of directors of these programs indicates that these PAs and NPs were used for clinical services to replace the service of physicians (Cawley, 1995):

- The Bureau of Labor Statistics career outlook projections for health care professionals indicate increased demand for PA services (Hecker, 2001).
- Estimates of the Bureau of Health Professions project future demand for nonphysician providers.
- State survey data of practicing PAs suggest increasing market demand for PAs (Henderson, 2001).
- Mandated cutbacks in hours worked for residents may increase the demand for PAs.

In response to the charge from the Council on Graduate Medical Education (COGME), the Advisory Group of Physician Assistants and the Workforce (AGPAW) developed a list of recommendations addressing PA education, PA practice characteristics, practice obstacles, and current and anticipated demand. The advisory group called for

- Increasing federal support for PA educational programs to expand the supply of PA graduates
- Increasing National Health Service Corps scholarships and loan repayment programs supporting PA students
- Developing federal policy to support and encourage increased representation from racial and ethnic minorities in the PA profession (Exhibit 14-3)

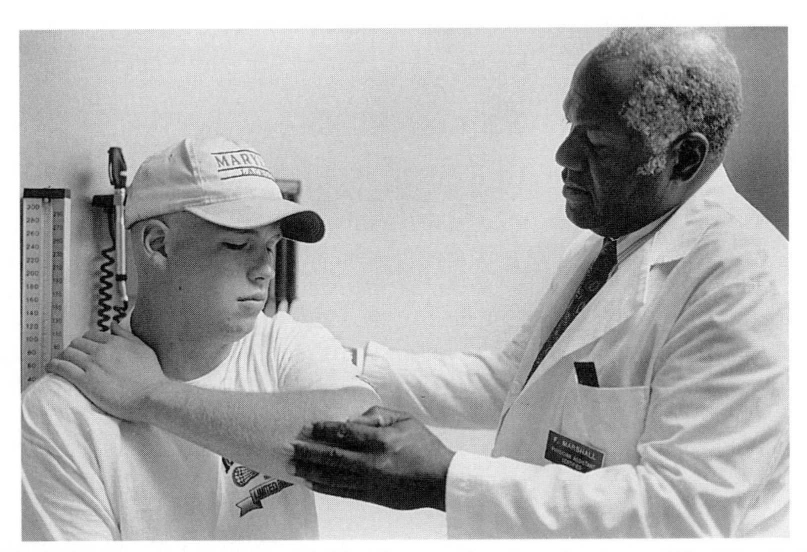

EXHIBIT 14-3 An occupational health PA. (Courtesy American Academy of Physician Assistants.)

- Including PAs in national and state health workforce planning activities
- Encouraging states to provide a more uniform regulatory climate for PAs

The Pew Health Professions Commission (1995) predicts that a number of forces will interact to produce a U.S. health care system that will be different from the one to which we are accustomed. The more obvious changes in health care will be as follows:

- More managed care with better integration of services and financing
- More accountability to those who purchase and use health care services
- More awareness of and responsiveness to the needs of enrolled populations
- Ability to use fewer resources more effectively
- More innovation and diversity in providing health care
- Less focus on treatment and more concern about education, prevention, and care management
- Orientation to improving the health of the entire population
- Reliance on outcomes data and evidence

Demand-side innovation, which addresses both old and new markets, requires increasing marketing sophistication and awareness. Strategies toward this goal include creation of new opportunities in the form of new specialties and subspecialties. Emerging new roles for PAs are wellness and disease prevention; clinical, biologic, and health services research; legal; genetics; toxicology; and medical administration. Expanded roles are in geriatrics, oncology, molecular biology, genetics, and protracted disease management. A major challenge to society and the health care system is to provide effective, humane, and economical care to the millions of individuals with chronic disease. PAs and NPs are probably in a better position to do this than physicians because patients will increasingly be absorbed by managed care organizations and their medical care will require intensive efforts to contain costs through innovative forms of labor.

In 1975 Rick Carlson wrote a book titled *The End of Medicine* (Carlson, 1975). At the time, the author (a lawyer) and his thesis were regarded as being on the radical fringe of health care policy. In this futuristic polemic, he asserted that eventually the medical profession, partly because of its arrogant stance of self-regulation, the rise of consumerism and preventive care, and the corporitization of health delivery, would become obsolete. While actual physician obsolescence is unlikely anytime soon, it is clear that in today's health system, the medical profession is not what it used to be. Over the past decade in particular, physician power and influence over the health system has eroded to the degree that applicants to medical schools are now falling, state medical boards are now led by nonphysicians and consumers, and NPs are asserting their roles as independent providers of primary care services. Medicine's power and prestige reached their zenith in the 1960's, the so-called "Golden Age of Medicine," and has since declined, substantially in the minds of some.

There are a multitude of reasons explaining the decline in physician influence over the health system, but without question an important consequence has been the steady growth over the past quarter century in the numbers and clinical activities of nonphysician providers like nurse practitioners and physician assistants. Medical sociologists spend time examining the characteristics of the delivery of health services and the nature and distribution of medical work. Some specialize in analyzing and debating the evolving changes in the status of the medical profession. Those asserting a decline in the power and prestige of the medical profession in the U.S. refer to this trend as "deprofessionalization" (Hafferty and McKinley, 1993). John McKinlay is among the more outspoken of the deprofessionalization theorists, and observes that the growing corporitization and bureaucratization of medicine has resulted in effectively eliminating physician self-employment and reduced physician autonomy. As the medical workplace becomes more and more bureaucratized, physicians are increasingly subject to the rules and systems of hierarchical structures that are not of their own making. Physicians are no longer professionally dominant because traditional elements of classic professionalism have been lost. Prerogatives such as control over training content, work autonomy, and the means and remuneration of labor have eroded. Today, the federal government, insurance companies, and consumer groups now hold considerable sway over medical training and practice and the methods by which physicians are paid for their work.

Another important factor in the decline of medicine as a profession is that physicians no longer have a monopoly over medical knowledge. Health consumers and a wide variety of other providers now approach or even exceed physician knowledge in specific areas. The days of the all knowing paternalistic physician dispensing medical directives to a subservient patient are gone. And as they have become more sophisticated, patients cum consumers now view medical care much as they view other services, and are demanding more control, choice, and convenience.

Delivering medical services in a patient convenient manner is a relatively new concept to many physicians Understandably, accustomed as they are to dealing with life and death situations, physicians in the past have not placed a high priority on customer service and convenience considerations, yet such adjustments may be required in the future health care delivery market.

The nature of physician roles in medical work is also changing. It is now clear that health providers like NPs and PAs can deliver a wide range of medical services as effectively and safely as physicians and at a lower cost. Nonphysicians may be equally knowledgeable in certain clinical disciplines, for example primary care, and have been shown to be as capable as physicians in performing technical procedures in a number of specialty areas, i.e., sigmoidoscopy. Consumers and others have come to the realization that physicians may be overtrained for what they do most of the time. Advances in technology now permit great accuracy and precision in diagnosis placing less emphasis on physician differential diagnostic and cognitive capabilities. Washington health pundit Daniel Greenberg once said that the system of medical education in the U.S. was akin to putting all bus drivers through astronaut training. The point is that it may not require 12 years of expensive and federally subsidized education to prepare the medical practitioner of the future, and perhaps this is particularly true in primary care. Physicians have reverted to a movement toward increasing specialization and appear to be abandoning primary care to other providers.

In 2000, for the third straight year, fewer U.S. medical school seniors chose primary care residency positions. Among internists, the hospitalist movement has become increasingly popular, driven in part by a desire by physicians to better control the circumstances of their work. It would be a mistake to believe that physicians as we know them are going to fade from the health delivery scene, yet it is clear that their roles are changing in the division of medical labor.

As economics and technology continue to drive medical care, portions of the work that once were exclusively in the domain of physicians will be passed on to others. Familiar examples of this work shifting are already evident with psychologists and psychiatric social workers in place of psychiatrists, and nurse midwives instead of obstetricians. It may very well be that in the future, should such trends continue, that NPs and PAs will take on an increasing share of the work of primary care. This occurrence could come about due to a combination of factors: (1) practice economics in the delivery system, (2) aggressive tactics mounted by some nonphysicians to wrest from physicians dominance in primary care, and (3) physicians abrogating primary care and instead seeking inpatient and specialty roles. It is possible that such a scenario could result in one in which more physicians assume a more medical managerial and care oversight role with actual clinical care being provided by nonphysicians. If such a redistribution of medical work were to transpire, a key question will be to what degree will nonphysicians be granted autonomy in their practices. And an even more intriguing question would be whether physicians would voluntarily grant such practice prerogatives.

Many of the restrictions on NPs in both mobility and time are likely to affect PAs as well. NPs, and nurses in general, have evidence of increasing need for part-time employment and ability to determine work time. As the composition of PAs shifts to be younger and female, these restrictions will affect PA (and physicians) even more than they do now (Exhibit 14-4).

SELF-ACTUALIZATION

Responsibility for administering the profession belongs to the profession. When PAs emerged in the late 1960s, the laws governing the practice of medicine were amended to recognize the physician's ability to delegate tasks to supervised individuals. Most of these laws have been modified

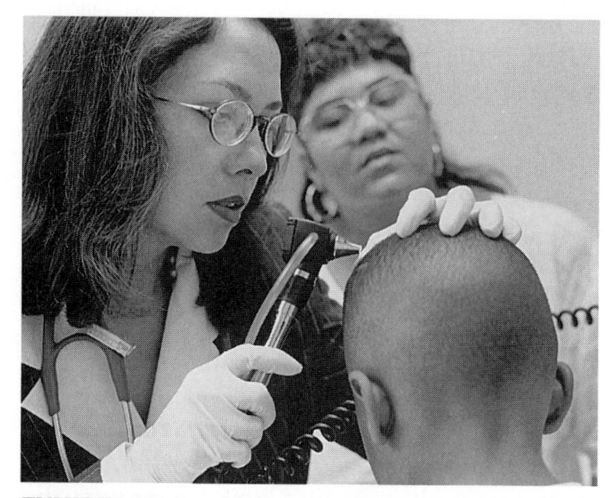

EXHIBIT 14-4 A family medicine PA. (Courtesy American Academy of Physician Assistants.)

and expanded, but the power to regulate PAs has remained, with only a few exceptions in the hands of the licensing board members who tend to be predominantly controlled by physicians. If PAs are to seek their own destiny, they must overcome these shortcomings in self-actualization and begin seeking avenues to educate their regulators.

On the other hand, if formal participation of PAs in the regulatory process is a worthy goal, it is not a panacea for problems that may exist between physician licensing boards and PAs. Once a PA becomes a board member or sits on a committee that is set up to ensure the benefit of citizens, he or she assumes the role of protector of the public health and safety. The responsibilities of that person are to the citizens of the state, not to the profession. Advocacy of professional concerns at the state level still rests with state PA associations, often aided by the national organization.

The ability of PAs to effectively identify, attract, and efficiently serve the varieties of consumers will largely determine their professional survival. Both organization and financing services will be key variables in these efforts. This will require understanding the microeconomics and macroeconomics, as well as the health care changes to maintain their demand. Macroeconomics, such as creative, aggressive, and effective marketing of the quality that PAs bring to society, and the recruitment of social scientists into education programs to undertake sorely need research on the profession. Research must be done on the economic use of PAs and expansion in specific client areas such as home health and genomics. In the area of microeconomics, increasing demand may expand into geriatrics, pediatrics, and gynecology in greater numbers. These strategies are outlined in Exhibit 14-5.

One area of self-actualization is to constantly update the knowledge base of what roles PAs play and how well they do them. Collecting demographic data is not enough; research on the health care workforce is constantly in demand and needs to be continuously updated.

RESEARCH

The research community will continue to evaluate the effects PA employment has on quality, cost, access, and other aspects of health care delivery. Only by carefully documenting the capabilities using acceptable research methodologies will we be able to measure the profession's ability to meet the needs of the medical marketplace. Staffing currently remains a function of physician attitudes instead of administrative rationale (Hooker, 1994). Radical changes

EXHIBIT 14-5

Areas to Increase Demand for PAs

Macro (on the professional organizational level)	Micro (on the individual level)
Aggressive, creative marketing	Aggressive, creative individual marketing
Research on economic use	Creative self-employment or group employment
Creative organization and financing	Expansion of client areas and contact
Expansion of client areas and contact (scope of practice)	Use of advanced technologies
Use of advanced technologies	Inclusion in policy making
Other	Administrative rank high enough to cause change

in health care staffing will not happen soon unless the data proving that PAs can function safely and effectively in almost all health care roles are placed before policymakers and managers.

Undoubtedly, there will be encroachments on the homeostasis of the PA in the area of finances, choice, and professional domain. The girders of physician support of PAs are linked to being less successful and more dependent, regardless of skill and outcome. Relative to PAs, economics is the overwhelming determinant of essential functions.

Formulating Research Questions

The PA profession must seek to formulate questions that will guide research in ways not only theoretically fruitful but also historically appropriate.

As part of this process the following research questions are offered:

- Will the market forces remain sufficient to create a long-term demand for PAs?
- Should the profession try to recruit more gifted trainees into the PA profession that might stimulate areas of research?
- Should the American Association of Physician Assistants (AAPA) contribute to funding research by supporting proactive, innovative studies that would enhance health care delivery?
- Should the AAPA help educate and nurture institutional leadership within organizations that have sufficient vision to recognize the pivotal role that PAs can play to more cost-effective health care delivery?
- How can the profession document the efficacy, efficiency, and economy of PAs as primary care providers for Americans?
- How can PAs continue to demonstrate innovation, high quality, and technical sophistication in primary care medicine?

Some changes are underway that show promise. The Association of Physician Assistant Programs (APAP) has created a mechanism to stimulate and fund research. The APAP Research Institute is organized to use the proceedings of investments to fund small grants for research ideas that examine PA behavior and education.

Areas for Further Research

Research activity on the clinical and professional activities of PAs and other nonphysician providers is now experiencing some resurgence since the extensive health professions investigations conducted in the 1970s. Although much knowledge about PA use and clinical potentials has been learned from this past body of research, as well as widespread empirical observations, many aspects of PA clinical roles and capabilities remain to be explored. For instance, what is the optimal mix of health care providers to deliver primary care? How can the economic advantages of these providers be best used in health care systems of the future? No data exist to determine how many PAs and NPs, along with physicians and other health professionals, would be required to staff newly emerging types of managed health care systems or to meet anticipated health workforce needs in either primary care or GME-related areas. Planning activities regarding the health professions should assess the present capacities of the United States in the health care workforce, consider the short-term and long-term population-based need for medical services, and articulate these estimates of need with national goals for providing services required to improve citizen health status. The present lack of reliable information on activities in the health care workforce places policymakers at a disadvantage in attempts to either promote the more effective use of PAs or better coordinate their supply and use with those of physicians.

Research on PA practice should focus on (1) determination of physician/PA substitutability ratios and task delegation levels in primary care, managed care, and GME settings and on maximal PA/physician substitution potentials and optimal staffing mix in using PAs in GME positions, (2) description of current practice characteristics and content of care delivered by PAs in primary care including clinical preventive services, measurement of PA levels of clinical productivity and patient care outcomes determined in various settings, comparisons of PA practice performance, and contributions in primary care delivery with those of physicians and other health practitioners, (3) description of the economic aspects of PA practice, including revenue generation, practice costs, and potential for savings, and (4) educational aspects contributing to minority attrition in PA educational programs.

LESSONS FROM AND FOR OTHER SYSTEMS

As changes take place there are lessons to be learned. These lessons are in what has happened to other systems that installed assistants to physicians and lessons that other systems can learn from the U.S. model of PAs.

Lessons From Other Systems

In projecting the future for PAs in the U.S. health care system, it is useful to consider the experiences of similar types of health practitioners in the medical systems of other countries. Practitioners similar to PAs have been used in a number of other nations. Examples include the feldsher in Russia, the barefoot doctor in China, the assistant medical officer in parts of Africa, and a wide range of the variously named health care providers working primarily in developing countries throughout the world. (See chapter 2.)

The natural history and pertinent experiences of these practitioners have been examined, and when compared with the American experience with nonphysician providers, it is clear that only a few parallels exist. Experience with NPCs and their successful or unsuccessful integration into a country's health care delivery system are based primarily on how these providers fit into the medical, economic, and cultural systems of the nations that employ them. Rarely are experiences with these types of providers exportable to other countries. Each nation that has created and used NPCs has fashioned them and their roles to meet specific needs and requirements in that country's systems. However, some overriding patterns do exist that are relevant in the assessment of the American PA.

Nonphysician practitioners are created by the existing cadre of medical providers in a country and emerge from specific perceived needs in health care delivery. In nearly all cases these needs involve a shortage of fully trained physicians to provide adequate medical services to the population. This was in fact the fundamental rationale for the creation of PAs in the United States.

Once nonphysicians enter the delivery system, evolving circumstances and changes in the system affect the roles and perceptions of these providers. As the supply of a country's physician population rises, and as experience with these practitioners accumulates, new perceptions of the roles that these providers can assume often develop. In some instances, there is no further need for these providers in the health care system. In others, the role of the nonphysician provider changes and becomes more technically oriented. In still other systems, nonphysician clinicians evolve into well-established members of a health care delivery team, participating with physicians in a wide variety of clinical functions. The broadest generalization that can be made is that nonphysicians must adjust and adapt to changing forces within the health delivery system in which they work once they outlive the rationale of their initial creation.

As we have seen, this is what has occurred with PAs in the United States.

Lessons for Other Systems

As we look to other systems to avoid the pitfalls of history lessons ignored, PAs must be cognizant that movements are underway to expand the notion of PAs to other countries. PAs in many ways represent a health care workforce innovation that has met a number of important needs in the U.S. health systems as a unique American creation. However, other countries are looking to PAs in American medicine as exportable models to address their own shortages.

Since the 1990s there have been a scattering of reports about the use of PAs in England. The editor in chief of the *British Journal of Nursing* reviews the use of PAs in North America and writes:

> With the emphasis on reducing doctors' hours and recent concerns about future shortages of doctors and nurses, it could be argued that we should be looking at the feasibility of such a development in the UK. As we do not have a large body of redundant military personnel from which to recruit, perhaps we could gradually convert operating department assistants, technicians and paramedics to the role. It may also be possible to encourage more medically oriented nurse practitioners to enlist! [However, problems exist within a small country with an expanding NP pres-

> ence, where conflict already exists with physicians resenting NPs, much less] introduction of a new species within an established healthcare system generating uncertainty and confusion. (Castledine, 1996)

Already, nurses are being tasked with new roles, and "the introduction of PAs could cause chaos." Castledine (1996) concludes his editorial by stating, "We must not increase the number of personnel the patient currently comes into contact with. Patients are already confused about the variety of roles that nurses undertake; to add more roles into the health-care team without proper evaluation of the benefits to the patient would be disastrous."

In another editorial in the same journal a solicitor and principal lecturer at the Centre of Advanced Litigation, Nottingham Law School in England, writes as a dedicated fan of the television series *ER* he was intrigued by the conflict between the nurse, the physician, and the PA and observed that the nurse "works with the doctors, often with equal responsibility, while the PA works for the doctors on specific tasks" (Peysner, 1996).

The author reflects that this debate is not unique to the United States or the health field because solicitors have "traditionally worked with legal executives who are often highly competent generalists." The news that "doctor's assistants" are being employed at a hospital in England suggests that a "potential conflict has now arrived." Instead of pursuing the PA role, the author then shifts to the controversy of "an extended role for nurses" and discusses some cases of alleged negligence:

> The test is in the Court of Appeal case of Wilsher vs Essex Area Health Authority (1986), which involved alleged negligence by a junior doctor who catheterized a premature baby, resulting in over-oxygenation and blindness. The doctor's lack of experience could not be a defense to an action for negligence: The test was to judge the appropriate standard of competence required for the specific job—inexperience had to be discounted. (Peysner, 1996)

Our impressions from discussions with nurses and observers of nurses in the United Kingdom is that the registered nurse (RN) is already tasked with a very high level of responsibility, particularly inpatient, nursing homes, and visiting nurses. The NP role is in considerable flux as inroads of advanced nursing are being met with widespread physician resentment. Exporting the PA concept to Canada, the Neatherlands, or Mexico may be a more logical step than trying it out in the United Kingdom.

As of 2002 the expansion of the Canadian PAs to both serve the nation's forces and enter into the civilian realm is underway. The Canadian Academy of Physician Assistants in Borden, Ontario, is developing under capable leadership. Although PAs in the Canadian Forces are warrant officers, their role is considered valuable and a possible solution to physician shortages throughout the providences (Hooker, 2002).

Interest is expanding in other countries as well. England, frustrated with physician and nurse shortages, considers PAs from time to time as evidenced in various editorials contemplating expanding nurses into NPs or adopting a PA model. Australia too is experiencing workforce shortages, both in physicians and in nurses, and has been examining NP and PA models as well. The AAPA Committee on International Affairs reports that 83 countries have expressed some interest in the PA model.

FUTURE ISSUES

No futurist is ever confident of his or her predictions. Making predictions is based on lessons learned, the sciences of history, economics, demographics, and politics, and observing changes based on technology and sociology. However, every prediction is subject to "wild cards," which are events and movements that are not expected but when they happen often produce unanticipated changes. Two potential wild cards are PA independence and international medical graduates (IMGs). Each could change the attitude of society toward PAs.

Independence and Professional Recognition

Issues of whether PAs should seek practice independence arise from time to time, often when there are issues about professional recognition. To some PAs professional recognition will come only if they gain the legal right to full independence of practice. That means they would be free to contract and negotiate for services similar to what a small number of NPs have in certain states. To some extent this is already underway as PAs find that there are opportunities to be entrepreneurs and independent owners of health care systems (Barnes and Hooker, 2001). Although the push for recognition comes from the PA profession, increased financial pressure on the health care industry is also an important substrate for change. A partial list of advantages and disadvantages of independent practice for PAs is listed in Exhibit 14-6.

International Medical Graduates as Physician Assistants

There are two types of IMGs: those who are U.S. citizens and have been to medical school outside of the United States and those who are non-U.S. citizens and not educated in the United States. When the latter immigrate to the United States and would like to practice as physicians, sometimes those skills are difficult to market. For some this means undertaking or even repeating a postgraduate training period (residency). Not all can qualify to work as a physician, and some IMGs for whom the door has been closed have sought to attain recognition as a PA as an alternative. This has caused some consternation because the National Commission on Certification of Physician Assistants (NCCPA) will not allow some IMGs to take the national certifying examination unless they are graduates of an accredited PA program. Studies performed in two states with high proportions of IMGs have demonstrated that cohorts of IMGs cannot pass the same examinations given to second-year PA students (Fowkes et al., 1996).

IMGs represent an issue because there is some evidence that IMGs will accept employment in the health sector that may not be desirable to physicians and NPCs such as corrections medicine and remote rural health. Furthermore, fewer U.S. medical school seniors are choosing primary care residency positions in family practice, pediatrics, internal medicine, and obstetrics and gynecology. This is continuing a parallel trend since the mid 1990s as non-U.S. citizen international medical graduates match in fewer numbers while U.S. citizen IMGs match in record numbers. The two trends are somewhat linked, because non-U.S. citizen IMGs are more likely to choose primary care positions than specialty programs such as surgery, dermatology, or urology. As fewer non-U.S. citizen IMGs enter residency programs over the next several years, and as more U.S. medical school seniors and U.S. citizen IMGs seek specialty slots, the number of primary care positions filled is expected to further decline. Specialties such as surgery, anesthesiology, and radiology are beginning to attract more U.S. medical school seniors because the rewards of primary care may not be as rewarding as it was once perceived. As U.S. medical school seniors began to flee primary care for the more lucrative specialties during the past two decades, primary care residencies began filling open slots with IMGs. Now, however, with fewer IMGs entering the system, there are fewer opportunities for residency programs in pediatrics, internal medicine,

EXHIBIT 14-6

Advantages and Disadvantages of PA Independent Practice

Advantages	Disadvantages
Able to seek employment and negotiate terms more easily	If physicians are not employers, jobs may not be as readily available
Supervising physician can help share the responsibility and fallout in malpractice cases	May be seen as more vulnerable to plaintiff lawyers
Will have a greater say in standards of care and educational levels	Will have to improve standards of care, seek legislative changes, and improve educational levels constantly on own
Can negotiate salary with more independence	Physicians are increasingly opting for salaried work instead of independence
Can form a business and work for the business and reap the rewards	Businesses are increasingly regulated with compliance consuming large amounts of time and resources
Independent reimbursement from insurance companies will improve return for work	Many third-party payers may resist another group seeking reimbursement

and family practice to fill open slots that U.S. medical school seniors continue to avoid. PAs may be the only viable alternative for this widening void.

SUMMARY

Growth and opportunity will be the catchwords for the PA profession as it moves along in the new century. Numerous changes can be expected, along with stimulating challenges. It is an exciting time to be a PA, and it is difficult for a profession to be too concerned about the future when it is riding the wave crest of demand. Current focus is on the expansion of the profession to meet the demand of the changing health care environment that wants more PAs. For the first time PAs are part of the health policy equation as planners estimate what the health workforce should be like in the years ahead. Like all waves, however, the crest will break and supply will exceed demand. When this will occur is difficult to predict. An expanding population and an aging population mean greater demand for services. Furthermore, an uninsured population that needs care tends to create demand for services that are unexpected. Excessive health care costs, poor access for some citizens, and uneven quality of care bodes well for the PA profession because PAs can help meet this demand quickly. However, increased penetration and the fickle nature of managed care, coupled with efforts to improve efficiency in delivery, have begun to dampen physician salaries. If rising PA salaries come close to physician salaries, then the surge of new graduates may produce the supply side of the equation that catches up with the demand side sooner than expected.

The quality of U.S.-trained physicians, PAs, and medical care in the United States has never been higher. If PAs want to remain in the great debate about what the health care workforce should look like, they must meet the challenge with science that shows they are viable players.

APPENDIX 1

PHYSICIAN ASSISTANT PROFESSIONAL ORGANIZATIONS

Two lists are presented here. The first is a list of Constituent Chapters of the American Academy of Physician Assistants (AAPA). These are state and federal organizations that constitute the AAPA House of Delegates. The second is a list of Physician assistants (PA) specialty organizations. This list was updated July 15, 2002.

CONSTITUENT CHAPTERS OF THE AMERICAN ACADEMY OF PHYSICIAN ASSISTANTS

Alabama Society of Physician Assistants
PO Box 550274, Birmingham, AL 35255-0274
Phone: (205) 408-5757; fax: (205) 933-2905
E-mail: alpasociety@aol.com
http://www.alabamapasociety.org

Alaska Academy of Physician Assistants
PO Box 74187, Fairbanks, AK 99707-4187
Phone: (800) 478-8684; fax: (907) 452-8373
E-mail: akapa@gci.net
http://www.akapa.org

Arizona State Association of Physician Assistants
PO Box 12307, Glendale, AZ 85318-2307
Toll free: (800) 595-6721
Phone: (623) 582-1246; fax: (800) 582-1246
E-mail: darr@primenet.com
http://www.asapa.org

Arkansas Academy of Physician Assistants
950 N. Washington St., Alexandria, VA 22314-1534
Phone: (877) 466-2272; fax: (703) 684-1924
E-mail: arapa@aapa.org
http://www.aapa.org/states/arapa.html

Society of Army Physician Assistants
6762 Candlewood Dr., Fort Myers, FL 33919-6402
Phone: (941) 482-2162; fax: (941) 482-2162
E-mail: hal.slusher@juno.com
http://www.sapa.org

California Academy of Physician Assistants
3100 W. Warner Ave., Ste. 3, Santa Ana, CA 92704-5331
Phone: (714) 427-0321; fax: (714) 427-0324
E-mail: capa@capanet.org
http://www.capanet.org

Colorado Academy of Physician Assistants
PO Box 4834, Englewood, CO 80155-4834
Phone: (303) 770-6048; fax: (303) 771-2550
E-mail: carol@goddardassociates.com
http://www.coloradopas.org

Connecticut Academy of Physician Assistants
PO Box 81362, Wellesley, MA 02481-0004
Phone: (800) 493-9200; fax: (781) 239-3259
E-mail: assnadv@tiac.net
http://www.connapa.org

Delaware Academy of Physician Assistants
704 Dorcaster Dr., Wilmington, DE 19808-2214
Phone: (302) 856-4360
E-mail: rfalcioni@zoominternet.net
http://www.delawarepas.org

District of Columbia Academy of Physician Assistants
PO Box 50147, 800 K St. NW, Washington, DC 20091-0147
E-mail: padcchapter@hotmail.com

Florida Academy of Physician Assistants
PO Box 150127, Altamonte Springs, FL 32715-0127
Phone: (407) 774-7880; fax: (407) 774-6440
E-mail: fapa@fapaonline.org
http://www.fapaonline.org

Georgia Association of Physician Assistants
980 Canton St., Bldg. 1, Ste. B, Roswell, GA 30075
Toll free: (888) 811-4192
Phone: (770) 640-1920; fax: (770) 640-1095
E-mail: gapa@gapaonline.org
http://www.gapaonline.org

Guam Association of Physician Assistants
PO Box 6578, Tamuning, GU 96931-6578
Phone: (671) 646-5825; fax: (671) 646-3120
E-mail: skipcherry@kuentos.guam.net

Hawaii Academy of Physician Assistants
PO Box 30355, Honolulu, HI 96820-0355
Phone: (808) 668-4864; fax: (808) 432-8330
E-mail: opa79@aol.com

Idaho Academy of Physician Assistants
PO Box 2668, 305 W. Jefferson, Boise, ID 83701-2668
Phone: (208) 344-7888; fax: (208) 344-7903
E-mail: ssass@idmed.org
http://www.IdahoPA.org

Illinois Academy of Physician Assistants
625 S. 2nd St., Springfield, IL 62704-2500
Toll free: (800) 975-9344
Phone: (800) 975-9344; fax: (217) 789-4664
E-mail: iapa@ampka.com
http://www.ampka.com/iapa

Indiana Academy of Physician Assistants
950 N. Washington St., Alexandria, VA 22314-1534
Phone: (888) 441-0423; fax: (703) 684-1924
E-mail: iapa@aapa.org
http://www.aapa.org/iapa.htm

Iowa Physician Assistant Society
200 10th St., Fl. 5, Des Moines, IA 50309-3609
Toll free: (877) 837-6982
Phone: (515) 243-2000; fax: (515) 243-5941
E-mail: ipas@netins.net
http://showcase.netins.net/web/ipas/

Kansas Academy of Physician Assistants
PO Box 597, Topeka, KS 66601-0597
Phone: (785) 235-5065; fax: (785) 235-8676
E-mail: dsmith@cjnetworks.com
http://www.kansaspa.com

Kentucky Academy of Physician Assistants
PO Box 23251, Lexington, KY 40523-3251
Toll free: (888) 884-5272
Phone: (606) 432-5532; fax: (606) 433-0110
E-mail: jchpac@se-tel.com
http://www.kyapa.org

Louisiana Academy of Physician Assistants
8550 United Plaza Blvd., Ste. 1001, Baton Rouge, LA 70809-0200
Phone: (225) 922-4630; fax: (225) 408-4424
E-mail: lapa@pncpa.com
http://www.louisianapa.org

Maine
Downeast Association of PAs
PO Box 2027, Augusta, ME 04338-2027
Phone: (207) 629-9417; fax: (207) 629-9243
E-mail: lindaroberts@bigplanet.com
http://www.deapa.com

Maryland Academy of Physician Assistants
8207 Selwin Ct., Rosedale, MD 21237-3362
Phone: (410) 661-6637
E-mail: vkmanning@comcast.net
http://www.mdapa.org

Massachusetts Association of Physician Assistants
950 N. Washington St., Alexandria, VA 22314-1534
Phone: (800) 441-2692; fax: (703) 684-1924
E-mail: mass-pa@aapa.org
http://www.mass-pa.com

Michigan Academy of Physician Assistants
120 W. Saginaw St., East Lansing, MI 48823-2605
Toll free: (887) 937-6272
Phone: (517) 336-1498; fax: (517) 337-2590
E-mail: mapa@michiganpa.org
http://www.michiganpa.org

Minnesota Academy of Physician Assistants
4248 Park Glen Rd., Minneapolis, MN 55416-4758
Phone: (612) 928-4666; fax: (612) 929-1318
E-mail: mtheisen@harringtonxcompany.com
http://www.mnacadpa.org

Mississippi Academy of Physician Assistants
PO Box 5128, Biloxi, MS 39534-0128
Phone: (800) 844-4902; fax: (703) 684-1924
E-mail: missipas@aapa.org
http://www.aapa.org/msapa.htm

Missouri Academy of Physician Assistants
950 N. Washington St., Alexandria, VA 22314-1534
Phone: (800) 844-4902; fax: (703) 684-1924
E-mail: mapa@aapa.org
http://www.moapa.org

Montana Academy of Physician Assistants
950 N. Washington St., Alexandria, VA 22314-1534
Phone: (406) 248-6038; fax: (703) 684-1924
E-mail: montanapas@aapa.org
http://www.aapa.org/mapa.htm

Naval Association of Physician Assistants
950 N. Washington St., Alexandria, VA 22314-1534
Phone: (888) 836-4169; fax: (703) 684-1924
E-mail: napa@aapa.org
http://www.aapa.org/napa.html

Nebraska Academy of Physician Assistants
7906 Davenport St., Omaha, NE 68114-3631
Phone: (402) 393-1415; fax: (402) 393-3216
E-mail: tgrothe@unmc.edu
http://MEMBERS.AOL.COM/NEACDPAS

Nevada Academy of Physician Assistants
PO Box 28877, Las Vegas, NV 89126-2877
Phone: (702) 451-4578
E-mail: mcppac@aol.com
http://www.nevada-pa-academy.org/

New Hampshire Society of Physician Assistants
PO Box 325, Manchester, NH 03105-0325
Phone: (603) 644-2262; fax: (603) 663-6350
E-mail: joam401@aol.com
http://www.nh-spa.org

New Jersey State Society of Physician Assistants
PO Box 1, Princeton, NJ 08543-0001
Phone: (609) 275-4123; fax: (609) 734-0065
E-mail: njsspa@njha.com
http://www.njsspa.org

New Mexico Academy of Physician Assistants
160 Washington St. SE #1, Albuquerque, NM 87108-2731
Phone: (505) 342-8023; fax: (505) 260-1919
E-mail: nmpa@nmapa.com
http://www.nmapa.com

New York State Society of Physician Assistants
251 New Karner Rd., Ste. 10A, Albany, NY 12205-4617
Phone: (212) 206-8300; fax: (212) 645-1147
E-mail: kdolci@msn.com
http://www.nysspa.org

North Carolina Academy of Physician Assistants
3209 Guess Rd., Ste. 105, Durham, NC
27705-2692
Toll free: (800) 352-2271
Phone: (919) 479-1995; fax: (919) 479-9726
E-mail: ncapa@ncapa.org
http://www.ncapa.org

North Dakota Academy of Physician Assistants
1412 Cottonwood Ave., Minot, ND 58707-0001
Phone: (701) 838-6394; fax: (701) 839-0967
E-mail: terri_lang@und.nodak.edu

Ohio Association of Physician Assistants
4683 Winterset Dr., Columbus, OH 43220-8113
Toll free: (800) 292-4997
Phone: (614) 292-4997; fax: (614) 459-4524
E-mail: oapa@infinet.com
http://www.ohiopa.com

Oklahoma Academy of Physician Assistants
PO Box 1132, Oklahoma City, OK 73101-1132
Phone: (405) 271-2058; fax: (405) 271-3621
E-mail: susan-andreatta@ouhsc.edu

Oregon Society of Physician Assistants
PO Box 514, Oregon City, OR 97045-0029
Phone: (503) 650-5864; fax: (503) 650-5864
E-mail: ospa@oregonpa.org
http://www.oregonpa.org

Pennsylvania Society of PAs
PO Box 128, Greensburg, PA 15601-0128
Phone: (724) 836-6411; fax: (724) 836-4449
E-mail: pspa@usaor.net
http://www.pspa.net

Public Health Service Academy of Physician
Assistants
950 N. Washington St., Alexandria, VA
22314-1534
Phone: (800) 441-3716; fax: (703) 684-1924
E-mail: phs@aapa.org
http://www.aapa.org/phs.htm

Rhode Island Academy of Physician Assistants
106 Francis St., Providence, RI 02903-1117
Phone: (401) 331-3207; fax: (703) 684-1924
http://www.aapa.org/states/riapa.html

South Carolina Academy of Physician Assistants
PO Box 2054, Lexington, SC 29071-2054
Phone: (803) 356-6809; fax: (803) 356-6826
E-mail: association@sc.rr.com
http://www.scapapartners.org/

South Dakota Academy of Physician Assistants
3708 W. Brooks Pl., Ste. 1, Sioux Falls, SD
57106-4207
Phone: (605) 361-2281; fax: (605) 361-5175
E-mail: cradduck@sdaho.org
http://www.sdapa.net

Tennessee Academy of Physician Assistants
1483 N. Mount Juliet Rd., PMB #203, Mount
Juliet, TN 37122-3315
Phone: (615) 443-3052; fax: (615) 453-9639
E-mail: tapadirector@msn.com
http://www.tnpa.com

Utah Academy of Physician Assistants
50 N Medical Dr., Bldg. 528, Salt Lake City, UT
84132-0001
Phone: (801) 581-7764; fax: (801) 374-1902
E-mail: d.robinson@upap.utah.edu
http://www.utahapa.org

Physician Assistant Academy of Vermont
68 Overlook Dr., South Burlington, VT
05403-7887
Phone: (802) 457-5000
E-mail: paav@cyberportal.net
http://www.paav.org

Veterans Affairs Physician Assistant Association
PO Box 128, Iron Mountain, MI 49801-0128
Phone: (866) 828-2722
E-mail: vapaa@aapa.org
http://www.vapaa.org

Virginia Academy of Physician Assistants
10366 Democracy Ln., Ste. B, Fairfax, VA
22030-2522
Phone: (703) 691-8515; fax: (703) 691-0896
E-mail: vapa@vapa.org
http://www.vapa.org

Washington State Academy of Physician Assistants
2033 6th Ave., Ste. 1100, Seattle, WA 98121-2590
Phone: (206) 956-3624; fax: (206) 441-5863
E-mail: LMK@wama.org
http://www.wapa.com

West Virginia Association of Physician Assistants
PO Box 3625, Charleston, WV 25336-3625
Phone: (304) 984-0308; fax: (304) 984-3718
E-mail: exedir@wvapa.com
http://www.wvapa.com

Wisconsin Academy of Physician Assistants
PO Box 1109, Madison, WI 53701-1109
Toll free: (800) 762-8965 ; fax: (608) 283-5424
E-mail: wapa@wismed.org
http://www.wapa.org

Wyoming Association of Physician Assistants
1260 W. 5th St., # 62, Sheridan, WY 82801-2702
Phone: (307) 674-6166; fax: (307) 672-8687
E-mail: mtrentpa@fiberpipe.net
http://www.wapa.net

PA SPECIALTY ORGANIZATIONS

AAPAs in Allergy, Asthma, and Immunology
10470 Vista del Sol Dr., Ste. 100, El Paso, TX 79925-7928
Phone: (559) 994-0714; fax: (559) 325-1375
E-mail: aapaaai99@netscape.net
http://www.aapa.org/spec/aapa-aai.html

American Academy of Nephrology PAs
http://www.aanpa.org

American Academy of PAs in Occupational Medicine
950 N. Washington St., Alexandria, VA 22314-1534
Phone: (800) 596-4398; fax: (703) 683-1924
E-mail: aaapom@aapa.org
http://www.aapa.org/paom.html

American Association of Plastic & Reconstructive Surgery PAs
18 Henry Harris St., Fl. 2, Chicopee, MA 01013-2508
Phone: (413) 732-7115
E-mail: leahkenney@hotmail.com

American Association of Surgical PAs
PO Box 867, Bernardsville, NJ 07924-0867
Phone: (888) 882-2772; fax: (732) 805-9582
E-mail: theaaspa@aol.com
http://www.aaspa.com

American Society of Endocrine Physician Assistants
950 N. Washington St., Alexandria, VA 22314-1534
Phone: (888) 441-0428; fax: (703) 683-1924
E-mail: asepa@aapa.org
http://www.asepa.com

Association of Family Practice PAs
7443 Legend Point Dr., San Antonio, TX 78244-2412
Toll free: (877) 890-0181 ; fax: (210) 805-9847
E-mail: afppa@afppa.org
http://www.afppa.org

Association of Neurosurgical PAs
PO Box 559, Bernardsville, NJ 07924-0559
Phone: (888) 942-6772; fax: (732) 805-9582
E-mail: neuropac@aol.com
http://www.anspa.org

Association of PAs in Cardiovascular Surgery
PO Box 4834, Englewood, CO 80155-4834
Phone: (877) 221-5651; fax: (303) 771-2550
E-mail: cagoddard@aol.com
http://WWW.APACVS.ORG

Association of PAs in Obstetrics & Gynecology
PO Box 1109, Madison, WI 53701-1109
Phone: (800) 545-0636; fax: (608) 283-5424
E-mail: kathym@wismed.org
http://www.paobgyn.org/

Association of Psychiatric PAs
3737 Southern Blvd., Kettering College of Medical Arts/Medical Center, Dayton, OH 45429-1225
Phone: (937) 298-3399 x55625; fax: (937) 297-8095
E-mail: willmosiereddpa@yahoo.com
http://communities.msn.com/ASSOCIATION-OFPSYCHIATRICPHYSICIANASSISTANTSINC

Gastrointestinal Physician Assistants
1346 Madison St., Mandeville, LA 70448-6034
Phone: (985) 626-4880
E-mail: rodbranch@yahoo.com

PAs in Orthopedic Surgery
PO Box 10781, Glendale, AZ 85318-0781
Phone: (800) 804-7267; fax: (602) 301-8674
E-mail: darr@primenet.com
http://www.paos.org

Society for PAs in Pediatrics
950 N. Washington St., Alexandria, VA 22314-1534
Phone: (800) 596-4398; fax: (703) 684-1924
E-mail: spap@aapa.org
http://www.aapa.org/spec/SPAP/

Society of Dermatology PAs
8301 Broadway St., Ste. 401, San Antonio, TX 78209-2067
Phone: (800) 380-3992; fax: (210) 822-8845
E-mail: sdpa@emsisa.com
http://home.pacifier.com/~jomonroe

Society of Emergency Medicine PAs
950 N. Washington St., Alexandria, VA 22314-1534
Phone: (703) 519-7334; fax: (703) 684-1924
E-mail: info@sempa.org
http://www.sempa.org

Society of PAs Caring for the Elderly
PO Box 639, Lizella, GA 31052-0639
Phone: (478) 784-3500
E-mail: tivolikw@aol.com

Society of PAs in Addiction Medicine
1157 Union Lake Rd., White Lake, MI 48386-4348
Phone: (248) 335-2288
E-mail: mickiepa@aol.com

Society of PAs in Otorhinolaryngology/Head & Neck Surgery
950 N. Washington St., Alexandria, VA 22314-1534
Phone: (713) 745-0495; fax: (713) 794-4662
E-mail: spao@aapa.org
Http://www.entpa.org

Urology Association of PAs
PO Box 11000, Mesa, AZ 85214-1000
Phone: (602) 926-6237
http://www.aapa.org/spec/uapa.html

Society of Air Force Physician Assistants
950 N. Washington St., Alexandria, VA 22314-1534
Phone: (888) 903-2272; fax: (703) 684-1924
E-mail: safpa@aapa.org
http://www.safpa.org

APPENDIX 2

PHYSICIAN ASSISTANT PROGRAMS

The following is a list of physician assistant programs with mailing addresses and telephone numbers. For further information about the status of a program's accreditation, please contact the program directly.*

ALABAMA

University of Alabama at Birmingham†
Surgical Physician Assistant Program
School of Health Related Professions
RMSB 481
1530 3rd Avenue South
Birmingham, AL 35294-1270
Telephone: (205) 934-4605
Fax: (205) 934-3780
www.uab.edu

University of South Alabama†
College of Allied Health Professions
Department of Physician Assistant Studies
1504 Springhill Ave., Room 4410
Mobile, AL 36604-3273
Telephone: (251) 434-3641
Fax: (251) 434-3646
E-mail: pastudies@usamail.usouthal.edu
www.southalabama.edu/allhealth/pa.htm

*These physician assistant programs have provisional accreditation from ARC-PA. Provisional accreditation is a time-limited accreditation status that is awarded to new programs prior to admission of their first class. Applicants should contact each program to discuss its accreditation status.

ARIZONA

Arizona School of Health Sciences†
A Division of Kirksville College of Osteopathic Medicine
Physician Assistant Program
5850 E. Still Cir.
Mesa, AZ 85206
Telephone: (480) 219-6040
Fax: (480) 219-6100
www.ashs.edu

Midwestern University*
Physician Assistant Program
19555 N. 59th Ave.
Glendale, AZ 85308
Telephone: (888) 247-9277; (623) 572-3311
Fax: (623) 572-3227

CALIFORNIA

Charles R. Drew University of Medicine and Science†
College of Allied Health
Physician Assistant Program
1731 East 120th St., MP42
Los Angeles, CA 90059
Telephone: (323) 563-5950
Fax: (323) 563-4833

†These physician assistant programs have been accredited by the Accreditation Review Commission on Education for the Physician Assistant, Inc (ARC-PA).

Loma Linda University*
School of Allied Health Professions
PA Program
Nichol Hall, Room 2033
Loma Linda, CA 92350
Telephone: (909) 558-7295
Fax: (909) 558-0495
www.llu.edu

Riverside County Regional Medical†
Center/Riverside Community College
PA Program
16130 Lasselle St.
Moreno Valley, CA 92551-2045
Telephone: (909) 571-6166
Fax: (909) 571-6221
www.rccd.cc.ca.us

Samuel Merritt College*
PA Program
450 30th St., Suite 4708
Oakland, CA 94609
Telephone: (510) 869-6623
Fax: (510) 869-6951
E-mail: dnakamura@smuelmerritt.edu
www.samuelmerritt.edu

Stanford University Medical Center/Foothill College†
Primary Care Associate Program
703 Welch Rd., Suite G-1
Palo Alto, CA 94304-1760
Telephone: (650) 725-6959
Fax: (650) 723-9692
www.stanford.edu/dept/medfm.pca/tofc.html

University of California, Davis Medical Center†
FNP/PA Program
2516 Stockton Blvd., #254
Sacramento, CA 95817-2208
Telephone: (916) 734-3551
Fax: (916) 452-2112
E-mail: patty.frank@ucdmc.ucdavis.edu
fnppa.ucdavis.edu

University of Southern California†
Keck School of Medicine
Primary Care PA Program
1000 South Fremont Ave.
Unit 7, Bldg. A6, Room 6249
Alhambra, CA 91803
Telephone: (626) 457-4240
Fax: (626) 457-4245
www.usc.edu/hsc/medicine/family_med/pa/index.html

Western University of Health Sciences†
Primary Care Physician Assistant Program
450 East Second St.
Pomona, CA 91766
Telephone: (909) 469-5378
Fax: (909) 469-5407
E-mail: admissions@westernu.edu
www.westernu.edu

COLORADO

Red Rocks Community College†
PA Program
13300 West Sixth Ave.
Lakewood, CO 80228
Telephone: (303) 914-6386
Fax: (303) 914-6806
E-mail: Arlene.duran@rrcc.cccoes.edu

University of Colorado†
Health Sciences Center
Child Health Associate/PA Program
PO Box 6508
Mailstop F543
Aurora, CO 80045-0508
Telephone: (303) 724-1350
Fax: (303) 315-6976
E-mail: Chapa-info@uchsc.edu
www.uchsc.edu/sm/chapa

CONNECTICUT

Quinnipiac University†
Physician Assistant Program
275 Mt. Carmel Ave.
Hamden, CT 06518-1961
Telephone: (203) 582-8704
Fax: (203) 582-5303

Yale University†
School of Medicine
PA Program
47 College St., Suite 220
New Haven, CT 06510-3209
Telephone: (203) 785-2860
Fax: (203) 785-3601
E-mail: Janet.liscio@yale.edu
www.info.med.yale.edu/phyassoc

DISTRICT OF COLUMBIA

George Washington University†
Physician Assistant Program
2175 K St., NW, Suite 820
Washington, DC 20037-1809
Telephone: (202) 530-2390
Fax: (202) 530-2360
E-mail: npalan@gwumc.edu
www.gwu.edu/~gwu_pa

Howard University†
Division of Allied Health Sciences
Physician Assistant Program
Sixth & Bryant St., NW
Washington, DC 20060
Telephone: (202) 806-7536
Fax: (202) 806-4476
www.cpnahs.howard.edu

FLORIDA

Barry University†
School of Graduate Medical Sciences
PA Program
11300 NE Second Ave., Box SGMS
Miami, FL 33161-6695
Telephone: (305) 899-4065
Fax: (305) 899-4038
E-mail: Dparkhurst@mail.barry.edu
www.barry.edu

Miami-Dade Community College†
Physician Assistant Program
950 NW 20th St.
Miami, FL 33127-4622
Telephone: (305) 237-4051
Fax: (305) 237-4278
E-mail: wtaylor@mdcc.edu
www.mdcc.edu/medical/PA/pa.htm

Nova Southeastern University†
College of Allied Health
Health Professions Division
Physician Assistant Program
3200 South University Dr.
Ft. Lauderdale, FL 33328
Telephone: (954) 262-1250
Fax: (954) 262-2285
E-mail: jkeena@nova.edu
www.nova.edu/pa

University of Florida†
Physician Assistant Program
Box 100176
Gainesville, FL 32610-0176
Telephone: (352) 265-7955
Fax: (352) 265-7996
E-mail: heikkpj@pap.ufl.edu
www.med.ufl.edu/pap/apply

GEORGIA

Emory University†
School of Medicine
Physician Assistant Program
1462 Clifton Rd. NE, Suite 280
Atlanta, GA 30322-1063
Telephone: (404) 727-7825
Fax: (404) 727-7836
www.pa.emory.edu

Emory University
School of Medicine
Anesthesiology Assistant/Anesthesiology PA Program
617 Woodruff Memorial Bldg.
1639 Pierce Dr.
Atlanta, GA 30322
Telephone: (404) 727-5910
Fax: (404) 727-3021
www.emory.edu/whsc/med/anesthesiology

Medical College of Georgia†
Physician Assistant Program, AE 1032
Augusta, GA 30912
Telephone: (706) 721-3246
Fax: (706) 721-3990
E-mail: bdadig@mail.mcg.edu
www.mcg.edu

South College†
Physician Assistant Program
709 Mall Blvd.
Savannah, GA 31406
Telephone: (912) 691-6023
Fax: (912) 691-6082
www.southcollege.edu

IDAHO

Idaho State University†
1021 Red Hill Rd.
Pocatello, ID 83209
Telephone: (208) 282-4726
Fax: (208) 282-4969
E-mail: kingnore@isu.edu
www.isu.edu/PAProg

ILLINOIS

Cook County Hospital/Malcolm X College†
Physician Assistant Program
1900 West Van Buren St., Suite 3241
Chicago, IL 60612-3197
Telephone: (312) 850-7268
Fax: (312) 850-3538

Finch University of Health Sciences/The Chicago Medical School†
Physician Assistant Program
3333 Green Bay Rd.
North Chicago, IL 60064-3095
Telephone: (847) 578-8511
Fax: (847) 578-8690
E-mail: Sharon.stewart@finch.cms.edu
www.finchcms.edu

Midwestern University†
PA Program-Downer's Grove Campus
555 31st St.
Downers Grove, IL 60515-1235
Telephone: (630) 515-6034
Fax: (630) 971-6402
E-mail: admiss@midwestern.edu
www.midwestern.edu

Southern Illinois University at Carbondale†
Physician Assistant Program
Mail Code 6516, Lindegren Hall 129
Carbondale, IL 62901
Telephone: (618) 453-1151
Fax: (618) 453-7216
E-mail: jbanning@siumed.edu
paserver3.som.siu.edu

INDIANA

Butler University†
College of Pharmacy and Health Sciences
Physician Assistant Program
4600 Sunset Ave.
Indianapolis, IN 46208-3485
Telephone: (317) 940-9969
Fax: (317) 940-6172
E-mail: canagel@butler.edu
www.butler.edu

University of Saint Frances†
Physician Assistant Program
2701 Spring St.
Fort Wayne, IN 46808
Telephone: (219) 434-3100
Fax: (219) 458-7695
E-mail: dunde@sf.edu
www.sf.edu/aliied/pa.html

IOWA

Des Moines University-Osteopathic Medical Center†
Physician Assistant Program
3200 Grand Ave.
Des Moines, IA 50312-4104
Telephone: (515) 271-1603
Fax: (515) 271-1410
E-mail: paadmit@dmu.edu
www.dmu.edu

University of Iowa†
College of Medicine
Physician Assistant Program
5167 Westlawn
Iowa City, IA 52242-1100
Telephone: (319) 335-8922
Fax: (319) 335-8923
E-mail: paprogram@uiowa.edu
www.medicine.uiowa.edu/pa/pa.htm

KANSAS

Wichita State University†
College of Health Professions
Physician Assistant Program
1845 N. Fairmount
Wichita, KS 67260-0043
Telephone: (316) 978-3011
Fax: (316) 978-3025
www.wichita.edu

KENTUCKY

University of Kentucky†
College of Allied Health
Physician Assistant Program
103 CAHP Building
121 Washington Ave.
Lexington, KY 40536
Telephone: (859) 323-1100, ext 273
Fax: (859) 257-2454
www.uky.edu

LOUISIANA

Louisiana State University Health Sciences Center†
School of Allied health Professions
Physician Assistant Program
1501 Kings Highway, PO Box 33932
Shreveport, LA 71130-3932
Telephone: (318) 675-7317
Fax: (318) 675-6937
www.lsuhsc.edu

MAINE

University of New England†
College of Health Professionals
Physician Assistant Program
716 Stevens Ave.
Portland, ME 04103-7688
Telephone: (207) 797-7688, x4529
Fax: (207) 286-9493
www.une.edu/chp/pa

MARYLAND

Anne Arundel Community College†
Physician Assistant Program
101 College Pkwy.
Arnold, MD 21012-1895
Telephone: (410) 777-7310
Fax: (410) 777-7099
www.aacc.cc.md.us

The Community College of Baltimore County
Essex Campus†
Physician Assistant Program
7201 Rossville Blvd.
Baltimore, MD 21237-3855
Telephone: (410) 780-6159
Fax: (410) 780-6405
E-mail: sshaw@ccbc.cc.md.us
www.ccbc.cc.md.us

University of Maryland-Eastern Shore*
Physician Assistant Program
Modular 934-5
Princess Anne, MD 21853
Telephone: (410) 651-7584
Fax: (410) 651-7586
E-mail: bjjaster@mail.umes.edu

MASSACHUSETTS

Massachusetts College of Pharmacy and Health Sciences†
Physician Assistant Program
179 Longwood Ave., WB01
Boston, MA 02115-5896
Telephone: (617) 732-2140
Fax: (617) 732-2075

Northeastern University†
Physician Assistant Program
202 Robinson Hall
360 Huntington Ave.
Boston, MA 02115-5005
Telephone: (617) 373-3195
Fax: (617) 373-3338
www.neu.edu/bouve/department/pa/pap.html

Springfield College/Baystate Health Systems†
Physician Assistant Program
263 Alden St.
Springfield, MA 01109-3797
Telephone: (413) 748-3554
Fax: (413) 739-5211
www.springfieldcollege.edu

MICHIGAN

Central Michigan University†
Physician Assistant Program
101 Foust
Mt. Pleasant, MI 48859
Telephone: (989) 774-1730
Fax: (989) 774-2433

Grand Valley State University†
Medical Education and Research Center
PA Studies Program
1000 Monroe NW
Grand Rapids, MI 49503
Telephone: (616) 233-6500
Fax: (616) 233-6525
E-mail: pas@gvsu.edu
www.gvsu.edu/pas

University of Detroit Mercy†
Physician Assistant Program
8200 W. Outer Drive, Box 13000
Detroit, MI 48219-0900
Telephone: (313) 993-6057
Fax: (313) 993-6175
E-mail: abdelno@udmercy.edu
ids.udmercy.edu/paprogram

Wayne State University†
College of Pharmacy & Allied Health Professions
PA Studies Program
60 E. Farnsworth
Rackham Bldg. 102
Detroit, MI 48202
Telephone: (313) 577-1368
Fax: (313) 577-5467
E-mail: Ab2278@wayne.edu
www.pa.wayne.edu

Western Michigan University†
Physician Assistant Program
Kalamazoo, MI 49008-5138
Telephone: (616) 387-5311
Fax: (616) 387-5319
E-mail: cindy.stineback@wmich.edu
www.wmich.edu/hhs/pa

MINNESOTA

Augsburg College†
Physician Assistant Program
2211 Riverside Ave., Box 149
Minneapolis, MN 55454-1350
Telephone: (612) 330-1039
Fax: (612) 330-1757
E-mail: paprog@augsburg.edu/pap
www.augsburg.edu/pap

MISSOURI

Saint Louis University†
School of Allied Health Professions
Physician Assistant Program
3437 Caroline St.
St. Louis, MO 63104
Telephone: (314) 577-8521
Fax: (314) 577-8503
E-mail: mayj@slu.edu
www.slu.edu/colleges/ah

Southwest Missouri State*
Physician Assistant Program
901 S. National Ave.
Springfield, MO 65804-0089
Telephone: (417) 836-6151
Fax: (417) 836-6406
E-mail: physicianasststudies@msn.edu
www.smsu.edu/pas

MONTANA

Rocky Mountain College†
Physician Assistant Program
1511 Poly Dr.
Billings, MT 59102-1739
Telephone: (406) 657-1190
Fax: (406) 657-1194
E-mail: mc@rocky.edu
jade.rocky.edu

NEBRASKA

Union College†
Physician Assistant Program
3800 S 48th St.
Lincoln, NE 68506
Telephone: (402) 486-2527
Fax: (402) 486-2559
E-mail: paprog@ucollege.edu
www.ucollege.edu/pa

University of Nebraska Medical Center†
Physician Assistant Program
984300 Nebraska Medical Center
Omaha, NE 68198-4300
Telephone: (402) 559-9495
Fax: (402) 559-5356
E-mail: dklandon@unmc.edu
www.unmc.edu/alliedhealth/pa

NEW HAMPSHIRE

Notre Dame College*
Master in Physician Assistant Studies
2321 Elm St.
Manchester, NH 03104-2299
Telephone: (603) 222-7100
Fax: (603) 222-7522

NEW JERSEY

The University of Medicine and Dentistry of New Jersey and Rutgers University†
Robert Woods Johnson Medical School
Physician Assistant Program
675 Hoes Ln.
Piscataway, NJ 08854-5635
Telephone: (732) 235-4445
Fax: (732) 235-4820
www.2umdnj.edu/paweb

Seton Hall University*
School of Graduate Medical Education
400 S. Orange Ave.
S. Orange, NJ 07079
Telephone: (973) 275-2596
Fax: (973) 275-2370
E-mail: gradmeded@hu.edu
gradmeded.shu.edu

NEW MEXICO

University of New Mexico†
School of Medicine/Department of Family & Community Medicine
Physician Assistant Program
2400 Tucker Ave., NE
Albuquerque, NM 87131-0001
Telephone: (505) 272-9678
Fax: (505) 272-9828
E-mail: paprogram@salud.unm.edu
hsc.unm.edu/pap

University of Saint Francis*
Physician Assistant Program
4401 Silver Ave., SE, Suite B
Albuquerque, NM 87108-2856
Telephone: (505) 266-5565
Fax: (505) 266-5585

NEW YORK

Albany Medical College Albany-Hudson Valley†
Physician Assistant Program
47 New Scotland Ave.
Mail Code 4
Albany, NY 12208-3412
Telephone: (518) 262-5251
Fax: (518) 262-6698
E-mail: irvined@mail.amc.edu
www.hvcc.edu/paprogram

Bronx Lebanon Hospital Center†
Physician Assistant Program
1650 Selwyn Ave., Suite 11D
Bronx, NY 10457-7628
Telephone: (718) 960-1255
Fax: (718) 960-1329

Brooklyn Hospital Center/Long Island University†
Physician Assistant Program
121 DeKalb Ave.
Brooklyn, NY 11201-5425
Telephone: (718) 260-2780
Fax: (718) 260-2790
E-mail: TBHCPAP@aol.com
www.liu.edu

City University of New York Medical School/
Harlem Hospital Center†
Sophie Davis School of Biomedical Education
Physician Assistant Program
506 Lenox Ave., WP, 619
New York, NY 10037
Telephone: (212) 939-2525
Fax: (212) 939-2529
E-mail: paprog@ccny.cuny.edu

D'Youville College†
Physician Assistant Program
320 Porter Ave.
Buffalo, NY 14201-1032
Telephone: (716) 881-7713
Fax: (716) 881-7732

Daemen College†
Physician Assistant Program
4380 Main St., Box 800
Amherst, NY 14226-3544
Telephone: (800) 462-7652, (716) 839-8563
Fax: (716) 839-8252
E-mail: admissions@daemen.edu
www.daemen.edu/departments/pa

LeMoyne College†
Physician Assistant Program
126 Coyne Science Center
1419 Salt Springs Rd.
Syracuse, NY 13214
Telephone: (800) 333-4733, (315) 445-4745
Fax: (315) 445-4602
E-mail: faulknsa@lemoyne.edu
www.lemoyne.edu

Mercy College*
Graduate Program in Physician Assistant Studies
555 Broadway
Dobbs Ferry, NY 10522
Telephone: (914) 674-7635
Fax: (914) 674-7623
E-mail: paprogram@mercy.edu
grad.mercynet.edu/physicianassistant

New York Institute of Technology*
Department of PA Studies
Physician Assistant Program
PO Box 8000, Northern Blvd.
Old Westbury, NY 11568-8000
Telephone: (516) 686-3881
Fax: (516) 686-3795
E-mail: sbarese@nyit.edu
www.nyit.edu

Pace University-Lenox Hill Hospital†
Physician Assistant Program
1 Pace Plaza, Room Y-31
New York, NY 10038-1502
Telephone: (212) 346-1357
Fax: (212) 346-1503
E-mail: paprogram@pace.edu
www.pace.edu/dyson/paprogram

Rochester Institute of Technology†
Department of Allied Health Sciences
Physician Assistant Program
85 Lomb Memorial Dr.
Rochester, NY 14623-5603
Telephone: (716) 475-2978
Fax: (716) 475-5809
E-mail: Ckhsc@rit.edu
www.rit.edu/~676www/main_pa.html

Saint Vincent's Catholic Medical Centers of New York†
Staten Island Region
Physician Assistant Program
75 Vanderbilt Ave.
Staten Island, NY 10304-3850
Telephone: (718) 818-5570
Fax: (718) 818-6146

Saint Vincent's Catholic Medical Centers of New York-Brooklyn/Queens Region†
Saint Anthony's Health Professions & Nursing Institute
Physician Assistant Program
175-05 Horace Harding Expy.
Fresh Meadows, NY 11365-1535
Telephone: (718) 357-0500
Fax: (718) 357-4588
E-mail: tsimone@cmcny.com

State University of New York Downstate Medical Center†
Physician Assistant Program
450 Clarkson Ave., Box 1222
Brooklyn, NY 11203-2012
Telephone: (718) 270-2324
Fax: (718) 270-7459
www.downstate.edu

State University of New York at Stony Brook†
School of Health Technology & Management
Physician Assistant Program
SHTM-HSC L2-052
Stony Brook, NY 11794-8202
Telephone: (631) 444-3190 x6
Fax: (631) 444-7621
E-mail: paprogram@sunysb.edu
www.uhmc.sunysb.edu/shtm

Touro College† (Bay Shore)
School of Health Sciences
Physician Assistant Program
1700 Union Blvd.
Bay Shore, NY 11706-7955
Telephone: (631) 665-1600
Fax: (631) 665-6086
E-mail: Jennyg1955@aol.com
www.touro.edu

Touro College* (Manhattan)
Manhattan Physician Assistant Program
27 W. 23rd St.
New York, NY 10010-4202
Telephone: (212) 463-0400, ext 792
Fax: (212) 741-0195
E-mail: ngraff@touro.edu
www.touro.edu/shs

Wagner College/Staten Island†
University Hospital
Physician Assistant Program
74 Melville St.
Staten Island, NY 10309-4035
Telephone: (718) 226-2928
Fax: (718) 226-2464

Weill Medical College of Cornell University†
Physician Assistant ("A Surgical Focus")
1300 York Ave., Box 195
New York, NY 10021
Telephone: (212) 746-5133, (212) 746-5134
Fax: (212) 746-0407
www.med.cornell.edu/pa

NORTH CAROLINA

Duke University Medical Center†
Physician Assistant Program
DUMC 3848
Durham, NC 27710-0001
Telephone: (919) 681-3161
Fax: (919) 681-3371
E-mail: Wanne001@mc.duke.edu
pa.mc.duke.edu

East Carolina University†
Scholl of Allied Health Sciences
Department of PA Studies
West Research Campus
1157 VOA SITE "C" Rd.
Greenville, NC 27834
Telephone: (252) 744-1100
Fax: (252) 744-1110
E-mail: huechtkere@mail.ecu.edu
www.ecu.edu/pa

Methodist College†
Physician Assistant Program
5107B College Centre Dr.
Fayetteville, NC 28311
Telephone: (910) 630-7495
Fax: (910) 630-7218

Wake Forest University†
School of Medicine
Physician Assistant Program
111 N. Chestnut St.
Winston Salem, NC 27101
Telephone: (336) 716-4356
Fax: (336) 716-4432
www.wfubmc.edu

NORTH DAKOTA

University of North Dakota School of Medicine & Health Sciences
Department of Community Medicine/Rural Health†
Physician Assistant Program
PO Box 9037
501 N. Columbia Rd.
Grand Forks, ND 58202
Telephone: (701) 777-2344
Fax: (701) 777-2389
E-mail: paapps@medicine.nodak.edu
www.med.und.nodak.edu

OHIO

Case Western Reserve University
Department of Anesthesiology
Anesthesiology Assistant Program
11100 Euclid Ave.
Cleveland, OH 44106-5007
Telephone: (216) 844-8077
Fax: (216) 844-7349
E-mail: Lms14@pocwru.edu
www.anesthesiaprogram.com

Cuyahoga Community College†
Physician/Surgical PA Programs
11000 Pleasant Valley Rd.
Parma, OH 44130-5114
Telephone: (216) 987-5363
Fax: (216) 987-5066
E-mail: Joyce.janicek@tri-c.cc.oh.us
www.tri-c.cc.oh.us

Kettering College of Medical Arts†
Physician Assistant Program
3737 Southern Blvd.
Kettering, OH 45429-1299
Telephone: (800) 433-5262, (937) 395-8638
Fax: (937) 395-8130/8095

Medical College of Ohio†
School of Allied Health Physician Assistant Program
3015 Arlington Ave.
Toledo, OH 43614-2570
Telephone: (419) 383-5408
Fax: (419) 383-5880
E-mail: pfrancis@mco.edu
www.mco.edu/allh/pa

University of Findlay†
Physician Assistant Program
1000 N. Main St.
Findlay, OH 45840-3695
Telephone: (419) 434-4529
Fax: (419) 434-6775
E-mail: Courtney@mail.findlay.edu
www.findlay.edu/academic/science/pa

OKLAHOMA

University of Oklahoma†
Physician Associate Program; Graduate PA Program: Occupational Health
900 NE Tenth St.
PO Box 26901
Oklahoma City, OK 73190-0001
Telephone: (405) 271-2058
Fax: (405) 271-3621
E-mail: Amber-hicks@ouhsc.edu
www.okpa.org

OREGON

Oregon Health Science University†
Physician Assistant Program
3181 SW Sam Jackson Park Rd., GH219
Portland, OR 97201-3098
Telephone: (503) 494-1484
Fax: (503) 494-1409
E-mail: Paprgm@ohsu.edu
www.ohsu.edu/pa

Pacific University†
School of Physician Assistant Studies
Physician Assistant Program
2043 College Way, UC Box 677
Forest Grove, OR 97116-1756
Telephone: (503) 359-2898
Fax: (503) 359-2977
E-mail: pa@pacificu.edu
www.pacificu.edu/academics/pa.html

PENNSYLVANIA

Arcadia University†
Physician Assistant Program
450 S Easton Rd.
Glenside, PA 19038-3215
Telephone: (215) 572-2888
Fax: (215) 881-8746
E-mail: dryer@arcadia.edu
www.arcadia.edu

Chatham College†
Physician Assistant Program
Woodland Rd.
Pittsburgh, PA 15232
Telephone: (800) 837-1290
Fax: (412) 365-1623
E-mail: admissions@chatham.edu
www.chatham.edu

DeSales University†
Physician Assistant Program
2755 Station Ave.
Center Valley, PA 18034-9565
Telephone: (610) 282-1100
Fax: (610) 282-1893
E-mail: Andrew.moyer@desales.edu
www.desales.edu

Duquesne University†
J.G. Rangos, Sr., School of Health Sciences
Physician Assistant Program
Suite 323, Health Sciences Bldg.
Pittsburgh, PA 15282-0001
Telephone: (412) 396-5914
Fax: (412) 396-5554
E-mail: essig@duq.edu
www.duq.edu/healthsciences

Gannon University†
Physician Assistant Program
109 University Sq.
Erie, PA 16541-0001
Telephone: (800) 426-6668, (814) 871-7240
Fax: (814) 871-5662
E-mail: Samuel001@gannon.edu
www.gannon.edu

King's College†
Physician Assistant Program
133 North River St.
Wilkes-Barre, PA 18711-0851
Telephone: (570) 208-5853
Fax: (570) 208-6018
E-mail: sesedon@kings.edu
www.kings.edu/~paprog

Lock Haven University†
Physician Assistant Program
G22 Stevenson Library
Lock Haven, PA 17745
Telephone: (570) 893-2541
Fax: (570) 893-2540
E-mail: lbeers@eagle.lhup.edu
www.lhup.edu/academic/acad_affairs/physician/academ_grad_phyas.html

MCP Hahnemann University†
School of health Professions
Physician Assistant Program
1505 Race St., 8th floor, MS504
Philadelphia, PA 19102-1194
Telephone: (215) 762-7135
Fax: (215) 762-1164
E-mail: Janet.stern@drexel.edu
World Wide Web: www.mcphu.edu

Pennsylvania College of Technology†
Physician Assistant Program
One College Ave.
Williamsport, PA 17701-5799
Telephone: (800) 637-9222, (570) 327-4779
Fax: (570) 321-5557
E-mail: jtrapp@pct.edu
www.pct.edu

Philadelphia College of Osteopathic Medicine†
Department of PA Studies
4170 City Ave.
Evans Hall, Suite 005
Philadelphia, PA 19131
Telephone: (215) 871-6772
Fax: (215) 871-6702
World Wide Web: www.pcom.edu

Philadelphia University†
Physician Assistant Program
School House Lane & Henry Ave.
Philadelphia, PA 19144
Telephone: (215) 951-2908
Fax: (215) 951-2526
E-mail: admissions@philau.edu
www.philau.edu

Saint Francis University†
Department of PA Sciences
PO Box 600
Loretto, PA 15940-0600
Telephone: (814) 472-3130
Fax: (814) 472-3137
E-mail: admissions@sfcpa.edu
www.francis.edu

Seton Hill College†
Physician Assistant Program
Seton Hill Dr.
Greensburg, PA 15601
Telephone: (724) 830-1097
Fax: (724) 838-7846
E-mail: fondy@setonhill.edu
www.setonhil.edu/~physasst

SOUTH CAROLINA

Medical University of South Carolina†
College of Health Professions
Physician Assistant Program
PO Box 250856
Charleston, SC 29425-0856
Telephone: (843) 792-0376
Fax: (843) 792-0506
E-mail: pastaff@musc.edu
www.musc.edu/pa_program

SOUTH DAKOTA

University of South Dakota†
School of Medicine
Physician Assistant Program
414 E. Clark St.
Vermillion, SD 57069-2307
Telephone: (605) 677-5128
Fax: (605) 677-6569
E-mail: usdpa@isd/edi
www.usd.edu/pa

TENNESSEE

Bethel College*
Physician Assistant Department
Physician Assistant Master of Science
325 Cherry Ave.
McKenzie, TN 38201
Telephone: (901) 352-4247
Fax: (901) 352-4069
E-mail: pa@bethel-college.edu or
taylore@bethel-college.edu
www.bethel-college.edu

Trevecca Nazarene College†
Physician Assistant Program
333 Murfreesboro Rd.
Nashville, TN 37210
Telephone: (615) 248-1225
Fax: (615) 248-1622
E-mail: dlennon@trevecca.edu

TEXAS

Baylor College of Medicine†
Physician Assistant Program
One Baylor Plaza, Room 633E
Houston, TX 77030
Telephone: (713) 798-3663
Fax: (713) 798-6128
E-mail: Pa01@bcmtmc.edu
bcm.tmc.edu

Brooke Army Medical Center
Department of Emergency Medicine
Emergency Medicine PA Residency Program
3851 Roger Brooke Dr.
Fort Sam Houston, TX 78234
Telephone: (210) 916-3598
Fax: (210) 916-2265
gergory.goodwiler@cen.amedd.ary.mil

Texas Tech University Health Sciences Center*
Physician Assistant Program
3600 N. Garfield
Midland, TX 79705
Telephone: (915) 620-9905
Fax: (915) 620-8605
E-mail: Christine.price@ttmcod.ttuhsc.edu
www.ttuhsc.edu/pages/alh

University of North Texas Health Science Center†
MPAS Program
3500 Camp Bowie Blvd.
Forth Worth, TX 76107-2699
Telephone: (817) 735-2301
Fax: (817) 735-2529
www.hcs.unt.edu/education/pasp

University of Texas Health Science Center at San Antonio*
Physician Assistant Program
7703 Floyd Curl Dr. MC6249
San Antonio, TX 78229-3900
Telephone: (210) 567-8810
Fax: (210) 567-8846
E-mail: pastudies@uthscsa.edu
www.uthscsa.edu/pastudies

University of Texas Medical Branch
Correctional Managed Care
PA Psychiatric Residency Program
Skyview Unit, PO Box 999
Rusk, TX 75785
Telephone: (903) 683-5781
Fax: (903) 683-6230
E-mail: hcariker@flash.net
www2.utmb.edu/managedcare

University of Texas Medical Branch†
School of Allied Health Services
Physician Assistant Program
301 University Blvd.
Galveston, TX 77555-1028
Telephone: (409) 772-3048
Fax: (409) 772-9710
www.sahs.utmb.edu/programs/pas

University of Texas-Pan American†
College of Health Sciences & Human Services
PA Studies Program
1201 W. University Dr.
Edinburg, TX 78539-2909
Telephone: (956) 381-2292
Fax: (956) 381-2438
E-mail: frankambriz@panam.edu
www.panam.edu/dept/pasp

University of Texas Southwestern Medical Center at Dallas†
Department of PA Studies
6011 Harry Hines Blvd., Suite V4.114
Dallas, TX 75390-9090
Telephone: (214) 648-1701
Fax: (214) 648-1003
E-mail: Pa.sahss@utsouthwestern.edu
www.utosuthwestern.edu

U.S. Army Medical Department Center and School†
Academy of Health Sciences
Interservice PA Program/Attn: MCCS HMP
3151 Scott Rd.
Fort Sam Houston, TX 78234-7579
Telephone: (210) 221-8004, (210) 221-8765
Fax: (210) 221-8493

UTAH

University of Utah†
School of Medicine
Physician Assistant Program
375 Chipeta Way, Suite A
Salt Lake City, UT 84108-1261
Telephone: (801) 581-7766
Fax: (801) 581-5807
www.utah.edu/upap

VIRGINIA

College of Health Sciences†
Physician Assistant Program
920 S. Jefferson Ct.
PO Box 13186
Roanoke, VA 24031-3186
Telephone: (540) 985-4016
Fax: (540) 224-4551
E-mail: pa@chs.edu
www.chs.edu

Eastern Virginia Medical School†
Physician Assistant Program
Lewis Hall Health Profession Programs
700 W Olney Rd., PO Box 1980
Norfolk, VA 23501-1980
Telephone: (757) 446-7158
Fax: (757) 446-7403
E-mail: paprog@evms.edu
www.evms.edu

James Madison University*
Department of Health Sciences
Physician Assistant Program
MSC 4301
Harrisonburg, VA 22807
Telephone: (540) 568-2395
Fax: (540) 568-3336
www.jmu.edu/healthsci/paweb.htm

Shenandoah University*
Division of Physician Assistant Studies
1460 University Dr.
Winchester, VA 22601
Telephone: (540) 545-7381
Fax: (540) 542-6210
www.su.edu/pa

WASHINGTON

Madigan Army Medical Center
Emergency Medicine PA Residency Program
Madigan Army Medical Center
Dept of Emergency Medicine
Tacoma, WA 98431
Telephone: (253) 968-1250
Fax: (253) 968-2550
E-mail: David.della-giustina@ne.amedd.army.mil
depts.washington.edu/muwemres

University of Washington†
School of Medicine/MEDEX Northwest
Physician Assistant Program
4245 Roosevelt Way NE
Seattle, WA 98105-6008
Telephone: (206) 598-2600
Fax: (206) 598-5195
E-mail: medex@u.washington.edu
www.washington.eud/medical/som/depts/medex

WEST VIRGINIA

Alderson-Broaddus College†
Physician Assistant Program
500 College Hill Dr.
PO Box 2036
Philippi, WV 26416
Telephone: (304) 457-6290
Fax: (304) 457-6308
E-mail: rus@ab.edu
www.ab.edu

Alderson-Broaddus College
Postgraduate PA Programs: Emergency Medicine, Rural Primary Care, Surgery
500 College Hill Dr.
PO Box 2036
Philippi, WV 26416
Telephone: (304) 457-6356
Fax: (304) 457-6308
E-mail: mercer@ab.edu
www.ab.edu

Mountain State University (formerly The College of West Virginia)†
Physician Assistant Program
PO Box 9003
609 S Kanawah St.
Beckley, WV 25802-2830
Telephone: (304) 253-7351, ext 1436
Fax: (304) 256-5571
E-mail: jamesmc@mountainstate.edu
www.mountainstate.edu

WISCONSIN

Marquette University†
Department of PA Studies
PO Box 1881
Milwaukee, WI 53201-1881
Telephone: (414) 288-5688
Fax: (414) 288-7951

University of Wisconsin-LaCross†
Gundersen Lutheran Medical Foundation, May School of Health-Related Sciences
Physician Assistant Program
1725 State St., 4046 HSC
La Crosse, WI 54601-3767
Telephone: (608) 785-6620
Fax: (608) 785-6647
E-mail: paprogram@uwlax.edu
www.uwlas.edu/pastudies

University of Wisconsin/Madison†
Physician Assistant Program
1300 University Ave.
Room 1050 Medical Sciences Center
Madison, WI 53706
Telephone: (608) 263-5620
Fax: (608) 263-6434
www.medsch.wisc.edu/pa

APPENDIX 3

MODEL STATE LEGISLATION REGARDING PHYSICIAN ASSISTANTS

INTRODUCTION

The model legislation reflects two principal concepts: that physician assistants (PAs) should be licensed to practice medicine with physician supervision and that PA scope of practice should be determined by supervising physicians.

Licensure is the most appropriate level of PA regulation to protect the public health and safety. Many states have been using a de facto licensing system; that is, permission to practice is dependent on presentation of appropriate qualifications and approval by the state regulatory agency. However, rather than calling this *licensure,* it has been called *certification* or *registration.*

Experts have defined *state certification* as regulation of the use of a specific occupational title. It is illegal to use a professional title without state approval, but anyone may deliver the service.

Registration creates an official list of persons. Registration presumes the existence of the right to engage in activity and makes it illegal to practice in a regulated occupation without being registered. It generally is not intended to ensure the public of qualified practitioners.

The Pew Health Commission's Task Force on Health Care Workforce Regulation issued a report in December 1995 recommending, among other things, that the term *licensure* be used for state regulation of health professions. The task force stated that the term *certification* should be reserved for voluntary private sector programs that attest to the competency of individual health professionals. For PAs, such a system is administered by the National Commission on Certification of Physician Assistants (NCCPA).

Thus to eliminate confusion between private and state certification and to identify the true level of regulation, the American Academy of Physician Assistants (AAPA) recommends that state laws use the term *license.* Most state laws conform to this recommendation. More than three quarters of states use *licensure* as the regulatory term for physician assistants; most of the others use the term *certification,* with a handful "registering" physician assistants. (See Exhibit 11-1, page 223.)

The model state legislation proposes an administrative process in which a PA presents his or her credentials to a state regulatory agency and receives a license in return. The license is renewable, based on meeting state requirements. Obtaining a license should occur independently of a PA's employment status. One analogy is a driver's license; you get one before you buy a car so that you can start driving as soon as you are ready. This system should be attractive to state licensing boards because it eliminates a lot of paperwork. Many of the early statutes either granted permission to physicians to use specific PAs or required PAs to submit all transcripts, test scores, references, and other like items, every time they changed employers or supervisors. Under such systems, PAs legally ceased to exist between jobs.

The model legislation does not propose a rigorous procedure for state approval of supervising physicians. It does recommend that licensed physicians and licensed PAs notify the state regulatory board of their intent to work together.

In addition, the scope of PA practice under the model legislation is dependent on what the supervising physician wishes to delegate. This is consistent with the original concept of PA use and reflects a movement away from a regulatory micromanagement of physician-PA practices.

The model legislation allows physicians to delegate prescriptive authority, including controlled substances in Schedules II through V, as well as limited dispensing authority. Also included is language clarifying a PA's authority to request, receive, and distribute professional samples. PAs who are delegated prescribers of controlled medications are required to register with the federal Drug Enforcement Administration.

It is stated quite clearly that a physician need not be physically on the premises as long as the PA and physician can contact each other easily. The details of supervision are left to the physician-PA team.

The Optional Replacement Parts are offered as substitutes for some of the provisions just described. If the delegatory system contained in the model legislation is not feasible, language is provided to give a licensing board more control over the supervising physician and PA. The Practice Agreement section would be inserted in place of Supervising Physician and Notification of Intent to Practice, and possibly other language.

If a description of PA scope of practice must be included, an alternative section is proposed that is intended to discourage the development of lists of tasks. This optional replacement section would take the place of Scope of Practice—Delegatory Authority, although it is recommended that the paragraph that describes PAs as agents of physicians be retained.

Locum tenens language is not necessary in the model legislation, because the proposed licensure system allows for easy substitution of one licensed PA for another. However, if the Practice Agreement concept is included, then the recommended section on locum tenens may be needed. The definition of *locum tenens* should be inserted in the Definitions section and the rest of the locum tenens provision placed elsewhere in the bill.

The final set of Optional Replacement Parts deals with the regulatory structure—control by a medical licensing board without PA input; a voting PA on the medical board; a separate PA board; and the most popular model, regulation by a medical board with a PA committee.

This model law was first drafted in 1991 and was revised in 1994, 1998, and 2001 to reflect changes in the PA program accrediting agencies and to incorporate other new provisions. The AAPA's government affairs staff is available to assist with revisions and additions as needed and to explain what and why the model bill contains what it does. We hope the ideas are clear and can be transformed into the appropriate style and format to be compatible with your existing state code.

The following model state legislation was first developed by Nicole Gara, Vice President for Government Affairs at the AAPA.

DEFINITIONS

Physician assistant means a health professional who meets the qualifications defined in this chapter and is licensed under this chapter to practice medicine with physician supervision.

Board means the Medical Licensing Board.

Supervising physician means an M.D. or D.O. physician licensed by the board who supervises physician assistants.

Supervision means overseeing the activities of, and accepting responsibility for, the medical services rendered by a physician assistant. The constant physical presence of the supervising physician is not required as long as the supervising physician and physician assistant are or can be easily in contact with each other by radio, telephone, or other telecommunications device.

QUALIFICATIONS FOR LICENSURE

Except as otherwise provided in this chapter, an individual shall be licensed by the board before the individual may practice as a physician assistant.

The board may grant a license as a physician assistant to an applicant who:

1. Submits an application on forms approved by the board
2. Pays the appropriate fee as determined by the board
3. Has successfully completed an educational program for physician assistants accredited by the Accreditation Review Commission on Education for the Physician Assistant or, prior to 2001, by either the Committee on Allied Health Education and Accreditation [or] the Commission on Accreditation of Allied Health Education Programs
4. Has passed the Physician Assistant National Certifying Examination administered by the National Commission on Certification of Physician Assistants
5. Certifies that he or she is mentally and physically able to engage safely in practice as a physician assistant
6. Has no licensure, certification, or registration as a physician assistant under current discipline, revocation, suspension, or probation for cause resulting from the applicant's practice as a physician assistant, unless the board considers such condition and agrees to licensure
7. Is of good moral character
8. Submits to the board any other information the board deems necessary to evaluate the applicant's qualifications
9. Has been approved by the board

The board may also grant a license to an applicant who does not meet the educational requirement specified in subsection 3, but who passed the Physician Assistant National Certifying Examination administered by the National Commission on Certification of Physician Assistants prior to 1986.

Graduate License

The board may grant a graduate license to an applicant who meets the qualifications for licensure except that the applicant has not yet taken the national certifying examination or the applicant has taken the national certifying examination and is awaiting the results.

A graduate license is valid:

1. For one year from the date of issuance
2. Until the results of an applicant's examination are available
3. Until the board makes a final decision on the applicant's request for licensure, whichever comes first. A graduate licensee who has not yet taken the examination is required to take the next available examination. Failure to do so is grounds for revocation of the graduate license unless the graduate licensee is unable to take the examination due to an emergency circumstance accepted as such by the board. The board may extend a graduate license, upon a majority vote of the board members, for a period not to exceed one year. Under no circumstances may the board grant more than one extension of a graduate license.

Temporary License

A temporary license may be granted to an applicant who meets all the qualifications for licensure but is awaiting the next scheduled meeting of the board.

Inactive License

Any physician assistant who notifies the board in writing on forms prescribed by the board may elect to place his or her license on an inactive status. A physician assistant with an inactive license shall be excused from payment of renewal fees and shall not practice as a physician assistant. Any licensee who engages in practice while his or her license is lapsed or on inactive status shall be considered to be practicing without a license, which shall be grounds for discipline. A physician assistant requesting restoration from inactive status shall be required to pay the current renewal fee and shall be required to meet the criteria for renewal.

Renewal

Each person who holds a license as a physician assistant in this state will, upon notification from the board, renew said license by:

1. Submitting the appropriate fee as determined by the board
2. Completing the appropriate forms

3. Meeting any other requirements set forth by the board

Exemption From Licensure

Nothing herein shall be construed to require licensure:

1. A physician assistant student enrolled in a physician assistant educational program accredited by the Accreditation Review Commission on Education for the Physician Assistant
2. A physician assistant employed in the service of the federal government while performing duties incident to that employment
3. Technicians or other assistants or employees of physicians who perform physician delegated tasks but who are not rendering services as a physician assistant or identifying themselves as a physician assistant.

SCOPE OF PRACTICE—DELEGATORY AUTHORITY—AGENT OF SUPERVISING PHYSICIAN

Physician assistants practice medicine with physician supervision. Physician assistants may perform those duties and responsibilities including the ordering, prescribing, dispensing, and administering drugs and medical devices that are delegated by their supervising physician(s).

Physician assistants may provide any medical service that is delegated by the supervising physician when the service is within the PA's skills, forms a component of the physician's scope of practice, and is provided with supervision. A physician assistant may perform a task not within the scope of practice of the supervising physician as long as the supervising physician has adequate training, oversight skills, and supervisory and referral arrangement to ensure competent provision of the service by the PA.

Physician assistants may pronounce death and may authenticate with their signature any form that may be authenticated by a physician's signature.

Physician assistants shall be considered the agents of their supervising physicians in the performance of all practice-related activities including, but not limited to, the ordering of diagnostic, therapeutic, and other medical services.

PRESCRIPTIVE AUTHORITY

A physician assistant may prescribe, dispense, and administer drugs and medical devices to the extent delegated by the supervising physician.

Prescribing and dispensing of drugs may include Schedule II through V substances as described in [the state controlled drug act] and all legend drugs.

All dispensing activities of physician assistants shall:

1. Comply with appropriate federal and state regulations
2. Occur when pharmacy services are not reasonably available, or when it is in the best interest of the patient, or when it is an emergency

Physician assistants may request, receive, and sign for professional samples and may distribute professional samples to patients.

Physician assistants authorized to prescribe and/or dispense controlled substances must register with the federal Drug Enforcement Administration (and any applicable state controlled substance regulatory authority).

SUPERVISION

Supervision shall be continuous but shall not be construed as necessarily requiring the physical presence of the supervising physician at the time and place that the services are rendered.

It is the obligation of each team of physician(s) and physician assistant(s) to ensure that the physician assistant's scope of practice is identified; that delegation of medical tasks is appropriate to the physician assistant's level of competence; that the relationship of, and access to, the supervising physician is defined; and that a process for evaluation of the physician assistant's performance is established.

Supervising Physician

A physician wishing to supervise a physician assistant must:

1. Be licensed in this state
2. Notify the board of his or her intent to supervise a physician assistant
3. Submit a statement to the board that he will exercise supervision over the physician assis-

tant in accordance with any rules adopted by the board and that he or she will retain professional and legal responsibility for the care rendered by the physician assistant

NOTIFICATION OF INTENT TO PRACTICE

A physician assistant licensed in this state, prior to initiating practice, will submit, on forms approved by the board, notification of such intent. Such notification shall include:

1. The name, business address, and telephone number of the supervising physician(s)
2. The name, business address, and telephone number of the physician assistant

A physician assistant will notify the board of any changes or additions in supervising physicians within _____ days.

SATELLITE SETTINGS

Nothing contained herein shall be construed to prohibit the rendering of services by a physician assistant in a setting geographically remote from the supervising physician.

EXCLUSIONS OF LIMITATIONS ON EMPLOYMENT

Nothing herein shall be construed to limit the employment arrangement of a physician assistant licensed under this act.

ASSUMPTION OF PROFESSIONAL LIABILITY

If a physician assistant is employed by a physician or group of physicians, the physician assistant shall be supervised by and be the legal responsibility of the employing physician(s). The legal responsibility for the physician assistant's patient care activities shall remain that of the employing physician(s), including when the physician assistant provides care and treatment for patients in health care facilities.

If a physician assistant is employed by a health care facility or other entity, the legal responsibility for the physician assistant's actions or omissions shall be that of the employing facility or entity. Physician assistants employed by such facilities shall be supervised by licensed physicians.

VIOLATIONS

The board may, following the exercise of due process, discipline any physician assistant who:

1. Fraudulently or deceptively obtains or attempts to obtain a license
2. Fraudulently or deceptively uses a license
3. Violates any provision of this chapter or any regulations adopted by the board pertaining to this chapter or any other laws or regulations governing licensed health professionals or any stipulation or agreement of the board
4. Is convicted of a felony
5. Is a habitual user of intoxicants or drugs to such an extent that he or she is unable to safely perform as a physician assistant
6. Has been adjudicated as mentally incompetent
7. Is physically or mentally unable to engage safely in practice as a physician assistant
8. Is negligent in practice as a physician assistant or demonstrates professional incompetence
9. Violates patient confidentiality except as required by law
10. Prescribes, sells, administers, distributes, orders, or gives away any drug classified as a controlled substance for other than medically accepted therapeutic purposes
11. Has committed an act of moral turpitude
12. Is disciplined or has been disciplined by another state or jurisdiction based upon acts or conduct similar to acts or conduct that would constitute grounds for disciplinary action as defined in this section
13. Fails to cooperate with an investigation conducted by the board
14. Represents himself or herself as a physician

DISCIPLINARY AUTHORITY

The board, upon finding that a physician assistant has committed any offense may

1. Refuse to grant a license
2. Administer a public or private reprimand
3. Revoke, suspend, limit, or otherwise restrict a license
4. Require a physician assistant to submit to the care or counseling or treatment of a physician or physicians designated by the board
5. Impose corrective measures
6. Suspend enforcement of its finding thereof and place the physician assistant on probation with the right to vacate the probationary order for noncompliance
7. Restore or reissue, at its discretion, a license and remove any disciplinary or corrective measure that it may have imposed

IMPAIRED PHYSICIAN ASSISTANT PROGRAM

The board shall establish and administer a program for the rehabilitation of physician assistants whose competency is impaired due to the abuse of drugs or alcohol. The board may contract with any other state agency or private corporation to perform duties under this section. The program shall be similar to that available to other health professionals licensed in this state.

TITLE AND PRACTICE PROTECTION

Any person not licensed under this act is guilty of a [felony or misdemeanor] and is subject to penalties applicable to the unlicensed practice of medicine if he or she:

1. Holds himself or herself out as a physician assistant
2. Uses any combination or abbreviation of the term "physician assistant" to indicate or imply that he or she is a physician assistant
3. Acts as a physician assistant without being licensed by the board.

An unlicensed physician shall not be permitted to use the title of "physician assistant" or to practice as a physician assistant unless he or she fulfills the requirements of this [act].

IDENTIFICATION REQUIREMENTS

Physician assistants licensed under this act shall keep their license available for inspection at their primary place of business and shall, when engaged in their professional activities, identify themselves as a "physician assistant."

PARTICIPATION IN DISASTER AND EMERGENCY CARE

A physician assistant licensed in this state or licensed or authorized to practice in any other state of the United States who is responding to a need for medical care created by an emergency or a state or local disaster (not to be defined as an emergency situation that occurs in the place of one's employment) may render such care that they are able to provide without supervision as it is defined in this section of law, or with such supervision as is available.

Any physician who supervises a physician assistant providing medical care in response to such an emergency or state or local disaster shall not be required to meet the requirements set forth in this section of law for an approved supervising physician.

No physician assistant licensed in this state or licensed or authorized to practice in other states of the United States who voluntarily and gratuitously, and other than in the ordinary course of employment or practice, renders emergency medical assistance shall be liable for civil damages for any personal injuries that result from acts or omissions by those persons in rendering emergency care that may constitute ordinary negligence. The immunity granted by this section shall not apply to acts or omissions constituting gross, willful, or wanton negligence or when the medical assistance is rendered at any hospital, physician's office, or other health care delivery entity where those services are normally rendered. No physician who supervises a physician assistant voluntarily and gratuitously providing emergency care as described in this subsection shall be liable for civil damages for any personal injuries that result from acts or omissions by the physician assistant rendering emergency care.

RULE-MAKING AUTHORITY

The board shall promulgate, in accordance with the provisions of the [state] Administrative Procedures Act, all rules that are reasonable and necessary for the performance of the various duties imposed upon the board by the provisions of this act, including but not limited to:

1. Setting licensure fees
2. Establishing renewal dates

OPTIONAL REPLACEMENT PARTS FOR MODEL LEGISLATION

Supervising Physician Practice Agreement

Any physician licensed in this state may apply to the board for permission to supervise a physician assistant. The application shall be jointly submitted by the physician and the physician assistant(s) and may be accompanied by a fee as determined by the board.

The joint application shall describe the manner and extent to which the physician assistant will practice and be supervised, including identification of additional licensed physicians who will supervise the physician assistant; the education, training, and experience of the primary supervisor and the physician assistant; and other such information as the board may require.

The board may approve, modify, or reject such applications.

Whenever it is determined that a physician or physician assistant is practicing in a manner inconsistent with the approval granted, the board may demand modification of the practice, withdraw approval of the practice agreement, or take other disciplinary action.

Physician Assistant Scope of Practice

The practice of a physician assistant shall include medical services within the education, training, and experience of the physician assistant that are delegated by the supervising physician.

Medical services rendered by physician assistants may include but are not limited to:

1. Obtaining patient histories and performing physical examinations
2. Ordering and/or performing diagnostic and therapeutic procedures
3. Formulating a diagnosis
4. Developing and implementing a treatment plan
5. Monitoring the effectiveness of therapeutic interventions
6. Assisting at surgery
7. Offering counseling and education to meet patient needs
8. Making appropriate referrals

The activities listed above may be performed in any setting authorized by the supervising physician, including but not limited to clinics, hospitals, ambulatory surgical centers, patient homes, nursing homes, and other institutional settings.

Locum Tenens Permit

The board may grant a locum tenens permit to any applicant who is licensed in the state. The permit may be granted by an authorized representative of the board. Such applications for locum tenens permits will be reviewed at the next scheduled board meeting. The maximum duration of a locum tenens permit is one year. The permit may be renewed annually on a date set by the board.

Definition: "Locum tenens means the temporary provision of services by a substitute provider."

REGULATORY OPTIONS

I. Regulation by the Medical Board

The state board of medical examiners shall administer the provisions of this act under such procedures as it considers advisable and may adopt rules that are reasonable and necessary to implement the provisions of this act.

II. Regulation by a Physician Assistant Board

To administer this act, there is hereby established a Board of Physician Assistant Examiners. The board shall consist of five members appointed by the governor, each of whom shall be residents of this state, four of whom shall be physician assistants who meet the criteria for licensure as established by this act, and one of whom shall be a licensed physician experienced in supervising physician assistants.

Initial appointments shall be made as follows:

1. Two members shall be appointed for terms of four years
2. One member shall be appointed for a term of three years
3. One member shall be appointed for a term of two years
4. One member shall be appointed for a term of one year.

Each regular appointment thereafter shall be for a term of four years. Any vacant term shall be filled by the governor for the balance of the unexpired term. No member shall serve more than two consecutive four-year terms, and each member shall serve on the board until his or her successor is appointed.

While engaged in the business of the board, each member shall receive a per diem of $_____ and shall also receive compensation for actual expenses paid in accordance with [other state regulations].

The board shall elect a chair and a secretary from among its members at the first meeting of each fiscal year. The board shall meet on a regular basis. A board meeting may be called, upon reasonable notice, at the discretion of the chair and shall be called at any time, upon reasonable notice, by a petition of three board members to the chair.

Powers and duties of the board shall include the following:

1. Promulgation of all rules reasonable and necessary to implement the provisions of this act
2. Review and approval or rejection of applications for licensure
3. Review and approval or rejection of applications for renewal
4. Issuance of all licenses
5. Denial, suspension, revocation, or other discipline of a licensee
6. Determination of the amount and collection of all fees

III. Regulation by a Medical Board With a PA Advisory Committee

There is hereby created a physician assistant committee that shall review and make recommendations to the board regarding all matters relating to physician assistants [who] come before the board. Such matters shall include but not be limited to:

1. Applications for licensure
2. Practice agreements
3. Disciplinary proceedings
4. Renewal requirements
5. Any other issues pertaining to the regulation and practice of physician assistants in this state

Committee Membership

The committee shall consist of three physician assistants, one physician experienced in supervising physician assistants, and one member of the board. All committee members must be residents of this state and hold a license in good standing in their respective disciplines.

The chair of the committee shall be elected by a majority vote of the committee members.

Committee members shall receive reimbursement for time and travel expenditures [consistent with usual state practices].

Appointments

The physician assistant and supervising physician members of the committee shall be appointed by the governor. The board of medical examiners shall designate one member to serve on the board. All appointments shall be made within 60 days of the effective date of this act. All appointments shall be for four-year terms, at staggered intervals. Members shall serve no more than two consecutive terms. Reappointments of the physician assistant and supervising physician members of the committee shall be made by the governor.

Meetings

The committee shall meet on a regular basis. A committee meeting may be called, upon reasonable notice, at the discretion of the chair and shall be called at any time, upon reasonable notice, by petition of three committee members to the chair.

IV. Adding a Physician Assistant to the Medical Board

To assist in the administration of this act, the governor shall appoint a licensed physician assistant to the Board of Medical Examiners for a term of _____ years, [in accordance with existing law]. The physician assistant member will have full voting privileges.

APPENDIX 4

GUIDELINES FOR ETHICAL CONDUCT FOR THE PHYSICIAN ASSISTANT

INTRODUCTION

The physician assistant profession has revised its code of ethics several times since the profession began. Although the fundamental principles underlying the ethical care of patients have not changed, the societal framework in which those principles are applied has. Economic pressures of the health care system, social pressures of church and state, technological advances, and changing patient demographics continually transform the landscape in which PAs practice.

Previous codes of the profession were brief lists of tenets for PAs to live by in their professional lives. This document departs from that format by attempting to describe ways in which those tenets apply. Each situation is unique. Individual PAs must use their best judgment in a given situation while considering the preferences of the patient and the supervising physician, clinical information, ethical concepts, and legal obligations.

Four main bioethical principles broadly guided the development of these guidelines: autonomy, beneficence, nonmaleficence, and justice.

Autonomy, strictly speaking, means self-rule. Patients have the right to make autonomous decisions and choices, and physician assistants should respect these decisions and choices.

Beneficence means that PAs should act in the patient's best interest. In certain cases, respecting the patient's autonomy and acting in their best interests may be difficult to balance.

Nonmaleficence means to do no harm, to impose no unnecessary or unacceptable burden upon the patient.

Justice means that patients in similar circumstances should receive similar care. Justice also applies to norms for the fair distribution of resources, risks, and costs.

Physician assistants are expected to behave both legally and morally. They should know and understand the laws governing their practice. Likewise, they should understand the ethical responsibilities of being a health care professional. Legal requirements and ethical expectations will not always be in agreement. Generally speaking, the law describes minimum standards of acceptable behavior, and ethical principles delineate the highest moral standards of behavior.

When faced with an ethical dilemma, PAs may find the guidance they need in this document. If not, they may wish to seek guidance elsewhere—possibly from a supervising physician, a hospital

*Courtesy American Academy of Physician Assistants: *JAAPA* 14:10, 12, 15-16, 19-20, 2001. Profession policy of the American Academy of Physician Assistants, adopted May 2000.

ethics committee, an ethicist, trusted colleagues, or other AAPA policies. PAs should seek legal counsel when they are concerned about the potential legal consequences of their decisions.

The following sections discuss ethical conduct of PAs in their professional interactions with patients, physicians, colleagues, other health professionals, and the public. The "Statement of Values" within this document defines the fundamental values that the PA profession strives to uphold. These values provide the foundation upon which the guidelines rest. The guidelines were written with the understanding that no document can encompass all actual and potential ethical responsibilities, and PAs should not regard them as comprehensive.

STATEMENT OF VALUES OF THE PHYSICIAN ASSISTANT PROFESSION

- Physician assistants hold as their primary responsibility the health, safety, welfare, and dignity of all human beings.
- Physician assistants uphold the tenets of patient autonomy, beneficence, nonmaleficence, and justice.
- Physician assistants recognize and promote the value of diversity.
- Physician assistants treat equally all persons who seek their care.
- Physician assistants hold in confidence the information shared in the course of practicing medicine.
- Physician assistants assess their personal capabilities and limitations, striving always to improve their medical practice.
- Physician assistants actively seek to expand their knowledge and skills, keeping abreast of advances in medicine.
- Physician assistants work with other members of the health care team to provide compassionate and effective care of patients.
- Physician assistants use their knowledge and experience to contribute to an improved community.
- Physician assistants respect their professional relationship with physicians.
- Physician assistants share and expand knowledge within the profession.

THE PA AND THE PATIENT

PA Role and Responsibilities

Physician assistant practice flows out of a unique relationship that involves the PA, the physician, and the patient. The individual patient-PA relationship is based on mutual respect and an agreement to work together regarding medical care. In addition, PAs practice medicine with physician supervision; therefore the care that a PA provides is an extension of the care of the supervising physician. The patient-PA relationship is also a patient-PA-physician relationship.

The principal value of the physician assistant profession is to respect the health, safety, welfare, and dignity of all human beings. This concept is the foundation of the patient-PA relationship. Physician assistants have an ethical obligation to see that each of their patients receives appropriate care. PAs should recognize that each patient is unique and has an ethical right to self-determination. PAs should be sensitive to the beliefs and expectations of the patient but are not expected to ignore their own personal values, scientific or ethical standards, or the law.

A PA has an ethical duty to offer patients the full range of information on relevant options for their health care. If personal moral, religious, or ethical beliefs prevent a PA from offering the full range of treatments available or care the patient desires, the PA has an ethical duty to refer an established patient to another qualified provider. PAs are obligated to care for patients in emergency situations and to responsibly transfer established patients if they cannot care for them.

The PA and Diversity

The physician assistant should respect the culture, values, beliefs, and expectations of the patient.

Discrimination

Physician assistants should not discriminate against classes or categories of patients in the delivery of needed health care. Such classes and categories include gender, color, creed, race, religion, age, ethnic or national origin, political beliefs, nature of illness, disability, socioeconomic status, or sexual orientation.

Initiation and Discontinuation of Care

In the absence of a preexisting patient-PA relationship, the physician assistant is under no ethical obligation to care for a person unless no other provider is available. A PA is morally bound to provide care in emergency situations and to arrange proper follow-up. PAs should keep in mind that contracts with health insurance plans might define a legal obligation to provide care to certain patients.

A physician assistant and supervising physician may discontinue their professional relationship with an established patient as long as proper procedures are followed. The PA and physician should provide the patient with adequate notice, offer to transfer records, and arrange for continuity of care if the patient has an ongoing medical condition. Discontinuation of the professional relationship should be undertaken only after a serious attempt has been made to clarify and understand the expectations and concerns of all involved parties.

If the patient decides to terminate the relationship, he or she is entitled to access appropriate information contained within their medical record.

Informed Consent

Physician assistants have a duty to protect and foster an individual patient's free and informed choices. The doctrine of informed consent means that a PA provides adequate information that is comprehendible to a competent patient or patient surrogate. At a minimum, this should include the nature of the medical condition, the objectives of the proposed treatment, treatment options, possible outcomes, and the risks involved. PAs should be committed to the concept of shared decision making, which involves assisting patients in making decisions that account for medical, situational, and personal factors.

In caring for adolescents, the PA should understand all of the laws and regulations in his or her jurisdiction that are related to the ability of minors to consent to or refuse health care. Adolescents should be encouraged to involve their families in health care decision making. The PA should also understand consent laws pertaining to emancipated or mature minors. (See the next section on confidentiality.)

When the person giving consent is a patient's surrogate, a family member, or other legally authorized representative, the PA should take reasonable care to assure that the decisions made are consistent with the patient's best interests and personal preferences, if known. If the PA believes the surrogate's choices do not reflect the patient's wishes or best interests, the PA should work to resolve the conflict. This may require the use of additional resources, such as an ethics committee.

Confidentiality

Physician assistants should maintain confidentiality. By maintaining confidentiality, PAs respect patient privacy and help to prevent discrimination based on medical conditions. If patients are confident that their privacy is protected, they are more likely to seek medical care and more likely to discuss their problems candidly.

In cases of adolescent patients, family support is important but should be balanced with the patient's need for confidentiality and the PA's obligation to respect their emerging autonomy. Adolescents may not be of age to make independent decisions about their health, but providers should respect that they soon will be. To the extent they can, PAs should allow these emerging adults to participate as fully as possible in decisions about their care. It is important that PAs be familiar with and understand the laws and regulations in their jurisdictions that relate to the confidentiality rights of adolescent patients. (See the section on informed consent.)

Any communication about a patient conducted in a manner that violates confidentiality is unethical. Because written, electronic, and verbal information may be intercepted or overheard, the PA should always be aware of anyone who might be monitoring communication about a patient.

PAs should choose methods of storage and transmission of patient information that minimize the likelihood of data becoming available to unauthorized persons or organizations. Modern technologies such as computerized record keeping and electronic data transmission present unique challenges that can make the maintenance of patient confidentiality difficult. PAs should advocate for policies and procedures that secure the confidentiality of patient information.

Patient and the Medical Record

Physician assistants have an obligation to keep information in the patient's medical record confidential. Information should be released only with the written permission of the patient or the patient's legally authorized representative. Specific exceptions to this general rule may exist (e.g., workers compensation, communicable disease, HIV, knife/gunshot wounds, abuse, substance abuse). It is important that a PA be familiar with and understand the laws and regulations in his or her jurisdiction that relate to the release of information. For example, stringent legal restrictions on release of genetic test results and mental health records often exist.

Both ethically and legally, a patient has certain rights to know the information contained in his or her medical record. While the chart is legally the property of the practice or the institution, the information in the chart is the property of the patient. Most states have laws that provide patients access to their medical records. The PA should know the laws and facilitate patient access to the information.

Disclosure

A physician assistant should disclose to his or her supervising physician information about errors made in the course of caring for a patient. The supervising physician and PA should disclose the error to the patient if such information is significant to the patient's interests and well being. Errors do not always constitute improper, negligent or unethical behavior, but failure to disclose them may.

Care of Family Members and Co-Workers

Treating oneself, co-workers, close friends, family members, or students whom the physician assistant supervises or teaches may be unethical or create conflicts of interest. PAs should be aware that their judgment might be less than objective in cases involving friends, family members, students, and colleagues and that providing "curbside" care might sway the individual from establishing an ongoing relationship with a provider. If it becomes necessary to treat a family member or close associate, a formal patient-provider relationship should be established, and the PA should consider transferring the patient's care to another provider as soon as it is practical. If a close associate requests care, the PA may wish to assist by helping them find an appropriate provider.

There may be exceptions to this guideline, for example, when a PA runs an employee health center or works in occupational medicine. Even in those situations, PAs should be sure they do not provide informal treatment, but provide appropriate medical care in a formally established patient-provider relationship.

Genetic Testing

Evaluating the risk of disease and performing diagnostic genetic tests raise significant ethical concerns. Physician assistants should be knowledgeable about the benefits and risks of genetic tests. Testing should be undertaken only after the patient's informed consent is obtained. If PAs order or conduct the tests, they should assure that appropriate pre- and post-test counseling is provided.

PAs should be sure that patients understand the potential consequences of undergoing genetic tests—from impact on patients themselves, possible implications for other family members, and potential use of the information by insurance companies or others who might have access to the information. Because of the potential for discrimination by insurers, employers, or others, PAs should be particularly aware of the need for confidentiality concerning genetic test results.

Reproductive Decision Making

Patients have a right to access the full range of reproductive health care services, including fertility treatments, contraception, sterilization, and abortion. Physician assistants have an ethical obligation to provide balanced and unbiased clinical information about reproductive health care.

When the PA's personal values conflict with providing full disclosure or providing certain services such as sterilization or abortion, the PA need not become involved in that aspect of the patient's care. By referring the patient to a qualified provider, the PA fulfills their ethical obligation to ensure the patient access to all legal options.

End of Life

Physician assistants have an obligation to optimize care and maximize quality of life for patients at the end of life. PAs are encouraged to facilitate open discussion with patients and their family members concerning end of life treatment choices.

PAs should involve the physician in all near-death planning. The PA should only withdraw life support with the supervising physician's agreement and in accordance with the policies of the health care institution.

PAs should be aware of the medical, legal, social, and ethical issues in end of life decision making.

Advance directives, living wills, and organ donation should be discussed during routine patient visits.

THE PA AND INDIVIDUAL PROFESSIONALISM

Conflict of Interest

Physician assistants should place service to patients before personal material gain and should avoid undue influence on their clinical judgment. Trust can be undermined by even the appearance of improper influence. Examples of excessive or undue influence on clinical judgment can take several forms. These may include financial incentives, pharmaceutical or other industry gifts, and business arrangements involving referrals. PAs should disclose any actual or potential conflict of interest to their patients.

Acceptance of gifts, trips, hospitality, or other items is discouraged. Before accepting a gift or financial arrangement, PAs might consider the guidelines of the Royal College of Physicians, "Would I be willing to have this arrangement generally known?" or of the American College of Physicians-American Society of Internal Medicine, "What would the public or my patients think of this arrangement?"

Professional Identity

Physician assistants should not misrepresent directly or indirectly their skills, training, professional credentials, or identity. Physician assistants should uphold the dignity of the PA profession and accept its ethical values.

Competency

Physician assistants should commit themselves to providing competent medical care and extend to each patient the full measure of their professional ability as dedicated, empathetic health care providers. PAs should also strive to maintain and increase the quality of their health care knowledge, cultural sensitivity, and cultural competence through individual study and continuing education.

Sexual Relationships

It is unethical for physician assistants to become sexually involved with patients. It also may be unethical for PAs to become sexually involved with former patients or key third parties. Key third parties are individuals who have influence over the patient. These might include spouses or partners, parents, guardians, or surrogates.

Such relationships generally are unethical because of the PA's position of authority and the inherent imbalance of knowledge, expertise, and status. Issues such as dependence, trust, transference, and inequalities of power may lead to increased vulnerability on the part of the current or former patients or key third parties.

Gender Discrimination and Sexual Harassment

It is unethical for physician assistants to engage in or condone any form of gender discrimination. Gender discrimination is defined as any behavior, action, or policy that adversely affects an individual or group of individuals due to disparate treatment, disparate impact, or the creation of a hostile or intimidating work or learning environment.

It is unethical for PAs to engage in or condone any form of sexual harassment. Sexual harassment is defined as unwelcome sexual advances, requests for sexual favors, or other verbal or physical conduct of a sexual nature when:

- Such conduct has the purpose or effect of interfering with an individual's work or academic performance or creating an intimidating, hostile, or offensive work or academic environment, or
- Accepting or rejecting such conduct affects or may be perceived to affect professional decisions concerning an individual, or
- Submission to such conduct is made either explicitly or implicitly a term or condition of an individual's training or professional position.

THE PA AND OTHER PROFESSIONALS

Team Practice

Physician assistants should be committed to working collegially with other members of the health care team to ensure integrated, well-managed, and effective care of patients. PAs should strive to maintain a spirit of cooperation with other health care professionals, their organizations, and the general public.

Illegal and Unethical Conduct

Physician assistants should not participate in or conceal any activity that will bring discredit or dishonor to the PA profession. They should report illegal or unethical conduct by health care professionals to the appropriate authorities.

Impairment

Physician assistants have an ethical responsibility to protect patients and the public by identifying and assisting impaired colleagues. "Impaired" means being unable to practice medicine with reasonable skill and safety because of physical or mental illness, loss of motor skills, or excessive use or abuse of drugs and alcohol.

PAs should be able to recognize impairment in physician supervisors, PAs, and other health care providers and should seek assistance from appropriate resources to encourage these individuals to obtain treatment.

PA-Physician Relationship

Supervision should include ongoing communication between the physician and the physician assistant regarding patient care. The PA should consult the supervising physician whenever it will safeguard or advance the welfare of the patient. This includes seeking assistance in situations of conflict with a patient or another health care professional.

Complementary and Alternative Medicine

A patient's request for alternative therapy may create conflict between the physician assistant and the patient. Though physician assistants are under no obligation to provide an alternative therapy, they do have a responsibility to be sensitive to the patient's needs and beliefs and to help the patient understand their medical condition. The PA should gain an understanding of the alternative therapy being considered or being used, the expected outcome, and whether the treatment would clearly be harmful to the patient. If the treatment would harm the patient, the PA should work diligently to dissuade the patient from using it and advise other treatment.

THE PA AND THE HEALTH CARE SYSTEM

Workplace Actions

Physician assistants may face difficult personal decisions to withhold medical services when workplace actions (e.g., strikes, sick-outs, slowdowns, etc.) occur. The potential harm to patients should be carefully weighed against the potential improvements to working conditions and, ultimately, patient care that could result. In general, PAs should individually and collectively work to find alternatives to such actions in addressing workplace concerns.

Managed Care

The focus of managed care organizations on cost containment and resource allocation can present particular ethical challenges to clinicians. When practicing in managed care systems, physician assistants should always act in the best interests of their patients and as an advocate when necessary. PAs should actively resist managed care policies that restrict free exchange of medical information. For example, a PA should not withhold information about treatment options simply because the option is not covered by a particular managed care organization.

PAs should inform patients of financial incentives to limit care, use resources in a fair and efficient way, and avoid arrangements or financial incentives that conflict with the patient's best interests.

PAs as Educators

All physician assistants have a responsibility to share knowledge and information with patients, other health professionals, students, and the public. The ethical duty to teach includes effective communication with patients so that they will have the information necessary to participate in their health care and wellness.

PAs and Research

The most important ethical principle in research is honesty. This includes assuring subjects' informed consent, following treatment protocols, and accurately reporting findings. Fraud and dishonesty in research should be reported so that the appropriate authorities can take action.

Physician assistants involved in research must be aware of potential conflicts of interest. The patient's welfare takes precedence over the desired research outcome. Any conflict of interest should be disclosed.

In scientific writing, PAs should report information honestly and accurately. Sources of funding for the research must be included in the published reports.

Plagiarism is unethical. Incorporating the words of others, either verbatim or by paraphrasing, without appropriate attribution is unethical and may have legal consequences. When submitting a document for publication, any previous publication of any portion of the document must be fully disclosed.

PAs as Expert Witnesses

The physician assistant expert witness should testify to what he or she believes to be the truth. The PA's review of medical facts should be thorough, fair, and impartial.

The PA expert witness should be fairly compensated for time spent preparing, appearing, and testifying. The PA should not accept a contingency fee based on the outcome of a case in which testimony is given or derive personal, financial, or professional favor in addition to compensation.

THE PA AND SOCIETY

Lawfulness

Physician assistants have the dual duty to respect the law and to work for positive change to laws that will enhance the health and well being of the community.

Executions

Physician assistants, as health care professionals, should not participate in executions because to do so would violate the ethical principle of beneficence.

Access to Care/Resource Allocation

Physician assistants have a responsibility to use health care resources in an appropriate and efficient manner so that all patients have access to needed health care. Resource allocation should be based on societal needs and policies, not the circumstances of an individual patient-PA encounter. PAs participating in policy decisions about resource allocation should consider medical need, cost-effectiveness, efficacy, and equitable distribution of benefits and burdens in society.

Community Well-Being

Physician assistants should work for the health, well-being, and the best interest of both the patient and the community. Sometimes there is a dynamic moral tension between the well being of the community in general and the individual patient. Conflict between an individual patient's best interest and the common good is not always easily resolved. In general, PAs should be committed to upholding and enhancing community values, be aware of the needs of the community, and use the knowledge and experience acquired as professionals to contribute to an improved community.

CONCLUSION

The American Academy of Physician Assistants recognizes its responsibility to aid the PA profession as it strives to provide high quality, accessible health care. Physician assistants wrote these guidelines for themselves and other physician assistants. The ultimate goal is to honor patients and earn their trust while providing the best and most appropriate care possible. At the same time, PAs must understand their personal values and beliefs and recognize the ways in which those values and beliefs can impact the care they provide.

APPENDIX 5

ACCREDITATION STANDARDS FOR PHYSICIAN ASSISTANT EDUCATION*

These *Standards* were initially adopted in 1971, revised in 1978, 1985, 1990, 1997, and 2000, and approved by the following:

- American Academy of Family Physicians
- American Academy of Pediatrics
- American Academy of Physician Assistants
- American College of Physicians-American Society of Internal Medicine
- American College of Surgeons
- American Medical Association
- Association of Physician Assistant Programs

These *Standards* constitute the minimum requirements to which an accredited program is held accountable and provide the basis on which the Accreditation Review Commission on Education for the Physician Assistant (ARC-PA) will confer or deny program accreditation.

The *Standards* apply to all program locations, regardless of geographical location or the method by which instruction is delivered.

INTRODUCTION

The American Academy of Family Physicians, the American Academy of Pediatrics, the American Academy of Physician Assistants, the American College of Physicians-American Society of Internal Medicine, the American College of Surgeons, the American Medical Association, and the Association of Physician Assistant Programs cooperate with the ARC-PA to establish, maintain, and promote appropriate standards of quality for entry-level education of physician assistants (PAs) and to provide recognition for educational programs that meet the minimum requirements outlined in these *Standards*. These *Standards* are to be used for the development, evaluation, and self-analysis of physician assistant programs.

Physician assistants are academically and clinically prepared to provide health care services with the direction and responsible supervision of a doctor of medicine or osteopathy. The physician-PA team relationship is fundamental to the PA profession and enhances the delivery of high-quality health care. Within the physician-PA relationship, PAs make clinical decisions and provide a broad range of diagnostic, therapeutic, preventive, and health maintenance services. The clinical role of PAs includes primary and specialty care in medical and surgical practice settings. PA practice is centered on patient care and may include educational, research, and administrative activities.

*Modified from ARC-PA, second edition, January 1, 2001.

The role of the PA demands intelligence, sound judgment, intellectual honesty, appropriate interpersonal skills, and the capacity to react to emergencies in a calm and reasoned manner. An attitude of respect for self and others, adherence to the concepts of privilege and confidentiality in communicating with patients, and a commitment to the patient's welfare are essential attributes of the graduate PA. The professional curriculum for PA education includes basic medical, behavioral, and social sciences; introduction to clinical medicine and patient assessment; supervised clinical practice; and health policy and professional practice issues.

These *Standards* acknowledge the evolution of the PA profession and endorse a fundamental tenet of PA education: competency-based education. While the opportunity for creativity and innovation in program design remains, this version of the *Standards* reflects the realization that a commonality in the core curriculum of programs has become not only desirable, but also necessary in order to offer curricula of sufficient depth and breadth to prepare PA graduates for practice in a dynamic and competitive health care arena. Additionally, the *Standards* reflect a graduate level of curricular intensity. Institutions that sponsor PA programs should endeavor to incorporate this higher level of academic rigor into their programs and acknowledge it with an appropriate degree.

PROGRAM REVIEW

Accreditation of PA programs is a voluntary process that includes a comprehensive review of the program relative to the *Standards*. Accreditation decisions are based on the ARC-PA's review of information contained in the accreditation application and self-study report, the report of site visit evaluation teams, any additional requested reports or documents submitted to the ARC-PA by the PA program, and the program's past accreditation history. Additional data to clarify information submitted with the application may be requested at the time of the site visit associated with the comprehensive review. New information submitted after a site visit will not be accepted or considered by the ARC-PA.

GENERAL REQUIREMENTS FOR ACCREDITATION

SECTION A: ADMINISTRATION

A1 Sponsorship

Institution Accreditation

A1.1 The sponsoring institution must be accredited as an institution of higher education by a recognized regional or national accrediting agency.

Program Location[1]

A1.2 Accredited PA programs must be established in

a) Schools of allopathic or osteopathic medicine
b) Colleges and universities affiliated with appropriate clinical teaching facilities
c) Medical education facilities of the federal government.

Institution Responsibilities

A1.3 One sponsor must be clearly identified as being ultimately responsible for the program.

A1.4 The sponsoring institution, together with its affiliates, must be capable of providing clinically oriented basic science education, as well as clinical instruction and experience requisite to PA education.

A1.5 The sponsoring institution assumes primary responsibility for:

a) student admission, including receiving and processing applications
b) curriculum planning and selection of course content
c) coordination of classroom teaching and supervised clinical practice
d) appointment of faculty
e) granting the credential documenting satisfactory completion of the educational program.

A1.6 In programs in which more than one institution is involved in the provision of academic and clinical education, responsibilities of the respective institutions for

[1]*Programs established before January 1, 2001, "should" be established in the settings indicated. Programs established on or after January 1, 2001, "must" be established in the settings indicated.*

instruction and supervision must be clearly described and documented in a manner signifying agreement by the involved institutions.

A2 Personnel

Core Program Faculty

A2.1 The program must have effective leadership and management.

A2.2 Program officials must possess the necessary qualifications to perform the functions identified in documented job descriptions.

A2.3 The program must have a designated program director, medical director, faculty, and administrative staff. The program director also may be the medical director.

A2.4 The program must have core program faculty responsible for the administration and coordination of didactic and clinical portions of the curriculum.

A2.5 Core program faculty must include, at a minimum, the program director, medical director, and two additional faculty positions for individuals currently certified as PAs. The latter two FTE positions cannot be occupied by more than four individuals.

A2.6 The core program faculty should have appointments and privileges comparable to other faculty who have similar responsibilities within the institution.

A2.7 Core program faculty are responsible for:
- a) teaching
- b) evaluating student performance
- c) identifying and counseling students who are not achieving the defined course or program objectives
- d) assuring the availability of remedial instruction
- e) developing, implementing, and evaluating curriculum
- f) administering and evaluating the program.

Program Director

A2.8 The program director must be a PA or a physician and must have the requisite knowledge and skills to administer the program effectively.[2] If the program director is a PA, he should hold current national certification. If the program director is a physician, he must be a licensed allopathic or osteopathic physician and should be board certified.

A2.9 The program director should be assigned to the program on a full time basis.

A2.10 The program director must be knowledgeable about the accreditation process and responsible for the organization, administration, continuous review and analysis, planning, and development of the program.

A2.11 The program director must supervise the medical director, faculty, and staff in all activities that directly relate to the PA program.

Medical Director

A2.12 The medical director must be a licensed allopathic or osteopathic physician who should be board certified.

A2.13 The medical director must support the program director in assuring that competent medical guidance is provided, so that both didactic and supervised instruction meets current acceptable practice.

A2.14 The medical director should be an advocate for the program within the medical and academic community.

Professional Development

A2.15 The program must assure continuing professional growth of the core faculty by supporting their clinical, teaching, scholarly, and management responsibilities. Programs must support core PA faculty in maintaining their national certification status.

Instructional Faculty

A2.16 In addition to the core program faculty, there must be additional faculty and instructors to provide students with the necessary attention, instruction, and supervised practice experiences to acquire the knowledge and competence needed for entry to the profession.

A2.17 Faculty and instructors must be qualified through academic preparation and experience to teach assigned subjects.

[2] *Programs established on or after January 1, 2001, must have a PA, MD, or DO as director. Programs established before January 1, 2001, will be held to this Standard only when a new program director is appointed.*

A2.18 Faculty and instructors must be knowledgeable in course content and effective in teaching assigned subjects.

A2.19 Faculty and instructors for the supervised clinical practice portion of the educational program must consist primarily of practicing physicians and PAs.

A2.20 The program should not rely principally on resident physicians for didactic or clinical instruction.

A2.21 All faculty and instructors assigned to teach students should be responsible for evaluating student performance and identifying students who are not achieving course and program objectives.

A2.22 In each location to which a student is assigned for didactic or supervised practice instruction, there must be an individual designated to supervise and make frequent assessments of the student's progress in achieving program requirements.

Administrative Support Staff

A2.23 The institution must provide administrative and technical support staff to meet the needs of the program.

A2.24 At a minimum, there must be one full-time support staff person assigned to the program to assist the core program faculty.

A3 Financial Resources

A3.1 Financial resources to operate an educational program must be sufficient to fulfill obligations to matriculating and enrolled students.

A4 Physical Resources

Classrooms and Laboratories

A4.1 Classrooms and laboratories must have sufficient seating to accommodate the class size. The seating, lighting, heating, and ventilation must be sufficient to facilitate the learning process.

Office and Meeting Space

A4.2 There must be designated space for confidential counseling of students by core faculty.

A4.3 There must be sufficient office space for core faculty to perform their program duties.

A4.4 Facilities should include meeting space for faculty meetings, program committees, and any other meeting space relevant to the program.

A4.5 There must be secure storage space for student files and records.

Office Equipment

A4.6 Sufficient computer hardware and software, office equipment, and supplies must be readily available for program faculty and staff.

Academic Resources

A4.7 Convenient and timely access to the full text of current books, journals, periodicals, and other reference materials related to the curriculum must be available to students and faculty.

Instructional Resources

A4.8 Instructional models, computer hardware and software, reference materials, and audio and visual resources must be available to facilitate faculty teaching and student learning.

Technology Resources

A4.9 The institution must provide access to and training in the use of the Internet, including medical and other health-related electronic databases.

A5 Operations

Fair Practices

A5.1 Announcements and advertising must accurately reflect the program offered.

A5.2 All personnel and student policies must be nondiscriminatory and consistent with federal and state statutes, rules, and regulations.

A5.3 At a minimum, the following must be defined, published, and readily available to prospective and enrolled students:

a) institutional policies and practices that favor specific groups of applicants

b) academic credit and costs to the student.

A5.4 Policies and procedures for processing student grievances must be defined, published, and readily available to students and faculty.

A5.5 Policies and procedures for processing faculty grievances must be defined, published, and readily available to faculty.

A5.6 Policies and procedures for student withdrawal and for refunds of tuition and fees must be published and readily available to all students.

A5.7 Policies that limit or prevent students from working must be made known to the students in advance of enrollment.

A5.8 Policies by which students may work within the program or institution while enrolled in the program must be published and made available to all students.

A5.9 Students must not be required to perform clerical or administrative work for the program.

A5.10 During clinical experiences, students must not be used to substitute for regular clinical or administrative staff.

A5.11 Appropriate security and personal safety measures must be provided to students in all locations in which instruction occurs.

Student Records

A5.12 Student files must include the following:
- a) data and information indicating that students have met published admission criteria
- b) documentation reflecting the evaluation of student performance while enrolled
- c) documentation of remediation and/or disciplinary action.

A5.13 The sponsoring institution must retain student transcripts permanently.

Faculty Records

A5.14 Records of core program faculty members must include a current curriculum vitae (CV) and current job description.

A5.15 The program must have a current CV for each course director.

Admission Policies and Procedures

A5.16 Admission of students must be made in accordance with clearly defined and published practices of the institution and program.

A5.17 At a minimum, the following information must be clearly defined, published, and readily available to prospective students:
- a) requirements for prior education or work experience
- b) policies regarding advanced placement, transfer of credit, and credit for experiential learning
- c) specific academic and technical standards.

SECTION B: CURRICULUM REQUIREMENTS

B1 Instructional Process

B1.1 The program is responsible for the curriculum design and implementation.

B1.2 The curriculum design must reflect learning experiences and sequencing that enable students to develop the clinical competence necessary for practice.

B1.3 The program must provide students with written program objectives, learning goals, and competencies required for successful completion of the program.

B1.4 For each didactic and clinical course, the program must provide a clearly written course syllabus that includes measurable instructional objectives and expected student competencies.

B1.5 The program must orient instructional faculty and preceptors to the specific educational competencies expected of PA students.

B2 Basic Medical Sciences

B2.1 Instruction in the basic medical sciences must include:
- a) human anatomy
- b) physiology
- c) pathophysiology
- d) pharmacology.

B2.2 While programs may require basic sciences as prerequisites to enrollment, those prerequisites do not substitute for the basic medical sciences education of the professional component of the program as required above.

B3 Behavioral and Social Sciences

B3.1 Programs must provide instruction in:
- a) personality development
- b) child development
- c) normative responses to stress
- d) psychosomatic manifestations of illness and injury
- e) sexuality
- f) responses to death and dying.

B3.2 Programs must provide instruction in basic counseling skills necessary to help patients and families cope with illness and injury, follow prescribed treatment regimens, and modify their behaviors to more healthful patterns.

B3.3 Programs must provide instruction in the counseling of patients regarding:
a) issues of health care management, including compliance with prescribed therapeutic regimens
b) normal growth and development
c) family planning
d) emotional problems of daily living.

B3.4 Programs must provide instruction in advance directives and end-of-life decisions.

B3.5 Programs must provide instruction on the influence of multicultural issues and their impact on the delivery of patient care.

B3.6 Programs must provide instruction in medical ethics and professional responsibility, including the concepts of privilege, confidentiality, and informed consent.

B3.7 Programs must provide instruction in effective interpersonal communication.

B4 Health Policy

B4.1 Programs must provide instruction on:
a) the impact of socioeconomic issues affecting health care
b) health care delivery systems
c) reimbursement, including documentation, coding, and billing
d) quality assurance and risk management in medical practice
e) legal issues of health care.

B5 Clinical Preparatory Sciences

B5.1 Program must provide students with instruction in assessment, including:
a) techniques of interviewing and eliciting a medical history
b) performing a physical examination across the life span
c) ordering and interpreting diagnostic studies
d) presenting patient data in oral and written form.

B5.2 The program must provide instruction covering the pathology of all organ systems and include the important aspects of preventive, acute, chronic, continuing, rehabilitative, and end-of-life care.

B5.3 Programs must provide instruction in technical procedures based on current professional practice.

B5.4 Programs must prepare students for prescriptive practice.

B5.5 Programs must assist students in becoming critical thinkers who can apply the concepts of medical decision making and problem solving.

B5.6 Programs must provide instruction in development and implementation of patient management and treatment plans that include patient education.

B5.7 Programs must provide instruction in evaluation and management of life-threatening situations.

B5.8 Programs must provide instruction in the referral of patients to other health care providers or agencies.

B5.9 Programs must provide instruction that stresses the examination of evidence from clinical research as a basis for clinical decision making.

B5.10 Programs must provide instruction to equip students with the necessary skills to search and interpret the medical literature and its application to patient care, in order to maintain a critical, current, and operational knowledge of new medical findings.

B6 Supervised Clinical Practice

B6.1 Programs must provide medical and surgical clinical practice experiences that enable students to meet program objectives and acquire the competencies needed for clinical PA practice.

B6.2 While specific clinical rotations are not required for each clinical discipline listed below, the program must document that every student has clinical experiences in:
a) family medicine
b) general internal medicine
c) pediatrics
d) prenatal care and gynecology
e) general surgery
f) emergency medicine
g) psychiatry/behavioral medicine
h) geriatrics.

B6.3 Clinical experience should be provided in ambulatory, emergency, inpatient, and long-term care settings.

B7 Professional Practice Issues

B7.1 Instruction must emphasize the attributes of respect for self and others, adherence to the concepts of privilege and confidentiality in communicating with patients, and a commitment to the patient's welfare.

B7.2 The program must provide students an historical perspective of the PA profession, as well as content related to current trends and the political and legal issues that affect PA practice.

B7.3 The program must provide instruction on the physician-PA team relationship.

B7.4 Instruction must include content relating to:

a) PA professional organizations
b) PA program accreditation.
c) graduate certification and recertification
d) licensure
e) credentialing
f) professional liability.

SECTION C: EVALUATION

C1 Program Evaluation

C1.1 The program must have a formal self-evaluation process for continually and systematically reviewing the effectiveness of the education it provides and for assessing its compliance with the *Standards*.

C2 Educational Effectiveness

C2.1 Programs must routinely secure qualitative and quantitative information regarding student and recent graduate outcomes.

C2.2 Critical analysis of outcome data must be incorporated in self-study reports and must include:

a) student attrition, deceleration, and remediation
b) faculty attrition
c) student failure rates in individual courses and rotations
d) student evaluations of individual didactic courses, clinical experiences, and faculty
e) timely surveys of graduates evaluating curriculum and program effectiveness
f) surveys of employers on such matters as employment settings, scope of practice, graduate competence, and suggestions for curriculum improvement
g) evaluation of the most recent five-year aggregate student performance on the national certifying examination.

C3 Program Modification

C3.1 Results of ongoing program evaluation must be reflected in the curriculum and other dimensions of the program.

C4 Self-Study Reports

C4.1 The program must prepare self-study reports that accurately and succinctly document the process of self-evaluation. Reports must document:

a) process and results of continuous evaluation
b) outcome data analysis
c) self-identified program strengths, weaknesses, and opportunities for improvement
d) modifications that occurred as a result of self-evaluation
e) plans for addressing weaknesses and areas needing improvement
f) response to the last accreditation citations
g) compliance with the *Standards*.

C5 Student Evaluation

C5.1 Written criteria for successful progression to and completion of each segment of the curriculum and for graduation must be given to each student upon enrollment.

C5.2 Objective evaluation methods must be equitable and include content related to the objectives and competencies described in the curriculum for both didactic and supervised clinical education components.

C5.3 The program must conduct frequent, objective, and documented formative evaluations of students to assess their acquisition of knowledge, problem-solving skills, psychomotor and clinical competencies, and behavioral performance.

C5.4 Progress of students must be monitored in such a way that deficiencies are promptly identified and a means for correction established.

C5.5 A summative evaluation of each student should be completed and documented prior to program completion to assure that students meet defined program objectives for the knowledge, skills, and attitudes that demonstrate suitability for practice.

C6 Clinical Site Evaluation

C6.1 The program must define and maintain a process to routinely evaluate sites for the students' clinical practice experiences.

C6.2 Equivalent evaluation processes must be applied to all clinical sites regardless of geographical location.

C6.3 The program must ensure and document that each clinical site provides the student access to the physical facilities, patient populations, and supervision necessary to fulfill the rotation objectives.

SECTION D: STUDENTS

D1 Health

D1.1 Documentation verifying that each student has completed health screening and meets program health requirements must be in program files.

D1.2 The student health records are confidential documents and must not be kept in program files.

D1.3 Health screening should include an annual PPD (tuberculosis skin test), should be consistent with institutional policies, and should occur at program entry and annually thereafter.

D1.4 Student immunization status should meet the current recommendations of the Advisory Committee on Immunization Practices of the federal Centers for Disease Control and Prevention.

D1.5 Students must be informed of and have access to the same student health care services that the sponsoring institution makes available to students enrolled in other courses of instruction.

D1.6 Core program faculty must not participate as the primary health care providers for students in the program.

D2 Guidance

D2.1 Guidance must be available to assist students in understanding and abiding by program policies and practices.

D2.2 Students must have timely access to faculty for assistance and counseling regarding their academic concerns and problems.

D2.3 The program must provide referral for counseling of students with personal problems that may interfere with their progress in the program.

D3 Student Identification

D3.1 PA students must be clearly identified as such to distinguish them from physicians, medical students, and other health profession students and graduates.

SECTION E: EDUCATIONAL EQUIVALENCY

E1 Instruction

E1.1 When courses in the basic medical sciences, behavioral and social sciences, health policy, clinical preparatory sciences, the PA role, and any other didactic courses are conducted on geographically separate campuses, or instruction is provided by different means on separate campuses, the program must assure educational equivalency of course content, student experience, and access to didactic and laboratory materials upon which course learning objectives are based.

E1.2 Regardless of location, sites used for students during supervised clinical practice must meet the program's prescribed clinical course learning objectives and performance evaluation measures.

E2 Administration

E2.1 Program policies must apply to all students and faculty regardless of the location of their campus.

E2.2 Students and faculty at campuses geographically distant from a main program campus must have access to services and resources equivalent to those on the main campus.

SECTION F: PROVISIONAL ACCREDITATION

Provisional accreditation is recognition granted for a limited period of time to a new program that at the time of the initial provisional site visit has demonstrated to the ARC-PA's satisfaction its preparedness to initiate a program in accordance with the *Standards*. The provisional accreditation process involves a thorough review of the planning, organization, and proposed content of a program that is in the advanced planning stages, but not yet operational. Provisional accreditation status indicates the ARC-PA's determination that the plans and resources allocated for the program demonstrate an ability to meet the *Standards* if fully implemented as proposed. In all cases, provisional accreditation of the program must precede the matriculation of students.

Initial provisional accreditation visits are conducted during the year prior to enrollment of the charter class of students.

Follow-up provisional visits are conducted at programs that have successfully achieved provisional accreditation. Follow-up visits must occur no sooner than four months after students have entered the clinical phase of the program and no later than six months after graduation of the first class.

Failure of a program to achieve accreditation after its follow-up provisional visit requires that the program enter the accrediation process again via the provisional pathway.

F1 Provisional Accreditation Requirements

F1.1 The parent institution must authorize the development of the PA program.

F1.2 There must be a program director and a medical director responsible for the development of the program. These individuals must meet the qualifications for their roles.

F1.3 If provisional accreditation status is granted, the program must not admit more students than the number for which it has been approved by the ARC-PA, based on its application.

F1.4 The program must agree to inform, in writing, everyone who requests information, applies, or plans to enroll that the program is not yet accredited and must convey the implications of nonaccreditation to applicants.

F1.5 The program must submit, with its application for provisional accreditation, a descriptive narrative report as described in the application materials.

F1.6 The chief academic officer of the sponsoring institution, or his designee, must sign the provisional accreditation application and descriptive narrative report, thus approving its content and verifying the institution's intent to implement and support the program as planned.

F1.7 A detailed line item budget for the first 3 years of the program must be provided.

F1.8 A copy of current or proposed promotional literature including the course of study and course descriptions, proposed tuition, and fees is required. Documentation should include the date that the information will be included in the institution's literature and should describe the current method for disseminating the information.

F1.9 The curriculum design, sequencing, and evaluation methods must be complete for all clinical and didactic components of the program.

F1.10 Course syllabi (course descriptions, learning objectives, and instruction methods) must be provided for the first 12 months of the program.

F1.11 Methods of student evaluation must be articulated for each course in the first 12 months of the program.

F1.12 Examples of evaluation instruments must be provided for each course in the first 12 months of the program.

F1.13 Qualified faculty must be identified in sufficient number to provide instruction for the first 12 months of the program.

F1.14 While all aspects of the program beyond the first 12 months are not required to be in place at the time of the site visit for provisional accreditation, plans and mechanisms for bringing the program into compliance with the *Standards* must be clearly articulated as required within the application.

F1.15 The program must have identified prospective clinical sites sufficient in number to meet the needs of students.

F1.16 The program must develop a written plan for an analytical self-study process.

F1.17 Although no outcome data will be available at the time of the initial review of materials, the program must submit a full plan for comprehensive program evaluation, including an assessment of outcomes.

F1.18 An application and self-study report must be submitted to the ARC-PA at least 6 weeks before the follow-up site visit for accreditation occurs.

SECTION G: MAINTAINING ACCREDITATION

G1 Program and Sponsoring Institution Responsibilities

G1.1 In accordance with ARC-PA policy, failure of a program to meet administrative requirements for maintaining accreditation will result in the program being placed on Administrative Probation and if not corrected as directed by the ARC-PA, ultimately to an accreditation action of Accreditation Withdrawn.

G1.2 The program must agree to a comprehensive review that may include a site visit as determined by the ARC-PA.

G1.3 The program must submit self-study reports or progress reports as required by the ARC-PA.

G1.4 The program must inform the ARC-PA in writing of changes in the program director, medical director, or core program faculty within 30 days of the date of the effective change.

G1.5 The program must inform the ARC-PA in writing, no less than six months prior to implementation, of any proposed change in the maximum aggregate student enrollment that will result in an increase of 15 percent or greater in maximum aggregate student enrollment, as compared to the program's most recent application for accreditation or as approved by the ARC-PA.

G1.6 The program must inform the ARC-PA in writing of any intended program expansion to a different primary geographic location or of any additional secondary, geographically separate educational sites (satellite program).

G1.7 The program must inform the ARC-PA in writing, no less than six months prior to implementation, of changes in the following:

a) degrees or certificate granted at program completion
b) requirements for graduation
c) program length.

G1.8 The sponsoring institution must inform the ARC-PA in writing of the intent to transfer program sponsorship in accordance with ARC-PA policy.

G1.9 The program and the sponsoring institution must pay ARC-PA accreditation fees as determined by the ARC-PA.

DEFINITIONS

NOTE: Where evaluative terms are not defined, their definitions are at the discretion of the ARC-PA.

Core Faculty: the program director, medical director, and at least 2 additional FTE positions occupied by no more than 4 individuals certified as PAs.

Distant Campus: a campus geographically separate from the main PA program at which didactic or preclinical instruction occurs for all or some of the students enrolled.

Formative Evaluation: intermediate or continuous evaluation that may include feedback to help in achieving goals.

Instructional Objective: a statement that describes what the learner will be able to do after completing a unit of instruction. Instructional objectives are related to intended outcomes not to the process for achieving those outcomes.

Maximum Aggregate Student Enrollment: the maximum total number of students enrolled in the program, as recorded on the program's most recent accreditation application or as approved by the ARC-PA, regardless of the geographic location of the campus.

Must: a term used to designate requirements that are compelled or mandatory. "Must" indicates an absolute requirement.

Physician Assistant (PA): individuals who practice medicine with supervision by licensed physicians. As members of the health care team, PAs provide a broad range of medical services that would otherwise be provided by physicians. Physician assistants are qualified by graduation from an accredited physician assistant education program and/or certification by the

National Commission on Certification of Physician Assistants. [Adopted 1980, reaffirmed 1990, reaffirmed by acclamation in 1993, amended 1991 and 1996; American Academy of Physician Assistants.]

Prospective Students: any individual who has requested information about the program or submitted information to the program.

Published: (material) presented in written or electronic (Web) format.

Readily Available: made accessible to others in a timely fashion via defined program or institution procedures.

Recognized Regional or National Accrediting Agencies:

Liaison Committee on Medical Education
American Osteopathic Association
Middle States Association of Colleges and Schools
New England Association of Schools and Colleges
New York State Education Department
North Central Association of Colleges and Schools
Northwest Association of Schools and Colleges
Southern Association of Colleges and Schools
Western Association of Schools and Colleges

Should: term used to designate requirements that are so important that their absence must be justified.

Sufficient: enough to meet the needs of a situation or proposed end.

Student(s): individuals enrolled in the professional phase of a PA program

Summative Evaluation: a written objective assessment by the program of the learner toward the end of the program. This comprehensive review is intended to document the learner's integration of the knowledge, skills and attitudes necessary for professional practice.

APPENDIX 6

MEDICAL PROFESSIONAL OATHS

INTRODUCTION

Like medical schools, most physician assistant (PA) programs do not use the original Oath of Hippocrates. They have dropped it altogether or rewritten it to apply to their own particular standards. One reason is that it is not enforceable and therefore is more ceremonial. Other documents and procedures provide official licensure, certification, and credentialing. Some PA programs have developed their own oaths and charges as to how they want to charge their graduates with health care responsibility. We provide some of the more common professional oaths that are administered to PAs, the *Oath of Geneva*, the original *Hippocratic Oath*, and the *Oath for Physician Assistants*. Other oaths are included to allow the reader to consider alternatives.

OATH OF GENEVA

At the time of being admitted as a member of the medical profession:

I solemnly pledge myself to consecrate my life to the service of humanity;

I will give to my teachers the respect and gratitude which is their due;

I will practice my profession with conscience and dignity;

The health of my patient will be my first consideration;

I will respect the secrets which are confided in me;

I will maintain by all means in my power, the honor and the noble traditions of the medical profession;

My colleagues will be my brothers and sisters;

I will not permit considerations of religion, nationality, race, party politics, or social standing to intervene between my duty and my patient;

I will maintain the utmost respect for human life, even under threat;

I will not use my medical knowledge contrary to the laws of humanity.

I make these promises solemnly, freely and upon my honor.

OATH OF HIPPOCRATES

I swear by Apollo, the physician, and Asclepius, and Health, and All-heal, and all the gods and goddesses, that according to my ability and judgment, I will keep this oath and stipulation; to reckon him who taught me this art equally dear to me as my parents, to share my substance with him and relieve his necessities if required; to regard his offspring as on the same footing with my own brothers, and to teach them this art if they should wish to learn it, without fee or stipulation, and that by precept, lecture and every other mode of instruction, I will impart a knowledge of the art to my own sons and to those of my teachers, and to disciples bound by a stipulation and oath, according to the law of medicine, but to none others.

I will follow that method of treatment, which, according to my ability and judgment, I consider for the benefit of my patients, and abstain, from whatever is deleterious and mischievous. I will give no deadly medicine to anyone if asked nor suggest any such counsel; furthermore, I will not give to a woman an instrument to produce abortion.

With purity and with holiness I will pass my life and practice my art. I will not cut a person who is suffering with a stone, but will leave this to be done by practitioners of this work. Into whatever houses I enter I will go into them for the benefit of the sick and will abstain from every voluntary act of mischief and corruption; and further from the seduction of females and males, bond or free.

Whatever, in connection with my professional practice, or not in connection with it, I may see or hear in the lives of men which ought not to be spoken abroad, I will not divulge, as reckoning that all such should be kept secret.

While I continue to keep this oath inviolate, may it be granted to me to enjoy life and the practice of the art, respected by all men at all times, but should I trespass and violate this oath, may the reverse be my lot.

AN OATH FOR PHYSICIAN ASSISTANTS

In 1999, the Association of Physician Assistant Programs Board of Directors voted to endorse the oath by the Student Academy of the American Academy of Physician Assistants (SAAAPA). The board recognized that many programs already have graduation oaths: This one is offered as a suggestion, to be modified if desired, to those programs that do not currently have an oath and would like to include one in their graduation ceremonies.

The SAAAPA oath is the result of many months of work and a good deal of fruitful collaboration. In 1999 a resolution was brought to the Student Assembly of Representatives charging the SAAAPA with developing an oath specific to the PA profession. The SAAAPA took on the project and began the process by collecting about 20 oaths currently used by different PA programs. An open comment period was held after the first draft was written, from which almost all suggestions were included. The final product was developed in collaboration with the AAPA's Professional Practice Council and Judicial Affairs Committee, to ensure consistency among the profession's ethical guides.

Oath for Physician Assistants

I pledge to perform the following duties with honesty, integrity, and dedication, remembering always that my primary responsibility is to the health, safety, welfare, and dignity of all human beings:

I recognize and promote the value of diversity and I will treat equally all persons who seek my care.

I will uphold the tenets of patient autonomy, beneficence, non-maleficence, justice, and the principle of informed consent.

I will hold in confidence the information shared with me in the course of practicing medicine, except where I am authorized to impart such knowledge.

I will be diligent in understanding both my personal capabilities and my limitations, striving always to improve my practice of medicine.

I will actively seek to expand my intellectual knowledge and skills, keeping abreast of advances in medical art and science.

I will work with other members of the health care team to assure compassionate and effective care of patients.

I will uphold and enhance community values and use the knowledge and experience acquired as a PA to contribute to an improved community.

I will respect my professional relationship with the physician and act always with the guidance and supervision provided by that physician, except where to do so would cause harm.

I recognize my duty to perpetuate knowledge within the profession.

These duties are pledged with sincerity and on my honor.

OTHER OATHS

*Oath of Asaph and Yohanan (Sixth Century)**

[1] This is the pact which Asaph ben Berakhyahu and Yohanan ben Zabda made with their pupils, and they adjured them with the following words:
[2] Do not attempt to kill any soul by means of a potion of herbs,
[3] Do not make a woman [who is] pregnant [as a result of] of whoring take a drink with a view to causing abortion,
[4] Do not covet beauty of form in women with a view to fornicating with them,
[5] Do not divulge the secret of a man who has trusted you,
[6] Do not take any reward [which may be offered in order to induce you] to destroy and to ruin,
[7] Do not harden your heart [and turn it away] from pitying the poor and healing the needy,
[8] Do not say of [what is] good, it is bad; nor of [what is] bad, it is good,
[9] Do not adopt the ways of the sorcerers using [as they do] charms, augury, and sorcery in order to separate a man from the wife of his bosom or a woman from the companion of her youth,
[10] You shall not covet any wealth or reward [which may be offered in order to induce you] to help in a lustful desire,
[11] You shall not seek help in any idolatrous [worship] so as to heal through [a recourse to idols], and you shall not heal with anything [pertaining] to their worship,
[12] But on the contrary detest and abhor and hate all those who worship them, put their trust in them, and give assurance [referring] to them,
[13] For they are all naught, useless, for they are nothing, demons, spirits of the dead; they cannot help their own corpses, how then could they help those who live?
[14] Now [then] put your trust in the Lord, your God, [who is] a true God, a living God,
[15] For [it is] He who kills and makes alive, who wounds and heals,
[16] Who teaches men knowledge and also to profit,
[17] Who wounds with justice and righteousness, and who heals with pity and compassion,
[18] No designs of [His] sagacity are beyond His [power]
[19] And nothing is hidden from His eyes.
[20] Who causes curative plants to grow,
[21] Who puts sagacity into the hearts of the wise in order that they should heal through the abundance of His loving-kindness, and that they should recount wonders in the congregation of many; so that every living [being] knows that He made him and that there is no saviour [other] than He.
[22] For the nations trust in their idols, who [are supposed] to save them from their distress and will not deliver them from their misfortunes
[23] For their trust and hope is in the dead.
[24] For this [reason] it is fitting to keep yourselves separate from them; to remove yourselves and keep far away from all the abominations of their idols,
[25] And to cleave to the name of the Lord God of spirits for all flesh,
[26] And the soul of every living being is in His hand to kill and to make live,
[27] And there is none that can deliver out of His hand.
[28] Remember Him always and seek Him in truth, in righteousness in an upright way, in order that you should prosper in all your works
[29] And He will give you help to make you prosper in [what you are doing], and you shall be [said to be] happy in the mouth of all flesh.
[30] And the nations will abandon their idols and images and will desire to worship God like you,
[31] For they will know that their trust is in vain and their endeavor fruitless,
[32] For they implore a god, who will not do good [to them], who will not save [them].
[33] As for you, be strong, do not let your hands be weak, for your work shall be rewarded,

*From Shlomo Pines. (1975) "The Oath of Asaph the Physician and Yohanan Ben Zabda. Its Relation to the Hippocratic Oath and the Doctrina Duarum Viarum of the Didache." Proceedings of the Israel Academy of Sciences and Humanities 9, 223-264.

[34] The Lord is with you, while you are with Him,
[35] If you keep His pact, follow His commandments, cleaving to them,
[36] You will be regarded as His saints in the eyes of all flesh, and they will say:
[37] Happy the people whose [lot] is such, happy the people whose God is the Lord.
[38] Their pupils answered saying:
[39] We will do all that you exhorted and ordered us [to do],
[40] For it is a commandment of the Torah,
[41] And we must do it with all our heart, with all our soul and with all our might, To do and to obey
[42] ***** Number List 42 Missing ****
[43] Not to swerve or turn aside to the right hand or the left
[44] And they [Asaph and Yohanan] blessed them in the name of God most high, maker of heaven and earth.
[45] And they continued to charge them, and said:
[46] The Lord God, His saints and His Torah [bear] witness, that you should fear Him, that you should not turn aside from His commandments, and that you should follow His laws with an upright heart,
[47] You shall not incline after lucre [so as] to help a godless [man in shedding] innocent blood. You shall not mix a deadly drug for any man or woman so that he [or she] should kill their fellow man,
[48] ***** Number List 48 Missing ****
[49] You shall not speak of the herbs [out of which such drugs are made]. You shall not hand them over to any man,
[50] And you shall not talk about any matter [connected] with this,
[51] you shall not use blood in any work of medicine,
[52] You shall not attempt to provoke an ailment in a human soul through [the use of] iron instruments or searing with fire before making an examination two or three times; then [only] should you give your advice.†

†Bodleian MS variant of [52]: You shall not provoke an ailment in a human soul. Do not cause a defect in a man through haste in breaking open the flesh of man with an iron instrument or with searing by fire before making an yexamination two or three times; then you should give your advice.

[53] You shall not be ruled – your eyes and your heart being lifted up – by a haughty spirit.
[54] Do not keep [in your hearts] the vindictiveness of hatred with regard to a sick man,
[55] You shall not change your words in anything,
[56] The Lord our God hates [?] [this?] being done,
[57] But keep His orders and commandments, and follow all His ways, in order to please Him, [and] to be pure, true and upright.
[58] Thus did Asaph and Yohanan exhort and adjure their pupils.

My Pledge to My Patients

I will treat the sick according to my best ability and judgment, always striving to do no harm. I will never give a deadly drug to anyone even if asked, nor will I suggest suicide.

Whenever I care for a terminally ill patient, I will give comfort care until natural death. I will also support my patients' wishes not to prolong the dying process with futile care.

Whatever I see or hear in the course of medical practice, I will keep private and confidential. I will always avoid sexual involvement with my patients.

I will always affirm and guard these ethical principles with integrity, recognizing that every human life is inherently valuable.‡

Fellowship Pledge of the American College of Obstetricians and Gynecologists

I will maintain the traditions, the dignity, the standards, and the ethics of The American College of Obstetricians and Gynecologists. I will devote myself to those medical activities, which properly come within the scope of obstetrics and gynecology. I will follow those methods of diagnosis and treatment, which, according to my ability and judgment, are consistent with the principles of the College. When in doubt, I will seek the counsel of my colleagues. I shall willingly assist others and advance knowledge in obstetrics and gynecology to the best of my ability.

‡From Physicians for Compassionate Care, 1996, Oregon.

From the Oath According to Hippocrates Insofar as a Christian May Swear It (Urbinus 64 mss)

Blessed be God the Father of our Lord Jesus Christ, who is blessed for ever and ever; I lie not.

I will bring no stain upon the learning of the medical art. Neither will I give poison to anybody though asked to do so, nor will I suggest such a plan. Similarly I will not give treatment to women to cause abortion, treatment neither from above nor from below. But I will teach this art, to those who require to learn it, without grudging and without an indenture. I will use treatment to help the sick according to my ability and judgment. And in purity and in holiness I will guard my art. Into whatsoever houses I enter, I will do so to help the sick, keeping myself free from all wrong-doing, intentional or unintentional, tending to death or to injury, and from fornication with bond or free, man or woman. Whatsoever in the course of practice I see or hear (or outside my practice in social intercourse) that ought not to be published abroad, I will not divulge, but consider such things to be holy secrets. Now if I keep this oath and break it not, may God be my helper in my life and art, and may I be honoured among all men for all time. If I keep faith, well; but if I forswear myself may the opposite befall me.[§]

[§]From Jones, W.H.S. (1924) *The Doctor's Oath.* Cambridge University Press, Cambridge, U.K.

BIBLIOGRAPHY

Aaronson, W.E. (1991) The use of physician extenders in nursing homes: a review. *Med.Care Rev.* 48, 411-447.

Aaronson, W.E. (1992) Is there a role for physician extenders in nursing homes? *J. Long. Term. Care Adm.* 20, 18-22.

Abbott, A. (1981) Status and status strain in the professions. *Am. J. Sociol.* 86, 819-835.

Ackermann, R.J. & Kemle, K.A. (1998) The effect of a physician assistant on the hospitalization of nursing home residents. *J. Am. Geriatr. Soc.* 46, 610-614.

Acuna, H.R. (1977) The physician's assistant and extension of health services. *Bull. Pan Am. Health Organ* 11, 189-194.

Alexander, B.J. & Lipscomb, J. (1992) Nonphysician practitioners panel report. In: Lipscomb, J. & Alexander, B.J., eds. *Physician Staffing for the VA.* National Academy Press, Washington, D.C.

AMA & American Medical Association. (2002) Physician Trends. In: Pasko, T. & Seidman, B., eds. *Physician Characteristics and Distribution in the US: 2002-2003 Edition.* American Medical Association, Chicago, Ill.

Amann, H.J. (1973) Physician's assistants: an extension of the physician. *U.S. Navy Med.* 62, 36-38.

American Academy of Pediatrics, Committee on Fetus and Newborn. (1982) Neonatal nurse clinicians. *Pediatrics* 70, 1004.

American Academy of Pediatrics, Committee on Hospital Care. (1999) The role of the nurse practitioner and physician assistant in the care of hospitalized children. *Pediatrics* 103, 1050-1052.

American Academy of Physician Assistants. (1999) *American Academy of Physician Assistants 1999-2000 Directory of Members & Information Resources.* American Academy of Physician Assistants, Alexandria, Va.

American Academy of Physician Assistants. (1999) *1999 AAPA Census Report.* American Academy of Physician Assistants, Alexandria, Va.

American Academy of Physician Assistants. (2000) AAPA's 28th annual physician assistant conference: presented at the American Academy of Physician Assistants 28th Annual Conference, May 29th, 2000, Chicago, IL. *Perspect. Physician Assist. Educ.* 11, 116-119.

American Academy of Physician Assitants. (2000) *2000 AAPA Census Report.* American Academy of Physician Assistants, Alexandria, Va.

American Academy of Physician Assitants. (2001) *2001 AAPA Census Report.* American Academy of Physician Assistants, Alexandria, Va.

American Academy of Physician Assitants. (2002) *2002 AAPA Census Report.* American Academy of Physician Assistants, Alexandria, Va.

American Association of Colleges of Nursing. (1996) *The Essentials of Master's Education for Advanced Nursing.* American Association of Colleges of Nursing, Washington, D.C.

American Association of Colleges of Nursing and National Organization of Nurse Practitioner Faculties. (Fall 1998) *National Survey of NP Programs.* National Organization of Nurse Practitioner Faculties, Washington, D.C. Available at: www.nonpf.org.

American College of Surgeons. (1973) Statement on surgeon's assistants. *American College of Surgeons Bulletin.*

American Hospital Association. (1992) *Job Description Manual: Vol. II. American Society for Healthcare Human Resources Administration of the American Hospital Association and the Wyatt Company.* American Hospital Association, Chicago, Ill.

American Nurses Association. (1993) *Executive summary. Meta-analysis of process of care, clinical outcomes, and cost-effectiveness: nurse practitioners and certified nurse midwives.* American Nurses Association, Washington, D.C.

Anderson, K.H. & Powers, L. (1970) The pediatric assistant. *N.C. Med. J.* 31, 1-8.

Anonymous. (1973) PAs branch out into insurance exams on their own. *Medical World News* 14, 17-19.

Anthony, M. (2000) It's all in the name: the case for associate physicians. *Adv. Physician Assist.* 8, 16.

Aparasu, R.R. & Hegge, M. (2001) Autonomous ambulatory care by nurse practitioners and physician assistants in office-based settings. *J. Allied Health* 30, 153-159.

Arnopolin, S.L. & Smithline, H.A. (2000) Patient care by physician assistants and by physicians in an emergency department. *JAAPA* 13, 39-40, 49-50, 53-54, 81.

Asprey, D.P. (2000) A description of physician assistant postgraduate training: The resident's perspective. *Perspect. Physician Asst. Educ.* 11, 79–86.
Asprey, D.P. & Helms, L. (1999) A description of physician assistant postgraduate residency training: the director's perspective. *Perspect. Physician Assist. Educ.* 10, 124-131.
Association of Perioperative Registered Nurses. Revised AORN official statement on RN first assistants. Available at: www.aorn.org/clinical/rnfaste.htm.
Association of Physician Assistant Programs. (2000) *2000 Physician Assistant Programs Directory*. Association of Physician Assistant Programs, Alexandria, Va.
Atwater, J.B. (1980) Must local health officers be physicians? *Am. J. Public Health.* 70, 11.
Atwater, R.E. (1993) Recruiting relationships: Q & A. *PA Career* 11, 7.
Austin, G., Foster, W., & Richards, J.C. (1968) Pediatric screening examinations in private practice. *Pediatrics* 41, 115-119.
Baker, J.A., Oliver, D., Donahue, W., et al. (1989) Predicting role satisfaction among practicing physician assistants. *JAAPA* 2, 461-470.
Ballenger, M.D. (1971) The physician's assistant: legal considerations. *Hospitals* 45, 58-61.
Ballenger, M.D. & Estes, E.H., Jr. (1971) Licensure of responsible delegation? *N. Engl. J. Med.* 284, 330-332.
Ballweg, R.M., Cawley, J., Crane, S.C., et al. (1998) Physician Assistant Task Force on the Impact of Managed Care. A Joint Report of the Pew Health Professions Commission and the Center for the Health Professions. University of California, San Francisco, Center for the Health Professions.
Ballweg, R.M. & Wick, K.H. (1999) Decentralized didactic training for physician assistants: academic performance across training sites. *J. Allied Health* 28, 220-225.
Barnes, D., & Hooker, R.S. (2001) Physician assistant entrepreneurs. *Physician Assist.* 25, 36-41.
Barnes, W. & Magnuson, L. (1971) An important untapped resource of health manpower for the seventies. *Arch. Environ. Health* 23, 82-87.
Begely, B. (1993) PA-C: PA-SEE or passe. *JAAPA* 4, 297.
Beinfield, M.S. (1991) Postgraduate surgical education versus on-the-job training [Editorial]? *JAAPA* 4, 451-452.
Bellin, L.E. (1982) The politics of ambulatory care. In: Pascarelli, E., ed. *Hospital-Based Ambulatory Care.* Appleton-Century-Crofts, Norwalk, Conn.
Benjamin, R., Bigby, J.A., Blessing, D., et al., for the Bureau of Health Professions (1999). Into the Future: Physician Assistants Look to the 21st Century, A Strategic Plan for the Physician Assistant Profession. *Perspec. Physic. Asst. Educ.* 10(2), 73–81.
Berg, R.H. (1966) More than a nurse, less than a doctor. *Look* 30, 58-61.
Bergeson, J., Cash, R., Boulger, J., et al. (1997) The attitudes of rural Minnesota family physicians toward nurse practitioners and physician assistants. *J. Rural Health* 13, 196-205.
Bergman, A.B. (1971) Two views on the latest health manpower issue: physician's assistants belong in the nursing profession. *Am. J. Nurs.* 71, 975.
Bernzweig, J., Takayama, J.I., Phibbs, C., et al. (1997) Gender differences in physician-patient communication: evidence from pediatric visits. *Arch. Pediatr. Adolesc. Med.* 151, 586-591.
Billingsley, M.C. & Harper, D.C. (1982) The extinction of the nurse practitioner: threat or reality? *Nurse Pract.* 7, 22-30.
Blaser, L. (1993) The business of clinical practice. *JAAPA* 6, 402-406.
Blendon, R.J. (1979) Can China's health care be transplanted without China's economic policies? *N. Engl. J. Med.* 300, 1453-1458.
Blessing, J.D., Askins, D.G., Jr., Cook, P.A., et al. (1998) Physician views on the PA profession. *Physician Assist.* 22, 100, 102-103, 106-108, 110, 116.
Borland, B.L., Williams, F.E., & Taylor, D. (1972) A survey of attitudes of physicians on proper use of physician's assistants. *Health Serv. Rep.* 87, 467-472.
Bottom, W.D. (1988) Geriatric medicine in the United States: new roles for physician assistants. *J. Community Health* 13, 95-103.
Bottom, W.D. & Evans, H.A. (1994) Who should be called "physician assistants?" *JAAPA* 7, 19A-20A.
Brady, G.F. (1980) Job to career satisfaction spillover among physician's assistants. *Med. Care* 18, 1057-1062.
Brandt, L.B., Beinfield, M.S., Laffaye, H.A., et al. (1989) The training and utilization of surgical physician assistants. A retrospective study. *Arch. Surg.* 124, 348-351.
Breslau, N. & Novack, A.H. (1979) Public attitudes toward some changes in the division of labor in medicine. *Med. Care* 17, 859-867.
Briggs, R.M., Schneidman, B.S., Thorson, E.N., & Deisher, R.D. (1978) Education and integration of midlevel health-care practitioners in obstetrics and gynecology: experience of a training program in Washington state. *Am. J. Obstet. Gynecol.* 132, 68-77.
Brock, R. (1998) The malpractice experience: how PAs fare. *JAAPA* 11, 93-94.
Brotherton, P. (2000) Administrator, consultant credit PA background for success. *AAPA News* 21, 7-7.
Broughton, B. (1996) A delineative study of physician assistants in orthopaedic surgery: tasks, professional relationships, and satisfaction [PhD dissertation]. Columbia Pacific University, California.
Brutsche, R.L. (1986) Utilization of PAs in federal correctional institutions. *Physician Assist.* 10, 60-66.
Buchanan, J.L., Kane, R.L., & Garrard, J. (1989) *Results of the Massachusetts Nursing Home Connection.* RAND Corporation, Santa Monica, Calif.
Buppert, C. (1998) Reimbursement for nurse practitioner services. *Nurse Pract.* 23, 67-81.
Bureau of Health Manpower Education. (1971) *Selected Training Programs for Physician Support Personnel.* National Institutes of Health, Department of Health, Education and Welfare, Washington, D.C.

Burnett, W.H. (1980) Building the primary health care team: the state of California approach. *Fam. Community Health* 3, 49-61.

Bush, T., Cherkin, D., & Barlow, W. (1993) The impact of physician attitudes on patient satisfaction with care for low back pain. *Arch. Fam. Med.* 2, 301-305.

Byrnes, J.F., Jr. (1991) The evolution of surgical PAs . . . physician assistants. *JAAPA* 4, 449-451.

Calabrese, W.J., Crane, S.C., & Legler, C.F. (1997) Issues in quality care. The two-sided coin of PA credentialing. *JAAPA* 10, 121-122.

Camp, B. (1984) PA prescriptive privileges: an ongoing controversy. *Physician Assist.* 8, 11, 14.

Campbell, J.C. & Soeken, K.L. (1999) Women's responses to battering: a test of the model. *Res. Nurs. Health* 22, 49-58.

Cardenas, A.P. (1993) Forensic pathology and the PA [Letter to the editor]. *Journal of the American Academy of Physician Assistants* 6, 77.

Cargill, V.A., Conti, M., Neuhauser, D., & McClish, D. (1991) Improving the effectiveness of screening for colorectal cancer by involving nurse clinicians. *Medical Care.* 29, 1-5.

Carlson, R. (1975) *The End of Medicine.* John Wiley and Sons, New York.

Carter, R., Emelio, J., & Perry, H. (1984) Enrollment and demographic characteristics of physician's assistant students. *J. Med. Educ.* 59, 316-322.

Carter, R.D. (1992) Sociocultural origins of the PA profession. *JAAPA* 5, 655-662.

Carter, R.D. (2000) An office to study, preserve, and present the history of the physician assistant profession. *Perspect. Physician Assist. Educ.* 11, 185-187.

Carter, R.D. & Strand, J. (2000) Physician assistants: a young profession celebrates the 35th anniversary of its birth in North Carolina. *N.C. Med. J.* 61(5), 249–256.

Carzoli, R.P., Martinez-Cruz, M., Cuevas, L.L., et al. (1994) Comparison of neonatal nurse practitioners, physician assistants, and residents in the neonatal intensive care unit. *Arch. Pediatr. Adolesc. Med.* 148, 1271-1276.

Cassard, S.D., Weisman, C.S., Plichta, S.B., & Johnson, T.L. (1997) Physician gender and women's preventive services. *Journal Womens Health* 6, 199-207.

Castledine, G. (1996) Do we need physician assistants in the UK? *Br. J. Nurs.* 5, 124.

Cawley, J.F. (1985) Medical writing [Editorial]. *PA Drug Update* 2, 10.

Cawley, J.F. (1988) Physician assistants as alternatives to foreign medical graduates [Letter]. *Health Affairs* 7, 152-156.

Cawley, J.F. (1992) Federal health policy and PAs. *JAAPA* 5, 679-688.

Cawley, J.F. (1995) *Physician assistants in the health workforce, 1994: final report of the Advisory Group on Physician Assistants and the Workforce submitted to Council on Graduate Medical Education (COGME).* Rockville, MD, Health Resources and Services Administration, Council on Graduate Medical Education, Rockville, Md.

Cawley, J.F. (2000) Prescriptive authority and the physician assistant. In: Edmunds, M.W. & Mayhew, M.S., eds. *Pharmacology for the Primary Care Provider.* Mosby, St. Louis, Mo.

Cawley, J.F., (2002) The major trends of 2001: women fill the ranks of the health professions. *Clinician News* [Editorial] 6, 3-19.

Cawley, J.F., Andrews, M.D., Barnhill, G.C., et al. (2001) What makes the day: an analysis of the content of physician assistant's practice. *JAAPA* 14, 41-42, 44, 47-50, 55-56.

Cawley, J.F., Combs, G.E., & Curry, R.H. (1986) Nonphysician providers [Letter]. *Am. J. Public Health* 76, 1360.

Cawley, J.F. & Golden, A.S. (1983) Nonphysicians in the United States: manpower policy in primary care. *J. Public Health Policy* 4, 69-82.

Cawley, J.F. & Jones, P.E. (1997) The possibility of an impending health professions glut. *JAAPA* 10, 80-92.

Cawley, J.F., Ott, J.E., & DeAtley, C.A. (1983) The future for physician assistants. *Ann. Intern. Med.* 98, 993-997.

Cawley, J.F., Rohrs, R., & Hooker, R.S. (1998) Physician assistants and malpractice risk: findings from the National Practitioner Data Bank. *Federal Bulletin* 85, 242-247.

Cawley, J.F., Simon, A., Blessing, J.D., et al. (2000) Marketplace demand for physician assistants: results of a national survey of 1998 graduates. *Perspect. Physician Assist. Educ.* 11, 12-17.

Chaffee, D. (1988) Do PAs have a future in cardiothoracic surgery? *Physician Assist.* 12, 107-108.

Chaikin, E.J., Thornby, J.I., & Merrill, J. (2000) Caring for terminally ill patients: a comparative analysis of physician assistant and medical students' attitude. *Perspect. Physician Assist. Educ.* 11, 87-94.

Chavez, R.S. (1989) Why PAs should endorse registered care technologists . . . physician assistants. *JAAPA* 2, 79-81.

Chernichovsky, D.E., Potapchik, H., Barnum, et al. (1996) *The Russian Health System in Transition: Coping with New and Old Challenges.* World Bank, Moscow.

Cherry, D.K., Burt, C.W., & Woodwell, D.A. (2001) *National Ambulatory Medical Care Survey: 1999 Summary.* National Center for Health Statistics, Hyattsville, Md. Advance Data from Vital and Health Statistics.

Cherry D.K. & Woodwell, D.A. (2002) *National Ambulatory Medical Care Survey: 2000 Summary.* National Center for Health Statistics, Hyattsville, Md. Advance data from vital and health statistics.

Chidley, E. (1997a) PA profiles: a New York PA directs a clinic in Kenya. *PA Today* 5, 10-13.

Chidley, E. (1997b) PA profile: a career in forensic medicine. *PA Today* 5, 8-10.

Christman, L. (1998) Advanced practice nursing: is the physician's assistant an accident of history or a failure to act? [see Comments]. *Nurs. Outlook* 46, 56-59.

Clark, A.R., Monroe, J., Feldman, S.R., et al. (1999) The emerging role of physician assistants in the delivery of dermatological health care. *Dermatol. Clin.* 18, 297-302.

Conant, L., Jr., Robertson, L.S., Kosa, J., et al. (1971) Anticipated patient acceptance of new nursing roles and physicians' assistants. *Am. J. Dis. Child.* 122, 202-205.

Condit, D. (1977) PAs: Russian style. *Health Pract. Physician Assist.* 1, 37-40.

Condit, D. (1992) A quarter century of surgical physician assistants. *Physician Assist.* 15, 3-3.

Condit, D. (1993) Our military heritage. *Physician Assist.* 17, 58.

Condit, D. (2000) Credentialing. *Surg. Physician Assist.* 6, 7-8.

Cooper, J.K. & Willig, S.H. (1971) Nonphysicians for coronary care delivery: are they legal? *Am. J. Cardiol.* 28, 363-365.

Cooper, R.A., Getzen, T.E., McKee, H.J., et al. (2002) Economic and demographic trends signal an impending physician shortage. *Health Affairs* 21, 141-154.

Cooper, R.A., Henderson, T., & Dietrich, C.L. (1998) Roles of nonphysician clinicians as autonomous providers of patient care. *JAMA* 280, 795-802.

Cooper, R.A., Laud, P., & Dietrich, C.L. (1998) Current and projected workforce of nonphysician clinicians. *JAMA* 280, 788-794.

Cornell, S. (1998) You say assistant, I say associate, we can't call the whole thing off. *Adv. Physician Assist.* 6, 12.

Cornell, S. (2000a) Care and convictions: PA practice in corrections medicine. *Adv. Physician Assist.* 8, 60-61.

Cornell, S. (2000b) A dinosaur on the ticket: PA Rick Hillegas bids for state senate seat. *Adv. Physician Assist.* 8, 58-59.

Coryell, W., Cloninger, C.R., & Reich, T. (1978) Clinical assessment: use of nonphysician interviewers. *Journal of Nervous & Mental Disease* 166, 599-606.

Coulter, I., Jacobson, P., & Parker, L.E. (2000) Sharing the mantle of primary female care: physicians, nurse practitioners, and physician assistants. *J. Am. Med. Womens Assoc.* 55, 100-103.

Council on Graduate Medical Education. (1994) *Recommendations to Improve Access to Health Care through Physician Workforce Reform. Fourth Report to Congress and Health and Human Services Secretary.* US Department of Health and Human Services, Rockville, Md.

Council on Graduate Medical Education. (1996) *Eighth Report: Patient Care Physician Supply and Requirements: Testing COGME Recommendations.* Council on Graduate Medical Education, Rockville, Md.

Council on Professional Practices & American Academy of Physician Assistants. (1994) Hospital privileges for physician assistants. *JAAPA* 7, 183-190.

Counselman, F.L., Graffeo, C.A., & Hill, J.T. (2000) Patient satisfaction with physician assistants (PAs) in an ED fast track. *Am. J. Emerg. Med.* 18, 661-665.

Coye, R.D. & Hansen, M.F. (1969) The "doctor's assistant:" a survey of physicians' expectations. *JAMA* 209, 529-533.

Crandall, L.A., Haas, W.H., & Radelet, M.L. (1986) Socioeconomic influences in patient assignment to PA or MD providers. *Physician Assist.* 10, 164, 167-168, 170.

Crandall, L.A., Santulli, W.P., Radelet, M.L., et al. (1984) Physician assistants in primary care. Patient assignment and task delegation. *Med. Care* 22, 268-282.

Crane, S.C. (1995) PAs/NPs: forging effective partnerships in managed care systems. *Physician Exec.* 21, 23-27.

Creating a body of knowledge. (2000) *Perspect. Physician Assist. Educ.* 11, 151.

Crile, G., Jr. (1987) Cleveland Clinic: the supporting cast 1920-1940. *Cleve. Clin. J. Med.* 54, 344-347.

Cultural perspectives. (2000) Treating patients from other cultures. *Perspect. Physician Assist. Educ.* 11, 129-130.

Curran, W.J. (1972) Legal responsibility for actions of physicians' assistants. *N. Engl. J. Med.* 286, 254.

Currey, C.J. & Bottom, W.D. (1988) A survey of PA educators . . . physician assistants. *JAAPA* 1, 141-147.

Currey, R. (1992) *Medicine for Sale: Commercialism vs Professionalism.* Grand Rounds Press, Knoxville, Tenn.

Cyr, K.A. (1985) Physician-PA practice in a military clinic: a statistical comparison of productivity/availability. *Physician Assist.* 9, 112-114.

Davis, A. (2002) State regulations of the physician assistant profession. *JAAPA* 15(10), 27–32.

Davis, K.M., Koch, K.E., Harvey, J.K., et al. (2000) Effects of hospitalists on cost, outcomes, and patient satisfaction in a rural health system [see Comments]. *Am. J. Med.* 108, 621-626.

DeBarth, K. (1996) Outer banks PA: medicine at the edge. *Clinician Reviews* 6, 148-158.

D'Ercole, A., Skodol, A.E., Struening, E., Curtis, J., & Millman, J. (1991) Diagnosis of physical illness in psychiatric patients using axis III and a standardized medical history. *Hosp.Community Psychiatry* 42, 395-400.

Dehn, R. & Hooker, R.S. (1999) Procedures performed by Iowa family practice physician assistants. *JAAPA*12, 63-77.

DeMaria, W.J., Cherry, W.A., & Treusdell, D.H. (1971) Evaluation of the marine physician assistant program. *HSMHA. Health Rep.* 86, 195-201.

Demory-Luce, D.K. & McPherson, R.S. (1999) Current clinical nutrition issues. Nutrition knowledge and attitudes of physician assistants. *Top. Clin. Nutr.* 14, 71-82.

DeMots, H., Coombs, B., Murphy, E., et al. (1987) Coronary arteriography performed by a physician assistant. *Am. J. Cardiol.* 60, 784-787.

DeNicola, L., Kleid, D., Brink, L., et al. (1994) Use of pediatric physician extenders in pediatric and neonatal intensive care units [see Comments]. *Crit. Care Med.* 22, 1856-1864.

Department of Health, Education and Welfare. (1977) *An Evaluation of Physician Assistants in Diagnostic Radiology.* U.S.Public Health Service, Health Resources Administration, National Center for Health Services, Research Digest Series, Rockville, Md.

Detmer, D.E., Toth, P.S., Thompson, L.K., III, Howard, D.R., & Sabiston, D.C., Jr. (1972) Surgical trainees in the Duke Physician's Associate program. *Surgery* 72, 142-148.

DeVore, L. & Shapiro, S. (1978) The physicians assistant: a new breed of dental educator. *J. Dent. Educ.* 42, 568-571.

Dial, T.H., Palsbo, S.E., Bergsten, C., et al. (1995) Clinical staffing in staff- and group-model HMOs. *Health Affairs (Milwood)* 14, 168-180.

Diekema, D.J., Ferguson, K.J., & Doebbeling, B.N. (1995) Motivation for hepatitis B vaccine acceptance among medical and physician assistant students. *J. Gen. Intern. Med.* 10, 1-6.

Diekema, D.J., Schuldt, S.S., Albanese, M.A., et al. (1995) Universal precautions training of preclinical students: impact on knowledge, attitudes, and compliance. *Prev. Med.* 24, 580-585.

Dieter, P.M. & Fasser, C.E. (1989) Physician assistants in geriatrics: meeting the demand. *JAAPA* 2, 49-51.

Donaldson, M.A., Yordy, K.D., Lohr, K.N., et al. (1996a) The primary care workforce. In: Donaldson, M.A., Yordy, K.D., Lohr, K.N., et al., eds. *Primary Care: America's Health in a New Era.* National Academy Press, Washington, D.C.

Donaldson, M.A., Yordy, K.D., Lohr, K.N., et al. (1996b) The delivery of primary care. In: Donaldson, M.S., Yordy, K.D., Lohr, K.N., et al., eds. *Primary Care: America's Health in a New Era.* National Academy Press, Washington, D.C.

Donovan, P. (1992) Vermont physician assistants perform abortions, train residents. *Fam. Plann. Perspect.* 24, 225.

Dracup, K., DeBusk, R.F., De Mots, H., et al. (1994) Task force 3: partnerships in delivery of cardiovascular care. *J. Am. Coll. Cardiol.* 24, 296-304.

Drozda, P.F. (1992) Physician extenders increase healthcare access. *Health Prog.* 73, 46-48, 74.

Dubaybo, B.A., Samson, M.K., & Carlson, R.W. (1991) The role of physician-assistants in critical care units [see Comments]. *Chest* 99, 89-91.

Dungy, C.I. (1974) The child health associate in a rural setting. *J. Natl. Med. Assoc.* 66, 32-34.

Dungy, C.I. (1975) The child health associate. The new image in the nursery. *Am. J. Public Health* 65, 1179-1183.

Dungy, C.I. & Silver, H.K. (1977) Pediatricians' perceptions: competence of child health associates. *Rocky Mt. Med. J.* 74, 25-27.

Duryea, W.R. & Hooker, R.S. (2000) Elder physician assistants and their practices. *JAAPA* 13, 67-68, 71-72, 74, 80, 82, 85.

Duttera, M.J. & Harlan, W.R. (1978) Evaluation of physician assistants in rural primary care. *Arch. Intern. Med.* 138, 224-228.

Dychtwald, K. & Zitter, M. (1988) Changes during the next decade will alter the way elder-care is provided, financed. *Mod.Healthc.* 18, 38.

Edmunds, M. (1991) Lack of evidence could exclude NPs from reimbursement reform legislation. *Nurse Pract.* 16, 8.

Edmunds, M. (2000) *Nurse practitioners: remembering the past, planning the future.* Medscape. http://www.medscape.com/viewarticle/408388. Retrieved September 17, 2002.

Edmunds, M.W. (1978) Evaluation of nurse practitioner effectiveness: an overview of the literature. *Eval. Health Prof.* 1, 69-82.

Edmunds, M.W. (1994) Time of risk. *Nurse Pract.* 8, 7-10.

Edmunds, M.W. (1999) Nursing leaders consider reactions to policy. *Nurse Pract.* 24, 73-76.

Ekwo, E., Daniels, M., Oliver, D., et al. (1979) The physician assistant in rural primary care practices: physician assistant activities and physician supervision at satellite and non-satellite practice sites. *Med. Care* 17, 787-795.

Elizondo, E. & Blessing, J.D. (1990) The ability of PAs to solve patients' psychosocial problems. A preliminary report on patient expectations. *Physician Assist.* 14, 75-82.

Elliott, C.H. (1984a) The physician assistant—newest member of the corporate health care team: a guide to hiring a PA and cutting health care costs. *Pers. Adm.* 29, 87-92.

Elliott, C.H. (1984b) The physician assistant in occupational medicine. *PA Drug Update* 4, 42-48.

Ellis, B.I. (1991) Physician's assistants in radiology: has the time come? [Letter; comments]. *Radiology* 180, 880-881.

Ellis, G.L. & Brandt, T.E. (1997) Use of physician extenders and fast tracks in United States emergency departments. *Am. J. Emerg. Med.* 15, 229-232.

Emelio, J. (1994) Barriers to physician assistant practice. In: Bureau of Health Professions, ed. *Health Personnel in the United States: Ninth Report to Congress.* US Department of Health and Human Services, Health Resources and Services Administration, Washington, D.C.

Enns, S.M., Muma, R.D., & Lary, M.J. (2000) Examining referral practices of primary care physician assistants. *JAAPA*13, 81-82, 84, 86, 118.

Erkert, J.D. (1985) Nurses' attitudes toward PAs. *Physician Assist.* 9, 41-44.

Estes, E.H. (1993) Training doctors for the future: lessons from 25 years of physician assistant education. In: Clawson, D.K. & Osterweis, M., eds. *The Roles of Physician Assistants and Nurse Practitioners in Primary Care.* Association of Academic Health Centers, Washington, D.C.

Estes, E.H., Jr. (1968a) The critical shortage—physicians and supporting personnel. *Ann. Intern. Med.* 69, 957-962.

Estes, E.H., Jr. (1968b) The Duke Physician Assistant Program: a progress report. *Arch. Environ. Health* 17, 690-691.

Estes, E.H., Jr. & Howard, D.R. (1969) The physician's assistant in the university center. *Ann. N. Y. Acad. Sci.* 166, 903-910.

Estes, E.H., Jr. & Howard, D.R. (1970) Potential for newer classes of personnel: experiences of the Duke physician's assistant program. *J. Med. Educ.* 45, 149-155.

Ewing, G.B., Selassie, A.W., Lopez, C.H., & McCutcheon, E.P. (1999) Self-report of delivery of clinical preventive services by U.S. physicians: comparing specialty, gender, age, setting of practice, and area of practice. *Am. J. Prev. Med.* 17, 62-72.

Expert Committee on Professional and Technical Education of Medical and Auxillary Personnel (WHO). (1968) *Training of medical assistants and similar personnel.* World Health Organization, Technician Report Service, Geneva.

Fahringer, D., Assell, R., Harrington, N., et al. (2000) Integrating service-learning as a course into a university curriculum. *Perspect. Physician Assist. Educ.* 11, 161-164.

Fasser, C.E. (1987) Educating physician assistants: the past ten years. *Physician Assist.* 11, 152-154.

Fasser, C.E., Andrus, P., & Smith, Q. (1984) Certification, registration and licensure of physician assistants. In: Carter, R.D. & Perry, H.B., III, eds. *Alternatives in Health Care Delivery.* Warren H. Green, St. Louis, Mo.

Fawcett, J. (1994) *Analysis and Evaluation of Conceptual Models of Nursing,* 3rd ed. F.A. Davis, Philadelphia.

Feldstein, P.J. (1988) *Health Care Economics.* Delmar Publishers, Albany, N.Y.

Fenn, P.A. (1987) Acceptance of physician assistants in Western North Carolina. *Physician Assist.* 11, 161-162.

Ferraro, K.F. & Southerland, T. (1989) Domains of medical practice: physicians' assessment of the role of physician extenders. *J. Health Soc. Behav.* 30, 192-205.

Fincham, J.E. (1986) How pharmacists are rated as a source of drug information by physician assistants. *Drug Intell. Clin. Pharm.* 20, 379-383.

Fine, L.L. (1977a) Pediatrician receives more than a helping hand from child health associate. *Commitment* 3, 14-18.

Fine, L.L. (1977b) The pediatric practice of the child health associate. *Am. J. Dis. Child.* 131, 634-637.

Fine, L.L. & Machotka, P. (1973) Role identity development of the child health associate. *J. Med. Educ.* 48, 670-675.

Fine, L.L. & Scriven, S.S. (1977) The child health associate: a nonphysician primary care practitioner for children. *PA J.* 7, 137-142.

Fine, L.L. & Silver, H.K. (1973) Comparative diagnostic abilities of child health associate interns and practicing pediatricians. *J. Pediatr.* 83, 332-335.

Fischer, J. (1995) PAs committed to practice with physician supervision [Letter; comment]. *Tex. Med.* 91, 7.

Fisher, D.W. & Horowitz, S.M. (1977) The physician's assistant: profile of a new health profession. In: Bliss, A.A. & Cohen, E. eds. *The New Health Professionals: Nurse Practitioners and Physician's Assistants.* Aspen System Corporation, Germantown, Md.

Fisher, L.A. (1995) I loved our new physician assistant—for 13 days. *Med. Econ.* 72, 75-77.

Ford, L.C. (1979) A nurse for all settings: the nurse practitioner. *Outlook* 27, 516-521.

Ford, L.C. (1979a) Nurse practitioner education. In: Hamburg, J., ed. *Review of Allied Health Education.* University Press of Kentucky, Lexington, Ky.

Ford, L.C. & Silver, H.K. (1967) Expanded role of the nurse in child care. *Nurs. Outlook* 15, 43-45.

Foreman, S. (1993) *Oral Testimony before the Physician Payment Review Commission.* Physician Payment Review Commission, Washington, D.C.

Fottler, M.D. (1979) Physician attitudes toward physician extenders: a comparison of nurse practitioners and physician assistants. *Med. Care* 17, 536-549.

Fowkes, V., Cawley, J.F., Herlihy, N., et al. (1996) Evaluating the potential of international medical graduates as physician assistants in primary care. *Acad. Med.* 71, 886-892.

Fowkes, V. & Gamel, N. (2000) The California physician assistant workforce: a 10-year perspective. *Perspect. Physician Assist. Educ.* 11, 152-156.

Fowkes, V.K., Hafferty, F.W., Goldberg, H.I., et al. (1983) Educational decentralization and deployment of physician's assistants. *J. Med. Educ.* 58, 194-200.

Fox, D.P. & Whittaker, R.G. (1983) PAs in the Veterans Administration: a report of a national survey. *Physician Assist.* 7, 106-106.

Frampton, J. & Wall, S. (1994) Exploring the use of NPs and PAs in primary care [see Comments]. *HMO Pract.* 8, 165-170.

Frary, T. (1996) A new definition of "physician assistant." *JAAPA* 9, 22-27.

Freeborn, D.K. & Hooker, R.S. (1995) Satisfaction of physician assistants and other nonphysician providers in a managed care setting. *Public Health Rep.* 110, 714-719.

Freeborn, D.K., Hooker, R.S., & Pope, C.R. (2002) Satisfaction and well-being of primary care providers in managed care. *Eval. Health Prof.* 25.

Freeborn, D.K. & Pope, C.R. (1994) *Promise and Performance in Managed Care: The Prepaid Group Practice Model.* Johns Hopkins University Press, Washington, D.C.

Freedman, M.A., Jillson, D.A., Coffin, R.R., & Novick, L.F. (1986) Comparison of complication rates in first trimester abortions performed by physician assistants and physicians. *Am. J. Public Health* 76, 550-554.

Freeman, G.M. & Rose, C.P. (1981) Vicarious liability and the ophthalmologist. *Can. J. Ophthalmol.* 16, 203-204.

Freidson, E. (1970) *The Profession of Medicine.* Dodd, Mead, N.Y.

Frick, J.C. (1983) Physician assistants as house officers: our experience. *Physician Assist.* 7, 13.

Frick, J.C. (1986) The urban health care setting: the Harper-Grace hospital experience. In: Zarbock,

S.F. & Harbert, K., eds. *Physician Assistants: Present and Future Models of Utilization*. Praeger, New York.

Friedman, E. (1978) Staff privileges for nonphysicians. Part 2: A sampling of hospital programs and privileges for nurse practitioners and physician's assistants. *Hosp. Med. Staff* 7, 22-28.

Fuchs, V. (1974) *Who Shall Live?* Basic Books, New York.

Fulop, T. & Roemer, M.I. (1982) International development of health manpower policy. *WHO Offset Publication* 61, 1-168.

Gambert, S.R., Rosenkranz, W.E., Basu, S.N., Jewell, K.E., & Winga, E.R. (1983) Role of the physician extender in the long-term care setting. *Wis. Med. J.* 82, 30-32.

Gara, N. (1989) State laws for physician assistants. *JAAPA* 2, 303-313.

Gara, N. (1995) AMA adopts guidelines on PA practice. *AAPA News* 3, 303-313.

Gaudry, C.L., Jr. & Nicholas, N.C. (1977) The USAF/USN physician assistant program. *Milit. Med.* 142, 29-31.

Gelrud, S.J. (1985) Why we need the National Alliance of Nurse Practitioners. *Nurse Pract.* 10, 8.

General Accounting Office. (1993) *Health care access: innovative programs using nonphysicians.* GAO/HRD-93-128, General Accounting Office.

Genova, N.J. (1995) The influence of market factors on physician assistant practice settings [Master's thesis]. University of Southern Maine, Edmund S. Muskie Institute of Public Affairs.

Gentile, C.A. (1976) Development of an emergency medical physician's assistant program in North Carolina. *Emerg. Med. Serv.* 5, 36-37, 64.

Giardino, A.P., Giardino, E.R., & Burns, K.M. (1994) Same place, different experience: nurses and residents on pediatric emergency transport. *Holist. Nurs. Pract.* 8, 54-63.

Gifford, J.F., Jr. (1987a) Prototype PA (Amos Johnson and Henry Treadwell). *N.C. Med. J.* 48, 601-603.

Gifford, J.F., Jr. (1987b) The fate of America's prototype PA. *Physician Assist.* 11, 95-96.

Gittins, P. (1996) Physician assistants in plastic and reconstructive surgery. *NEWS-Line for Physician Assistants* 5, 4-7.

Glazer-Waldman, H.R. (1984) Perceptions of patient-provider relationships in allied health education textbooks. *J. Allied Health* 13, 104-111.

Glenn, J.K. & Hofmeister, R.W. (1976) Will physicians rush out and get physician extenders? *Health Serv. Res.* 11, 69-74.

Goldberg, G.A., Jolly, D.M. Hosek, S., et al. (1981) Physician's extenders' performance in Air Force clinics. *Med. Care* 19, 951-965.

Golden, A.S. & Cawley, J.F. (1983) A national survey of performance objectives of physician's assistant training programs. *J. Med. Educ.* 58, 418-424.

Golden, A.S., Hagan, J.L., & Carlson, D. (1981) *The Art of Teaching Primary Care.* Springer Publishers, New York.

Golden, R.M. (1986) Physician assistants in forensic pathology. *Physician Assist.* 10, 101-102.

Goldfrank, L., Corso, T., & Squillacote, D. (1980) The emergency services physician assistant: results of two years' experience. *Ann. Emerg. Med.* 9, 96-99.

Golladay, F.L., Miller, M., & Smith, K.R. (1973) Allied health manpower strategies: estimates of the potential gains from efficient task delegation. *Med. Care* 11, 457-469.

Goode, W. (1960) Encroachment, charlatanism, and the emerging profession: psychology, sociology, and medicine. *Am. Sociol. Rev.* 25, 902-914.

Gore, C.L. (2000) A physician's liability for mistakes of a physician assistant. *J. Leg. Med.* 21, 125-142.

Gould, S.H. & Gould, J.S. (1984) The microsurgical assistant. *J.Reconstr.Microsurg.* 1, 113-117.

Grabenkort, W.R. & Ramsay, J.G. (1991) Role of physician assistants in critical care units. *Chest* 99, 89-91.

Gray, D. (1997) What is the Association of PAs in Cardiovascular Surgery. *Surg. Physician Assist.* 3, 38.

Gray, J., Lacey, C., Alexander, S., et al. (1995) Do PAs use the procedures and skills they learn? *JAAPA* 8, 45-51.

Green, B.A. & Johnson, T. (1995) Replacing residents with midlevel practitioners: a New York City-area analysis. *Health Affairs (Milwood)* 14, 192-198.

Green, H. (2000) Student forum. Physician assistant students' guide to paying for school. *Perspect. Physician Assist. Educ.* 11, 131-133.

Greene, J. (2000) Match Day 2000: primary care still passed over. *AMA News*

Greenfield, S., Komaroff, A.L., Pass, T.M., et al. (1978) Efficiency and cost of primary care by nurses and physician assistants. *N. Engl. J. Med.* 298, 305-309.

Greenlee, R.L., Levy, J.W., & Allen, A.J. (1977) Utilization of a physician assistant in a comprehensive community mental health center. *PA J.* 7, 143-147.

Grumbach, K., Selby, J.V., Schmittdiel, J.A., et al. (1999) Quality of primary care practice in a large HMO according to physician specialty. *Health Serv. Res.* 34, 485-502.

Grzybicki, D., Galvis, C., & Raab, S. (1999) The usefulness of pathologists' assistants. *Am. J. Clin. Pathol.* 112, 619-626.

Gunderson, C.H. & Kampen, D. (1988) Utilization of nurse clinicians and physician assistants by active members and fellows of the American Academy of Neurology. *Neurology* 38, 156-160.

Gunneson, T.J., Menon, K.V., & Wiesner, R.H., et al. (2002) Ultrasound-assisted percutaneous liver biospy performed by a physician assistant. *Am. J. Gastroenterol.* 97(6), 1472-1475.

Gwinn, D.H. & Keller, J.E. (1999) Military medicine. In: Ballweg, R.M., Stolberg, S., & Sullivan, E., eds. *Physician Assistant: A Guide to Clinical Practice,* 2nd ed. W.B. Saunders, Philadelphia.

Hallerty, F.W. & McKinley, J.B. (1993). Oxford University Press, New York.

Hankins, G.D., Shaw, S.B., Cruess, D.F., et al. (1996) Patient satisfaction with collaborative practice. *Obstet. Gynecol.* 88, 1011-1015.

Hanna, K.M. (1993) Effect of nu rse-client transaction on female adolescents' oral contraceptive adherence. *Image J. Nurs. Scholarship* 25, 285-290.

Hansen, J.P., Stinson, J.A., & Herpok, F.J. (1980) Cost effectiveness of physician extenders as compared to family physicians in a university health clinic. *J. Am. Coll. Health Assoc.* 28, 211-214.

Harbert, K. (1991) Past becomes future: portraits of PAs in Operation Desert Storm. *Physician Assist.* 15, 30-34.

Harbert, K. (1993) The role of physician assistants as health educators: a national study [PhD dissertation]. Pennsylvania State University.

Harbert, K., Shipman, R.A., & Conrad, W. (1994) The utilization of physician extenders. Mid-level providers in a large group practice within a tertiary health care setting. *Med. Group Manage. J.* 41, 26.

Harbert, K.R. (1978) PAs and the coke oven industry. *Newsl. Maryland Academy of Physician Assistants* 5(2), 6-8.

Harper, D.C. & Johnson, J. (1996) *NONPF Workforce Project: Analysis of Nurse Practitioner Educational Programs, 1988-1995.* National Organization of Nurse Practitioner Faculty, Washington, D.C.

Harty-Golder, B. (1995) Physician extenders. *J. Fla. Med. Assoc.* 82, 417-420.

Haug Associates, Inc., for the Board of Medical Examiners. (1973) *Attitudes Toward the Physician's Assistant Program Among the Public, Physicians, and Allied Health Professionals.* Board of Medical Examiners, California.

Hayden, R.J., Salley, M.A., Brasseur, J., et al. (1995) Provider-assisted suicide: a survey of PA attitudes. Results of the 1994 Michigan survey conducted by the Michigan Academy of Physician Assistants Public Policy Committee. *Physician Assist.* 19, 73-76, 78.

Health Resources and Services Administration, Department of Health and Human Services, Division of Nursing, Bureau of Health Professionals. (1996) *National Sample Survey of Nurses.* US Department of Health and Human Services.

Hecker, D. (2001) Occupational employment projections to 2010. *Monthly Labor Review* 124, 57-84.

Heinerich, J. (2000) International rotations: an informal survey of PA schools. *Adv. Physician Assist.* 8, 30.

Heinrich, J.J., Fichandler, B.C., Beinfield, M., et al. (1980) The physician's assistant as resident on surgical service. An example of creative problem solving in surgical manpower. *Arch. Surg.* 115, 310-314.

Heller, L.E. & Fasser, C. (1978) Physicians' assistants: the new prescribers. *Am. Pharm.* 18, 12-17.

Henderson, T. (2001) *The Health Care Workforce in Ten States: Education, Practice and Policy.* National Conference of State Legislature, Washington, D.C.

Henry, R.A. (1974) Evaluation of physician's assistants in Gilchrist County, Florida. *Public Health Rep.* 89, 428-432.

Henson, K.E. (1999) In Kosovo, making a difference. *JAAPA* 12, 77-79.

Herrera, J., Gendron, B.P., & Rice, M.M. (1994) Military emergency medicine physician assistants. *Mil. Med.* 159, 241-242.

Herrick, T. (2000a) NPs/PAs get "short-scripted" in market research: prescription audit numbers off by millions. *Clinician News* 4, 1, 8, 14.

Herrick, T. (2000b) PA union movement flourishes in NY. *Clinician News* 4, 19-20.

Hillman, B.J., Fajardo, L.L., Hunter, T.B., et al. (1987) Mammogram interpretation by physician assistants. *AJR Am. J. Roentgenol.* 149, 907-912.

Hoffman, C. (1994) Medicaid payment for nonphysician practitioners: an access issue. *Health Affairs (Milwood)* 13, 140-152.

Hoffman, E. & Redmon, J. (1995) Physician assistants and nurse practitioners in Louisiana. *J. La. State Med. Soc.* 147, 267-279.

Holmes, S.E. & Fasser, C.E. (1993) Occupational stress among physician assistants. *JAAPA* 6, 172-178.

Holt, N. (1998) "Confusion's masterpiece:" the development of the physician assistant profession. *Bull. Hist. Med.* 72, 246-278.

Homan, T.C. (1994) Use of physician extenders by cardiothoracic surgery groups. *AORN J.* 59, 1073-1075.

Hooker, R.S. (1986) Medical care utilization: MD-PA/NP comparisons in an HMO. In: Zarbock, S.F. & Harbert, K., eds. *Physician Assistants: Present and Future Models of Utilization*. Praeger, New York.

Hooker, R.S. (1987) Coast Guard Physician Assistants. *AAPA News* 8(7).

Hooker, R.S. (1989) A comparison of rank and pay structure for military physician assistants. *JAAPA* 2, 293-300.

Hooker, R.S. (1991a) The military physician assistant. *Mil. Med.* 156, 657-660.

Hooker, R.S. (1991b) The Coast Guard Medical Service. *Navy Med.* 82, 18-21.

Hooker, R.S. (1992) Employment specialization in the PA profession. *JAAPA* 5, 695-704.

Hooker, R.S. (1993) The roles of physician assistants and nurse practitioners in a managed care organization. In: Clawson, D.K. & Osterweis, M., eds. *The Roles of Physician Assistants and Nurse Practitioners in Primary Care.* Association of Academic Health Centers, Washington, D.C.

Hooker, R.S. (1994) PAs and NPs in HMOs [Editorial]. *HMO Pract.* 8, 148-150.

Hooker, R.S. (1997) Is there an undersupply of PAs? *JAAPA* 10, 81, 94, 97-98, 101-102.

Hooker, R.S. (1999) Cost-benefit analysis of physician assistants [Dissertation]. Portland State University.

Hooker, R.S. (2000) The economics of physician assistant employment. *Physician Assist.* 24, 67-85.

Hooker, R.S. (2001a) Comparative analysis of physician assistant and nurse practitioner demographics. *Clinician Reviews* 11, 31-34.

Hooker, R.S. (2001b) "Women Physician Assistants: Trends and Projections." Presented to: Association of Physician Assistant Programs, October 20, 2001, Albuquerque, M.M.

Hooker, R.S. (2002) A cost analysis of physician assistants in primary care. *JAAPA* 15(11), 6-12.

Hooker, R.S. & Berlin, L. (2002) Trends in the supply of physician assistants and nurse practitioners in the American health care system. *Health Affairs* 21, 5.

Hooker, R.S. & Brown, J.B. (1985) Rheumatology referrals. *HMO. Pract.* 4, 61-65.

Hooker, R.S. & Cawley, J.F. (1995) Clinical staffing in HMOs [Letter to the editor]. *Health Affairs (Milwood)* 14, 282.

Hooker, R.S. & Cawley, J.F. (1997) *Physician Assistants in American Medicine*. Churchill Livingstone, New York.

Hooker, R.S., Cipher, D., & Hess, B. (2002) Physician assistant education program attributes as predictors of national certifying examinations. In presss.

Hooker, R.S. & Freeborn, D.K. (1991) Use of physician assistants in a managed health care system. *Public Health Rep.* 106, 90-94.

Hooker, R.S. & McCaig, L. (1996) Emergency department uses of physician assistants and nurse practitioners: a national survey. *Am. J. Emerg. Med.* 14(3), 245-249.

Hooker, R.S. & McCaig, L.F. (2001) Use of physician assistants and nurse practitioners in primary care, 1995-1999. *Health Affairs* 20, 231-238.

Hooker, R. S., MacDonald, K., Shea, J., & Ashman, T. (2002). Canadian physician assistants. *Military Medicine*, accepted for publication.

Hooker, R.S., Potts, R., & Ray, W. (1997) Patient satisfaction: comparing physician assistants, nurse practitioners and physicians. *Permanente J.* 1, 38-42.

Hooker, R.S. & Warren, J. (2001) Comparison of physician assistant programs by tuition costs. *Perspect. Physician Assist. Educ.* 12, 87-91.

Houston, E.A., et al. (2001) How physician assistants use and perceive complementary and alternative medicine. *JAAPA* 14, 29-30, 33-34, 39-40, 44-46.

Howard, D.R. (1969) The physician's assistant. *J. Kans. Med. Soc.* 70, 411-416.

Howard, D.R. (1971) The physician's associate in occupational medicine. *Occup. Health Nurs.* 19, 14-17.

Howard, P. (2000) PA clinical analyst and researcher find nonclinical jobs rewarding. *AAPA News* 21, 4-10.

Hsiao, W.C. (1984) Transformation of health care in China. *N. Engl. J. Med.* 310, 932-936.

Hsu, R.C. (1974) The barefoot doctors of the People's Republic of China—some problems. *N. Engl. J. Med.* 291, 124-127.

Huch, M.H. (1992) Nurse practitioners and physician assistants: are they the same? *Nurs. Sci. Q.* 5, 52-53.

Hudson, C.L. (1961) Expansion of medical professional services with nonprofessional personnel. *JAMA* 176, 839-841.

Hughes, N. (2000) PA on bargaining team for Kaiser Permanente strike. *AAPA News* 21, 1-10.

Hummel, J. & Pirzada, S. (1994) Estimating the cost of using non-physician providers in primary care teams in an HMO: where would the savings begin? *HMO Pract.* 8, 162-164.

Huntington, S. & Warnick, J.S. (1987) Pharmacists' attitudes toward PAs. Results of a Wisconsin study. *Physician Assist.* 11, 108, 110-111, 114.

Hutchinson, M.K. (1999) Individual, family, and relationship predictors of young women's sexual risk perceptions. *J Obstet. Gynecol. Neonatal Nurs.* 28, 60-67.

Institute of Medicine. (1978) *A Manpower Policy for Primary Health Care: Report of a Study/Institute of Medicine*. National Academy of Sciences, Division of Health Manpower and Resources Development, Washington, D.C.

Ippolito, R. (2000) APAP Consortium policy update. *Perspect. Physician Assist. Educ.* 11, 168.

Isiadinso, O.O. (1979) Physician's assistant in geriatric medicine. *N. Y. State J. Med.* 79, 1069-1071.

Jacobson, P.D., Parker, L.E., & Coulter, I.D. (1998) Nurse practitioners and physician assistants as primary care providers in institutional settings. *Inquiry* 35, 432-446.

Jameson, K.P. (2000) Contemplative page. Address to the 1995 graduating class of the Utah PA program. *Perspect. Physician Assist. Educ.* 11, 125-128.

Janis, I.L. (1980) An analysis of psychological and sociological ambivalence: nonadherence to courses of action prescribed by health-care professionals. *Trans. N.Y. Acad. Sci.* 39, 91-110.

Jarmul, D.B. & Chavez, R.S. (1991) On "Ethics of PAs' work" . . . role in cavity searches within a correctional facility. *JAAPA* 4, 602-603.

Jarski, R.W. (1988) An investigation of physician assistant and medical student empathic skills. *J. Allied Health* 17, 211-219.

Jarski, R.W. (2001) PAs are recommending, and using, CAM [Editorial]. *JAAPA* 14, 6-12.

Jekel, J.F., Dunaye, T.M., Siker, E., & Rossetti, M. (1980) The impact of non-physician health directors on full-time public health coverage in Connecticut. *Am. J. Public Health* 70, 73-74.

Johnson, B.X. (1998) The 5 *R*'s of becoming a psychiatric nurse practitioner: rationale, readying, roles, rules, and reality. *J. Psychosoc. Nurs. Ment. Health Serv.* 36, 20-24, 38-39.

Johnson, J., Evans, H., Grant, E., et al. (1998) The central application service for physician assistants (CASPA): an update. *Perspect. Physician Assist. Educ.* 9, 83-86.

Johnson, R., Driggers, D.A., & Huff, C.W. (1983) PA utilization in a family practice residency program. *Physician Assist. Health Pract.* 7, 68-70.

Johnson, R.E. & Freeborn, D.K. (1986) Comparing HMO physicians' attitudes towards NPs and PAs. *Nurse Pract.* 11, 39, 43-46, 49.

Johnson, R.E., Hooker, R.S., & Freeborn, D.K. (1988) The future role of physician assistants in prepaid group practice health maintenance organizations. *JAAPA* 1, 88-90.

Joiner, C.L. (1974) Attitudes of primary care physicians in the state of Alabama toward physician assistants: a preliminary report. *Ala. J. Med. Sci.* 11, 363-365.

Jones, P.E. (1994) A descriptive study of doctorally prepared physician assistants. *JAAPA* 7, 353.

Jones, P.E. (1995) Market forces and the shape of primary care to come [Editorial]. *JAAPA* 8, 13-17.

Joyner, S.L. & Easley, D. (1984) Organ donation: who holds the key? *Physician Assist.* 8, 106, 119

Judd, C.R. & Hooker, R.S. (2001) Physician assistant education in substance abuse. *Perspect. Physician Assist. Educ.* 12, 172-176.

Kane, R.L., Gardner, J., Wright, D.D., et al. (1978) Differences in the outcomes of acute episodes of care provided by various types of family practitioners. *J. Fam. Pract.* 6, 133-138.

Kane, R.L., Garrard, J., Buchanan, J.L., et al. (1991) Improving primary care in nursing homes. *J. Am. Geriatr. Soc.* 39, 359-367.

Kane, R.L., Olsen, D.M., & Castle, C.H. (1978) Effects of adding a Medex on practice costs and productivity. *J. Community Health* 3, 216-226.

Kane, R.L., Olsen, D.M., Wilson, W.M., et al. (1976) Adding a Medex to the medical mix: an evaluation. *Med. Care* 14, 996-1003.

Kappes, T.J. (1992) PA-C vs OPA-C . . . "Physician Assistant-Certified" . . . American Society of Orthopaedic Physician Assistants. *JAAPA* 5, 70-71.

Katterjohn, K.R. (1982) Dermatologic physician assistants [Letter]. *J. Am. Acad. Dermatol.* 6, 950-951.

Katz, H.P., Cushman, I., Brooks, W., et al. (1994) A physician assistant laceration management program. *HMO. Pract.* 8, 187-189.

Kearns, P.J., Wang, C.C., Morris, W.J., et al. (2001) Hospital care by hospital-based and clinic-based faculty: a prospective, controlled trial. *Arch. Intern. Med.* 22, 161, 235-241.

Keene, M.G., Petrusa, E.R., Jr., Carter, R.D., et al. (2000) Is faculty review of applications worth the effort? *Perspect. Physician Assist. Educ.* 11, 157-160.

Keith, C. (1974) Auxillary utilization in dentistry. *PA J.* 4, 14-20.

Kelly, P. (2000) Determining the influence of pre-admission health care experience on measures of entry-level clinical competence in a cohort of physician assistant graduates [Dissertation]. Nova Southeastern University, Fort Lauderdale, Fla.

Kelvin, J.F. & Moore-Higgs, G.J. (1999) Description of the role of nonphysician practitioners in radiation oncology. *Int. J. Radiat. Oncol. Biol. Phys.* 45, 163-169.

Kelvin, J.F., Moore-Higgs, G.J., Maher, K.E., et al. (1999) Non-physician practitioners in radiation oncology: advanced practice nurses and physician assistants. *Int. J. Radiat. Oncol. Biol. Phys.* 45, 255-263.

Kessler, R. & Berlin, A. (1999) Physician assistants as inpatient caregivers. A new role for mid-level practitioners. *Cost Quality* 5, 32-33.

Kiernan, B. & Rosenbaum, H.D. (1977) The impact of a physician assistant in diagnostic radiology [PA-DR] on the delivery of diagnostic radiologic clinical services. *Invest. Radiol.* 12, 7-14.

Knaus, W.A. (1981) *Inside Russian Medicine: An American Doctor's First Hand Report.* Everst House, New York.

Knickman, J.R., Lipkin, M., Finkler, S.A., et al. (1992) The potential for using nonphysicians to compensate for the reduced availability of residents. *Acad. Med.* 67, 429-438.

Koenig, J.D., Tapias, M.P., Hoff, T., et al. (2000) Are US health professionals likely to prescribe mifepristone or methotrexate? *J. Am. Med. Womens Assoc.* 55, 155-160.

Kole, L.A. (1988) A new incarnation. *JAAPA* 1, 1-2.

Kole, L.A. (1991) Speculating on the specialization of PAs . . . physician assistants. *JAAPA* 4, 542-543.

Kossoy, E. & Ohry, A. (1992) *The feldshers: medical, sociological and historical aspects of practitioners with below university level education.* Jerusalem Magnes Press, Hebrew University, Jerusalem.

Kraak, W. (1979) Institutional elderly—more than a success in geriatrics. *Physician Assist. Health Pract.* 3, 70-72.

Kraft, J., Alexander, L.A., & Rowlands, D.T., Jr. (1992) Tissue transplantation. Quality assurance in the banking and utilization of musculoskeletal allografts. *Physician Assist.* 16, 49-46.

Krasner, M., Ramsay, D.L., Weary, P.E., & Johnson, M.L. (1977) New health practitioners and dermatology manpower planning. *Arch. Dermatol.* 113, 1280-1282.

Krein, S.L. (1997a) The employment and use of nurse practitioners and physician assistants by rural hospitals. *J. Rural Health* 13, 45-58.

Krein, S.L. (1997b) Rural hospitals and provider-based rural health clinics: the influence of market and institutional forces (nurse practitioner, physician assistant). *DAI* 58, 2381.

Kress, L.M. (1971) Let's look at the P.A. A new member of the health team. *Q. Rev. DC. Nurses Assoc.* 39, 9-11.

Lairson, P.D., Record, J.C., & James, J.C. (1974) Physician assistants at Kaiser: distinctive patterns of practice. *Inquiry* 11, 207-219.

Lane, S. & Evans, E. (2000) *2000 Physician Assistant Programs Directory*. Association of Physician Assistant Programs, Alexandria, Va.

Lapius, S.K. (1983) Physicians and midlevel practitioners. Can the conflict be resolved? *Postgrad. Med.* 73, 94-95.

Larson, E.H., Hart, L.G., & Ballweg, R.M. (2001) National Estimates of Physician Assistant Productivity. *J. Allied Health* 30(3), 146-152.

Larson, E.H., Hart, L.G., & Hummel, J. (1994) Rural physician assistants: a survey of graduates of MEDEX Northwest. *Public Health Rep.* 109, 266-274.

Larson, E.H., Hart, L.G., Goodwin, M.K., et al. (1999) Dimensions of retention: a national study of the locational histories of physician assistants. *J. Rural Health* 15, 391-402.

Larson, L.W. (2000) Are RNFAs a threat to PAs? *JAAPA* 13, 20, 26, 29.

Larson, M.S. (1977) *The Rise of Professionalism.* University of California Press, Berkeley.

Laur, W.E., Posey, R.E., & Waller, J.D. (1981) The dermatologic physician's assistant: an overview of one year's experience. *J. Am. Acad. Dermatol.* 5, 367-372.

Lawrence, D. (1978) Physician assistants & nurse practitioners: their impact on health care access, costs, and quality. *Health Med. Care Serv. Rev.* 1, 1, 3-12.

Lee, J., Cooper, J., Lopez, E.C., et al. (2000) Survey on utilization of nonsurgeon practitioners in cardiothoracic surgery (SUNPICS). *Surg. Physician Assist.* 6, 14-21.

Legler, C.F. (1983) A survey of physician attitudes toward the PA. *Physician Assist.* 7, 98, 101-104, 109.

Leiken, A.M. (1985) Factors affecting the distribution of physician assistants in New York State: policy implications. *J. Public Health Policy* 6, 236-243.

Li, L.B., Williams, S.D., & Scammon, S.L. (1995) Practicing with the urban underserved. A qualitative analysis of motivations, incentives, and disincentives. *Arch. Fam. Med.* 4, 124-133.

Liaison Committee on Medical Education. (2001) Medical schools in the United States. *JAMA* 286, 1085-1093.

Lichter, P.R. (1995) Confusing licensure with education: medicine's slippery slope. *Federal Bulletin* 82, 16-20.

Lieberman, D. & Lalwani, A. (1994) Physician-only and physician assistant statutes: a case of perceived but unfounded conflict. *J. Am. Med. Womens Assoc.* 49, 146-149.

Lieberman, D.A. & Ghormley, J.M. (1992) Physician assistants in gastroenterology: should they perform endoscopy? *Am. J. Gastroenterol.* 87, 940-943.

Lillquist, D.R., Suruda, A., Stephenson, D., et al. (2000) Remember to ask—what is your occupation? *Perspect. Physician Assist. Educ.* 11, 165-167.

Litman, T.J. (1972) Public perceptions of the physicians' assistant—a survey of the attitudes and opinions of rural Iowa and Minnesota residents. *Am. J. Public Health* 62, 343-346.

Little, G.A. & Buus-Frank, M.E. (1996) Transition from housestaff in the neonatal intensive care unit: a time to review, revise, and reconfirm [Editorial; comment]. *Am. J. Perinatol.* 13, 127-129.

Lohrenz, F.N., Payne, R.A., Intress, R.C., et al. 1976 Placement of primary care physician's assistants in small rural communities. *Wis. Med. J.* 75(10):93-94.

Lombness, P.M. (1994) Difference in length of stay with care managed by clinical nurse specialists or physician assistants. *Clin. Nurse Spec.* 8, 253-260.

Lowe, D. (1971) The training and use of physician's assistants in industry. *Med Today* 5, 77-81.

Lurie, N., Rank, B., Parenti, C., et al. (1989) How do house officers spend their nights? A time study of internal medicine house staff on call. *N. Engl. J. Med.* 22, 320, 1673-1677.

Ly, N., McCaig, L., & Burt, C.W. (2001) *National Ambulatory Medical Care Survey: 1999 Outpatient Department Summary.* National Center for Health Statistics, Hyattsville, Md. Advance Data from Vital and Health Statistics. No. 321.

Lyman, P., Elli, L., & Gebhart, R. (1999) Physician assistants in the Department of Veterans Affairs. *Veterans Health Syst. J.* 4, 25-29.

Lynch, J. (1971) Allied health personnel in occupational medicine: report of the long range planning committee. *J. Occup. Med.* 13, 232-237.

Machotka, P., Ott, J.E., Moon, J.B., et al. (1973) Competence of child health associates, I: comparison of their basic science and clinical knowledge with that of medical students and pediatric residents. *Am. J. Dis. Child.* 125, 199-203.

Mahon, J. & Batrus, J. (2000) A day in the life of a psych PA. *Adv. Physician Assist.* 8, 66.

Mainous, A.G., III, Bertolino, J.G., & Harrell, P.L. (1992) Physician extenders: who is using them? *Fam. Med.* 24, 201-204.

Manpower and Primary Health Care: Guidelines for Improving/Expanding Health Services Coverage in Developing Countries. (1978) The University Press of Hawaii, Honolulu, Hawaii.

Marsters, C.E. (2000) Pneumothorax as a complication of central venous cannulation performed by physician assistants. *Surg. Physician Assist.* 6, 18-24.

Marvelle, K. & Kraditor, K. (1999) Do PAs in clinical practice find their work satisfying? *JAAPA* 12, 43-50.

Mastrangelo, R. (1993) The name game. *Adv. Physician Assist.* 2, 17-18.

Mathew, M.S. & Stevens, R. (1982) Medical evaluation of CMHC patients by a physician's assistant. *Hosp. Community Psychiatry* 33, 224-225.

Mathews, W.A. & Yohe, C.D. (1984) PAs in psychiatry: filling the gap. *Physician Assist.* 8, 26.

Mattingly, D.E. & Curtis, L.G. (1996) Physician assistant impairment. A peer review program for North Carolina. *N.C. Med. J.* 57, 233-235.

Mauney, F., Keller, C., & King, L. (1972) The physician's assistant to the cardiovascular and thoracic surgeon. *PA J.* 2, 148-151.

Mauney, F.M., Jr. (1980) Report on . . . "The matter of the saturation point for physician assistants in this state . . ." First of two parts. *N.C. Med. J.* 41, 585-589.

Maxfield, R.G. (1976) Use of physician's assistants in a general surgical practice. *Am. J. Surg.* 131, 504-508.

Maxfield, R.G., Lemire, M.D., Thomas, M., & Wansleben, O. (1975) Utilization of supervised physician's assistants in emergency room coverage in a small rural community hospital. *J. Trauma* 15, 795-799.

Mayer, R.P., Solomon, R.J., Trimbath, J., & Rohrs, R. (1988) Physician assistants as administrators. Opportunities in management. Panel discussion. *Physician Assist.* 12, 87, 90, 95-87, 90, 97 (passim).

Mayes, J.R. (1991) Reader disputes "Legislation" column [Letter]. *AORN J.* 53, 13-14.

McCaig, L.F., Hooker, R.S., Sekscenski, E.S., et al. (1998) Physician assistants and nurse practitioners in hospital outpatient departments, 1993-1994. *Public Health Rep.* 113, 75-82.

McCarty, J.E., Stuetzer, L., & Somers, J.E. (2001) Physician assistant program accreditation—history in the making. *Perspect. Physician Assist. Educ.* 12, 24-38.

McCowan, T.C., Goertzen, T.C., Lieberman, et al. (1992) Physician's assistants in vascular and interventional radiology [Letter; comment]. *Radiology* 184, 582.

McDowell, L., Clemens, D., & Frosch, D. (1999) Analysis of physician assistant program performance on the PANCE based on degree granted, length of curriculum, and duration of accreditation. *Perspect. Physician Assist. Educ.* 10, 180-183.

McGill, F., Kleiner, G.J., Vanderbilt, C., et al. (1990) Postgraduate internship in gynecology and obstetrics for physician assistants: a 4-year experience. *Obstet. Gynecol.* 76, 1135-1139.

McKelvey, P.A., Oliver, D.R., & Conboy, J.E. (1986) PA roles in a tertiary medical center. *Physician Assist.* 10, 149-152, 159.

McKibbin, R.C. (1978) Cost-effectiveness of physician assistants: a review of recent evidence. *PA J.* 8, 110-115.

Mechanic, D. (1974) *Politics, Medicine and Social Science.* Wiley, New York.

Medical Group Management Association. (2001) *Physician Compensation and Production Survey: 2001 Report Based on 2000.* Medical Group Management Association, Englewood, Co.

Meikle, T.H. (1992) *An Expanded Role for the Physician Assistant.* Association of Academic Health Centers, Washington, D.C.

Melby, C.S. & Edmunds, M.W. (1997) Negotiating the politics and policies of managed care. *Am. J. Nurs.* 11(suppl), 2-7.

Mendenhall, R.C., Repicky, P.A., & Neville, R.E. (1980) Assessing the utilization and productivity of nurse practitioners and physician's assistants: methodology and findings on productivity. *Med. Care* 18, 609-623.

Meyers, H. (1978) *The Physician's Assistant: A Baccalaureate Curriculum.* Alderson-Broaddus College, Philippi, W.Va.

Miles, D.L. & Rushing, W.A. (1976) A study of physicians' assistants in a rural setting. *Med. Care* 14, 987-995.

Miller, D.C. (1991) *Handbook of Research Design and Social Measurement,* 15th ed. Sage Publication, Newbury Park, Calif.

Miller, A.A., Allison, L., Asprey, D., et al. (2001) Programs Degree Task Force final paper September 28, 2000. *Perspect. Physician Assist. Educ.* 11, 157-160.

Miller, J.I., Craver, J.M., & Hatcher, C.R. (1978) Use of physicians' assistants in thoracic and cardiovascular surgery in the community hospital. *Am. Surg.* 44, 162-164.

Miller, J.I. & Hatcher, C.R. (1978) Physicians' assistants on a university cardiothoracic surgical service. A five-year update. *J. Thorac. Cardiovasc. Surg.* 76, 639-642.

Miller, W., Riehl, E., Napier, M., et al. (1998) Use of physician assistants as surgery/trauma house staff at an American College of Surgeons–verified level II trauma center. *J. Trauma* 44, 372-376.

Mishel, M.H. (1998) Uncertainty in Illness. *Image J. Nurs. Scholarship* 20, 225-232.

Mittman, D. (1995) Physician's assistant (PA) and CNS [Letter; comment]. *Clin. Nurse Spec.* 9, 121.

Mittman, D.E., Cawley, J.F., & Fenn, W.H. (2002) Physician assistants in the United States. *BMJ* 325, 485-487.

Mittman, D. & Mirotznik, J. (1984) PA prescribing behavior and attitudes: a profile. *Physician Assist.* 8, 15-24.

Mondy, L.W., Lutz, D.B., Heartwell, S.F., & Zetzman, M.R. (1986) Physician extender services in family planning agencies: issues in Medicaid reimbursement. *J. Public Health Policy* 7, 183-189.

More, E.S. (1999) *Restoring the Balance: Women Physicians and the Profession of Medicine, 1850-1995.* Harvard University Press, Cambridge, Mass.

Morian, J.P., Jr. (1986) The PA's role in medical research: implications for PA education. *Physician Assist.* 10, 141-142, 146, 161.

Morreale, J. & Chitradon, R. (1977) *A cost analysis of the use of physician's assistants providing primary medical care in a psychiatric setting.* Western Psychiatric Institute and Clinic and the University Center for Urban Research, University of Pittsburgh, Pittsburgh, Pa.

Mullan, F., Rivo, M.L., & Politzer, R.M. (1993) Doctors, dollars, and determination: making physician work-force policy. *Health Affairs (Milwood)* 12(suppl), 138-151.

Mundinger, M.O., Kane, R.L., Lenz, E.R., et al. (2000) Primary care outcomes in patients treated by nurse practitioners or physicians: a randomized trial. *JAMA* 283, 59-68.

Nasca, T.J., Veloski, J.J., Monnier, J.A., et al. (2001) Minimum instructional and program-specific administrative costs of educating residents in internal medicine. *Arch. Intern. Med.* 12, 161, 760-766.

Nelson, E.C., Jacobs, A.R., Breer, P.E., et al. (1975) Impact of physician's assistants on patient visits in ambulatory care practices. *Ann. Intern. Med.* 82, 608-612.

Nelson, E.C., Jacobs, A.R., Breer, P.E., & Johnson, K.G. (1975) Impact of physician's assistants on patient visits in ambulatory care practices. *Ann. Intern. Med.* 82, 608-612.

Nelson, E.C., Jacobs, A.R., Cordner, K., et al. (1975a) Financial impact of physician assistants on medical practice. *N. Engl. J. Med.* 293, 527-530.

Nelson, E.C., Jacobs, A.R., & Johnson, K.G. (1974) Patients' acceptance of physician's assistants. *JAMA* 228, 63-67.

Nelson, E.C., Johnson, K.G., & Jacobs, A.R. (1977) Impact of Medex on physician activities: redistribution of physician time after incorporating a Medex into the practice. *J. Fam. Pract.* 5, 607-612.

Nelson, L.B. (1982) New Jersey physician assistant graduates are successful practitioners. *J. Med. Soc. N.J.* 79, 829-833.

Nelson, R. (2000) AAPA physician assistant census results; fringe benefits. *AAPA News* 21, 4-4.

Neuman, B. (1989) *The Neuman Systems Model,* 2nd ed. Appleton & Lange, Norwalk, Conn.

Nichols, A.W. (1980) Physician extenders, the law, and the future. *J. Fam. Pract.* 11, 101-108.

NONPF to Initiate Review and Approval. (1999) *Nurse Pract.* 24, 78.

Oakes, D.L., MacLaren, L.M., Gorie, C.T., et al. (1999) Predicting success on the physician assistant national certifying examination. *Perspect. Physician Assist. Educ.* 10, 63-69.

Office of Inspector General, Office of Enhancement and Inspection. (1993) *Enhancing the Utilization of Nonphysician Services.* Department of Health and Human Services, New York.

Office of Technology Assessment. (1986) *Nurse practitioners, physician assistants, and certified nurse-midwives: an analysis [Case Study 37].* U.S. Congress, Government Printing Office, Washington, D.C.

Office of Technology Assessment. (1990) *Health Care in Rural America. Office of Technology Assessment and U.S. Congress.* Government Printing Office, Washington, D.C.

O'Hearn, C.J. (1991) Physician assistants' role in combat medicine [Letter; comment]. *Postgrad. Med.* 90, 48.

Oliver, D. (1993) Physician assistant education: a review of program characteristics by sponsoring institution. In: Clawson, D.K. & Osterweis, M., eds. *The Roles of Physician Assistants and Nurse Practitioners in Primary Care.* Association of Academic Health Centers, Washington, D.C.

Oliver, D.R., Conboy, J.E., Donahue, W.J., et al. (1986) Patients' satisfaction with physician assistant services. *Physician Assist.* 10, 51-60.

Oliver, D.R., Laube, D.W., Gerstbrein, J.J., et al. (1977) Distribution of primary care physician's assistants in the State of Iowa. *J. Iowa Med. Soc.* 67, 320-323.

Olsen, D.M., Kane, R.L., Manson, J., et al. (1978) Measuring impact of Medex using third-party payer claims. *Inquiry* 15, 160-165.

Olson, J.H. (1983) Geriatric medicine: a new horizon for the physician's assistant. *J. Am. Geriatr. Soc.* 31, 236-237.

Orem, D.E. (1995) *Concepts of Practice.* McGraw-Hill, New York.

O'Rourke, R.A. (1987) The specialized physician assistant: an alternative to the clinical cardiology trainee [Editorial]. *Am. J. Cardiol.* 60, 901-902.

Ortiz, D., Addari, G., Hastings-Schmidt, V., et al. (2000) *Factors Affecting Physicians Decisions to Hire Physician Assistants.* Presented at the American Academy of Physician Assistants 28th Annual Conference, 29 May 2000, Chicago. Poster presentation.

Orubuloye, I.O. & Oyeneye, O.Y. (1982) Primary health care in developing countries: the case of Nigeria, Sri Lanka and Tanzania. *Soc. Sci. Med.* 16, 675-686.

Ostergard, D.R., Gunning, J.E., & Marshall, J.R. (1975) Training and function of a women's health-care specialist, a physician's assistant, or nurse practitioner in obstetrics and gynecology. *Am. J. Obstet. Gynecol.* 121, 1029-1037.

Osterweis, M. & Garfinkel, S. (1993) Roles and functions of non-physician practitioners in primary care. In: Clawson, D.K. & Osterweis, M., eds. *The Roles of Physician Assistants and Nurse Practitioners in Primary Care.* Association of Academic Health Centers, Washington, D.C.

Ott, J.E., Bellaire, J., Machotka, P., et al. (1974) Patient management by telephone by child health associates and pediatric house officers. *J. Med. Educ.* 49, 596-600.

Otterbourg, E.J. (1986) The expanding role of physician assistants in neonatology. *Physician Assist.* 10, 116-118, 121.

Ottley, R.G., Agbontaen, J.X., & Wilkow, B.R. (2000) The hospitalist PA: an emerging opportunity. *JAAPA* 13, 21-22.

Page, R.R. (1975) *The Military Physician's Assistant. Study File 7.4.5 DASD (HA).* Office of the Assistant Secretary of Defense (Health and Environment), Pentagon City, Va.

Palmer, P.N. (1990) Latest expansion of physician assistants' scope of practice raises questions [Editorial]. *AORN J.* 51, 671-672.

Pan, S., Geller, J.M., Gullicks, J.N., et al. (1997) A comparative analysis of primary care nurse practitioners and physician assistants [Letter]. *Nurse Pract.* 22, 14-17.

Pan, S., Geller, J.M., Muus, K.J., et al. (1996) Predicting the degree of rurality of physician assistant practice location. *Hosp. Health Serv. Adm.* 41, 105-119.

Pantell, R.H., Reilly, T., & Liang, M.H. (1980) Analysis of the reasons for the high turnover of clinicians in neighborhood health centers. *Public Health Rep.* 95, 344-350.

Parker, H.J., McCoy, J.F., & Connor, R.B. (1972) Delegation of tasks in radiology to allied health personnel. Reaction of radiologists. *Radiology* 103, 257-261.

Parse, R.R. (1992) Human becoming: Parse's theory. *Nurs. Sci. Q.* 5, 35-42.

Pasko, T., Seidman, B. (2002) *Physician Characteristics and Distribution in the U.S.: 2002-2003 Edition*, AMA Press, Chicago.

Patterson, P.K. (1969) Parent reaction to the concept of pediatric assistants. *Pediatrics* 44, 69-75.

Pearson, L.J. (1999) Annual update of how each state stands on legislative issues affecting advanced practice. *Nurse Pract.* 24, 16-83.

Pelligrino, E.D. (1976) Prescribing and drug ingestion symbols and substances. *Drug Intell. Clin. Pharm.* 624-630.

Pender, N. & Pender, A.R. (1996) *Health Promotion in Nursing Practice.* Appleton & Lange, Norwalk, Conn.

Pereira, C., Bugalho, A., Bergstrom, S., et al. (1996) A comparative study of caesarean deliveries by assistant medical officers and obstetricians in Mozambique. *Br. J. Obstet. Gynaecol.* 103, 508-512.

Perry, H.B., III. (1977) Physician assistants: an empirical analysis of their general characteristics, job performance, and job satisfaction [Dissertation]. Johns Hopkins University, Baltimore, Md.

Perry, H.B., III. (1978) The job satisfaction of physician assistants: a causal analysis. *Soc. Sci. Med.* 12, 377-385.

Perry, H.B., III. (1980) An analysis of the effects of personal background and work setting variables upon selected job characteristics of physician assistants. *J. Community Health* 5, 228-243.

Perry, H.B., III. (1989) Role satisfaction: an important and neglected subject. *JAAPA* 2, 427-428.

Perry, H.B., III, Detmer, D.E., & Redmond, E.L. (1981) The current and future role of surgical physician assistants. Report of a national survey of surgical chairmen in large U.S. hospitals. *Ann. Surg.* 193, 132-137.

Perry, H.B., III, & Redmond, E.L. (1984) Career trends and attrition among PAs. *Physician Assist.* 8, 121-129.

Perry, K. (1995) Patient survey: physician extenders. Why patients love physician extenders. *Med. Econ.* 72, 58, 63, 67.

Peterson, M.L. (1980) The Institute of Medicine report, "a manpower policy for primary health care:" a commentary from the American College of Physicians. *Ann. Intern. Med.* 92, 843-851.

Pew Health Professions Commission (1993) *Health Professions Education in the Future: Schools in Service to the Nation.* Center for the Health Professions, San Francisco.

Pew Health Professions Commission. (1995) *Critical Challenges: Revitalizing the Health Professions for the Twenty-First Century.* University of California, San Francisco, Center for Health Professions.

Peysner, J. (1996) Physicians' assistants: legal implications of the extended role [Editorial]. *Br. J. Nurs.* 5, 592.

Physician Payment Review Commission. (1994) *Nonphysician Practitioners.* Physician Payment Review Commission, Washington, D.C.

Picot, S.J.F., Zauszniewski, J.A., Debanne, S.M., et al. (1999) Mood and blood pressure responses in black female caregivers and noncaregivers. *Nurs. Res.* 48, 150-161.

Pondy, L.R., Jones, J.M., & Braun, J.A. (1973) Utilization and productivity of the Duke Physician's Associate. *Socioecon. Plann. Sci.* 7, 327-352.

Poppen, C.F. (1996) Physician assistants in otorhinolaryngology—head and neck surgery. *NEWS-Line for Physician Assistants* 5, 8.

Power, L., Bakker, D.L., & Cooper, M.I. (1973) *Diabetes Outpatient Care Through Physician Assistants—A model for Health Maintenance Organizations.* Thomas Publishing, Springfield, Ill.

Pucillo, J.M. (2000) Welcome to the jungle: the Bolivia diaries. *PA Today* 8, 34-38.

Rabin, D.L. & Spector, K.K. (1980) Delegation potential of primary care visits by physician assistants, Medex and Primex. *Med. Care* 18, 1114-1125.

Rada-Sidinger, P. & Connor, P. (1992) Profiles in caring: PAs as primary care providers for poor and underserved children. *JAAPA* 5, 784-789.

Ramos, M. (1989) Occupational medicine. An overview for physician assistants. *Physician Assist.* 13, 79-6.

Ramos, M. (1999) Occupational and Environmental Medicine. In: Ballweg, R.M., Stolberg, S., & Sullivan, E. eds. *Physician Assistant: A Guide to Clinical Practice, Second Edition.* W.B. Saunders, Philadelphia.

Randall, G.B. (1997) *Don't Call Me Doctor.* Morris Publishing, Kearney, Neb.

Record, J.C. (1976) PAs in research: levels of involvement and responsibility. *PA J.* 6, 138-140.

Record, J.C. (1981a) Staffing primary care in 1990: the findings and policy implications. *Springer Ser. Health Care Soc.* 6, 131-153.

Record, J.C. (1981b) The productivity of new health practitioners. *Springer Ser. Health Care Soc.* 6, 37-52.

Record, J.C., Blomquist, R.H., McCabe, M.A., et al. (1981) Delegation in adult primary care: the generalizability of HMO data. *Springer Ser. Health Care Soc.* 6, 68-83.

Record, J.C. & Greenlick, M.R. (1975) New health professionals and the physician role: an hypothesis from Kaiser experience. *Public Health Rep.* 90, 241-246.

Record, J.C., McCally, M., Schweitzer, S.O., et al. (1980) New health professions after a decade and a half: delegation, productivity and costs in primary care. *J. Health Polit. Policy Law* 5, 470-497.

Record, J.C. & Schweitzer, S.O. (1981) Staffing primary care in 1990—potential effects on staffing and costs: estimates from the model. *Springer Ser. Health Care Soc.* 6, 87-114.

Record, J.C. & Schweitzer, S.O. (1981a) Staffing primary care in 1990: effects of national health insurance on staffing and costs. *Springer Ser. Health Care Soc.* 6, 115-127.

Regan, D.M. & Harbert, K.R. (1991) Measuring the financial productivity of physician assistants. *Med. Group Manage. J.* 38, 46, 48, 50-52.

Reinhardt, U.E. (1972) A production function for physician services. *Rev. Econ. Stat.* 54, 55-66.

Riess, J. & Lawrence, D. (1976) *Practitioners in Remote Practices: Summary of a Study of Training, Utilization, Financing and Provider Satisfaction.* Division of Medicine, Bureau of Health Manpower; Department of Health, Education, and Welfare, Washington, D.C.

Repicky, P.A., Mendenhall, R.C., & Neville, R.E. (1982) The professional role of physician's assistants in adult ambulatory care practices. *Eval. Health Prof.* 5, 283-301.

Richmond, H.W. (1974) Health care delivery in Cummins Engine Company. *Arch. Environ. Health* 29, 348-350.

Riportella-Muller, R., Libby, D., & Kindig, D. (1995) The substitution of physician assistants and urse practitioners for physician residents in teaching hospitals. *Health Affairs* 14, 181-191.

Rodican, A.J. (1998) *Getting into the PA School of Your Choice.* Appleton & Lange, Norwalk, Conn.

Roemer, M.I. (1977) Primary care and physician extenders in affluent countries. *Int. J. Health Serv.* 7, 545-555.

Rogers, B. (2000) Physician assistants in nonclinical roles put medical knowledge to work on a broader scale. *AAPA News* 6, 8-9.

Rogers, M. (1972) Nursing: to be or not to be? *Outlook* 20, 42-46.

Rogers, M.E., Malinski, V.M., & Barrett, E.A. (1994) *Martha E. Rogers: Her Life and Her Work.* F.A. Davis, Philadelphia.

Romeis, J.C., Schey, H.M., Marion, G.S., & Keith, J.F., Jr. (1985) Extending the extenders: compromise for the geriatric specialization-manpower debate. *J. Am. Geriatr. Soc.* 33, 559-565.

Romm, J., Berkowitz, A., Cahn, M.A., et al. (1979) The physician extender reimbursement experiment. *J. Ambulatory Care Manage.* 2, 1-12.

Rose, C. (2001) PA devotes career to psychiatric care. *NEWS-Line for Physician Assistants* 10(3), 4-7.

Rose, C.M. (1999) Physicians and non-physician practitioners: working together for improved patient care [Editorial]. *Int. J. Radiat. Oncol. Biol. Phys.* 45, 545-546.

Rosen, R.G. (1986) The Montefiore Medical Center experience. In: Zarbock, S.F. & Harbert, K., eds.

Physician Assistants: Present and Future Models of Utilization. Praeger, New York.
Rosevelt, J. & Frankl, H. (1984) Colorectal cancer screening by nurse practitioner using 60-cm flexible fiberoptic sigmoidoscope. *Digestive Diseases & Sciences* 29, 161-163.
Rothwell, W. (1993) PAs in cardiothoracic surgery. *JAAPA*6, 150-157.
Rousselot, L.M., Beard, S.E., & Berrey, B.H. (1971) The evolution of the physician's assistant: Brownian movement or coordinated progress. *Bull. N. Y. Acad. Med.* 47, 1473-1500.
Roy, S.C. & Andrews, H.A. (1998) *The Roy Adaptation Model*. Appleton & Lange, Norwalk, Conn.
Rudy, E.B., Davidson, L.J., Daly, B., et al. (1998) Care activities and outcomes of patients cared for by acute care nurse practitioners, physician assistants, and resident physicians: a comparison. *Am. J. Crit. Care* 7, 267-281.
Running, A., Calder, J., Mustain, B., et al. (2000) A survey of nurse practitioners across the United States. *Nurse Pract.* 25, 15, 16, 110-116.
Sadler, A.M., Jr., Sadler, B.L., & Bliss, A.A. (1972) *The Physician's Assistant: Today and Tomorrow.* Yale University Press, New Haven, Conn.
Safriet, B.J. (1992) Health care dollars and regulatory sense: the role of advanced practice nursing. *Yale J. Regul.* 9, 417-477.
Safriet, B.J. (1998) Still spending dollars, still searching for sense: advanced practice nursing in an era of regulatory and economic turmoil. *Adv. Pract. Nurs. Q.* 4, 24-33.
Salcido, R., Fisher, S.B., Reinstein, L., et al. (1993) Underutilization of physician assistants in physical medicine and rehabilitation. *Arch. Phys. Med. Rehabil.* 74, 826-829.
Salmon, M.A. & Stein, J. (1986) Distribution of nurse practitioners and physician assistants: are they meeting the need for primary care? *N.C. Med. J.* 47, 147-148.
Salmon, M.E. & Culbertson, R.A. (1985) Health manpower oversupply: implications for physicians, nurse practitioners and physician assistants. A model. *Hosp. Health Serv. Adm* 30, 100-115.
Salyer, S. (2002) Military physician assistants in the new millenium. *JAAPA* 15(10), 35-39.
Samarel, N., Fawcett, J., Piacentino, J.C., et al. (1998) Women's perceptions of group support and adaptation to breast cancer. *J. Adv. Nurs.* 28, 1259-1268.
Samsot, M. (1997) Learning something new about the brain every day. *Adv. Physician Assist.* 4-7.
Samsot, M. (1998) Innovations in dermatology. *NEWS-line for Physician Assistants* 7, 4-7.
Samsot, M. & Heinlein, M. (1996) Orthopaedic PA duties: extensive and on the increase. *NEWS-Line for Physician Assistants* 5, 4-7.
Scarborough, C. (1995) Filling the gaps. Mid-level practitioners try to find a niche. *Healthcare Ala.* 8, 4-9, 22.
Schaefer, K.M. & Potylycki, M.J.S. (1993) Fatigue associated with congestive heart failure. *J. Adv. Nurs.* 18, 260-268.
Schafft, G.E. & Cawley, J.F. (1987a) *The Physician Assistant in a Changing Health Care Environment.* Aspen Publishers, Rockville, Md.
Schafft, G.E. & Cawley, J.F. (1987b) Geriatric care and the physician assistant. *The Physician Assistant in a Changing Health Care Environment.* Aspen Publishers, Rockville, MD.
Scheffler, R.M. (1977) The employment, utilization, and earnings of physician extenders. *Soc. Sci. Med.* 11, 785-791.
Scheffler, R.M. (1979) The productivity of new health practitioners: physician assistants and Medex. *Res. Health Econ.* 1, 37-56.
Scheffler, R.M., Waitzman, N.J., & Hillman, J.M. (1996) The productivity of physician assistants and nurse practitioners and health work force policy in the era of managed health care. *J. Allied Health* 25, 207-217.
Schmittou, E.V. (1977) Cadaver kidney procurement: a unique role for a physician assistant. *PA J.* 7, 23-28.
Schneider, D.P. & Foley, W.J. (1977) A systems analysis of the impact of physician extenders on medical cost and manpower requirements. *Med. Care* 15, 277-297.
Schneider, J. (1972) Manpower problem in obstetrics and gynecology: statistics and possible solutions. *Clin. Obstet. Gynecol.* 15, 293-304.
Schneller, E.S. (1978) *The Physician's Assistant: Innovation in the Medical Division of Labor.* Lexington Books, Lexington, Mass.
Schneller, E.S. (1994) A PA by any other name. *JAAPA* 7, 689-692.
Schneller, E.S. & Simon, J.A. (1977) A profile of the backgrounds and expectations of the class of 1977. *PA J.* 7, 67-72.
Schneller, E.S. & Weiner, T.S. (1978) The black physician's assistant: problems and prospects. *J. Med. Educ.* 53, 661-666.
Schroeder, S.A. (1992) Must America look to non-doctors for primary care [Interview by Mark Holoweiko]? *Med. Econ.* 69, 82-87.
Schroy, P.C., Wiggins, T., Winawer, S.J., et al. (1988) Video endoscopy by nurse practitioners: a model for colorectal cancer screening. *Gastrointest. Endosc.* 34, 390-394.
Schulman, M., Lucchese, K.R., & Sullivan, A.C. (1995) Transition from housestaff to nonphysicians as neonatal intensive care providers: cost, impact on revenue, and quality of care [see Comments]. *Am. J. Perinatol.* 12, 442-446.
Scott-Levin Associates. (2000) Nurse practitioners and physician assistants: all about promotion, patients and prescribing. Available at: www.quintiles.com/products.
Sekscenski, E.S., Sansom, S., Bazell, C., et al. (1994) State practice environments and the supply of physician assistants, nurse practitioners, and certified nurse-midwives. *N. Engl. J. Med.* 331, 1266-1271.
Sells, C.J. & Herdener, R.S. (1975) Medex: a time-motion study. *Pediatrics* 56, 255-261.
Seto, T.B., Taira, D.A., Davis, R.B., et al. (1997) Effect of physician gender on the prescription of estrogen

replacement therapy. *J. Gen. Intern. Med.* 11, 197-203.

Sharp, N. (1998) From "incident to telehealth": new federal rules and regulations affect NPs. *Nurse Pract.* 23, 68-69.

Shi, L. & Samuels, M.E. (1997) Practice environment and the employment of nurse practitioners, physician assistants, and certified nurse midwives by community health centers. *J. Allied Health* 26, 105-111.

Shi, L., Samuels, M.E., Konrad, T.R., et al. (1993) The determinants of utilization of nonphysician providers in rural community and migrant health centers. *J. Rural Health* 9, 27-39.

Shi, L., Samuels, M.E., Ricketts, T.C., III, et al. (1994) A rural-urban comparative study of nonphysician providers in community and migrant health centers. *Public Health Rep.* 109, 809-815.

Shortell, S.M. (1974) Occupational prestige differences within the medical and allied health professions. *Soc. Sci. Med.* 8, 1-9.

Sidel, V.W. (1968a) Feldshers and "feldsherism": the role and training of the feldsher in the USSR. *N. Engl. J. Med.* 278, 987-992.

Sidel, V.W. (1968b) Feldshers and "feldsherism": the role and training of the feldsher in the USSR. [Review] [31 refs]. *N. Engl. J. Med.* 278, 934-939.

Sidel, V.W. (1969) Lessons from aboard: the feldsher in the USSR. *Ann. N. Y. Acad. Sci.* 166, 957-966.

Silver, H.K. (1971) New allied health professionals: implications of the Colorado child health associate law. *N. Engl. J. Med.* 284, 304-307.

Silver, H.K. (1973a) A blueprint for pediatric health manpower for the 1970's. The 1972 George Armstrong Lecture. *J. Pediatr.* 82, 149-156.

Silver, H.K. (1973b) A new primary-care medical practitioner. *Am. J. Dis. Child.* 126, 324-327.

Silver, H.K. & McAtee, P.A. (1984) On the use of nonphysician "associate residents" in overcrowded specialty-training programs. *N. Engl. J. Med.* 311, 326-328.

Silver, H.K. & McAtee, P.A. (1988) Additions to departments of medicine [Letter]. *N. Engl. J. Med.* 318, 645-646.

Silver, H.K. & Ott, J.E. (1973) The child health associate: a new professional to provide comprehensive health care to children. *Physician Assist.* 3, 21-26.

Silver, H.K., Ott, J.E., Dungy, C.I., et al. (1981) Assessment and evaluation of child health associates. *Pediatrics* 67, 47-52.

Simmer, T.L., Nerenz, D.R., Rutt, W.M., et al. (1991) A randomized, controlled trial of an attending staff service in general internal medicine. *Med. Care* 29, JS31-JS40.

Simmons, J. (2000) PAs become part of political process by running for public office. *AAPA News* 21, 1, 14.

Simon, A., Link, M.S., & Miko, A.S. (1999) *Fifteenth Annual Report on Physician Assistant Education in the United States, 1998-1999.* Association of Physician Assistant Programs, Alexandria, Va.

Simon, A., Link, M.S., & Miko, A.S. (2000) *Sixteenth Annual Report on Physician Assistant Education in the United States, 1999-2000.* Association of Physician Assistant Programs, Alexandria, Va.

Simon, A., Link, M.S., & Miko, A.S. (2001) *Seventeenth Annual Report on Physician Assistant Education in the United States, 2000-2001.* Association of Physician Assistant Programs, Alexandria, Va.

Singer, A.J., Hollander, J.E., Cassara, G., et al. (1995) Level of training, wound care practices, and infection rates. *Am. J. Emerg. Med.* 13, 265-268.

Singer, A.M. & Hooker, R.S. (1996) Determinants of specialty choice of physician assistants. *Acad. Med.* 71, 917-919.

Skinner, A.L. (1968) Parental acceptance of delegated pediatric services. *Pediatrics* 41, 1003-1004.

Sloop, P.R. (1995) Rheumatology PA in an HMO [Letter to the editor]. *HMO Pract.* 9, 7.

Smith, C.W., Jr. (1981) Patient attitudes toward physicians' assistants. *J. Fam. Pract.* 13, 201-204.

Smith, J.L. (1992) Physicians' assistants doing endoscopy? [Editorial]. *Am. J. Gastroenterol.* 87, 937-939.

Smith, M.O. (1996) Correctional medicine: an outstanding setting for the PA. *Physician Assist.* 20, 103-104.

Smith, R.A. (1969) Medex: a demonstration program in primary medical care. *Northwest. Med.* 68, 1023-1030.

Smith, R.A. (1974) Principal training programmes in the USA. MEDEX. *Public Health Pap.* 62-68.

Sonntag, V.K., Steiner, S., & Stein, B.M. (1977) Neurosurgery and the physician assistant. *Surg. Neurol.* 8, 207-208.

Sorem, K. R., & Portnoi, V. A. (1983) Decreased rates of polypharmacy, hospitalization and mortality through geriatric medical team involvement in a nursing home. Association of Physician Assistant Programs. American Academy of Physician Assistants, Alexandria, Va. Proceedings of the eleventh annual Physician Assistant Conference, St. Louis, Mo.

Sox, H.C., Jr. (1979) Quality of patient care by nurse practitioners and physician's assistants: a ten-year perspective. *Ann. Intern. Med.* 91, 459-468.

Sox, H.C., Jr., Sox, C.H., & Tompkins, R.K. (1973) The training of physician's assistants: the use of a clinical algorithm system for patient care, audit of performance and education. *N. Engl. J. Med.* 288, 818-824.

Spitzer, W.O. (1984) The nurse practitioner revisited: slow death of a good idea. *N. Engl. J. Med.* 310, 1049-1051.

Srba, L. (1981) *Nurse Practitioners and Physician Assistants in Substance Abuse Programs.* U.S. Department of Health and Human Services, Public Health Service, Alcohol, Drug Abuse, and Mental Health Administration, Rockville, Md.

Stanhope, W.D. (1992) The roots of the AAPA . . . American Academy of Physician Assistants. *JAAPA* 5, 671-678.

Stanhope, W.D., Fasser, C.E., & Cawley, J.F. (1992) The FMG debate continues . . . foreign medical graduate. *JAAPA* 5, 612-614.

Starfield, B.H. (1993) Roles and functions of nonphysician practitioners in primary care. In:

Clawson, D.K. & Osterweis, M., eds. *The Roles of Physician Assistants and Nurse Practitioners in Primary Care.* Association of Academic Health Centers, Washington, D.C.

Stark, R., Mann, R., DeJoseph, J.F., & Emery, M. (1984) The women's health care training project—an alternative for training midwives. *J. Nurse Midwifery* 29, 191-196.

Starr, P. (1982) *The Social Transformation of American Medicine*. Basic Books, New York.

Stead, E.A., Jr. (1966) Conserving costly talents—providing physicians' new assistants. *JAMA.* 198, 1108-1109.

Stead, E.A., Jr. (1971) Use of physicians' assistants in the delivery of medical care. *Annu. Rev. Med.* 22, 273-282.

Stead, E.A., Jr. (1979) New roles for personnel in hospitals: physician extenders. *Bull. N. Y. Acad. Med.* 55, 41-45.

Stead, E.A., Jr. (2001) A new way of making doctors: distance learning for nontraditional students. *N.C. Med. J.* 62, 326-327.

Steinwachs, D.M., Weiner, J.P., Shapiro, S., et al. (1986) A comparison of the requirements for primary care physicians in HMOs with projections made by the GMENAC. *N. Engl. J. Med.* 314, 217-222.

Stone, E.L. (1995) Nurse practitioners and physician assistants: do they have a role in your practice? *Pediatrics* 96, 844-850.

Storey, P.B. & Roth, R.B. (1971) Emergency medical care in the Soviet Union. A study of the Skoraya. *JAMA* 217, 588-592.

Storms, D.M. & Fox, J.G. (1979) The public's view of physicians' assistants and nurse practitioners: a survey of Baltimore urban residents. *Med. Care* 17, 526-535.

Stradtman, J.C. (1989) Utilizing physician's assistants in the medical intensive care unit: a pilot project. *Hosp. Top.* 67, 24-25.

Strand, J. (1994) Physician assistants don't participate in executions [Letter]. *Tex. Med.* 90, 7.

Strickland, W.J., Strickland, D.L., & Garretson, C. (1998) Rural and urban nonphysician providers in Georgia. *J. Rural Health* 14, 109-120.

Strunk, H.K. (1973) Patient attitudes toward physician's assistants. *Calif. Med.* 118, 73-77.

Stuart, R.B. & Blair, J.H. (1974) Army physicians' attitudes about physicians' assistants. *Milit. Med.* 141, 470-472.

Stuart, R.B., Robinson, H.A., Jr., & Reed, R.F. (1973) The training and role of physicians' assistants in the Army Medical Department. *Milit. Med.* 138, 227-230.

Sturmann, K.M., Ehrenberg, K., & Salzberg, M.R. (1990) Physician assistants in emergency medicine. *Ann. Emerg. Med.* 19, 304-308.

Swann, K. (2000) Las Vegas company makes house calls. *AAPA News* 6, 11.

Sylvester, P.A. (1996) Forensic medicine. *JAAPA*9, 53-65.

Synowiez, P.M. (1986) Utilization of physician assistants in group practice. *Coll. Rev.* 3, 57-67.

Synowiez, P.M., Fisher, R.L., & Royer, T.C. (1984) PAs in a tertiary medical center: a ten-year experience. *Physician Assist.* 8, 63-64, 69, 75.

Talbot, M. (1994) Canadian Forces physician assistants [Letter; comment]. *CMAJ* 150, 1058-1059.

Taft, J.M. & Hooker, R.S. (1999) Physician assistants in neurology practice. *Neurology* 52, 1513.

Taft, J.M. & Hooker, R.S. (2000) Physician assistants and the practice of neurology. *JAAPA* 13, 97-106.

Teaching tips. Giving feedback. (2000) *Perspect. Physician Assist. Educ.* 11, 134-135.

Terris, M. (1977) Issues in primary care: false starts and lesser alternatives. *Bull. N. Y. Acad. Med.* 53, 129-140.

Thompson, T. (1972) Utilization of specialty-trained physician's assiciates. *Physician's Associate* 2, 153-156.

Thompson, T.T. (1971) Radiologists look at physician's assistants in radiology. *Radiology* 100, 199-202.

Thompson, T.T. (1974) The evaluation of physician's assistants in radiology. *Radiology* 111, 603-606.

Thorpe, K.E. (1990) House staff supervision and working hours. Implications of regulatory change in New York State [see Comments]. *JAMA* 20, 263, 3177-3181.

Tideiksaar, R. (1982) Geriatric medicine—the place for PAs? *Physician Assist. Health Pract.* 6, 67-68.

Tideiksaar, R. (1984) The PA's role in the nursing home. *Physician Assist.* 8, 28-30.

Tideiksaar, R. (1986) The physician assistant and geriatrics: what does the future hold? *Physician Assist.* 10, 111-112.

Tiger, S. (1992) A brief history of Physician Assistant: an editor's retrospective. *Physician Assist.* 15, 54-55.

Tiger, S. (1993) Roots and radicals [Editorial]. *Physician Assist.* 17, 8, 11.

Todd, I.K. (2000) The last word . . . the devil's bargain . . . learning technologies. *Perspect. Physician Assist. Educ.* 11, 137-138.

Tompkins, R.K., Wood, R.W., Wolcott, B.W., et al. (1977) The effectiveness and cost of acute respiratory illness medical care provided by physicians and algorithm-assisted physicians' assistants. *Med. Care* 15, 991-1003.

Toth, P.S., Pickrell, K.L., & Thompson, L.K., III. (1978) Role of physician's assistant and the plastic surgeon. *South. Med. J.* 71, 430-431.

Trigg, M.E. (1990) PA utilization on a pediatric bone marrow transplant unit. *Physician Assist.* 14, 64, 67-68, 70.

Turner, J.G., Clark, A.J., Gauthier, D.K., et al. (1998) The effect of therapeutic touch on pain and anxiety in burn patients. *J. Adv. Nurs.* 28, 10-20.

Valentine, P. (1990) PA students reach out to the homeless. *JAAPA* 3, 504-510.

van Rhee, J. (1997) A study of the cost effectiveness of physician assistant service in comparison to an intern/resident service at a large teaching hospital [Dissertation]. Finch University of Health Sciences/ Chicago Medical School, Chicago.

Van Rhee, J., Ritchie, J., & Eward, A.M. (2002) Resource use by physician assistant services versus teaching services. *JAAPA* 15, 33-38, 40, 42 passim.

Vause, R.C., Beeler, A., & Miller-Blanks, M. (1997) Seeking a practice challenge? PAs in federal prisons. *JAAPA* 10, 59-62.

Vollmer, R.T. (1999) Pathologists' assistants in surgical pathology [Editorial]. *Am. J. Clin. Pathol.* 112, 597-598.

Wallace, K.W. (1995) Physician assistants in orthopedic surgery. *Surgical Physician Assistant* 1, 52-52.

Wallen, J., Davidson, S.M., Epstein, D., et al. (1982) Nonphysician health care providers in pediatrics. *Paediatrician* 11, 225-239.

Walters, R. (1986) Geisinger Medical Center tertiary care perspectives. In: Zarbock, S.F. & Harbert, K., eds. *Physician Assistants: Present and Future Models of Utilization*. Praeger, New York.

Wassenaar, J.D. & Tran, S.L. (2000) Trends in the physician market. In: Wassenaar, J.D. & Tran, S.L., eds. *Physician Socioeconomic Statistics: 2000-2002*. American Medical Association, Chicago.

Webster, B.S. & Snook, S.H. (1990) The cost of compensable low back pain. *J. Occup. Med.* 32, 13-15.

Weiner, J.P. (1994) Forecasting the effects of health reform on US physician workforce staffing patterns: evidence from HMO staffing patterns. *JAMA* 272, 222-230.

Weiner, J.P., Steinwachs, D.M., & Williamson, J.W. (1986) Nurse practitioner and physician assistant practices in three HMOs: implications for future US health manpower needs. *Am. J. Public Health* 76, 507-511.

Weisenberger, B.L. (1974) Occupational medicine's new resource. *J. Occup. Med.* 16, 676-677.

Weissman, G.S., Winawer, S.J., Baldwin,M.P., et al. (1987) Multicenter evaluation of training of non-endoscopists in 30-cm flexible sigmoidoscopy. *CA Cancer J. Clin.* 37, 26-30.

Wen, C.P. & Hays, C.W. (1975) Medical education in China in the postcultural Revolution era. *N. Engl. J. Med.* 292, 998-1005.

White, G.L. (1992) *The Medical School's Mission and The Population's Health*. Springer-Verlag, New York.

White, R.I., Jr., Denny, D.F., Jr., Osterman, F.A., et al. (1989) Logistics of a university interventional radiology practice. *Radiology* 170 , 951-954.

White, R.I., Jr., Rizer, D.M., Shuman, K.R., et al. (1988) Streamlining operation of an admitting service for interventional radiology. *Radiology* 168, 127-130.

Whitman, N.A. (2000) Whitman sampler. Is teaching a certifiable profession? *Perspect. Physician Assist. Educ.* 11, 136.

Willams, W.H., Kopchak, J., Yearby, L.G., et al. (1984) The surgical physician assistant as a member of the cardiovascular surgical team in the academic medical center. In: Carter, R.D. & Perry, H.H., III, eds. *Alternatives in Health Care Delivery*. Warren Green, St. Louis, Mo.

Williams, K. (1999) Where have all the feldshers gone? *Clinician News* March, 15-18.

Willis, J.B. (1992) Explaining the salary discrepancy between male and female PAs. *JAAPA* 5, 280-288.

Willis, J.B. (1993) Barriers to PA prescribing in primary care and rural medically underserved areas. *JAAPA* 6, 418-422.

Willis, J.B. & Reid, J. (1990) Prescriptive practice patterns of physician assistants. *J. Am. Acad.Physician Assist.* 3, 57-60.

Wilson, W.M., Pedersen, D.M., Ballweg, R., et al. (1995) PA training: shaping a model clinical therapeutics curriculum. *JAAPA* 8, 51-53.

Wilson, W.M., White, G.L., Jr., & Murdock, R.T. (1990) Physician assistants in ophthalmology: a national survey. *Physician Assist.* 14, 57-59.

World Health Organization. (1987) *Report on the Community-based Education of Health Personnel.* World Health Organization, Geneva.

World Health Organization. (1980) *The Primary Health Worker.* World Health Organization, Geneva.

World Health Organization. (1987) *The Primary Care Worker.* World Health Organization, Geneva.

Wright, D.D., Kane, R.L., Snell, G.F., et al. (1977) Costs and outcomes for different primary care providers. *JAMA* 238, 46-50.

Wright, W.K. & Hirsch, C.S. (1987) The physician assistant as forensic investigator. *J. Forensic Sci.* 32, 1059-1061.

Yackeren, T.F. (2000) Prescriber beware. *Clinician News* 4, 4, 7.

Yanni, F., Backman, P.F., & Potash, J. (1972) Physician's attitudes on the physician's assistant. *Physician's Associate* 2, 6-10.

Young, G.P. (1993) Status of clinical and academic emergency medicine at 111 Veterans Affairs medical centers. *Annals of Emergency Medicine* 22, 1304-1309.

Yturri-Byrd, K. & Glazer-Waldman, H. (1984) The physician assistant and care of the geriatric patient. *Gerontol. Geriatr. Educ.* 5, 33-41.

Zarbock, S.F. (1985) Unique experiences in hospice home care. The Danbury Hospice. *Am. J. Hosp. Care* 2, 24-26.

Zechauser, R. & Eliastam, M. (1974) The productivity potential of the physician assistant. *J. Hum. Resources* 9, 5-116.

Zellmer, M.R. (1992) A survey of Minnesota physicians regarding delegation of prescriptive practice to PAs. *JAAPA* 5, 582-586.

Zimmerly, J.G. & Norman, J.C. (1985) Physician assistants and malpractice liability. *Physician Assist. Consult.* 5, 11-13.

INDEX

Page numbers followed by e indicate exhibits.